PSYCHOSOCIAL FRAMES OF REFERENCE

CORE FOR OCCUPATION-BASED PRACTICE

Third Edition

Mary Ann Giroux Bruce, PhD, OTR
Washington University
St. Louis, Missouri

Barbara A. Borg, MA, OTR
Colorado State University
Fort Collins, Colorado

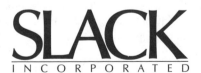

SLACK
INCORPORATED

An innovative information, education and management company
6900 Grove Road • Thorofare, NJ 08086

The procedures and practices described in this book should be implemented in a manner consistent with the professional standards set for the circumstances that apply in each specific situation. Every effort has been made to confirm the accuracy of the information presented and to correctly relate generally accepted practices. The author, editor, and publisher cannot accept responsibility for errors or exclusions or for the outcome of the application of the material presented herein. There is no expressed or implied warranty of this book or information imparted by it.

The work SLACK publishes is peer reviewed. Prior to publication, recognized leaders in the field, educators, and clinicians provide important feedback on the concepts and content that we publish. We welcome feedback on this work.

Printed in the United States of America.

Library of Congress Cataloging-in-Publication Data

Bruce, Mary Ann.
    Psychosocial frames of reference : core for occupation-based practice / Mary Ann
Giroux Bruce, Barbara A. Borg.--3rd ed.
        p. ; cm.
    Includes bibliographical references and index.
    ISBN 1-55642-494-9 (alk. paper)
    1. Occupational therapy. 2. Mentally ill--Rehabilitation. I. Borg, Barbara, 1948- II.
Bruce, Mary Ann. Psychosocial occupational therapy. III. Title.
    [DNLM: 1. Occupational Therapy--methods. 2. Mental Disorders--rehabilitation. WM
450.5.O2 B887p2001]
    RC487 .B78 2001
    616.89'165--dc21

                                                                        2001049066

Published by: SLACK Incorporated
                 6900 Grove Road
                 Thorofare, NJ 08086 USA
                 Telephone: 856-848-1000
                 Fax: 856-853-5991
                 www.slackbooks.com

Contact SLACK Incorporated for more information about other books in this field or about the availability of our books from distributors outside the United States.

Last digit is print number: 10   9   8   7   6   5   4   3

PSYCHOSOCIAL FRAMES OF REFERENCE

CORE FOR OCCUPATION-BASED PRACTICE

Third Edition

DEDICATION

To our parents, who have loved us unconditionally.

Our families—Andrew, Emily, John, and Juan Carlos—who bring balance to our lives.

Our students, who pose important questions and make teaching fun.

Our colleagues, who contribute immeasurably to our knowledge and challenge us to grow in our own thinking.

And to our patients and clients who have shared their lives and helped us learn from their experiences.

CONTENTS

ACKNOWLEDGMENTS

We wish to express appreciation to Peter Slack, for his belief in the occupational therapy profession and for supporting us since the first edition of this text; to Amy Drummond and John Bond for their enthusiasm and promotion of our work; and to April Johnson, Debra Toulson, and Lauren Plummer, for their excellent suggestions, flexibility, and hard work.

ABOUT THE AUTHORS

Since beginning her occupational therapy career in 1968, Mary Ann Giroux Bruce has enjoyed the challenges of practice, academia, management, and consultation. In her first position at Bethesda Hospital and Community Mental Health Center, Denver, Colorado, she developed an interest in psychosocial theory, established her foundation in client-centered practice, and began a career commitment to advocating for patients and families, as well as students and colleagues. In 1974, she moved to Hamden, Connecticut and assumed a faculty role (and later Program Chair) in the Occupational Therapy Program at Quinnipiac College. After 10 very meaningful years of learning with students and colleagues, she left Quinnipiac and joined the faculty in Occupational Therapy at the University of Texas Health Science Center, San Antonio where she pursued interests in group interventions, consultation, and gerontology. In 1989, she moved to Irvine, California, where she practiced in cognitive rehabilitation outpatient and community contexts and completed her PhD in Educational Psychology. In 1998, she became Associate Director of Professional Education, Program in Occupational Therapy, Washington University, St. Louis. In this dynamic environment of students, friends, and colleagues, she juggled interesting management, education, and research roles while pursuing her interests in problem-based learning, psychosocial and cognitive rehabilitation in occupational therapy, and learning and problem-solving in student and community contexts. In summer 2001, she moved to Irvine, California, where she is an independent contractor in occupational therapy.

Mary Ann has a bachelor's degree in occupational therapy and home economics from Colorado State University, a master's degree in counseling from Southern Connecticut State University, and a doctoral degree in educational psychology from the University of Southern California. She was an accreditation site visitor and Self-Study project reviewer for the American Occupational Therapy Association, a reviewer for the *American Journal of Occupational Therapy,* and a test item writer for certification and specialty certification exams. She has contributed chapters to edited texts and this is the fifth text she has co-authored with her friend and colleague Barbara Borg. Books include: *Psychosocial Occupational Therapy: Frames of Reference for Intervention* (1987, 1993); *The Group System: The Therapeutic Activity Group in Occupational Therapy* (1991); and *Occupational Therapy Stories: Psychosocial Interaction in Practice* (1997) (all published by SLACK Incorporated).

Barbara Borg, MA, OTR, has a bachelor's degree in occupational therapy from Colorado State University and a master's degree in counseling psychology from the University of Northern Colorado. She has engaged in occupational practice in inpatient, community, and home care settings; and in individual, couple, family and group counseling with children and adults of all ages. She has held the position of Director of Occupational Therapy and Fieldwork coordinator at Bethesda Hospital and Community Mental Health Center in Denver, Colorado. She is currently Assistant Professor at Colorado State University, where she has taught for 12 years, and consults in the community with Spirit Crossing Clubhouse and Gardening Angels. In 1995, she received the Gilfoyle Award for Teaching Excellence.

Barbara's articles have appeared in the *American Journal of Occupational Therapy,* and she has been a presenter at national and state professional conferences. She has been a reviewer for the *American Journal of Occupational Therapy* and the *Occupational Therapy Journal of Research,* and served on the Editorial Board for the American Occupational Therapy Association's *Cognitive Rehabilitation: Self Study Series* (1993). In addition to the previous editions of this text (1987, 1993), she and Mary Ann Giroux-Bruce have co-authored two other books in the area of psychosocial practice: *The Group System: The Therapeutic Activity Group in Occupational Therapy* (1991) and *Occupational Therapy Stories: Psychosocial Interaction in Practice* (1997). Barbara and Mary Ann also contributed a chapter to *Occupational Therapy: Overcoming Human Performance Deficits.*

Barbara lives in Colorado with her children, Andrew and Emily.

INTRODUCTION

The title and emphasis of this, our third edition, has been changed from that used for the first two editions—*Psychosocial Occupational Therapy: Frames of Reference for Intervention*—to better reflect our and the profession's belief that addressing the psychosocial concerns or psychological part of the person is vital in all occupational therapy practice. While the phrase "psychosocial occupational therapy" might seem to refer exclusively to working with persons having identified mental illness, in truth, the psychological self is an integral part of that whole person who therapists are committed to helping in all contexts, and psychosocial practice lies at the core of all occupational therapy. At the same time, we recognize the need to prepare students to intervene with persons whom have mental illness. We provide in this text models of practice (also called frames of reference) that enable the occupational therapist to address psychosocial issues across a continuum, with normal worry, anger, sadness, enthusiasm, confidence, or reluctance residing on one end of that psychological continuum and severe mental illness at the other.

The text is first a book that describes the theoretical basis for intervention in addressing these psychosocial constructs as they impact the client's ability to engage in meaningful occupation. It gives the reader multiple ways to understand the "person" in the person-environment-occupation relationship. Given this theoretical basis, it is second a text that describes application, providing guides for applying this knowledge in practice. Practice in this usage refers not only to direct care, but also to multiple roles that the therapist may take within diverse environments, whether through habilitation, rehabilitation, prevention, education, or consultation. Unlike the previous two editions, which addressed only intervention with adults, this new edition discusses the application of these occupational therapy practice models with persons across the life span. This is not a book about the clinical reasoning process, per se. It does, however, contribute to that basis of information with which the occupational therapist reasons. Likewise, it helps the reader identify bases for best evidence-based practice and avenues for future research and theory development.

As in the previous editions, this third edition describes multiple and diverse models of practice or frames of reference for occupational therapy. Many of these models have been generated by professionals within our field; other models use concepts that originated outside of the field of OT (e.g., from psychology, education, or cognition) and represent a mechanism through which these concepts have been brought into the field of OT. As we have worked on this third edition, we have been struck by the quantity of information that has been gleaned both nationally and internationally, and the wealth of knowledge from disciplines outside of OT that has been applied in our professional practice. Our challenge as authors was to select information and resources that were representative of the core of psychosocial practice in OT across a breadth of OT services. We have been selective and have chosen information that we believe to be central and especially useful in helping readers to understand the relationship of person-activity/occupation-environment from major and differing theoretical perspectives. As in the previous editions of this text, the theories summarized are comprehensive and are presented according to a similar format. Additionally, for each model, we continue to identify for whom each model was developed and believed to be best suited. Each of these frameworks for intervention helps us, as occupational therapists, to identify, select, and organize principles, which in turn gives coherence to our practice. When we recognize that each framework has strengths and limitations and clinical problems for which it is best suited, we have a basis for making decisions that promote client-centered practice. Rather than expecting that the client accommodate to fit the model, we can select a model that best fits the unique characteristics of the client as well as the environment of practice. We have strived to make our format clear and reader friendly, and one that enables readers to easily compare and contrast the various models. In addition to posing initial focus questions, in this third edition we have added learning activities, some of which have been especially designed to help the reader use what he or she knows or has experienced and integrate it with theoretical information. As in previous editions, we have identified significant terms with boldface type. These terms have been highlighted and defined in the context of the chapter so that they may be more easily understood.

This third edition retains and updates the models identified in the previous two editions with a couple of exceptions or modifications. Much of what was in the previous editions' "holistic" chapter (addressing intervention with persons having a head injury) is now discussed as part of Chapter Nine. This seemed especially appropriate given that Joan Toglia has continued to expand her model. It also helped dispel the idea that other models presented were not "holistic." We believe that all models when applied within the person-occupation-environment framework can help us more effectively work "holistically." Also, we no longer devote a separate chapter to development as a model for practice, but rather propose that principles of growth and development underlie and are consistent with multiple models in practice across the life span. These principles are elaborated upon within each chapter where they apply. The discussion of suicide, which was presented as an appendix in the first two editions, has been updated and now stands as the last chapter in our text. We realize that it incorporates and applies certain principles taken from other models in the text. We view information and concerns in the area of suicide and crisis intervention as unique and most clearly addressed in a separate chapter.

How psychological issues are viewed and one's therapeutic response is intimately tied to his or her theoretical and practice model. The reader is encouraged to evaluate each of the frameworks carefully; each frame of reference in this text places a different emphasis when addressing clinical problems or educational outreach and seeks different kinds of solutions. One shared conviction, common to all of these frameworks, is that it is through their engagement in occupation that people learn, enhance their skills, alter feelings and perceptions, and create meaning in their lives.

CHAPTER ONE

Evolution of Psychosocial Practice— Specialty and Core Occupational Therapy Contexts

KEY POINTS

✧ Psychosocial Concepts in Occupational Therapy
✧ Medications and the Remedicalization of Psychiatry
✧ Deinstitutionalization of State Hospitals
✧ Occupational Therapy Community Practice
✧ Re-Embracing Humanistic Philosophy—Basis for Client-Centered Practice
✧ Expanded Role for Occupational Therapists
✧ Impact of Economy and Health Care Changes
✧ Terminology in Occupational Therapy
✧ Evidence-Based Practice

FOCUS QUESTIONS

1. How is humanitarianism different from humanistic philosophy? What do they both share?
2. How has humanistic philosophy influenced occupational therapy theory and practice?
3. Identify some core beliefs that contribute to occupational therapy practice.
4. Identify several important social changes in the United States that have significantly impacted occupational therapy. What were the effects of these social changes on occupational therapy services?
5. Why was occupational therapy's pursuit of a stronger scientific base viewed as "reductionistic"?
6. What differences are suggested by the terms used to describe the persons in occupational therapy practice contexts (i.e., patient versus client versus consumer)?
7. What is subsumed within a frame of reference and model of practice? How does a frame of reference assist the therapist?
8. Identify the roles that occupational therapists assume in community practice.
9. What effect has the medicalization of psychiatry had on occupational therapy?
10. How have economic changes affected the provision of occupational therapy services in mental health?
11. What is meant by the term "evidence-based practice," and where does the therapist go to find this evidence?
12. Why is evidence so important in the current climate of health care and service delivery?
13. Describe the efficacy guides for descriptive, evaluative, and intervention studies.

INTRODUCTION

We begin our text by highlighting important marker events and trends in the development of occupational therapy in mental health. In our review we pay particular attention to the relationship between events and trends occurring in society and the mental health community and events occurring in our profession in order to provide a meaningful context for understanding the changes the profession has gone through.

We will see how concern for the mental and emotional health of those people we serve and the belief that participation in occupation contributes to one's mental health have not only developed into an area of specialty called psychosocial occupational therapy but have become an essential part, or "core," of all occupational therapy. As stated in the official position paper of the American Occupational Therapy Association (AOTA, 1998), "...psychosocial dimensions of human performance are... fundamental..." (p. 244) in all areas of occupational therapy practice. These dimensions contribute to our understanding of the relationship between the person's mind and body in all contexts of intervention. The mental health specialty area of practice uses the psychosocial core and "specific knowledge" needed to plan inter-ventions for populations with mental illness (p. 245). See Appendix A for the official AOTA document.

We will see how occupational therapy has contributed to improved function and enhanced quality of life for persons who have mental illness and will also see why it is critically important that we demonstrate the outcome of our intervention. Understanding the history of our profession brings insights similar to those gained from understanding each of our personal histories. We appreciate where we have come from, why we value what we do, and what will guide us in the future.

PSYCHOSOCIAL CONCEPTS IN OCCUPATIONAL THERAPY

Humanitarian Care

Throughout occupational therapy's history, whether viewed from within psychiatry and mental health systems or beyond these boundaries, the profession has been based upon a humanitarian philosophy. **Humanitarian** here refers to a concern for the human condition; a belief that society has an obligation to help those who are ill or disabled and a belief in the value and dignity of each person. Also evident in the earliest philosophical foundation is that of humanism. The use of the term **humanism** (and "humanistic") is more recent in occupational therapy. In many respects humanism overlaps with that of "humanitarian" but is not identical. To have a humanistic orientation implies not only a concern for the human condition, but the belief that each person lives and makes choices from the inside out or based upon one's unique, personal perspective. Humanistic orientation also implies that people can and do take responsibility for shaping their own lives through the actions they take. This is articulated, for example, in the inaugural issue of the field's first journal, *Archives of Occupational Therapy*, in which Adolph Meyer writes:

> Our conception of man... an organism that maintains and balances itself in the world of reality and actuality by being in active life and active use... in harmony with... nature and the nature about it... gives the ultimate stamp to our every organ. (Meyer, 1922, p. 1, and quoted from Kielhofner, 1992, p. 29)

As we take a cursory look at the development of occupational therapy in mental health, we find the interplay of both humanitarian and humanistic ideologies, and it becomes difficult, if not impossible at times, to separate one from the other because we seek to treat each client or patient as a valuable and unique individual. In our language we describe each client as a person **having** an illness or disability, rather than referring to him or her as a diagnostic label. The humanistic philosophy is most explicit today in the priority given to establishing client-centered therapeutic relationships in which the patient's or client's desires drive therapeutic goals. In order to simplify our discussion, we will in some instances refer to the profession's "humanistic" roots, using the term to connote both humanitarian and humanistic ideology. Bearing this in mind, we view the humanistic orientation as one that is compatible with other theories that are used in occupational therapy practice.

The profession's basis in humanitarian care arose from a "moral" concern for the mentally ill in the late 1800s and early 1900s. During this time, two hospitals in the eastern United States—McClean Asylum, MA, and Friend's Asylum, Frankfurt, PA—were recognized for having treatment programs based on a holistic philosophy in which patients were treated kindly and were involved in various tasks and activities that were believed to be capable of helping them to resume a more normal life. Those enacting this "moral treatment" believed that people became mentally ill because they had "succumbed to external pressures," developed faulty habits, and became disengaged from society (Kielhofner, 1992, p. 27). Re-engaging in normal activities was believed to be one way that these patients could regain control over their illness and their own lives.

Earliest Founder's Beliefs: Activities and Occupation

The idea that engaging in everyday activities could help one to resume a normal life became a core belief upon which the occupational therapy profession was and still is based. Promulgated by early writers in the field was the premise that a person's participation in activities and occupation influenced health, built competence (both in terms of life skills and beliefs about one's own efficacy), and was the medium for the development of habits and routines that enabled satisfactory engagement in life. Early postulates about rehabilitation include those from professional men and women generally recognized as the founders of the profession—Meyer, Tracy, Slagle, Dunton, Haas, and Bryan and Marsh—and are summarized in Founders' Contributions. These philosophies continue to be referenced in current professional literature.

Role of Activity and Occupation

After World War I, occupational therapy further developed to provide occupations for the mentally ill and to help them resolve what were viewed as "problems of living" (Hopkins, 1983; Tiffany, 1983). The occupational therapy used during this period was developed by Meyer and by others who were concerned about the person and wanted to help patients identify their capabilities and use them in productive occupations. Early proponents recognized that activities needed to be ones in which patients had an interest and could develop personal pride. Only in this way would participation in activities contribute to feelings of mastery and confidence in one's own ability to successfully resume partic-

FOUNDERS' CONTRIBUTIONS

- Adolph Meyer addressed the complex biological and psychological interactions of persons that influence their social performance in daily life and saw mental illness as a breakdown in normal living habits (1922).

- Susan Tracy emphasized the importance of using activities that would be of interest and were meaningful to the patient (1912).

- Eleanor Clarke Slagle recommended the use of purposeful activity to develop a person's habits, which in turn would support health and well-being (1922).

- William Rush Dunton focused on the formation of habits to help the patient work and socialize in the community; his writing brought many early moral treatment concepts into OT (1915, 1919, 1922).

- Louis J. Haas wrote about the importance of helping the person achieve competence and a sense of pride from activities completed in the workshop (1925).

- Bryan and Marsh used industrial therapy to help patients continue to be productive members of society (Kielhofner & Burke, 1977).

ipation in daily life. Activities included games, those that used music and those that emphasized craftsmanship, as well as work activities within the hospital setting.

The environment in which activities were carried out was also recognized as being critically important. It was in some instances strictly organized and regimented in order to encourage patients to establish and adhere to daily schedules and "good" habits, or it was made intentionally more playful and stimulating in order to attract the interest of withdrawn or regressed mentally ill individuals.

Presumed outcomes of the person's participation in this form of therapy included a building of morale and an engendering of interest in and commitment to the present and the future (Kielhofner, 1992, p. 29). Early founders recognized that the person's mental health, or "mind," was directly linked to physical health, or the body. This form of therapy was practiced in the medical setting and was seen as augmenting medical treatment.

During the 1930s and 1940s, the occupational therapist used activities to provide multiple services within mental health facilities. The therapist used specific activities to aid in diagnosis and facilitate patient adjustment to the hospital. Activities were also used to supplement other therapies that the patient received and continued to help patients develop constructive habits (Hopkins, 1983; Tiffany, 1983).

Throughout occupational therapy's history, activities have been modified to serve multiple intervention purposes and to be compatible with contemporary environments; however, the belief that participation in activity has value has endured. Today, the incorporation of activity into occupational therapy in multiple contexts reflects the central role of activity in practice. The literature has made possible a more comprehensive understanding of activity through activity analysis and thereby helped therapists discern how engagement in activity contributes to enhanced occupational performance. Currently, we see a continuum of intervention that identifies the many functions of activities. Interventions may include or emphasize any one or more of the following: adjunctive methods, enabling activities, purposeful activities, and occupation-based interventions (Chisholm, Dolhi, & Schreiber, 2000).

Expansion of Theory and Philosophical Shifts

During the late 1940s and throughout the 1950s in the United States, there was minimal new legislation advocating the rights of the mentally ill. During this period, the occupational therapy profession invested energy primarily in developing more scientific approaches to treatment and in expanding services to the physically disabled (Hopkins, 1983; Tiffany, 1983). If occupational therapists purported that their treatment philosophies and methods helped patients improve, they were now called upon to come up with objective evidence as to how this came about. Overall, the profession, along with that of medicine and other physical sciences, embraced what has been called a "reductionistic" approach in which observable phenomena are "reduced" into measurable units whose relationship to each other can be described (Kielhofner, 1992, p. 35). During this period, for example, occupational therapists carefully measured the strength, mobility, and endurance of physically impaired patients and used improvements in these parameters as indications that therapy was successful. In mental health, occupational therapists were particularly influenced by psychodynamics and behavioral theories, both of which were prevalent in psychiatric settings and reflected a more "scientific" approach to explaining behavior. Many viewed this "scientific" movement as a negation of humanism, a loss of holism, and a shift from the original philosophical base of the profession. Alternatively, however, this could be viewed as a time when scientific knowledge was expanded, later to be incorporated with humanistic ideology to create a holistic or biopsychosocial approach within occupational therapy.

Knowledge gained during the 1950s included that which occupational therapists take for granted today. The increased understanding of psychodynamics by psychiatry and principles of interpersonal relations from psychology broadened occupational therapists' understanding of the therapeutic relationship, strengthened their appreciation of the meaning of activities for patients and clients, and gave them a way to understand and respond to confused, chaotic, and otherwise non-productive behavior. This knowledge also increased the therapist's awareness of the critical role and importance of social and interpersonal communication and group process. This laid the foundation for the application of psychosocial occupational therapy within a therapeutic group setting or therapeutic milieu during the 1960s and thereafter (Fidler & Fidler, 1963). Principles related to the use of a therapeutic milieu are described in Chapter Four, "Psychodynamic Frame of Reference—Person Perspective and Meaning."

Today, the expansion of knowledge has grown into what has been a virtual explosion of knowledge in the physical and social sciences, medicine, health care, and rehabilitation science. The task for occupational therapy continues to be to develop knowledge within the field (to expand its own science) and to use what is being learned outside the field, while maintaining its commitment to a humanistic philosophical base.

Relationships Among Activity, Task, and Occupation

One significant negative outcome of the scientific movement was that it categorized patients and activities in a way that attempted to match a particular activity with the treatment of a particular diagnosis or to relieve specific symptoms. Activities began to be used in a restricted manner, and often an unrealistic attempt was made to cure a patient who had an illness rather than help the patient use capabilities to solve problems in living, adapt to his or her life situation, and increase participation in daily life.

Matching symptom with activity tended to eliminate the personalization of intervention and the appreciation of the interpersonal and cultural contexts in which activities occur; however, this negation of the interpersonal context of activity is minimized in contemporary practice. Today, the profession encourages clinicians to integrate scientific knowledge and the art of practice through client-centered assessment and occupation-based practice. Although certain activities are more (or less) appropriate given the limitations related to symptoms, activities are not like pills given to cure symptoms. Rather, activities have a purpose in a personal context, and they become meaningful and capable of enhancing function and promoting quality of life within that context.

MEDICATIONS AND THE REMEDICALIZATION OF PSYCHIATRY

The influence of science was also felt in psychiatry as psychopharmacology became more sophisticated, and psychiatrists sought to control patient symptoms through the use of medication. Since the 1940s, medications have been used in moderation or extensively in mental health depending on the philosophy of the attending physician or care setting. The expanded use of medication continues today for multiple reasons. Research based on sophisticated technology has identified structural and chemical abnormalities in the brains of persons having mental illness and continues to validate the benefits of medication for managing behavior and symptoms. When psychotropic medications enable persons with mental illnesses to manage their behavior and think clearly, they are more likely to be able to learn and carry out skills needed to function in the community. This does not mean, however, that they automatically have the skills they need. The real work of occupational therapy often begins once persons have been stabilized with medication.

The occupational therapist is sensitive to the effects of medication on daily function/occupational performance, reports findings to the attending physician and other team members, and may educate clients to the effects of medication on performance in daily life. As stated, in many instances, the use of medications minimizes the person's symptoms and makes the person more amenable to interventions. In other cases, however, when a person is overly or heavily medicated for long periods of time, detrimental side effects may occur. Today, given the advancements in psychopharmacology, medications are more effectively managed and can sometimes be used to prevent symptoms. This expanded use of psychotropic medications has been referred to as the **medicalization** or **remedicalization** of psychiatry (Palmer, 1988; Robertson, 1988).

DEINSTITUTIONALIZATION OF STATE HOSPITALS

Up to and throughout the 1950s, most mentally ill individuals were treated in inpatient settings: state hospitals; general, city, and county hospitals; and a few private institutions (Peters, 1988). The most severely disturbed individuals were institutionalized in state psychiatric hospitals, many for years or even most of their adult lives (Marcos, 1989).

Due in part to the ability to better control symptoms in persons who were mentally ill and bowing to economic and philosophical pressure, state agencies began to release these individuals. In 1955, 560,000 residents were in state institutions (today there are "roughly" 100,000 institutional beds) (Kaplan & Sadock, 1998, p. 178). Unfortunately, most of these residents were not prepared to live independently. Many became homeless or were imprisoned for crimes. The burden of caring for those who reappeared in need of mental health services fell largely to community mental health and other local service agencies. Persons in acute crisis were often hospitalized, but whenever feasible, outpatient treatment was used. During the 1990s, institutions continued to downsize and release patients/residents. Therefore, community agencies have found their resources depleted and have needed additional funding. One response by these community agencies has been to eliminate services and redefine clinician roles, which in turn has provided incentives for increased interagency networking and for the development of education and prevention approaches. This has also led to a shift to crisis intervention rather than ongoing support programming. Crisis intervention approaches vary with the individual need and the source of the crisis. In general, the intervention may vary from one to two sessions to a series of sessions for 1 to 2 months (Kaplan & Sadock, 1998, p. 896).

OCCUPATIONAL THERAPY COMMUNITY PRACTICE

Some people believe that occupational therapy's role in community practice began recently; however, occupational therapists have assumed varied roles in community practice for more than 50 years. From about the mid-1940s through the mid-1950s there was increased support from the community at large and from within occupational therapy to develop vocational rehabilitation programs for psychiatric patients. This support promoted prevocational evaluation and programming and led to patient employment within treatment settings (D. Dunton, 1963). The employment of patients in community treatment settings was furthered by the development of sheltered workshops and through contractual agreements made between mental health settings and community businesses during the 1960s. Patient work programs, however, were called into question during the 1970s as patient advocacy grew and as work unions classified jobs and limited the boundaries of employment to the confines of the institutional setting.

Today, the renewed interest in community services has been influenced by the factors previously cited, as well as the profession's commitment to return to the core of the profession—"occupation." As financial support for all health care services, and in particular those for mental health services, decreases, the inpatient and long-term hospital census in mental health has declined, and a continuum of care has developed for occupational therapy services. Patients having acute mental health problems (e.g., those who are psychotic or suicidal) may be initially hospitalized but are typically discharged as soon as their acute symptoms abate. An **acute** hospitalization period varies with the source of the mental health problems. It may vary from an average of 3 to 6 days to 6 to 12 weeks for severe illnesses or child mental disorders (Kaplan & Sadock, 1998, pp. 185, 485, 1276). The goals for the patient are the clarification of diagnosis, behavior, and functional assessment. Typically, mentally ill persons are stabilized on medication, the therapeutic relationship is initiated (Foto, 1988; Margo & Manring, 1989), and a crisis and initial intervention plan is developed. They then return to their homes or to the community to live in group homes or community residences designed to address specific and chronic problems, such as substance abuse, or those related to a need for shelter. Their problems and symptoms are often managed through community agencies and services or home care. Occupational therapists in these community environments may work in traditional clinical roles or, with increasing frequency, in new roles. New roles include that of case manager (see Case Manager), consultant, manager in a community service agency, and advocate at local and state levels (Dressler & MacRae, 1998; Kautzmann, 1998; Samuel, 1998; Smith, 1999; Tewfik & Precin, 1998).

CASE MANAGER

"A **case manager** or **care manager** coordinates services; analyzes fiscal benefits; advocates for essential services; advises the client, family, or caregiver; and monitors the use of resources."

"**Case management** is provided at all levels of care… elements of the case management process parallel elements of occupational therapy practice." Elements include: "…comprehensive assessment of skills, deficits, environmental demands, and available resources…"

"Case management decisions are based on ethical considerations, such as the long-term cost to the client; the family; and the health, education, and/or social system." (AOTA, 1998, pp. 333-335)

PATIENTS' RIGHTS

During the 1960s, the community mental health movement was a strong force that contributed to the growth and development of mental health practice, occupational therapy practice, and applied psychology in general. The community mental health movement introduced new terminology, expanded the scope of intervention settings and strategies, and established new responsibilities for mental health professionals (with some role blurring). It also heightened public awareness of mental health issues and requested an empathetic response from the general public to persons with mental illness. These changes helped bring about federal, state, and local legislation that called attention to patients' rights and the legal responsibilities of institutions. It influenced the standards criteria for patient care and quality assurance (Marcos, 1989).

An example of federal law is the Americans with Disabilities Act (ADA). It provides the guides that ensure that persons with a disability (mental or physical) have the same civil rights as other members of society. Compliance with this guideline integrates a person with a disability into main-

stream society and provides equal opportunities for employment, public accommodations and transportation, telecommunications, and access to state and local governments. The AOTA supports this law and encourages clinicians to play a key role in its implementation (Kornblau, 1990).

The economic changes of the past two decades continue to decrease the resources for mental health services to a point of national concern. Although there has been particular emphasis given to the increased incidence of depression in persons in the United States, there is a need to broadly support mental health research and services. Presently, occupational therapists advocate for patient rights and try to help mentally ill persons obtain quality mental health services. They also work to increase the opportunities for persons with a mental illness to participate in meaningful occupations. Therapists take active roles in national and state associations of the Alliance for Mental Health, participate in support groups for client populations, and interact with state Coalitions for Mental Health, to cite just a few of the many avenues for advocacy (Dressler & MacRae, 1998; Kautzmann, 1998; Samuel, 1998; Tewfik & Precin, 1998).

RE-EMBRACING HUMANISTIC PHILOSOPHY AND CLEAR ARTICULATION OF CLIENT-CENTERED BASIS FOR PRACTICE

During the 1960s and 1970s, there were many other changes going on within occupational therapy and the fields of psychiatry and psychology that led to changes in the direction that occupational therapy has taken. There emerged a powerful influence within psychiatry and psychology that is sometimes referred to as the "third force" (i.e., the "humanistic" movement). It rejected the reductionistic principles associated with psychodynamic and behavioral theory. Perhaps more fundamentally, humanistic philosophy argues that people need not be externally controlled; rather, they are internally motivated to develop their potential and have primary responsibility for how their lives can turn out. It was from humanistic philosophy that the principle of a client-centered therapy emerged. Leaders in the profession, like Elizabeth Yerxa (1966) and many who followed, recognized the parallel between what was being proposed by this "third force" in psychology and the basic tenets upon which the occupational therapy profession had been based.

Yerxa reminded therapists that being "professional" and committing themselves to developing science was not incompatible with a concern for the client as a human being (1966, p. 1). What therapists had to realize was that the outcome of therapy, like life, could not be fully understood or reduced to bits and pieces of observable phenomenon;

rather, meaningful therapy, like a meaningful life, is composed of occupations that must be understood in their context and from the patient's/client's point of view. Yerxa described people as being primarily responsible for making their choices and living according to their beliefs. To do otherwise meant that the person lived unauthentically. The mandate was for occupational therapy to establish collaboration between therapist and client/patient. Being humanistic meant not just being humanitarian (i.e., caring about the person), it meant giving clients information and trusting that the client could make healthy decisions for him- or herself. In other words, it meant creating and maintaining a client-centered relationship.

Yerxa's writing led the way for more reflection regarding the "art" of occupational therapy, including the importance of the therapist's ability to communicate concern and empathic understanding to the patient or client. The theoretical evolution and current expression of this idea of client-centered philosophy is addressed in more detail in Chapter Four.

Around the same time, occupational therapist and educator Mary Reilly (1962, 1966) called for a return to the roots of the profession and a reaffirmation of the importance of occupation to one's health and well-being. Neither Yerxa nor Reilly proposed that science be abandoned; to the contrary, they proposed that occupational therapy embodied ideas that were powerful change agents that needed to be further demonstrated.

Currently, as the support for returning to the occupational core of our profession grows (Christiansen, 1999), and theory and research support the provision of services in context, clinicians are increasingly emphasizing occupation and client-centered practice in context (i.e., in the client's or patient's home, school, work, or community environments). Therapists often help educate family, teachers, or employers about how best to support the person's participation at home or in the community. Clinicians also teach clients with chronic mental illnesses ways to manage their symptoms and disabilities. The expansion of occupational therapy in community practice is evident in preventive programs as well. These programs are based on the belief in the occupational nature of health and well-being. For example, the combination of occupational science and psychosocial practice principles comes together to support prevention through such programs as lifestyle redesign (see Lifestyle Redesign) (Clark et al., 1997).

EXPANDED ROLE FOR OCCUPATIONAL THERAPISTS

In mental health settings, occupational therapists have a history of assuming multiple roles. For example, they have developed occupational therapy services for day-treatment

LIFESTYLE REDESIGN

In response to the identified physical, psychosocial, cognitive, and economic needs of the elderly who are living longer and need support to maintain their quality of life, Clark and colleagues (1997) planned and implemented the Well Elderly Study. This randomized controlled study evaluated the effect of occupation-based intervention on the older adult's participation in activity and on the person's health and well-being. The study compared the responses of the adults of a multi-ethnic group consisting of persons aged 60 years or older and living independently in the community. The researchers compared the outcomes of an occupational therapy group that used both educational models and activities and tasks with the outcomes of an activity group and a non-treatment group. The activity group provided an opportunity for socialization during activities such as crafts, community outings, games, and arts and entertainment events. Participants in the occupational therapy group learned about safety, transportation resources, joint protection, energy conservation, exercise, nutrition, adaptive equipment, and managing barriers in their environment. The outcomes of the study suggest that the occupational therapy group is a preferred intervention and that older adults benefit from a prevention program. The outcome measures of the study suggest that the occupational therapy group positively influences the participant's sense of health and life satisfaction. The occupational therapy group also promotes and supports physical, mental, and social functioning in the everyday environments of the persons in the sample. The reader is referred to the original study for a detailed description and analysis of the study.

---

programs, for residential community living, and for transition centers. They provide clinical services, design prevention programs, train caregivers, and educate and consult with families, teachers, employers, and community agencies (AOTA, 1998; Learnard, Walsh, & Ward, 1999; Scott, 1999; Walens et al., 1998). Because persons with chronic mental illness so often are unable to consistently care for themselves and have difficulty sustaining involvement in daily activities, the expertise that the therapist offers in these expanded roles is vital in helping these persons participate in the community and to have an enhanced quality of life.

ACTIVITIES THERAPY

One outcome of role and service expansion was the evolution of activities therapy. Initially in an activities therapy program, occupational therapists, recreational therapists, dance therapists, art therapists, music therapists, and (sometimes) horticultural therapists worked together. These therapists came with their own professional training and offered a particular specialty, as suggested by their titles, that contributed to treatment within the therapeutic milieu. The therapists used a variety of experiences to improve psychosocial functioning (e.g., creative-expressive media, work-oriented experiences, recreational activities, activities of daily living, and interpersonal communication exercises).

The activities therapy movement had a significant impact on the growth and development of psychosocial occupational therapy, as well as on other specialties such as recreational therapy. It also influenced, and perhaps limited, occupational therapy's role. Each of the therapies identified can be viewed as one kind of activities therapy; therefore, the training for an activities therapist is varied. Since the initiation of this concept, community colleges in some states have developed programs for activities directors as well as activities therapists. Economic constraints and the limited resource pool of qualified occupational therapists during the 1970s and 1980s in some instances promoted the hiring of activities therapists rather than occupational therapists.

Today, those with specific activities expertise are integrated into mental health, physical rehabilitation, school, and community settings in varied capacities. The specific qualifications for these positions may vary within a state or the practice environment.

EXPANSION OF PRACTICE AND CONCERNS ABOUT RECRUITMENT

The literature of the past decade suggests that mental health practice has expanded to meet the psychosocial needs of children (Florey, 1998; Hahn, 2000; Hatje Kaufman et al., 1988; Kramer & Hinojosa, 1999; Lougher, 2001; Sholle-Martin & Alessi, 1990), the homeless, and persons with HIV disease (Gutterman, 1990; O'Rourke, 1990; Palmer, 1988).

While the literature describes multiple roles for the occupational therapist in providing mental health services, there has been increasing concern for the recruitment and retention of therapists in mental health. The question has been raised as to whether the specialty of psychosocial occupational therapy will survive (Bailey, 1990a, 1990b; Burnette-Beaulier, 1982; Cottrell, 1989; Fine, 1998).

We assume that provision of occupational therapy services within a mental health context will survive. We also strongly agree with the official statement of the occupational therapy profession that indicates that all practitioners are responsible for

> ...developing and maintaining professional competence and skill in psychosocial interventions... interventions are designed in considera-

tion of a whole person functioning in the context of an environment. Such consideration includes the psychosocial, physical, societal, cultural, environmental, and temporal aspects of a person's performance. (AOTA, 1998, p. 373)

As with other areas of occupational therapy practice, mental health practice must continue to evolve to meet the changing needs of persons and the changing environments in which care is provided. Having a broad understanding of how engagement in life's activities contributes to the creation and maintenance of mental health places the therapist in the best position to contribute in both current settings and those not yet foreseen.

REIMBURSEMENT FOR SERVICES—ECONOMIC CONSTRAINTS

Historically, private insurers paid for inpatient psychiatric care only to a limited extent (Peters, 1988). They were even more restrictive in their coverage of outpatient treatment. Additionally, state and federal reimbursing agencies such as Medicare and Medicaid, feeling the economic crunch, have demanded more careful accountability in the use of state and federal institutions (Foto, 1988; Hanft, 1988; Peters, 1988), and some states waive the coverage for mental health problems (Kautzmann, 1998). Professional peer review and cost accounting systems evolved in an effort to contain costs and to ensure that service providers delivered the outcomes promised. The managed care system and capitation reimbursement plans also resulted from the effort to contain cost. These changes challenged occupational therapists to contribute to client well-being through case management, consultation, education, and prevention (Kautzmann, 1998). Some feel, however, that the implementation of the system has evolved to a point that the current mental health environment undermines the ability of therapists to respond to the specific needs of their clients and impedes the enactment of the humanistic beliefs of the profession (Fine, 1998).

IMPACT OF HEALTH CARE CHANGES

Clearly, the economy and its effects in mental health care and rehabilitation have tremendously affected occupational therapy. Health care costs continue to skyrocket, consumers are more knowledgeable, and reimbursement is more limited. The occupational therapist, along with other health care professionals, has been asked to demonstrate and document the effectiveness of intervention and to contain costs. In years past, occupational therapy services were covered as part of the inpatient room rate or a type of program such as day rehabilitation per diem fee. Occupational therapy services are now identified and paid for separately by the reimbursing party. With the patient/client in treatment for shorter periods of time and with fewer available dollars, there is increased competition among service providers. The response from the profession has been to consult more closely with consumers in professional policy making and to partner with agencies that advocate for mental health and rehabilitation and their services.

As summarized by Foto (1988), insurers and reimbursement payers (and we would add clients, families, and the community at large) want health delivery systems that "promote wellness, provide appropriate care, reduce hospital days, treat patients at the lowest level of appropriate care, return patients to the healthiest state and most functional level possible, and keep patients satisfied and served" (Foto, 1988). Given this desire and the fact that many individuals suffer from chronic or recurring psychiatric problems, there is an impetus for occupational therapy to build functional skills that will help persons with mental illness care for themselves (Fine, 1988; Lang & Cara, 1989).

OTHER SOCIAL INFLUENCES

Countless other socioeconomic events have influenced and continue to affect mental health practice. Examples include the civil rights movement; the women's movement; changes in criminal law and an increased use of the "insanity" plea; and society's changing view about disease, mental health and illness, and deviance. These trends have led to legislation and legal decisions that support a person's rights and patient advocacy. Many witnessing the growing number of homeless, displaced persons and single-parent families predict an acceleration in the number of persons who will need mental health services, transitional support prevention programs, and health and wellness programs. These societal changes contribute to the heightened social conscience of occupational therapists as they strive to respond to the greater interests of society and they create new opportunities for occupational therapy practice in less traditional contexts (Bowen, 1999; Cunningham Piergrossi, 1999; Earle, 1999; Pierce, 1999a, 1999b; Smith, 1999; Starnes, 2000; Swarbrick & Duffy, 2000; Townsend, Birch, Langley, & Langille, 2000; Trump, 2000).

DEFINING TERMS IN OCCUPATIONAL THERAPY

Evolution of Theory—Theoretical Frameworks

Theory is always evolving. Theory development within occupational therapy has included the creation or development of knowledge within the field as well as the assimilation of information from related disciplines. Each time that we revise this text, we see the evolution of occupational therapy theory in the literature we review. An example of theoretical evolution and a major theoretical contribution to the occupational therapy profession is represented by the development of occupational science (Christiansen, 1999; Clark et al., 1991; Farnworth, 1999; Kellegrew, 2000; Larson, 1999; Pierce, 1999a, 1999b; Primeau, 1998; Wilcox, 1998; Yerxa et al., 1990; Zemke & Clark, 1996).

As theory evolves, it often introduces new terminology or uses existing terms in new ways. Since the previous editions of this text (1987, 1993), new terminology has been introduced into the professional literature and practice environment and continues to be refined. Throughout the text you will find recent terminology clarified. We have chosen to describe those terms that we believe most directly impact the frameworks described in our text. You will see that terms are not always used consistently, and we suggest that you not only read carefully but also listen to how therapists (and you yourself) use these terms with clients, peers, and in the larger professional community. The reader is referred to Reed and Sanderson (1999) for a detailed description of the constructs that influence occupational therapy practice. This reference also gives insight into the construction and the evolution of theory in occupational therapy.

Paradigm, Model, Frame of Reference

The profession of occupational therapy holds multiple definitions and interpretations of the following terms: **paradigm**, **model**, and **frame of reference**. Rather than repeat these definitions, we summarize the terms as they are used in this text.

Paradigm

The work of Kuhn (1974) is often cited in the discussion of the term **paradigm**. As applied to occupational therapy, a paradigm contains the guiding premises and theories behind the profession as a whole. As such, a paradigm identifies the theories that have been or need to be tested and that will lead to the creation and organization of knowledge.

Model of Practice or Frame of Reference

In her book entitled *Three Frames of Reference for Mental Health*, occupational therapist Anne Mosey (1970) used the term **frame of reference** to describe a set of internally consistent and related concepts, postulates, and principles that could be used to guide practice. According to Mosey, a comprehensive frame of reference includes:

1. A statement of the theoretical base (e.g., an explanation of how the person is viewed, the nature of the person, activity, and/or environment interaction)

2. A delineation of function and dysfunction continuums (what behaviors or attributes identify that there is or is not a problem)

3. Statements regarding evaluation (including the tools and techniques that will be used and what should be assessed)

4. Postulates regarding change (what the therapist pays attention to and how therapy is carried out) (Mosey, 1970, pp. 9-13)

Mosey viewed the frames of reference in occupational therapy as incorporating theories and assumptions from both inside and outside the field (e.g., from psychology, sociology, learning theory, or neurology) and then applied specifically to occupational therapy practice.

Dr. Gary Kielhofner (1992) used the term **conceptual model of practice** to refer to Mosey's frame of reference; however, he proposed that a conceptual model of practice for occupational therapy should articulate unique occupational therapy theory (p. 80). In addition to unique knowledge, occupational therapists may also need to use knowledge obtained from related disciplines such as medicine and psychology. It is important for the clinician to make a clear distinction between occupational therapy and related knowledge (Kielhofner, 1997, p. 25). The four tasks that the conceptual model performs are:

1. Identify the integrated theories that form the theoretical base

2. Describe the theoretical rationale that supports the descriptions of function and dysfunction

3. Recommend theory application for assessment and treatment approaches

4. Summarize the research that tests theory in practice and evaluates the outcomes of its application (Kielhofner, 1997, pp. 22-23)

In this text we use the terms "frame of reference" (or framework) and "model of practice" (or model) interchangeably. The reader will discern that some of the models presented in the text originated outside of the profession (e.g., the psychodynamic, behavioral, and cognitive-behavioral models) and then postulates were adapted for use by occupational therapy. Others models have been generated by occupational therapists (e.g., Allen's cognitive disabilities model and Toglia's dynamic interaction model). The reader is advised, however, that even when generated by occupational therapists for use in occupational therapy, these "OT" models incorporate information and ideas drawn from outside the field. In some instances, we refer the reader to these outside sources in order to provide additional perspective and help the reader trace the development of theory.

Today there are also models that emphasize occupation and describe how three factors or components interact to promote or limit function or occupational performance (Christiansen & Baum, 1997; Crepeau, 1998; Holm, Rogers, & Stone, 1998; Reed & Sanderson, 1999). These three factors are the person, the occupation, and the environment. Of these components, the "person" is the only one that is identified in a consistent way. In some models, "occupation" may be referred to as "task," and "environment" may be identified as "context." These occupational therapy models contribute to the knowledge base of the profession and are reproduced from Reed and Sanderson in Table 1-1.

We view these person-environment-occupation models as providing an overarching structure for intervention, but lacking specific guidelines for responding to identified clinical problems. We discuss the relationships between these three components in greater detail in Chapter Two.

The frames of reference (models) presented in this text contain explicit intervention guides. They tell the therapist what to pay attention to and how to implement therapy. Collectively, the frames of reference included in our text represent a diverse body of knowledge in occupational therapy. What they have in common is that all address psychosocial concerns in practice. Given the multiple arenas of practice in which psychosocial issues are a primary or secondary focus, we have chosen frameworks that are applicable in diverse settings, with persons of many ages and varied abilities. No framework is diagnostic-specific. The reader is advised, however, that with each model there are statements regarding the types of problems and issues the model seeks to address. The frameworks in this text are presented in a manner that allows the reader to see the evolution of psychosocial thinking in occupational therapy and to contrast and compare important ideas represented in each of the frameworks.

The Person and Disability

There are multiple definitions for describing the disability and the person who receives occupational therapy services. The terms are influenced by the philosophical beliefs of the profession, the theoretical models specific to populations, and the environments of practice. Some terms used in current literature include **client**, **patient**, **consumer**, **member** (from the Clubhouse Model), and **citizen** (Community Model).

Disability and International Classification of Impairments, Disabilities, and Handicaps

Deciding what term to use to describe the status of having illness or disabling conditions has been an international concern for more than 40 years. The work of Nagi (1976) produced a model that identified both emotional and physical attributes around the construct of "disability." The World Health Organization (1980, 1999) also published a classification system in which the terms "impairment," "disability," and "handicap" were defined. This guide is the *International Classification of Impairments, Disabilities, and Handicaps* (ICIDH) and is used internationally. This original classification was revised, *International Classification of Functioning and Disability Beta-2*, and is now being tested in field trials until 2001. The reader is referred to Chapter Two, in which the ICIDH classification is discussed in more detail.

Table 1-1

Models by Year of Major Publication

1910	Invalid occupation—Susan E. Tracy, nurse
	Graded occupation—Herbert Hall, MD
1911	Therapeutic occupation—William Rush Dunton Jr., MD
1918	Biomechanical or restoration model—Bird T. Baldwin (psychologist who started the OT department at Walter Reed General Hospital)
1919	Reconstruction therapy—William Rush Dunton Jr., MD
	Re-education—George E. Barton, architect
1922	Philosophy of occupation therapy—Adolph Meyer, MD
	Habit training—Eleanor Clarke Slagle, OT Reg
1925	Pre-industrial training—Thomas B. Kidner (manual education teacher and architect)
1934	Orthopedic model—Marjorie Taylor, OT Reg
1947	Kinetic model—Sidney Licht
1954	Sensorimotor therapy—Margaret Rood, OTR, RPT
1958	Perceptual motor development—A. Jean Ayres, OTR
1959	Object relations—H. Azima, MD
1961	Reflex development—Mary Fiorentino, OTR
1963	Communication process—Gail Fidler, OTR and Jay Fidler, MD
1966	Recapitualization of ontogenesis—Anne Mosey, OTR
	Occupational behavior—Mary Reilly, OTR
1968	Sensory integration—A. Jean Ayres, OTR
1970	Group development—Anne Mosey, OTR
1972	Prevention—Ruth Brunyate Weimer, OTR
1973	Activity therapy—Anne Mosey, OTR
1974	Play model—Mary Reilly, OTR
	Biopsychosocial model—Anne Mosey, OTR
	Program educator model—AOTA
1976	Human development through occupation—Patricia Nuse Clark (Allen), OTR
	Facilitating growth and development—Lela Llorens, OTR
1977	Temporal adaptation—Gary Kielhofner, OTR
1978	Activities model—Simme Cynkin, OTR
	Doing and becoming—Gail Fidler, OTR
	Individual adaptation—Lorna Jean King, OTR
1979	Neurobehavioral model—Barbara Banus
	Uniform terminology model—AOTA
1980	Model of human occupation—Gary Kielhofner, OTR
	Personal adaptation through occupation—Kathlyn Reed, OTR
1981	Spatiotemporal adaptation—Eleanor Gilfoyle, OTR and Ann Grady, OTR
1982	Clinical reasoning—Joan Rogers, OTR
	Ecological systems model—Margot Howe, OTR and Ann Briggs, OTR
1983	Client-centred practice—Task Force of the Canadian Association of Occupational Therapy

(continued)

Table 1-1 (Continued)	
1985	Perceptual cognitive rehabilitation—Beatriz Abreu, OTR
	Cognitive disability—Claudia Allen, OTR
	Group work—Sharon Schwartzberg, OTR and Margot Howe, OTR
1988	Occupational form and occupational performance—David Nelson, OTR
1989	Occupational science—Elizabeth J. Yerxa, OTR and Florence Clark, OTR
1991	Person-environment-occupational performance model—Charles Christiansen, OTR and Carolyn Baum, OTR
1992	Occupational adaptation—Jeanette Schkade, OTR and Sally Schulz, OTR
	Multicontext treatment approach—Janet Toglia, OTR
	Occupational competence model—Helen J. Polatajko, OT(C)
1994	Ecology of human performance—Winnie Dunn, OTR, Catana Brown, OTR, Linda H. McClain, OTR, and Kay Westman, OTR
	Contemporary task-oriented approach—Virgil Mathiowetz, OTR and Julie Bass Haugen, OTR
1995	The enablement model—Rose Martini, OT(C), Helene J. Polatajko, OT(C), and Ann Wilcox
	Model of occupational functioning (ends-means)—Catherine A. Trombly, OTR
1996	Person-environment-occupation model—Mary Law, OT(C), Barbara Cooper, OT(C), Susan Strong, OT(C), Debra Stewart, OT(C), Patricia Rigby, OT(C), and Lori Letts, OT(C)
1997	Occupational performance process model—Virginia Fearing, OT, Mary Law, OT(C), and Jo Clark, OT
	Playfulness—Anita Bundy, OTR

Patient, Client, or Consumer?

When occupational therapy began, recipients of services were typically seen in hospital settings and were referred to as **patients**. An outcome of the community mental health movement was to call into question the use of the term **patient**. Many mental health professionals felt that the term "patient" reinforced the sick role of the individual and supported the idea of pathology or illness and the individual's need to be taken care of by health professionals. Wishing to minimize the sick role, they chose the term **client** to focus on problems of living, not illness, and to encourage the individual to assume responsibility for his or her own health and care. A client is someone who "seeks a service but not a medical service" (Gillette, 1971). The reader should note that the use of the term client is inconsistent with a medical model of care.

In occupational therapy, both terms—client and patient—as well as other terms are used depending on the practice or intervention setting. The descriptor may also reflect the preference of the occupational therapist or the professional intervention team. In the mid-1980s, however, a controversy developed over which term was preferable. Until then, the choice of the term patient was probably made with little consideration given to legal, ethical, and moral issues. These issues, as well as the far-reaching implications for the profession, were brought to the occupational therapists' attention by Reilly (1984) and were researched and summarized by Sharrott and Yerxa (1985).

Sharrott and Yerxa justified the continued use of the term patient for the following reasons:
- The term is based on a moral-ethical tradition rather than an economic-legalistic foundation, and the occupational therapy profession has a moral-ethical base.
- The term is compatible with the Meyer-ian philosophy of the profession.
- The term connotes the ethical stance of moral treatment of the 19th century.

- The term supports opportunity for health care regardless of the patient's ability to provide financial remuneration (Sharrott & Yerxa, 1985).

Covenant Code

For those therapists who preferred to use the term client to equalize the responsibilities in intervention, Sharrott and Yerxa referred to Veatch's conceptualization of medical ethics to identify how responsibilities could be equalized in the patient/therapist relationship. Briefly, Veatch (1981) proposed that medical ethics be based on a **covenant code**. "A covenant is a contract that emphasizes moral bonds and fidelity and requires right action by both health professionals and the lay public." Medical ethics are designed to apply to "patient-health professional relationships" (see Principles of the Covenant).

PRINCIPLES OF THE COVENANT

The fundamental principles of the covenant are as follows:

1. Keep promises and commitments to one another.

2. Treat one another as autonomous members of the moral community free to make choices that do not violate other basic ethical requirements.

3. Interact honestly with one another.

4. Avoid actively and knowingly the taking of morally protected life.

5. Strive for equality in individual welfare and equality in the right of access to health care.

6. Produce good for one another and treat one another with respect, dignity, and compassion (Sharrott & Yerxa, 1985; Veatch, 1981).

Consumer

With the changes in the health care and occupational therapy practice arenas, another term began to be used—**consumer**. Peloquin (1997, 2000) asks, however, that before occupational therapists adopt this term they carefully consider its origin and meaning. She asks therapists to consider not only the definition from the point of view of the *Essentials and Guidelines for an Accredited Educational Program for the Occupational Therapist* (Accreditation Council for Occupational Therapy Education, 1998), which refers to "the recipient of therapeutic and educational services," but also the word origin. The term consumer arises from the marketplace, an environment with a **primary concern** for profit and a **secondary focus** on caring, empathy, quality, reliability, and the person as central (Peloquin, 1997, 2000).

Peloquin's choice is "persons" when "naming those we serve" (2000, p. 28). "Person" is also our choice.

Person in Context

This text predominantly refers to **person(s)** or **individual(s)**; however, **patient** or **client** is also used when the discussion or example relates to a specific environment or context. These terms continue to be congruent with occupational therapy's philosophy and history. They support a moral-ethical base for practice. They are compatible with mutuality of respect and responsibility vital to the collaborative relationship that exists in occupational therapy practice. They support occupational therapy's advocacy role for quality care for those we treat regardless of the disability or the practice setting.

We recognize, however, the need to function within one's environment and are aware that such terms as "student," "learner," "resident," "family," and "worker" may be appropriate to the service environment. We feel that regardless of the term applied, the material presented in the text is viable in practice in multiple contexts.

SUMMARY—HISTORY AND TERMINOLOGY IN PSYCHOSOCIAL PRACTICE

We have briefly considered some of the changes within society, medicine, and the mental health community in order to highlight their influence in the history of psychosocial occupational therapy. Historical events have consistently challenged occupational therapists to broaden their roles in the profession and increase the environments of practice. Occupational therapy history, both in theory and in practice, shows a continued commitment to humanitarian care, to the use of activities and occupations, and to respectful understanding of and responding to the needs of the "whole person." The commitment to these ideals challenges the occupational therapist to be aware and responsive to the psychosocial issues that influence the person's occupational performance, participation in daily life, and sense of well-being.

Commitment to these ideals, however, is not enough. We are now faced with our next challenge: evaluating and demonstrating the outcomes of our therapeutic intervention. To evaluate our theories and their effects on outcomes, current and future practitioners will more frequently assume the role of researcher and educator as well as clinician. With the blending of these roles, occupational therapists will be better able to improve the quality of client-centered and "holistic" practice. They will also be able to provide evidence-based practice. With the support of our national and international professional organizations, such as AOTA, the American Occupational Therapy Foundation, The World Federation of Occupational Therapy, and our collaborations with other national and international professional groups, we can pursue the evidence that supports quality practice of occupational therapy. This is our current professional priority (Holm, 2000).

EVIDENCE-BASED PRACTICE

Through its history, occupational therapy has developed and refined theories regarding the role of occupation in enabling people to achieve and maintain health. Further, it has delineated specific practice models that can be used to put patients' problems into perspective and guide the therapeutic response. Clinicians, educators, and researchers have been reflective as they made clinical decisions and again as they evaluated the outcome of therapy at its conclusion. While there has been some clinical research, clinicians have observed and listened carefully to clients, family members, and other team members in order to make sound clinical decisions. What has been learned has been shared through our professional literature, but what has been lacking is the systematic collection and reference to this literature.

Since 1998, occupational therapists, influenced by their colleagues in medicine (Sackett, Richardson, Rosenberg, & Haynes, 1997) and others, have begun to initiate the use of methods that would enable evidence-based practice. These methods do not specifically or narrowly describe assessment and treatment. The methods are integrated with client-centered reasoning to find the "best evidence" for making individual clinical decisions based on current and best evidence (see System to Organize and Evaluate Evidence).

SYSTEM TO ORGANIZE AND EVALUATE EVIDENCE

The medical community developed a specific system to evaluate and organize their evidence for practice. Organizations such as the Cochrane Collaboration (1998; Glanville, 1994; Hayes & McGrath, 1998) and the Journal Club (Partridge, 1996) follow an extensive process. The process is a multistep sequence that begins with identifying a problem or clinical question. The information related to the problem is then gathered from juried publications and unpublished evidence. The evidence is systematically reviewed, analyzed, and then synthesized. The review results identify the most efficient and cost-effective interventions (Greenhalgh, 1996; Greenhalgh & Macfarlane, 1997). These results are available on the Internet and on CD-ROMs (Greengold & Weingarten, 1996; Sharpe et al., 1996). Results are shared with experts who use the evidence to develop practice guidelines.

A "Toolbox" for the Practitioner

In the article that initiated the Evidence-Based Practice Forum in the *American Journal of Occupational Therapy*, Linda Tickle-Degnen, the author of this discussion section, provided a definition of evidence-based practice and described it as a clinical reasoning tool.

Tickle-Degnen (1999) defines evidence-based practice as a "toolbox of methods to aid clinical reasoning… a toolbox consisting primarily of methods designed to integrate research studies and evidence into the clinical reasoning process" (p. 537). When reasoning, the goal is for the therapist to use the most "current" and the "best" information to make clinical decisions.

The evidence for decisions can come from multiple sources:
- Clinical experts
- Continuing education courses
- Professional and related discipline literatures
- Expert opinion from peers
- Observations and perceptions of our clients

The reader should note that these represent multiple sources of evidence. Evidence-based practice uses research literature as well as that describing theory and clinical practice.

After gathering information from these varied sources, the clinician organizes and evaluates this information before selecting the assessment and intervention strategies he or she will use with a particular client.

Framework for Evidence-Based Practice

To support the efficient use of the evidence in daily practice, the information needs to be well organized so it can be easily accessed for the process of clinical reasoning. Tickle-Degnen (1999) describes a framework for the organization of evidence and its integration into practice. The framework has three parts:
1. A system for filing and categorizing data
2. An evaluation of information for its current validity
3. An evaluation of the data's relationship to occupational therapy practice for specific populations

Gathering and organizing data is a lifelong learning process. The therapist can gather information and validate his or her knowledge from new resources as well as those traditionally identified for professionals. When discussing her "toolbox" and possible ways for the clinician to make a "toolbox," Tickle-Degnen (2000a, pp. 103-104) suggests that practitioners and scholars attend continuing education courses, participate in listserv groups, do frequent periodical reviews and Internet searches, participate in study and journal groups, and gather knowledge from meta-analysis (see Meta-Analysis).

META-ANALYSIS

A **meta-analysis** is a synthesis of information from a group of related studies. The synthesis provides an analysis that is "...rigorous, comprehensive, and concise..." (Tickle-Degnen, 1998a, p. 527) to determine the effect size. The **effect size** is the estimate of the **effectiveness** of treatment and the evaluation of the relationship between treatment and outcome. The effectiveness of an intervention is based upon the evaluation of contrasting treatment groups and the evaluation of the difference between those who receive no help and those who participate in an intervention. The therapist translates this analysis into a summary that uses lay terms and can be used in a collaborative client effort for decision making in occupational therapy. The data can also be used to measure the effectiveness of occupational therapy (Ottenbacher & Maas, 1998; Tickle-Degnen, 1998a). The reader is referred to some original sources (Cook et al., 1992; Cooper & Hedges, 1994; Portney & Watkins, 2000) for more details that discuss meta-analysis and its design and use.

When reasoning, clinicians work within the *Guide to Occupational Therapy Practice* (Moyers, 1999), the *Standards of Practice* (AOTA, 1998), and AOTA's 2001 *The Practice Guidelines Series*, which is described in Chapter Three. While using these guides, the clinician chooses evidence from occupational therapy and other discipline literatures and from expert opinions or clinical observations. The professional guides and the evidence support the clinician's decisions that plan intervention and guide daily practice. When clinicians evaluate and choose from the available evidence, they also consider if the information is compatible with the individual needs of the clients and the specific environment in which intervention occurs.

Additionally, each clinician should establish a database for his or her practice environment. The database is a record of assessment information and intervention outcomes. This evidence is analyzed to identify the variables of the client population treated and the outcome of occupational therapy interventions in the clinician's practice environment. When making day-to-day decisions, the clinician can use this data from previous clients treated in his or her practice, or the therapist may compare current therapy outcomes with previous ones. These databases can also be a resource for future professional publications that can contribute to the evidence in the profession (Tickle-Degnen, 2000d).

The Development of Evidence-Based Practice

The system Tickle-Degnen describes has been influenced by current systems for evidence-based practice used by medicine and other health care professions. Tickle-Degnen (1999) refers to the system described by Sackett, Richardson, Rosenberg, and Haynes (1997) as one that can serve as a guide for organizing data around clinical tasks. The tasks in medicine include clinical evaluation, identifying causes of disease, making diagnoses, predicting outcomes, selecting tests and treatment, and developing prevention and health promotion programs. Occupational therapists have some similar tasks but the focus is on the unique contributions of occupational therapy. In occupational therapy, the focus in assessment, intervention, prevention, and health promotion is activities, tasks, and occupations for participation in daily life.

The model that Tickle-Degnen (1999, p. 538) uses has three central clinical tasks:
1. Describe the occupations and occupational performance that represent a population
2. Choose an assessment approach
3. Choose an intervention plan
   The three tasks are driven by clinical questions such as:
1. What are the patterns of occupational performance of an individual or population?
2. What are the reliable and valid methods of assessment for the client or the population?
3. What interventions support activity participation in activity and occupations?

These questions can be answered through multiple avenues. The answers can come from within and outside of occupational therapy literature, for example, in descriptions of strategies and outcomes of not only occupational therapy but also related therapies. They can be found within theoretical models that guide practice or come from specific research, including descriptive studies of populations, correlation studies, cross-sectional and longitudinal designs, analysis of qualitative and quantitative data, and experimental and quasi-experimental designs that relate to assessment and intervention (Tickle-Degnen, 1999, p. 539; 2000a, p. 103). Holm (2000) also gives an extensive guide for evaluating and selecting evidence that can be used to answer the previous practice questions and other practice questions specific to occupational therapy.

Considerations for Choosing Best Evidence

The challenge for practitioners is choosing evidence that addresses concerns specific to the client. In most instances, no one study will provide all the information sought. This is due in part to the complex individual nature of the client's occupational therapy needs and the limited database specific to occupational therapy theory and practice. To help the therapist sort out and evaluate research data, Tickle-Degnen (2000b) has provided some standards for evaluating the evidence in quantitative studies, which address three types of studies: descriptive, assessment, and intervention studies.

Evaluation of Descriptive Studies

When evaluating descriptive studies, the therapist should determine if the study "investigated a variable that is relevant to the specific occupation, occupational performance, or component of occupational performance variable in the evidence-based clinical question" (Tickle-Degnen, 2000b, p. 219). If the study meets these criteria, the therapist then looks for information to answer the following questions that relate to the standards for assessing descriptive studies:

- Does the variable relate to occupation?
- Was the variable assessment reliable and valid?
- Is your client a member of the population described?
- Does the study fully or adequately answer the clinical question?
- Does the study describe the individual differences within the population studied (Tickle-Degnen, 2000b, p. 219)?

Evaluation of Assessment Studies

In order to determine if a study used a reliable and valid measure for assessing occupations, occupational performance, and/or other variables, the therapist chooses evidence that answers the following standard-based questions for assessment:

- Does the assessment method measure individual clinical needs?
- Does the assessment measure the variables of occupation, occupational performance, and its components?
- Which form of validity and reliability of the assessment was tested: Evaluative validity? Test-retest reliability? Discriminative validity? Inter-rater reliability?
- Is your client a member of the population described in the study?
- Does the study describe the individual differences within the population studied (Tickle-Degnen, 2000b, p. 220)?

Evaluation of Intervention Studies

The therapist looks for evidence that identifies interventions that support the client's participation in daily life. Tickle-Degnen (2000b) applies the previous standards to single studies of varied sample size. The occupational therapist evaluates if the study evaluated the variables related to occupation, occupational performance, and its components in the context of a specific case. He or she poses the following questions for evaluating intervention (Tickle-Degnen, 2000b, pp. 220-221):

- Was the outcome assessed with a reliable and valid measure?
- Were the individuals of the sample members of the population described in the clinical question?
- Does the study describe the effects of the intervention?
- Does the study eliminate or describe the possible effects of conditions not specific to the intervention?
- Does the study describe the individual differences in outcomes of the intervention?

Communicating Evidence to the Client

The occupational therapist not only uses the evidence that he or she has for his or her own clinical reasoning, but shares this information with clients and their families and with colleagues in occupational therapy practice. When using evidence to describe the purpose or effectiveness of interventions to clients, the occupational therapist uses lay terminology and considers the client's ability to understand the rationale for intervention. The rationale shared with clients relates to the client's specific condition, function, and goals. For example, therapists may share examples of similar cases, or they may use lay terminology to describe the results of a study that relates to the client's condition. When sharing the results of a large study, the clinician may state that the intervention is effective in 95% of the cases with similar conditions. The clinician usually does not use the research terminology that describes the power or level of statistical significance of the data analysis. The reader is referred to resources in the area of research and statistics (Ottenbacher & Maas, 1999; Portney & Watkins, 2000) for details related to data analysis and interpretation of statistics. To understand the difference between large and small sample studies and to compare the outcomes of studies, clinicians need to be able to describe the meaning of frequencies, ranges, means, standard deviations, and correlations (Tickle-Degnen, 2000c, p. 342).

Therapists can also help the client understand evidence by relating research outcomes to the client's existing condition and experiences. Clinicians help the client relate his or her experience to single cases or the sample populations in the studies. Therapists can summarize the assessment data in studies and identify what the client can learn from his or her own occupational therapy assessment. They can also discuss the outcomes from occupational therapy intervention and identify the possible benefits from those in which the client will participate. If the client understands the evidence, then there can be collaboration for client-centered decision making (Tickle-Degnen, 1998b, 2000c).

SUMMARY—RELATIONSHIP BETWEEN EVIDENCE AND PRACTICE

As we bring closure to this chapter and summarize the focus of evidence in practice, we can see the past developments in the profession that have formed our current focus of development. Our history reflects a strong commitment to theory-based practice that is sensitive to the changes in society and integrates some of the developments from sciences, humanities, education, medicine, rehabilitation, and health. As theory evolves, practice expands to new populations while continuing to meet the current needs of the persons we serve in health care, education, industry, and community environments. As health care and policy systems change and theory and practice expand, occupational therapists have new challenges and assume new roles in practice, education, and research.

In occupational therapy and rehabilitation, there is a broad theoretical foundation for practice but limited evidence in support of specific intervention strategies. Thus, the next major challenge for the profession is identifying the evidence that supports our interventions or helps us revise them to meet the needs of individuals or populations. Currently, the occupational therapy literature contains discussions of the advantages and disadvantages of evidence-based practice (Law & Baum, 1998). It suggests approaches for identifying evidence (Hayes & McGrath, 1998; Holm, 2000; Law, 2000; Tickle-Degnen, 1998a, 1998b, 1999, 2000a, 2000b, 2000c) and ways to use evidence in clinical practice (Egan et al., 1998, Holm, 2000; Hunt, 1997; Law, 2000; Tickle-Degnen, 1999, 2000a, 2000b, 2000c, 2000d; Turner & Whitfield, 1997).

Like other health care professionals (Dowie, 1994; Partridge, 1996), occupational therapists want systems that gather and organize evidence and achieve three goals: clinicians want systems that will enhance their clinical effectiveness, provide information that can be given to clients about their health care, and give data that can justify their services to third-party payers and administrators. Currently, there remains a need for occupational therapists to initiate studies and build systems that will provide accessible information in regard to the person-activity-environment relationships and their effects on daily performance, quality of life, and a person's mental health. In particular, the profession needs evidence that addresses:

- The constructs of occupation and the many components of occupational performance
- Reliable and valid measures of occupation and performance component constructs
- Outcomes and effects of occupational therapy services
- Individual differences that affect intervention outcomes

We are confident that occupational therapists will successfully meet this challenge as they have met others in our history. We see evidence-based practice as providing growth and opportunities in practice, education, and research. Most important, evidence supports clinical reasoning and gives an occupational therapy outcome that improves the quality of services we provide to people who wish to increase their participation in daily life and have increased health and well-being.

REFERENCES

Accreditation Council for Occupational Therapy Education. (1998). Standards for an accredited educational program for the occupational therapist. *Am J Occup Ther, 53,* 575-582.

American Occupational Therapy Association. (1998). *The reference manual of the official documents of the American Occupational Therapy Association, Inc.* (7th ed.). Bethesda, MD: Author.

Bailey, D. (1990a). Reasons for attrition from occupational therapy. *Am J Occup Ther, 44*(3), 23-30.

Bailey, D. (1990b). Ways to retain or reactivate occupational therapists. *Am J Occup Ther, 44*(3), 31-38.

Bowen, J. E. (1999). Health promotion in the new millennium. *OT Practice, 4,* 14-19.

Burnette-Beaulier, S. (1982). Occupational therapy profession dropouts: Escape from the grief process. *American Journal of Occupational Therapy Mental Health, 2,* 45-55.

Chisholm, D., Dolhi, C., & Schreiber, J. (2000). Creating occupation-based opportunities in a medical model clinical practice setting. *Occupational Therapy Practice, 5*(11), 12-15.

Christiansen, C. (1999). Defining lives: Occupation as identity: An essay on competence, coherence, and the creation of meaning. *Am J Occup Ther, 53,* 547-558.

Christiansen, C., & Baum, C. (1997). *Occupational therapy: Enabling function and well-being* (2nd ed.). Thorofare, NJ: SLACK Incorporated.

Clark, F., Azen, S. P., Zemke, R., Jackson, J., Carlson, M., Mandel, D., Hay, J., Josephson, K., Cherry, B., Hessel, C., Palmer, J., & Lipson, L. (1997). Occupational therapy for independent-living older adults: A randomized controlled trial. *JAMA, 278,* 1321-1326.

Clark, F., Parham, D., Carlson, M., Frank, G., Jackson, J., Pierce, D., Wolf, R. J., & Zemke, R. (1991). Occupational science: Academic motivation in the service of occupational therapy's future. *Am J Occup Ther, 45,* 300-310.

Cochrane Collaboration. (1998). *Cochrane brochure.* Available at: http://www.cochrane.org.

Cook, T. D., Cooper, H., Cordray, D. D., Hartmann, H., Hedges, L. V., Light, R. J., Louis, T., & Mosteller, F. (Eds.). (1992). *Meta-analysis for explanation: A casebook.* New York, NY: Russell Sage Foundation.

Cooper, H. M., & Hedges, L. V. (Eds.). (1994). *The handbook of research synthesis.* New York, NY: Russell Sage Foundation.

Cottrell, R. F. (1989). Perceived competence among occupational therapists in mental health. *Am J Occup Ther, 44*(2), 118-124.

Crepeau, E. (1998). Activity analysis: A way of thinking about occupational performance. In M. E. Neistadt & E. B. Crepeau (Eds.), *Willard and Spackman's occupational therapy* (9th ed., pp. 135-147). Philadelphia, PA: Lippincott, Williams & Wilkins.

Cunningham Piergrossi, J. (1999). Using activities for consulting in community mental health. *World Federation of Occupational Therapist Bulletin, 40,* 44-49.

Dowie, J. (1994, October). *The research practice gap and the role of decision analysis in closing it.* Paper presented at the European Medicine Decision Making Conference, Lille, Norway.

Dressler, J., & MacRae, A. (1998). Advocacy, partnerships, and client-centered practice in California. *Occupational Therapy in Mental Health, 14,* 35-44.

Dunton, D. (1963). Psychiatric occupational therapy. In H. Willard & C. Spackman (Eds.), *Occupational therapy* (3rd ed., pp. 55-74). Philadelphia, PA: J. B. Lippincott.

Dunton, W. R. (1915). *Occupational therapy: A manual for nurses.* Philadelphia, PA: W. B. Saunders.

Dunton, W. R. (1919). *Reconstruction therapy.* Philadelphia, PA: W. B. Saunders.

Dunton, W. R. (1922). The educational possibilities of occupational therapy in state hospitals. *Archives of Occupational Therapy, 1,* 403.

Earle, G. K. (1999). OT's role in mental health home care. *OT Practice, 4,* 16-18.

Egan, M., Dubouloz, C. J., Von Zweck, C., & Vallerand, J. (1998). The client-centered evidence-based practice of occupational therapy. *Can J Occup Ther, 65,* 136-143.

Farnworth, L. (1999). Time use and leisure occupations of young offenders. *Am J Occup Ther, 54,* 315-325.

Fidler, G., & Fidler, J. (1963). *Occupational therapy—A communication process in psychiatry.* New York, NY: The Macmillan Co.

Fine, S. (1988). Working the system: A perspective for managing change. *Am J Occup Ther, 47*(7), 417-419.

Fine, S. B. (1998). Surviving the health care revolution: Rediscovering the meaning of "good work." *Occupational Therapy in Mental Health, 14,* 7-18.

Florey, L. (1998). Psychosocial dysfunction in childhood and adolescence. In M. E. Neistadt & E. B. Crepeau (Eds.), *Willard & Spackman's occupational therapy* (9th ed., pp. 622-635). Philadelphia, PA: Lippincott, Williams & Wilkins.

Foto, M. (1988). Managing change in reimbursement patterns. *Am J Occup Ther, 42*(9), 563-565.

Gillette, N. (1971). Occupational therapy and mental health. In H. Willard & C. Spackman (Eds.), *Occupational therapy* (4th ed., pp. 51-132). Philadelphia, PA: J. B. Lippincott.

Glanville, J. (1994). Evidence-based practice: The role of NHS centres for reviews and dissemination. *Health Library Review, 11,* 243-252.

Greengold, N. L., & Weingarten, S. R. (1996). Developing evidence-based practice guidelines and pathways: The experience at the local hospital level. *Jt Comm J Qual Improv, 22,* 391-402.

Greenhalgh, T. (1996). Is my practice evidence-based? (Editorial). *BMJ, 313,* 957-958.

Greenhalgh, T., & Macfarlane, F. (1997). Towards a competency grid for evidence-based practice. *J Eval Clin Pract, 3,* 161-165.

Gutterman, L. (1990). A day program for persons with AIDS. *Am J Occup Ther, 44*(3), 234-238.

Haas, L. (1925). *Occupational therapy for the mentally and nervously ill.* Milwaukee, WI: Bruce.

Hahn, C. (2000). Building mental health roles into school system practice. *OT Practice, 5,* 14-16.

Hanft, B. (1988). Prospective payment for psychiatric services. In S. Robertson (Ed.), *Mental health focus: Skills for assessment and treatment* (pp. 3.10-3.15). Rockville, MD: American Occupational Therapy Association.

Hatje Kaufman, C., Daniels, R., Laverdure, P., Moyer, R., & Campana, L. (1988). Pediatric occupational therapy within a cognitive behavioral setting. In D. Scott & N. Katz (Eds.), *Occupational therapy in mental health: Principles in practice.* London: Taylor & Francis.

Hayes, R., & McGrath, J. (1998). Evidence-based practice: The Cochrane Collaboration and occupational therapy. *Can J Occup Ther, 65,* 144-151.

Holm, M. B. (2000). Our mandate for the new millennium: Evidence-based practice. *Am J Occup Ther, 54,* 575-585.

Holm, M. B., Rogers, J. C., & Stone, R. G. (1998). Person-task-environment interventions: A decision-making guide. In M. E. Neistadt & E. B. Crepeau (Eds.), *Willard & Spackman's occupational therapy* (9th ed., pp. 471-498). Philadelphia, PA: Lippincott, Williams & Wilkins.

Hopkins, H. (1983). An historical perspective on occupational therapy. In H. Hopkins & H. Smith (Eds.), *Willard and Spackman's occupational therapy* (6th ed.). Philadelphia, PA: J. B. Lippincott.

Hunt, J. (1997). Towards evidence-based practice. *Nursing Manager, 4,* 14-17.

Kaplan, H. I., & Sadock, B. J. (1998). *Synopsis of psychiatry* (8th ed.). Philadelphia, PA: Lippincott, Williams & Wilkins.

Kautzmann, L. N. (1998). Contributing to a system change in Kentucky: Occupational therapy in an evolving program of Medicaid managed behavioral healthcare. *Occupational Therapy in Mental Health, 14,* 21-28.

Kellegrew, D. (2000). Constructing daily routines: A qualitative examination of mothers with young children with disabilities. *Am J Occup Ther, 54,* 252-259.

Kielhofner, G. (1992). *Conceptual foundations of occupational therapy.* Philadelphia, PA: F. A. Davis.

Kielhofner, G. (1997). *Conceptual foundations of occupational therapy* (2nd ed.). Philadelphia, PA: F. A. Davis.

Kielhofner, G., & Burke, J. (1977). Occupational therapy after 60 years: An account of changing identity and knowledge. *Am J Occup Ther, 31*(10), 675-689.

Kornblau, B. L. (1990). Occupational therapy and the Americans with Disabilities Act (ADA). In American Occupational Therapy Association, *The reference manual of the official documents.* Bethesda, MD: American Occupational Therapy Association.

Kramer, P., & Hinojosa, J. (1999). *Frames of reference for pediatric occupational therapy* (2nd ed.). Philadelphia, PA: Lippincott, Williams & Wilkins.

Kuhn, T. (1974). *The structure of scientific revolutions.* Chicago, IL: University of Chicago Press.

Lang, S., & Cara, E. (1989). Vocational integration for the psychiatrically disabled. *Hospital and Community Psychiatry, 40*(9), 890-892.

Larson, E. A. (1999). Mothering: Letting go of the past ideal and valuing the real. *Am J Occup Ther, 29,* 249-251.

Law, M. (2000). Evidence-based practice—What can it mean for me? *OT Practice, 5*(17), 16-18.

Law, M., & Baum, C. (1998). Evidence-based occupational therapy. *Can J Occup Ther, 65,* 131-135.

Learnard, L., Walsh, A., & Ward, J. D. (1999, November). *The establishment of a private psychosocial practice in a rural community.* Paper presented at the American Occupational Therapy Association SIS Practice Conference, Reno, NV.

Lougher, L. (Ed.). (2001). *Occupational therapy for child and adolescent mental health.* Edinburgh: Churchill Livingstone.

Marcos, L. (1989). Taking issue: Who profits from deinstitutionalization. *Hospital and Community Psychiatry, 40*(12), 1221.

Margo, G., & Manring, J. (1989). The current literature on inpatient psychotherapy. *Hospital and Community Psychiatry, 40*(9), 909-915.

Meyer, A. (1922). The philosophy of occupational therapy. *Archives of Occupational Therapy, 1,* 1.

Mosey, A. C. (1970). *Three frames of reference for mental health.* Thorofare, NJ: SLACK Incorporated.

Moyers, P. A. (1999). The guide to occupational therapy practice. *Am J Occup Ther, 53,* 247-322.

Nagi, S. (1976). An epidemiology of disability among adults in the USA. *MMFQ/Health and Society, 54,* 439-467.

O'Rourke, G. C. (1990). The HIV-positive intravenous drug abuser. *Am J Occup Ther, 44*(3), 280-293.

Ottenbacher, K. J., & Maas, F. (1998). How to detect effects: Statistical power and evidence-based practice in occupational therapy research. *Am J Occup Ther, 53,* 181-188.

Ottenbacher, K. J., & Maas, F. (1999). Quantitative research series—How to detect effects: Statistical power and evidence-based practice in occupational therapy research. *Am J Occup Ther, 53,* 181-188.

Palmer, F. (1988). The present context of service delivery. In S. Robertson (Ed.), *Mental health focus: Skills for assessment and treatment* (pp. 1.28-1.36). Rockville, MD: American Occupational Therapy Association.

Partridge, C. (1996). Evidence-based medicine—Implications for physiotherapy? *Physiotherapy Research International, 1,* 69-73.

Peloquin, S. M. (1997). The issue is—Should we trade person-centered service for a consumer-based model? *Am J Occup Ther, 51,* 612-615.

Peloquin, S. M. (2000). Do we really want to call them consumers? *OT Practice, Jan. 31,* 26-28.

Peters, M. (1988). Reimbursement for psychiatric occupational services. In S. Robertson (Ed.), *Mental health focus: Skills for assessment and treatment* (pp. 3.3-3.9). Rockville, MD: American Occupational Therapy Association.

Pierce, D. (1999a). Maternal management of the home as a developmental play space for infants and toddlers. *Am J Occup Ther, 29,* 290-299.

Pierce, D. (1999b). Putting occupation to work in occupational therapy curricula. *Education Special Interest Section Quarterly, 9*(3), 1-4.

Portney, L. C., & Watkins, M. P. (2000). *Foundations of clincial research—Applications to practice* (2nd ed.). Saddle River, NJ: Prentice Hall Health.

Primeau, L. A. (1998). Orchestration of work and play within families. *Am J Occup Ther, 52,* 188-195.

Reed, K., & Sanderson, N. (1999). *Concepts of occupational therapy* (4th ed.). Philadelphia, PA: Lippincott, Williams & Wilkins.

Reilly, M. (1962). Occupational therapy can be one of the great ideas of 20th century medicine. *Am J Occup Ther, 16,* 1.

Reilly, M. (1966). A psychiatric occupational therapy program as a teaching model. *Am J Occup Ther, 20,* 61.

Reilly, M. (1984). The importance of the client versus patient issue for occupational therapy. *Am J Occup Ther, 38*(6), 404-406.

Robertson, S. (1988). Factors influencing service delivery. In S. Robertson (Ed.), *Mental health focus: Skills for assessment and treatment* (pp. 1.24-1.27). Rockville, MD: American Occupational Therapy Association.

Sackett, D. L., Richardson, W. S., Rosenberg, W., & Haynes, R. B. (1997). *Evidence based medicine: How to practice and teach EBM.* New York, NY: Churchill Livingstone.

Samuel, L. (1998). Responsive changes in mental health practice in Wisconsin. In A. H. Scott (Ed.), New frontiers in psychosocial occupational therapy. *Occupational Therapy in Mental Health, 14,* 29-34.

Scott, A. H. (1999). Wellness works: Community service health promotion groups led by occupational therapy students. *Am J Occup Ther, 53,* 566-574.

Sharpe, M., Hawton, K., Simkin, S., Surawy, C., Hackmann, A., Klimes, I., Peto, T., Warrell, D., & Seagroatt, V. (1996). Cognitive behavior therapy for the chronic fatigue syndrome: A randomized controlled trial. *British Medical Journal, 312,* 22-26.

Sharrott, G., & Yerxa, E. (1985). Promises to keep: Implications of the referent "patient" versus "client" for those served by occupational therapy. *Am J Occup Ther, 39*(6), 401-405.

Sholle-Martin, S., & Alessi, N. E. (1990). Formulating a role for occupational therapy in child psychiatry: A clinical application. *Am J Occup Ther, 44*(10), 871-883.

Slagle, E. C. (1922). Training aides for mental patients. *Archives of Occupational Therapy, 1,* 11.

Smith, S. I. (1999). Occupational therapy—Practicing in the community. *World Federation of Occupational Therapy Bulletin, 40,* 6-11.

Starnes, W. (2000). Expanding to the community. *OT Practice, 5,* 14-19.

Swarbrick, P., & Duffy, M. (2000). Consumer-operated organization and programs: A role for occupational therapy programs. *Mental Health Special Interest Section Quarterly, 23,* 1-4.

Tewfik, D., & Precin, P. (1998). The New York experience: The remodeling of mental health practice. *Occupational Therapy in Mental Health, 14,* 45-54.

Tickle-Degnen, L. (1998a). Communicating with patients about treatment outcomes: The use of meta-analytic evidence in collaborative treatment planning. *Am J Occup Ther, 52*, 526-530.

Tickle-Degnen, L. (1998b). Using research evidence in planning treatment for the individual client. *Can J Occup Ther, 65*, 152-159.

Tickle-Degnen, L. (1999). Organizing, evaluating, and using evidence in occupational therapy practice. *Am J Occup Ther, 53*, 537-539.

Tickle-Degnen, L. (2000a). Gathering current research evidence to enhance clinical reasoning. *Am J Occup Ther, 54*, 102-105.

Tickle-Degnen, L. (2000b). What is the best evidence to use in practice? *Am J Occup Ther, 54*, 218-221.

Tickle-Degnen, L. (2000c). Communicating with clients, family members, and colleagues about research evidence. *Am J Occup Ther, 54*, 341-343.

Tickle-Degnen, L. (2000d). Monitoring and documenting evidence during assessment and intervention. *Am J Occup Ther, 54*, 343-436.

Tiffany, E. (1983). Psychiatry and mental health. In H. Hopkins & H. Smith (Eds.), *Willard and Spackman's occupational therapy* (6th ed., pp. 267-334). Philadelphia, PA: J. B. Lippincott.

Townsend, E., Birch, D., Langley, J., & Langille, L. (2000). Participatory research in a mental health clubhouse. *Occupational Therapy Journal of Research, 29*, 18-44.

Tracy, S. (1912). *Studies in invalid occupation*. Boston, MA: Whitcomb & Barrows.

Trump, S. M. (2000). The role of occupational therapy in hospice. *Home and Community Health Special Interest Section Quarterly, 7*, 1-4.

Turner, P., & Whitfield, T. W. A. (1997). Physiotherapists' use of evidence-based practice: A cross-national study. *Physiotherapy Resident International, 2*, 17-29.

Veatch, R. (1981). *A theory of medical ethics* (pp. 327-328). New York, NY: Basic Books.

Walens, D., Wittman, P., Dickie, V., Kannenberg, K., Tomlinson, J., & Raynor, O. (1998). Current and future education and practice: Issues for occupational therapy practitioners in mental health settings. *Occupational Therapy in Mental Health, 14*, 107-118.

Wilcox, A. A. (1998). *An occupation perspective of health*. Thorofare, NJ: SLACK Incorporated.

World Health Organization. (1980). *International classification of impairments, disabilities, and handicaps*. Geneva: Author.

World Health Organization. (1999). *International classification of functioning and disability beta-2 draft short version*. Geneva: Author, Assessment, Classification and Epidemiology Group.

Yerxa, E. (1966). Authentic occupational therapy. *Am J Occup Ther, XXI*(1), 1-9.

Yerxa, E., Clark, F., Frank, G., Jackson, J., Parham, D., Pierce, D., Stein, C., & Zemke, R. (1990). An introduction to occupational science: A foundation for occupational therapy in the 21st century. *Occupational Therapy in Health Care, 6*, 1-17.

Zemke, R., & Clark, F. (Eds.). (1996). *Occupational science: The evolving discipline*. Philadelphia, PA: F. A. Davis.

CHAPTER TWO

Person-Activity/Occupation-Environment/Context— Occupational Therapy Practice Variables

Authors' Note: Some of the definitions in this chapter are cited from a document that is being developed by the Commission on Practice, American Occupational Therapy Association. This new document, which is a revision of the terms in the Uniform Terminology of Occupational Therapy—Third Edition, *will be an official document that is compatible with ICIDH-2 and supports the* Guide to Occupational Therapy Practice. *The reader is referred to* www.aota.org *for future document drafts that are available for review and feedback by the members of the profession. The official document will be available in 2002.*

KEY POINTS

✧ The Person and Function
- Theoretical Concepts of Mental Health
- Universal Language in Mental Health Rehabilitation
- Occupational Therapy and Global Assessment of Function
- Psychosocial Components of Function
- Motivation—Multiple Perspectives

✧ Activity, Task, and Occupation
- Activity: Connects Mind, Body, Spirit, and Enables Participation in Life
- Activity: Means to Establish Habits and Carry Out Roles
- Occupational Performance Model of Activity
- Models of Practice Provide Criteria for Therapeutic Activity
- Activity Analysis—Clinical Reasoning for Client-Centered Intervention

✧ Environment/Context
- Types of Environments
- The Person's Place in the Environment
- The Psychosocial Impact of the Environment

FOCUS QUESTIONS

Person

1. What is mental health?
2. Why are mental health issues believed to be vital to all areas of practice?
3. What is a psychological construct?
4. Compare the official definitions of **mental health** and **mental disorder** in Canada and the United States. How are they similar? How are they different?
5. What are the four major classifications of disablement as defined by the World Health Organization?
6. What is the critical requirement for a child to be given the label **serious emotional disorder**?
7. How is the person's global level of function determined?
8. Describe the psychosocial components of performance.

Activity/Occupation

9. What is the relationship between **activity** and **occupation**?
10. How are "adjunctive" and "enabling" activities distinguished from purposeful activity?
11. Identify something you do in your own life that fulfills the three types of meaningful life goals described by Csikszentmihalyi.
12. Contrast the different functions of activity in psychosocial contexts.
13. Why do occupational therapists perform activity analysis? Describe the three types of activity analysis that the clinician uses during clinical reasoning.
14. What does it mean that engagement in activity contributes to one's "spirituality"?
15. How would you design a study in which the purpose was to better understand meaningful activity?

Environment

16. Describe the types of environments in which people participate.
17. How does the person's position in the environment influence occupational therapy?
18. Give examples of the cultural and psychosocial features of one of the environmental assessments used in occupational therapy.
19. Identify multiple ways in which the environment enhances and detracts from the person's mental health and well-being. How does it impact his or her occupational performance?

INTRODUCTION

Chapter One provided an overview of the important developments that have shaped our profession. In it we saw that we have been strongly influenced by events and trends outside our own field, such as those in medicine and education. Just as importantly, we have been shaped from within through the efforts made by occupational therapists and our professional organization, the American Occupational Therapy Association (AOTA), and its precursor, the American Occupational Therapy Foundation. These organizations have contributed to our theory base and philosophy of practice and supported the development of our science.

From the beginning of our profession, the value and importance of occupation and activity has been central in defining who we are and what we do. It is through occupation and activity that people connect to their environment and create the relationships that lead to satisfactory participation in daily life. It is the interrelationship of person-activity/occupation and environment that creates the occupational therapy practice structure.

In this chapter, we will discuss in more depth each of the major elements or components in this "person-activity-environment" relationship so that we might better understand how each contributes to the overall practice of occupational therapy, which has a mental health focus. Within our discussion of these components we will describe and, in some instances, define multiple additional variables that the occupational therapist may consider in his or her role as an educator, researcher, or practitioner.

Starting with this premise of the person-activity-environment triad will help ground your reasoning and problem solving as you think about what frame of reference or model of practice you wish to use in your intervention. These same components will be those you consider as you form hypotheses for further research. What you will find when you move further into the text and study each of the frames of reference for practice is that within each model, there are differing and specific beliefs about how the person-activity and environment can both contribute to and are changed by meaningful occupation. Consistent with these postulates, there are guidelines, logically developed and related, for carrying out intervention. Our conviction throughout the writing of this third edition has been that this overarching relationship of person-activity-environment helps us, as occupational therapists, pay attention to what is important, but is in itself incomplete as we reason through our therapeutic intervention. The frames of reference (also called models of practice) take the therapist to the next step in reasoning through evaluation, intervention, research, consultation, or other roles. This is true for the novice as well as the experienced therapist.

There is also a framework for practice created by the larger shared understanding of what is meant by mental health, mental disorder, and mental illness, and by the multiple psychiatric diagnoses that are used to describe individuals' symptoms and behaviors. While we recognize that these are addressed in the reader's education through other coursework, we believe it is important for the occupational therapist who is committed to promoting the "mental health" or addressing psychosocial concerns of his or her clients to have given considerable thought to what it means to "address mental health" issues and what it means to be "mentally healthy." Only with this as a basis can one proceed to respond to mental health concerns from the unique perspective of occupational therapy.

THE PERSON

In each of the three sections of this chapter we highlight those elements that are believed to interrelate in the unfolding of occupational performance. They are the **person**; the task, **activity**, or occupation; and the **environment**. Each of these components is taken into account by all of the models of practice for mental health in occupational therapy discussed in this text. In other words, each model has postulates about the person, attributes of the task or activity that make it a good match with the person's desires and abilities, and beliefs about what characterizes those environmental or contextual conditions to optimize the person's engagement in activity and occupations.

What Shall We Pay Attention To?

Having said that, one of the most critical questions that is addressed differently by each model presented in this text is, **"What is it about the person that should be our primary concern?"**

When we think about or describe individuals, whether children or adults, we may consider what they do; how they move; what and how they think; what they say, believe, and desire; and what they feel. In other words, we take into account the physical, sensorimotor, psychosocial, and cognitive aspects of the individual, group, or population. That is as true in psychosocial intervention as in any other area of occupational therapy practice. As an occupational therapist, what we attend to in daily practice is determined in part and framed by the practice model that frames our perception of the person, his or her environment, problems, strengths, and therapeutic use of occupation. Some models in this text pay particular attention to the *patient's or client's knowledge, thoughts, and beliefs*, assuming that these determine how successful his or her participation in meaningful life activities will be. Other models focus on *what the person does—his or her task behavior*—with the assumption that if we can enhance repertoires of behaviors and teach skills that can be generalized to multiple environments, then the person will develop more positive beliefs about the self and will be able to participate in a more personally satisfying and socially acceptable manner. Other models are especially concerned with the *person's physical attributes* (e.g., his or her *posture and manner of moving about*). These models believe that until one can adequately take in and physiologically process sensory information, he or she will not be able to function optimally in daily life activities.

Should We Expect To Change the Person?

Another question that inevitably must be raised and answered by each model is, **"To what extent can we expect the person to change as an outcome of occupational therapy?"** While all models strive to promote the optimum function of patients/clients, some models propose that we cannot expect to change the person. For example, *we may not be able to, or should not, change how he or she routinely performs tasks.* Rather, they suggest that we direct our efforts toward adapting tasks and home, work, or school environments so that the way the individual (or group or population) goes about performing on a daily basis makes the safest and most satisfying fit with daily life tasks and typical life settings.

Other models postulate that we can enhance functional performance by helping the person change. For example, *we may change function by challenging the person's beliefs in order to change his or her thoughts of efficacy.* We may change beliefs by enriching the person's knowledge base or facilitating his or her investment of energy in new roles or occupations. We change beliefs by teaching the person problem-solving strategies or by providing experiences that are designed to improve the ability to process information by his or her sensorimotor processing system. The unique characteristics of the person and his or her condition determine whether or not the goal of therapeutic intervention is to change something in the person. Within the discussion of each model, expect to read for whom the model is specifically intended. You will learn that *some models were developed out of the perceived need to address a particular client or patient population.* For example, Toglia's dynamic interactional model (Chapter Nine) was developed in response to the special circumstances and needs of adults with acquired brain injury and is seen as a viable option for clients with schizophrenia. Allen's cognitive disabilities model (Chapter Eight) developed from her work with chronic mentally ill adults but has since been used with special-needs adolescents and older adults with early dementia. Still other models adapt theories from psychology and are applied to occupational therapy with children and adults of virtually all ages and with a broad range of emotional, coping, and/or behavior problems.

Addressing the Person's Mental Health Needs—Basic Premises

All of the models included in this text are here because they address what we have identified as mental health issues.

We have already articulated a major premise of this book, which is that **the models presented in this text help us, as occupational therapists, address the mental health issues of not only persons with identified psychiatric disorders (e.g., those whom we might see within the mental health system), but also the mental health needs of all our clients throughout the life span.** Clearly, a person does not need to have an identified psychiatric disorder, nor does a child need to have an identified emotional disorder, in order to have issues related to his or her mental well-being.

A second premise is that **people's psychological health impacts whether or not they will be able to fully participate in and learn from activities and occupations that are important to them.** Some of the models that you will read propose that occupational therapy intervention can directly address and impact the mental health of our clients/patients. Other models will, in a sense, take us out of that role and suggest that we can improve the safety, life skills, and/or overall quality of life of persons with mental illness but not presume that we are impacting his or her "mental health." It is important to recognize that in the larger health delivery system in the United States, as well as in many other service delivery contexts, *the goal is improved functional performance of persons having mental health issues. The end goal is not that a person "feel better" or "think more clearly"—it is that the person's clarity of thinking or enhanced subjective feelings of well-being enable him or her to function in a more personally satisfying and socially acceptable way.* In that respect, occupational therapy's focus on occupational function is compatible with the goals of therapy in multiple contexts.

A third basic premise of this text is that **engaging in meaningful/purposeful occupation and activities contributes to one's mental health.** Therefore, even when the identified goal of intervention is to improve function within activities of daily life, we can expect that frequently a positive related outcome is an improvement in the individual's confidence, self-efficacy, and sense of well-being.

Because this text is intended to help you cope with mental health issues in practice, we ask you to pause before you read further and ask yourself, "What is mental health? How do I see it?"

What is Mental Health?

Take a moment and ask yourself, "What is mental health? What does it mean to be mentally healthy?" There are many ways you can approach this. You might begin by asking yourself, "What is a mentally healthy student? How do I know when I'm mentally healthy?" Next, ask yourself the following:

- How does the state of my mental health influence my ability to do my work and enjoy the company of others?
- How important is my ability to participate in work and daily life activities to the maintenance of my own mental health?
- Do others around me (friends, family, and community) see mental health the way I do?
- What are the mental health characteristics of a person with a spinal cord injury? Or with any disability?
- Do the characteristics of mental health change throughout a person's life span? If so, when do they

change? In childhood? During adolescence? In later adulthood?

- Have the therapists I have observed or worked with ever held a different view of what is mentally "healthy" as compared to that held by their patients or clients? If so, how does one decide who is correct?

Perhaps you'd like to read ahead and compare your answers and definition of "mental health" with that of various official position papers. Does your view of mental health agree with theirs?

You will find if you discuss these questions with your peers, there are multiple variables that contribute to our and the client's perception of mental health. For those of you who would like to contrast your description of mental health with a theoretical definition, we share our summary of a theoretical concept of mental health that comes from Jahonda (1958) and Berger (1977) and is described in the occupational therapy literature by Stein and Cutler (1998).

Theoretical Concept of Mental Health

As summarized by Stein and Cutler (1998), a person's **mental health** is reflected in his or her thoughts, emotions, and behavior and how these are expressed in daily life. The mentally healthy person has positive feelings about one's self. The person has a sense of autonomy but can empathize with others, imagining their perspective, and can work toward a common good. The person can define him- or herself as separate from others but does not feel isolated. The person has a perception of reality that is not distorted and can integrate a sense of hope or at least a willingness to use one's potential. The person can use his or her potential, yet has a sense of personal boundaries; he or she can use his or her abilities and available resources to master challenges in the environment. The person can manage and use stress to respond to daily situations, and the person has a sense of hope and a desire for self-fulfillment (pp. 209-214).

As you read this and other theoretical descriptions or listen to philosophical discussions about what it means to be "mentally healthy," we think you will begin to conceptualize a continuum for the many variables that contribute to this thing called "mental health." One who is mentally healthy is, for example, "autonomous" but not so autonomous that he or she cannot ask for or accept help with daily challenges and tasks. One should be able to listen and empathize with others and contribute to other's well-being, but not become lost in their stories nor constantly disregard one's own needs. One should develop and use one's skills, but skills and occupations change. The ability to learn and make mistakes and accept mediocre performance may at times be as healthy as striving for expertise. You will, we believe, also begin to understand the individual nature of mental health for each person. This leads us to another important premise of this book—**mental health is a subjective state.**

You will hear both professionals and the lay community describe various psychological constructs, or characteristics, that are associated with mental health. **Psychological constructs** are terms that are commonly used to describe mental states, but they have no universally agreed-upon definitions. These constructs include, for example, self-concept, self-esteem, autonomy, sense of culture, internal locus of control, well-being, motivation, self-efficacy, "stressed-out," and self-actualization. Psychological constructs give people a shared language to communicate and reflect upon feelings (Borg & Bruce, 1991, p. 547). To increase your understanding of psychological constructs frequently used in occupational therapy, perform the learning activity, Increase Your Understanding: Psychological Constructs, then share your ideas with your peers.

In the discussion of the frames of reference in this text, various definitions of these psychological constructs are used, sometimes in ways that are specific to the theory under discussion and in ways with which you may not be familiar. Other constructs are probably very familiar to you and fit comfortably with beliefs you have about mental health and how mental health can be best enhanced through occupational therapy.

Universal Language in Mental Health Rehabilitation

The external guidelines for conceptualizing mental health in health care and community contexts in the United States have their basis in publications and documents generated by many international and national organizations, including the AOTA. These published guidelines establish definitions or a working language through which professionals can address and communicate mental health issues and the impact of mental disorders on the person's ability to function in everyday life. Those documents that have had a significant impact on mental health intervention by occupational therapists are highlighted next.

International Classification of Impairments, Disabilities, and Handicaps

Since the previous edition of this text, occupational therapists more and more refer to information and terminology from the *International Classification of Impairments, Disabilities, and Handicaps (ICIDH-2)*, not just in mental health practice but in all areas of occupational therapy practice. You will hear clinicians use terms from the ICIDH-2 in dialogue with clients and other professionals. Medicare in the United States requires that billing codes for reimbursement follow the ICIDH-2.

The current ICIDH-2 document uses a biopsychosocial model to describe a continuum of function from complete participation in daily life through varied types of functional limitation. There are three kinds of disablement: (1) impairment, (2) activity limitations, and (3) restricted participation. Since the document considers both the variables that

INCREASE YOUR UNDERSTANDING: PSYCHOLOGICAL CONSTRUCTS

The popular magazines that we pick up at the grocery store or newsstand frequently have articles that address familiar psychological constructs such as self-esteem, sense of well-being, comfort, personal power, popularity, self-control, motivation, and mental health. Identify one or more of these constructs and see how they are described and given context within several of your favorite magazines. Look through those magazines that your children or nieces and nephews read or magazines popular with people different than yourself. An excellent place to find magazines that you do not ordinarily read is at the local community library. You could do the same exercise by browsing the World Wide Web, typing in some of these constructs as search words, and seeing what information you receive.

That so much attention is paid to psychological constructs, especially mental health and well-being, is a commentary on the importance of these in the United States. As you read and explore these articles, do you find that mental health constructs are defined or used in the same way as you would use them? If not, what is different? The following list includes some key terms that you can look for, but feel free to add to this list:

- Self-concept
- Self-esteem
- Confidence
- Independence
- Spirituality
- Self-control
- Well-being
- Motivation
- Mental or emotional health

contribute or interfere with function, it's descriptions can apply to anyone. It does not just assign a disablement label based upon disease or illness. The classification system considers all of the systems and structures of a person's body. It also is sensitive to the person's physical and mental conditions and the context of function. The document describes function related to (1) body structures and functions, (2) activities, (3) participation, and (4) environmental factors. For detailed descriptions of the attributes, measurement characteristics and the boundaries of function of ICIDH-2, see World Health Organization, 2001, *www.who.int.icidh.* See ICIDH-2 Terminology for basic concepts of function.

ICIDH-2 TERMINOLOGY

Impairment—The change in or loss of a body structure or system that results in a change in the person's health condition and a physical, psychological, or social change in function. For example, changes in a person's mental, sensory, or endocrine systems, or changes in muscle, skin, or joint structures can change or limit a person's function in daily life (World Health Organization, 2001).

Activity—The person's level of function includes the nature, extent, duration, and quality of performance. The level of activity is what the person does, not a person's possibilities for performance. For example, a person uses a computer to send an e-mail, or completes daily self care tasks with assistance and increased time. In previous classification editions, the "activity dimension" was named "disability" (World Health Organization, 2001).

Participation—A person's involvement in daily life with the identified facilitators for function or the environmental barriers to performance. Participation may be restricted by nature, duration, and quality of experience. Participation includes a person's social and physical function in an environment (e.g., at home or in the community) or in other contexts within the boundaries of his or her impairment. For example, a person uses public transportation to attend church on Sundays (World Health Organization, 2001).

Environmental factors—The physical and social variables that contribute to the context of a person's function. These factors may be a barrier to participation or facilitate performance. They include physical space, technology, society's support, attitudes, services, and policies that influence a person's activities and participation in daily life. For example, a person works half a day with the support of a job coach and electronic access to the building. Or, a person requires social and economic support to return to living in his/her one-bedroom apartment (World Health Organization, 2001).

Mental Health and Mental Health Problems and Disorders

Moving from the broad boundaries established by the World Health Organization to the more specific context of mental health we see that occupational therapy practice is also influenced by the language and recommendations of such major associations as the American Psychological Association ([APA], 1994, 2000), Canadian National Health and Welfare (1988), and the AOTA (1997, 1998b). Within the guides provided by these various organizations and governing bodies, specific terminology is used to describe mental health, mental illness, mental disorders, and associated problems of living.

Canadian Continuum of Mental Health

Through their contributions to the occupational therapy literature, Canadian occupational therapists have influenced both occupational therapy philosophy and practice in the United States as well throughout the world. Canadian occupational therapists function within a national mental health system whose policy is established in and by the national government of Canada. Within the literature of this governing body are definitions for the constructs **mental health**, **mental disorder**, and **mental health problem**. In the definition of all three constructs there is considerably more emphasis given to the interaction and mutuality of the individual, the group, and the environment than exists in the American position, as posited by the APA. The Canadians propose a continuum as related to mental health and mental disorder that would support intervention by occupational therapy practitioners to evaluate and monitor a person's sense of well-being and its relationship to a person's illness or disability (see Canadian Description of Mental Health and Mental Disorder).

CANADIAN DESCRIPTION OF MENTAL HEALTH AND MENTAL DISORDER

"**Mental health** is the capacity of the individual, the group, and the environment to interact with one another in ways that promote subjective well-being, the optimal development and use of mental abilities (cognitive, affective, and relational), the achievement of individual and collective goals consistent with justice, and the attainment and preservation of conditions of fundamental equality.

"**Mental disorder** may be defined as a recognized, medically diagnosable illness that results in the significant impairment of an individual's cognitive, affective, or relational abilities. Mental disorders result from biological, developmental, and/or psychosocial factors, and can—in principle, at least—be managed using approaches comparable to those applied to physical disease (i.e., prevention, diagnosis, treatment, and rehabilitation).

"A **mental health problem**, on the other hand, is a disruption in the interactions between the individual, the group, and the environment. Such a disruption may result from factors within the individual, including physical or mental illness or inadequate coping skills. It may also spring from external causes, such as the existence of harsh environmental conditions, unjust social structures, or tensions within the family or community. An effective response to mental health problems must therefore address a broader range of factors" (Canadian National Health and Welfare, 1988, pp. 7-8).

Classification of Mental Disorders in the United States

Occupational therapists employed within the mental health delivery system in the United Stated can expect to be influenced by the multi-axial, diagnostic system published by the APA (1994, 2000). This multi-axial categorization of mental illness is compatible with the ICIDH system. The APA also provides its definition of **mental disorder** (see How Mental Disorder Is Understood in DSM-IV-TR), which the reader will discern is significantly different than that of Canada.

Although a psychiatric diagnosis does not determine occupational therapy treatment, the occupational therapist does need a general understanding of what characterizes a diagnosis in order to evaluate the functional outcomes of a mental disorder.

The Diagnostic and Statistical Manual of Mental Disorders, Text Revision—A Clinical Tool

The DSM-IV-TR (APA, 2000) is the most recent update of the text material in the DSM-IV manual. In 1997, physicians and psychologists formed work groups to review the large amount of research that had been published since 1992 with the purpose of updating the fourth edition manual. The goals of the text revision were to make changes that reflect current literature: "...insure that the text is up to date... correct any errors... increase the educational value... [and] be compatible with ICD-9 and ICD-10 codes [draft to be realeased in 2004]..." (pp. xxvi-xxx). There are no changes in the criteria for a disorder or its subtypes. The reader is referred to the original source for descriptions of the changes in DSM-IV-TR and the comprehensive information that it provides for understanding mental disorders.

The manual is still a clinical tool developed and used by clinical experts, such as psychologists and psychiatrists, to make diagnoses. In the preparation of DSM-IV and DSM-IV-TR, those preparing the manual worked to make it compatible with the International Classification of Diseases (ICD). DSM-IV, like ICIDH, is cited for insurance reimbursement, to determine disability, and in forensic matters. The DSM-IV-TR manual categorizes observable symptoms that in turn constitute the various psychiatric illnesses. Expert clinicians evaluate the person's symptoms and use the manual as a tool or a guide for categorizing these symptoms and making diagnoses. The validity of a clinician's diagnosis depends on his or her clinical judgment. We emphasize that the DSM-IV-TR is a "tool" that frames a person's symptoms; it is not a prescription for intervention. The APA also recommends that when making a diagnosis, clinicians be sensitive to the person's culture, family, personal history, previous interventions, and the individual nature of symptoms. The person's diagnosis does not reflect the individual differences in function or disability. The text also states:

HOW MENTAL DISORDER IS UNDERSTOOD IN DSM-IV-TR

Prior to restating the definition of mental disorder from DSM-IV, the work groups for DSM-IV-TR state that:

"...the term mental disorder unfortunately implies a distinction between 'mental' disorders and 'physical' disorders that is a reductionistic anachronism of mind/body dualism. Compelling literature documents that there is much 'physical' in 'mental' disorders and much 'mental' in 'physical' disorders. The problem raised by the term 'mental' disorders has been much clearer than its solution, and, unfortunately, the term persists in the title of DSM-IV because we have not found an appropriate substitute" (APA, 2000, p. xxx).

Moreover, although this manual (DSM-IV-TR) provides a classification of mental disorders, it must be admitted that no definition adequately specifies precise boundaries for the concept of "mental disorder." The concept of mental disorder, like many other concepts in medicine and science, lacks a consistent operational definition that covers all situations (APA, 2000, p. xxx).

In DSM-IV (1994) and as reiterated in DSM-IV-TR (2000), the APA defined a mental disorder as a "behavioral, psychological, or biological dysfunction in the individual" (APA, 2000, pp. xxi-xxii).

A **mental disorder** is a "clinically significant behavioral or psychological syndrome or pattern that occurs in an individual and that is associated with present distress (i.e., a painful symptom) or disability (i.e., impairment in one or more important areas of function) or with a significantly increased risk of suffering death, pain, disability, or an important loss of freedom. In addition, this syndrome or pattern must not be merely an expectable or culturally sanctioned response to a particular event (e.g., the death of a loved one). Whatever its original cause, it must currently be considered a manifestation of behavioral, psychological, or biological dysfunction in the individual. Neither deviant behavior (e.g., political, religious, or sexual) nor conflicts that are primarily between the individual and society are mental disorders, unless the deviance or conflict is a symptom of a dysfunction in the individual as described above" (2000, p. xxxi).

A common misconception is that a classification of mental disorders classifies people, when actually what are being classified are disorders that people have... the text... avoids the use of such expressions as "a schizophrenic"... instead uses the more accurate but admittedly more cumbersome, "individual with schizophrenia"... (p. xxxi)

Just as we did in the previous editions of this text, we chose to avoid classification pejorative language.

The DSM-IV-TR multi-axial system for classifying a disorder has five axes, which are briefly summarized in Multi-Axial System in the DSM-IV Classification System.

Multi-Axial System in the DSM-IV Classification System

Axis I

- Clinical disorders—All classified mental disorders except those on Axis II. Other conditions that may be a focus of clinical attention—Factors related to the clinical disorder.

Axis II

- Mental retardation—Disorders that begin in childhood and persist throughout the life span.
- Personality disorders

Axis III

- General medical conditions—ICD-9 codes related to the mental disorder.

Axis IV

- Psychosocial and environmental problems—Life stressors that impact upon the mental disorder.

Axis V

- Global assessment of functioning—General level of psychosocial and occupational function of the last year.

Occupational Therapists Monitor Symptoms

Occupational therapists do not make diagnoses; however, they do identify and monitor symptoms and behaviors that patients demonstrate during occupational performance. Often individuals present perplexing symptoms, and they may be given a provisional diagnosis. Further assessment by professional staff makes possible the more accurate determination of a diagnosis. For example, the severity of a disorder is associated with the person's ability/inability to perform daily life tasks. Occupational therapy practitioners use initial and ongoing assessments to gather data about the person's participation in daily life and the effects of mental problems and disorders on activity and participation at home, school, work, or in social settings. By sharing and documenting these observations, occupational therapists can contribute to decisions that others make about diagnoses. They can help monitor the outcome and efficacy of their own as well as other mental health interventions.

Occupational Therapy and Global Assessment of Function

The therapist employed within a mental health facility typically needs to have a working understanding of the DSM-IV. Persons having an identified mental illness may also be patients or clients in other settings as well, and it is vital that therapists understand what the diagnostic information means.

In many mental health settings, professional and paraprofessional staff or "team" members use the common language of the DSM-IV-TR during discussions and when planning intervention. Additionally, the occupational therapist reports the results of occupational therapy assessment and intervention. There is one portion or axis of the DSM-IV-TR classification in which occupational therapy assessment data are particularly pertinent. This axis is referred to as Axis V, the Global Assessment of Functioning (GAF). The occupational therapist contributes to the GAF information about the person's:

1. Self-care, use of time, and performance during work, school, and leisure tasks
2. Participation in roles and relationships, and in home and community environments
3. Cognitive, psychosocial, and physical performance in varied contexts

Often the patient for whom treatment is beginning is given an initial GAF score, which is based on his or her presenting function or previous best level of function. This can then be compared to his or her ability to function at the time that intervention is terminated. Each frame of reference presented in this text identifies relevant occupational therapy procedures and instruments used by an occupational therapist to gather information that contributes to the determination of the person's global level of function.

Serious Emotional Disturbance: The School Vernacular

The Individuals with Disabilities Education Act, Public Law 101-47620 (1990), enacted by the United States Congress, provides for the education of school-aged children whose emotional disturbances interfere with their educational performance. (Note: These children need not have been given a psychiatric diagnosis from ICD or DSM-IV-TR.)

The term **serious emotional disturbance** (SED) is applied to the behavior of those children whose school performance is adversely affected by one or more of the following characteristics:

- An inability to learn that is not due to intellectual, sensory, or health factors
- An inability to maintain satisfactory peer or student-teacher relationships
- Inappropriate behavior or feelings

- A pervasive mood of unhappiness or depression
- A tendency to develop physical symptoms or fears associated with personal or school problems

SED also applies to children diagnosed with schizophrenia.

Language of the Occupational Therapy Profession in Describing Psychosocial Components

In addition to the international and national guidelines shared by all professionals who work in mental health, the occupational therapy profession has defined and published terminology used by occupational therapists to describe the areas, context, and components of occupational performance, including those components specific to psychosocial function. This document, *Uniform Terminology for Occupational Therapy* (3rd ed.) (AOTA, 1998b), has been in existence since 1979 and is currently undergoing revision. The revised document is not available at this writing.

Uniform terminology influences the description of a person's performance. It describes the activities of daily living, work and productive activities, and leisure or play that are the focus of evaluation and contribute to the intervention plan to improve occupational performance. It outlines the sensorimotor, cognitive and cognitive integration, and psychosocial components of function. It suggests temporal and environmental contexts of performance that are considered barriers to performance and increase the individualized approaches to evaluation and intervention (see Content Focus of AOTA Uniform Terminology). The reader is referred to Appendix B for comprehensive descriptions of the performance areas, components, and contexts. Uniform terminology can also guide the clinician's communication with clients (e.g., person in therapy, professionals, third-party payers, and families) when the therapist shares information about the person's performance during occupational therapy. The therapist's observations of occupational performance can contribute to the description of the person's GAF. The occupational therapist reports on the status of client's/patient's mental health or disorder as it is reflected in their functional performance.

Psychosocial Core of Practice—Psychosocial Components of Performance

In all practice environments, not just those specific to mental health, occupational therapists are concerned with the person-activity-environment fit and its effect on the client's wellbeing, mental health, and participation in daily life. Thus, during evaluation and intervention, the therapist does not isolate the three major components of performance (sensorimotor, cognitive, and psychosocial) but considers their mindbody relationships that influence occupational performance.

CONTENT FOCUS OF AOTA UNIFORM TERMINOLOGY

Uniform Terminology for Occupational Therapy (3rd ed.) describes:
- Areas of performance or the person's participation in activities of daily living, work or productive activity, and one's play and leisure pursuits.
- Components of function or the sensorimotor, cognitive, psychosocial, and psychological variables that contribute to a person's daily function.
- Context of the person's performance, the temporal and environmental contexts of a person's performance. The context gives performance boundaries based upon the developmental expectations for the person and one's chronological age, the person's health status and physical abilities, and the social and cultural variables in one's environment that influence participation in daily life (AOTA, 1998b).

For example, the psychosocial components as expressed during client function can interact with other functional components (e.g., physical, cognitive, sensorimotor) and support or interfere with client performance in daily life. They influence the goals that clients set to change their performance, and they influence the strategies a person uses to manage the interactions among the person, activity, and environment. The psychosocial components are highlighted in Psychosocial Components of Function.

PSYCHOSOCIAL COMPONENTS OF FUNCTION

The *Uniform Terminology for Occupational Therapy* (3rd ed.) document describes psychosocial components that influence occupational performance:
- **Psychological components and skills**—The person's values, interests, and self-concept.
- **Social components and skills**—The person's role performance, social conduct, interpersonal skills, and self-expression.
- **Self-management components and skills**—The person's coping skills, time management, and self-control (AOTA, 1994, 1998b).

Summary—Communicating with Psychosocial Language

In summary, documents provided by international, national, and professional groups give broad guidelines for understanding the person and the psychosocial issues that influence the person's participation in daily life. When occupational therapists use these guides along with psychosocial frames of reference, such as those described in this text, therapists are better able to communicate with others both within and outside of the profession.

While using a shared terminology, the therapist must describe each patient's or client's ability to function in such a way that it captures what is unique about the person (including his or her mental health, problems, strengths, and living or working environments). In other words, the therapist uses professional language to describe the individual nature of the relationship of **person-activity-environment** as these come together in performance.

Motivation: Examining a Psychological Construct from Multiple Perspectives

As we bring our discussion of the person to a close, we will use "motivation" as an example of a psychological construct that influences people's mental health, their ability to profit from occupational therapy, and ultimately their ability to participate in life. Motivation is not viewed identically by each of the occupational therapy models in this text, nor is the occupational therapist's response to perceived "motivation" problems identical in each model. We hope that this example will illustrate why psychological or mental health constructs must be taken into account when helping people participate in activity or occupation.

The following example is condensed and described in more detail in another text (Borg & Bruce, 1997).

A woman, whom we'll call Eva, was in her late 40s when she had a massive basilar stroke. Formerly a prominent lawyer and very active in her community, she now had severe upper extremity ataxia, poor sitting and standing balance, dependency in all self-care, and was limited in her ability to speak. She had received occupational therapy for about 6 months, but it was discontinued because she had failed to progress. That was when her family instituted a home therapy program for her. Recently, Eva had stopped cooperating in the home therapy program and was resisting eating. The family asked for professional help, and the occupational therapist was called in to help evaluate Eva's apparent lack of motivation (pp. 103-104).

The occupational therapist could look at Eva's motivational issue from multiple perspectives, as represented by the models for practice presented in this text.

The first possibility he or she would need to consider is that behavior like Eva's may be a direct outcome of the neurological impairment. One often sees, for example, that a head injury or other central nervous system (CNS) disorder adversely affects a person's modulation of drive, inhibition, arousal, level of anxiety, control of aggression, sexual response, perseverance, and motivation. These changes in neurobehavioral function are frequently identified by care providers as problems with motivation, as anger, willful noncompliance, or even passive aggressive behavior. Eva had previously been cooperative, so we will proceed under the assumption that something else is wrong.

Ways Motivation Problems Can Be Approached

Behavioral theory suggests that motivation is innate but is sustained when one is rewarded for his or her efforts. Rewards meet different types of needs—those that meet basic needs, such as for nourishment or sex, and those that meet secondary needs, such as that for love, attention, approval, or self-satisfaction. Perhaps Eva's efforts in the home therapy program have not been sufficiently rewarded or are no longer sufficiently rewarding, either by the attention or approval of others, which is something Eva desires, or by her own feelings of satisfaction. Why should she continue in therapy if she perceives she has nothing to gain? Perhaps she is getting more rewards from her noncompliance. Regarding her resistance to eat, perhaps what she is expected to eat does not taste good to her or requires more effort on her part than seems worthwhile to her.

Psychodynamic principles when applied in occupational therapy suggest that people are innately motivated by their own need to achieve and to master. For example, assume that people receive pleasure from investing in activity for activity's sake. Psychodynamic theory also proposes that engagement in activity takes energy and that people have a finite amount of energy to invest. These principles also indicate that individuals are more likely to take appropriate risks (i.e., try something at which they might fail) when they are in an environment in which they believe others will not be critical of them. Each person is also more likely to engage in activities that fit his or her mental picture of one's self. Perhaps Eva's family has been so anxious for Eva to improve that she fears they will be disappointed if she fails, so she stops trying. Perhaps she is disappointed with herself, and pulling back from home therapy is less emotionally painful than feeling like she has failed. One can wonder, too, do the family's efforts to engage her in therapy help her enjoy the world around her? What is the nature of the therapeutic activities in which she is being expected to engage? Perhaps she is depressed and lacks the energy to stay engaged or is too tired from other home activities and her energy is depleted by the time the home program begins. Should a referral to a physician for a medical evaluation be the first priority? Does the family need to be helped to accept that Eva is not expected to improve further? Are they most concerned for her welfare?

Cognitive and cognitive behavioral theory suggests that several sources of motivation exist at the same time, that novel and familiar experiences can motivate a person to learn and interact in the environment, and that personal satisfaction and competence become the motivator. Perhaps the challenges being posed to Eva are too great and need to be simplified or broken down so that she can succeed and gain self-confidence. Cognitive behavioral theory also emphasizes that it is one's thoughts about one's self as being capable that need to be in place if one is to stay motivated. What are Eva's thoughts? Maybe she does not clearly understand what she has accomplished. Does she believe she will be able to succeed in the future? What information has she been given about her disorder? Cognitive behavioral theory also proposes that it is satisfying for people to feel that they have control. Is Eva being asked what she would like to do in this home program? Is resisting involvement the only way she believes she can take control in her life? Is the family pushing Eva in a direction she no longer cares to go?

Toglia's dynamic interactional approach advises the therapist to take into account everything going on in relation to this home program—Eva herself, the cognitive demands of the tasks she is being asked to do, and the influence of the home environment. Is Eva cognitively able to understand what is expected? Does this issue with motivation represent a problem with comprehension? Attention? Memory? To what is she attending, and how well can she maintain her attention? Is the environment too distracting or not stimulating enough? How does the family communicate with Eva? What would help her to communicate? Are there adaptations in the task or environment that would enable her to be more successful or strategies that she could learn that might help her to become engaged or stay engaged in therapy? If the answer to this question proves to be "no," can the family be taught other ways in which to contribute to Eva's comfort and quality of life?

These are not the only questions that would be raised within these models, but they illustrate how reasoning through this perceived problem with the psychological construct of motivation would be approached differently depending on the psychosocial frame of reference. This example illustrates too the critical need for occupational therapists to address psychological constructs and consider issues related to the individual's mental health. If we fail to understand and address the mental health needs of the person in this person-activity-relationship, our best efforts may fall short.

ACTIVITY, TASK, AND OCCUPATION

We next consider "activity" as the second of the three factors that come together in the person-activity-environment relationship. In our practice and in our professional literature you will find that occupational therapists have multiple definitions for the terms **activity**, **task**, and **occupation**, and use these terms interchangeably. In the presentation of each of the frames of reference for practice, you will find that the "role of activity" is explicitly addressed and will also reflect the multiple uses of these terms (along with many other terms or phrases that refer to one's engagement in daily life tasks). In the discussion that follows, however, we highlight what are felt to be significant roles of activity/task/occupation in the maintenance or restoration of mental health, and we examine some of the differences in the way these terms are used.

Activity: Connects Mind and Body and Enables Participation in Life

The AOTA has defined both **activity** and **occupation** in a manner that implies a reciprocal relationship between the two. Activities are goal-directed behaviors and actions or "units" that make up an occupation (AOTA, 2000, p. 15).

The terms "activity" and "therapeutic activity" are used by occupational therapists in a way that is quite specific to our field. **Activities** are what we as people "do," but they are neither random nor isolated movements. To an occupational therapist, an activity might be combing one's hair, writing a term paper, or taking the family dog for a walk. Usually (but not always, as we shall discuss), there is something accomplished. Some special types of activities that are often referred to in the occupational therapy literature and in occupational therapy assessments are "activities of daily living" (ADLs). These are generally viewed as activities related to basic self-care. The term "instrumental activities of daily living" (IADLs) connotes more than basic care. These activities include budgeting activities, washing one's car, managing one's home or business, etc.

Occupation refers to "meaningful groupings of activities in which humans choose to engage" and is "typically extended over time; engagement in occupations allows for survival (self-maintenance), maintenance of roles, self-expression, development of identity, adaptation, enjoyment, meaning, and fulfillment" (AOTA, 2000, p. 26). Occupations include grooming and hygiene, participating in a favorite hobby, carrying out one's employment responsibilities, and participating with friends in an enjoyable social group. Occupations are built of related tasks or activities.

Pedretti (1996) blurs the demarcation between activity and **occupation,** as she describes occupation as a self-initiated, self-directed, and purposeful activity that joins the person's mind and body.

Difference Between Activity and Occupation

Although the term occupation is defined in many ways and is sometimes used interchangeably with the term "purposeful activity," Darnell and Heater (1994) remind us that an **occupation** is a purposeful activity but that a purposeful activity may not be a person's occupation. Occupations bring together the person's physical and mental abilities and provide the context for the person's growth and development throughout life. Because the person integrates the components of performance within a specific context during activities and occupations, the person has the opportunity to develop a sense of self, experience competence and control, and build self-esteem and a sense of well-being (Christiansen, 1999; Jackson, 1998).

Simultaneously, within occupation, the person can fulfill occupational roles. Sample occupational roles are student, worker, homemaker, volunteer, friend, spouse, parent, child, and community member. The knowledge, skills, and attitudes needed for these occupational roles can be developed or readdressed during occupational therapy interventions through use of sensorimotor, cognitive, and social learning experiences. The therapeutic experience is chosen for its potential to effectively integrate activities, tasks, and occupations in support of fulfilling occupational roles and meeting client goals.

Whether they are referred to as "activities" or "occupations," both are central in our lives because activities and occupations are the mediums for the transactions between the person and the environment. In addition, participating in activities and occupations enhances the meaning and quality of our lives.

Activity Theory

Activity theory (Cynkin & Robinson, 1990) suggests that participating in a variety of different activities, such as those that emphasize physical, social, cognitive, sensory, developmental, and cultural experiences, provides the breadth of experiences that a person needs to grow and change. Participating in a favorite activity or occupation can be quite exhilarating and something we look forward to when we arise on a given morning. Such participation can also teach each individual his or her limits. In a sense, activity and occupation are the means by which people create their lives. We have already articulated two critical premises on which occupational therapy in mental health rests: 1) when people have mental health disorders they may become less able to engage in activity/occupations in a satisfying way, and 2) engaging in activity/occupations can enhance or contribute to one's mental health. We know, for example, that people with mental health impairments are sometimes unable to enjoy activities they once enjoyed. They may lose confidence in their ability to be successful in activities, or they may have a very unrealistic picture of their capabilities. Individuals with mental illness sometimes have a history of being unable to carry out even the seemingly simplest activity.

Just as one's ability to participate in a range of activities helps him or her avoid boredom and creates challenge prior to a rehabilitation experience, therapists need to consider the importance of using a variety of therapeutic activities or creating novelty within an activity to help maintain clients' interest and sustain their motivation.

All of this presumes that the activities and occupations to which we refer are those that the person is interested and that have a purpose to him or her. The importance of incorporating "purposeful" activity and "meaningful" activity is also addressed by each of the models in this text, though coined in a variety of ways.

Activities as a Means to Establish Habits and Carry Out Roles

As suggested by early and current leaders of the profession (Christiansen & Baum, 1997; Kidner, 1924; Kielhofner, 1995; Neistadt & Crepeau, 1998; Slagle, 1922), activities can be used to establish habits and routines. In this way activities help to structure people's lives. Though individuals vary in their desire to have structure, you will read in many of the models that activities and occupation are important in helping establish routines. In some instances, such as with persons struggling with schizophrenia or anxiety, having a predictable structure to their daily life helps alleviate stress and assists many people to accomplish their goals. In this way, activities enhance mental health and promote a sense of well-being.

The totality of the person's activities and occupations and the individual way in which they are performed contributes to one's lifestyle. Through his or her roles in life, the individual not only meets his or her own physical needs (e.g., needs for social contact, satisfaction, and feelings of competence) but also contributes to the larger society. The person is more likely to know who they are and have a healthy lifestyle and therfore will not need occupational therapy services if his or her needs are met.

Occupational Performance Model

As we have indicated, occupational therapists generally value an activity that they believe to be "purposeful" to the client/patient—it is, for example, something the person believes is necessary, valuable, or enjoyable to do; it brings him or her closer to something that he or she wishes to accomplish. It is not just activity for activity's sake. Often, however, when therapists carry out interventions or help others design service delivery programs, they must consider using an activity that will eventually enable the client to do purposeful activity but that may be viewed as preparatory to this activity. Pedretti (1996) describes this in more detail in her discussion of the occupational performance model. She distinguishes the role of activity during each of four stages of intervention:

1. The adjunctive methods stage
2. The enabling activities stage
3. The purposeful activity stage
4. The occupational performance and role stage

During each of these stages the occupational therapist uses different types of activities for different purposes; in none of these stages would activity be regarded as "purposeless" (Pedretti, 1996, pp. 8-9).

During the adjunctive stage, methods or activities (**adjunctive activities**) are preparatory and may include, for example, physical exercise or range of motion that "warms the client up" for eventual participation in purposeful activities. **Enabling activities** engage clients in components or simulation of a purposeful activity and in this regard are also preparatory. For example, during work or driving simulations, clients can learn important skills that will enable them to return to actual driving or employment in the real-life setting. Learning to use adaptive equipment is also considered an enabling activity. The therapist may have to explain to the client the purpose of both adjunctive and enabling activities and their relationship to purposeful activity. **Purposeful activity** in this usage is that in which the client participates in real-life tasks that he or she wishes to do, often in his or her home or community environment. **Occupational performance and roles** are the focus of the fourth stage of the treatment continuum of the occupational performance model. The person performs activities and tasks that fulfill his or her roles in work, leisure, and ADL occupations in the person's living environment (e.g., home or community) (pp. 8-9). Pedretti's activity stages, which follow, give a more complete description of each.

Adjunctive activity stage: The clinician uses activities that give the context for assessing performance and remedial experiences for sensorimotor, cognitive, and psychosocial components of performance. These activity experiences prepare the client for participation in purposeful activity. The goal of adjunctive activities is maximum participation in a performance area. For example, a client participates in physical exercise to increase sensorimotor performance by building the strength and endurance needed for the purposeful activities chosen by the client. They also may be considered warm-up activities that prevent injury or prepare the mind and body for participation. When patients or clients can see their own progress, it contributes to their confidence, increases their sense of control, and helps them gain the sense of efficacy that can come from learning to use one's body and feeling good physically as one prepares to participate in purposeful activity.

For example, a client who has had a stroke and is participating in outpatient therapy might spend 10 minutes doing stretches, range of motion, and strength exercises to prepare for water volleyball. This 10-minute warm-up prepares the body for a leisure activity and is one that will help build endurance. It also allows the clinician to assess the quality of the client's performance, the level of recall, and mastery of a home program in which these exercises had been prescribed.

Enabling activities stage: Enabling activities have limited meaning for the person, but they facilitate and build the components of function. When clients are unable to understand the goal or purpose of these activities, the therapist will need to motivate the client to participate.

Frequently, a statement that explains the therapeutic value of an enabling activity motivates clients. This explanation usually describes the relationship of the activity to the client's goals and relates the activity to the assessment and remediation of components needed for function. The occupational therapist also uses enabling activities to assess and teach skills in varied contexts to enhance performance.

Enabling activities such as driver training activities, work task trials, and cognitive games can be used to identify and build components of function and to establish a behavioral baseline. Therapists can, for example, integrate the use of pegs, blocks, and cones into games in which clients can learn performance strategies and increase their own awareness of performance boundaries. Such games and simulations are more frequently used when intervention cannot be carried out in the actual home or community context, and they often provide a safer environment for initial learning. Games and simulations are more likely to be effective when clinicians relate them to client goals and use them to teach performance strategies.

Purposeful activity stage: Since the beginning of the profession, purposeful activity has been described as the core of occupational therapy intervention. Unlike adjunctive and enabling activities that emphasize the process of therapy, purposeful activity is distinguished by its emphasis on the outcome of the experience and its relationship to the client's values and interests in daily life. The client's goals are inherent in the activity and, thus, the activity is relevant and meaningful to the person. The activity integrates the mind and body through the integrated use of the components of function—the sensorimotor, cognitive, and psychosocial systems—during occupational performance. During purposeful activities, the person participates without hesitation and frequently and automatically sees its value and relationship to his or her goals. The activities are used during evaluation and intervention to do the following:

- Achieve multiple outcomes
- Evaluate current level of and potential for performance
- Enable practice and mastery of life skills
- Promote development and growth
- Increase participation in one's home or community
- Increase one's quality of daily life

The client, not the therapist, determines whether and how an activity has purpose. For example, a man who prior to his stroke had enjoyed a weekly golf game with a group of friends refused the offer to participate in an adaptive golf class in the community. The man explained to the occupational therapist that the game would "not be the same," because he wouldn't be able to compete with his colleagues and he was not interested in "just playing the game," whether it be for the challenge of mastering one-handed play or an opportunity for socialization. In his view, adapted golf was not a purposeful activity, and it was his perception that needed to be respected.

Occupational activity stage: Like purposeful activities, occupations are also described as the core of occupational therapy. The major difference is that occupations are performed in context of the person's actual role and/or in his or her own environment. They help clients resume or assume participation in the their home or community environments and support their roles in many contexts. Using occupational activities, the individual carries out self-care, work, and productive occupations, and pursues play and leisure. Clients can participate in occupations during both remedial and compensatory interventions in order to maintain or build performance abilities in home and community contexts.

Sample occupational activities include grooming and hygiene, arts and crafts, sports, computer work, office work, and volunteer activities. Just because these activities are occupations does not guarantee that they are meaningful to the client. For example, clients may prefer to have assistance with dressing (rather than independently performing the task) in order to conserve the energy needed for participating in one's work. Clients may wish to change their work roles rather than resume previous job activities.

Note: The description of activities is adapted from Pedretti, L. (1996). *Occupational therapy—Practice skills for physical dysfunction* (4th ed.). St. Louis, MO: Mosby and American Occupational Therapy Association. (1998a). *The reference manual of the official documents of the American Occupational Therapy Association, Inc.* (7th ed.). Bethesda, MD: Author. The examples and possible uses in occupational therapy contexts are based upon clinical experiences of Mary Ann Giroux-Bruce and Barbara Borg.

Although each of these activity stages is defined separately, the reader should keep in mind that these represent a sequence of stages that can and usually do overlap. These stages can occur within an intervention session or over a series of sessions. The clinician often uses all of the different types of activities throughout the therapy process. When observing therapy, it may appear as if the clinician is sliding along the continuum, forward or backward, as he or she uses activities to keep intervention client-centered. This will be evident in the discussion of activities in the models presented in this text. Although theorists may not say so, you will discern that they are referring to the use of activity in one or more of the ways that Pedretti has identified. Overall, adjunctive, enabling, and purposeful activities, tasks, and occupations are used for multiple purposes within the context of achieving goals that support the client's performance and participation in his or her chosen roles. The following example illustrates the importance of listening to and appreciating the individual's perception of what he or she experiences as "purposeful" when we recommend activities to be used within therapeutic intervention.

Example—Client-Centered versus Clinician Perspective

> I recall a client, a gentleman who had sustained a closed head injury. He disagreed with me about the amount of time we should spend doing warm-up exercises prior to the modified sports and cognitive activities that were planned for his occupational therapy intervention. He wanted more time for what I considered "stretching and warm-up." He reminded me that fitness activities were critical to the body-building program he had been carrying out at the gym before his injury. He was anxious about his current appearance and wanted to be more "buff" before he saw his friends again at the gym. I had viewed the sports activity as the purposeful activity in the session but had to consider what was most "purposeful" to this client while practicing within the context of safe performance. (Mary Ann Bruce, 2000)

Often we as therapists think of exercise as a means to increase strength, flexibility, or mobility in preparation for other activity, but this vignette reminds us that exercise can be "purposeful activity." In this and other similar instances, exercise programs within therapy are not only a means to enhance a client's physical prowess but can be the precursors to establishing wellness programs for clients with disabilities. They can also support return-to-fitness programs in one's community, which in turn provide opportunities for socialization and re-connecting to the person's environment. Also, they may be integral to the fitness culture of our clients or can be a means by which clients manage stress.

Meaning of Activities—Bringing Together Mind, Body, and Spirit

It is not only the type or stage of therapeutic activity but the client's perception of the meaning of activity that influences his or her desire to engage in that activity and its effectiveness as a vehicle for therapy. Meaning is considered the "invisible dimension of performance" that influences one's choice of and participation in activities (Hasselkus & Rosa, 1997, p. 375). It is because activity is "meaningful" that the person is motivated to participate (Trombly, 1995). How an activity takes on its meaning can relate to one's spirituality, to the rituals in one's culture (Crepeau, 1995), or to everyday life routines, plans, and goals. When activities have meaning to the individual, they contribute to the person's quality of life and general sense of well-being (Yerxa, 1998).

This implies that not all activity in which people engage needs to have accomplishment as its final goal. There are limitless numbers of activities in which one feels at peace, becomes curious, is profoundly satisfied, or emotionally

INCREASE YOUR UNDERSTANDING: MEANING

The Effect of Meaningful Activity

To understand the effect of meaningful activity and occupation on a person's quality of life, occupational therapists have conducted quantitative and qualitative studies. Two occupational therapy studies are highlighted here.

Quantitative Study

One such quantitative study was conducted by Christiansen, Backman, Little, and Nguyen (1999) in which they studied personal projects to identify the relationships between meaning, occupations, and well-being. The study found that stressful and difficult activities decreased the person's sense of well-being. In contrast, there was an increased experience of well-being related to the person's sense of efficacy that came from progress toward or completing personal goals through goal-directed activities. The study demonstrated significant relationships between meaning and well-being based upon the variables of "enjoyment," "absorption," and "personal identity" as descriptors of meaning. The relationship between meaning, occupation, and well-being was not as strongly related as the researchers had hoped.

However, the researchers suggest that the significance of meaning during a person's projects and activities would increase if the definition of "meaning" had included spirituality as a variable or the "spiritual" dimensions of meaning. Spiritual meaning does not refer only to religion. It comes from the person's beliefs about meaning in life, one's sense of control, and one's beliefs about personal power and possible supernatural power (Christiansen, 1997). For example, a person's spiritual sense can come from experiencing the arts or enjoying nature.

Qualitative Study

Occupational therapists also use qualitative methods to study meaning. The study conducted by Jacobs (1994) used the **experience sampling method** to identify the person's meaning of an experience. This method requires the person to wear a beeper and record what he or she was doing when beeped. Subjects were contacted at varied times of the day or night and were asked to record their current experience. They kept a journal/log that described the activity as well as the meaning of the experience. Csikszentmihalyi (1990, 1997) used this method to gain an understanding of the meaning of everyday activities and the roles identified with optimal experience. When a person functions at an optimal level, he or she is in a state of flow. **Flow** here refers to "enjoyment... a rewarding experience... [and a] state of mind" (Csikszentmihalyi, 1990, p. 111).

---

moved, but has not "accomplished" (made, produced) anything. This might happen, for example, when we stop to appreciate nature or take the time to really watch our children at play. Activities that touch people in this way are also important to the creation of quality of life. See Increase Your Understanding: Meaning for research approaches that study "meaning" and its relationship to occupation.

Not everyone may agree that to be mentally healthy one needs to feel that his or her life has "quality." Is it enough that we do what we need to do to get food on the table, feed ourselves and our families, and meet our commitments? Or is there an intangible something more that contributes to mental health? What does it mean to have a quality of life? Culturally speaking, is this idea of "quality of life" a very Western concept? These questions are not addressed equally by all of the models presented in this text, but they could be viewed as extremely important to the very heart of occupational therapy.

The "Spirit" of Activity and Quality of Life—Supports for Mental Health

Sometimes individuals participate in activity for the sake of activity itself, and they derive satisfaction from developing their own abilities, enhancing their sense of self, or heightening their awareness of the world and people around them. Something may be accomplished, but it is not necessarily observable or measurable. This is believed to contribute to a **quality of life**.

Mihalyi Csikszentmihalyi (1990, 1996, 1997) is a writer, researcher, and philosopher who has studied the "quality of life" construct. His writing is in the tradition of writers and philosophers who have preceded him, including Carl Jung and others who are identified as humanistic and/or existential in their thinking. In occupational therapy literature, their work is cited to shed light on the spiritual dimension of activity and occupation.

In the latter 1990s, Csikszentmihalyi's book *Flow—The Psychology of Optimal Experience* (1990) became popular reading in the United States. As he described it, the experience of quality of life is universal and is dependent upon one's participation in activities that provide an opportunity for concentrated effort, an increased sense of control, and feedback about his or her performance. Quality of life is not dependent on a person's social or financial status, possessions, achievement, or recognition. Rather it comes from the "just-right challenge" created by the activity itself, and it requires people to use their skills and resources to achieve chosen goals. Challenging activity promotes pleasure and can result in personal growth and a feeling of personal satisfaction, all of which enhances quality of life (Csikszentmihalyi, 1990, pp. 45-67).

Flow, the Person, and Activity

During their lifetime and contributing to this sense of a quality of life, according to Csikszentmihalyi, most people are capable of experiencing "flow." Like quality of life, **flow** is a subjective feeling or state of mind that results when the person functions at an optimum level and is totally absorbed in what he or she is doing. Flow combines the use of one's senses, one's physical abilities, and one's cognitive abilities. Picture a child or group of children building a castle from building blocks—notice how absorbed they are, unaware of what is going on outside their own play. Remember yourself totally engrossed in a heated discussion in which you felt passionately about the ideas you were expressing, and you can imagine this state of "flow." In occupational therapy, we could say that flow depends on the integration of sensorimotor, cognitive, and psychosocial components of performance. Flow can result from the person's daily experiences of self-care, work, or leisure activities (Emerson, 1998).

Csikszentmihalyi suggests that flow may be experienced when we watch a sunset, exercise and feel physically fit, go dancing or act in a play, read or write a novel, listen to or play music, or share a sexual experience. The reader should discern that not every purposeful activity (as occupational therapists use the term) engenders flow, which implies an intensity or "oneness" with activity. Flow comes from functioning in the "here and now" and from accomplishing short-term, not long-term, goals. The experience of flow is one way in which the meaningfulness of an activity can be experienced and contribute to quality of life.

Flow is interrupted when a person is unable to concentrate, unable to attend to activities, and unable to set goals; any of these in turn can be the outcome of life disruptions brought about by illness, accident, or trauma. Flow is also compromised when one's goals and investment of energy in activity results in boredom, conflict, or anxiety (Csikszentmihalyi, 1990).

Re-Embracing Simple Pleasures and Commitment to What We Do

Another well-known writer who addresses the meaningfulness of everyday activity is Thomas Moore (1992, 1996, 1997). He proposes that when people allow themselves to take time for and truly pay attention to everyday events, it nurtures that spirit inside each person, which he refers to as the "soul." Spirit here does not refer exclusively to its use within religion, rather to that part of the self that relates to the bigger universe or experiences the meaning of life. He points to what he calls the early "wisdom" of the Shakers in America who believed that any work done with care and

commitment could nurture this spirit and contribute to an enhanced quality of life (Moore, 1997). Activities become meaningful not only because something is accomplished but because of the very process of participation.

It is this "spiritual" meaning of activity, occupation, and life's everyday roles that has received increased attention in the popular literature and public media in the United States. Not only Moore and Csikszentmihalyi, but many others, including Zukav (1980, 1989, 2000), Ram Dass (2000), Levey and Levey (1998), Breathnach (1995), and Ciulla (2000), encourage the public to examine how it spends time and to evaluate whether or not the way one divides time between work, leisure, daily chores, and other activities promotes his or her well-being and that of the people in his or her life, and whether it nurtures the spirit within each person. As noted by Ciulla (2000), there has been a press toward simplifying one's life and taking pleasure from the simple things in order to enhance one's quality of life. She adds that while this may sound reasonable and perhaps helpful for many people, it is not necessarily "simple" and cannot be treated in a cavalier fashion. What these and other authors point out is that how individuals spend their time engaged in activity and occupation reflects basic personal values about what is important in their lives and influences life satisfaction. The role of activity in nurturing the spirit is explored in the occupational therapy literature (Enquist, Short-DeGraff, Gliner, & Oltjenbruns, 1997; Gutterman, 1990; Howard & Howard, 1997; Kirsch, 1996; Schkade & Schultz, 1992; Toomey, 1999; Urbanowski & Vargo, 1994), particularly in the psychodynamic model and model of human occupation in this text. Regardless of their theoretical orientation, it seems vital that occupational therapists never lose sight of the many ways in which activities take on importance and meaning to their clients. **Meaningful activity** is not predicated on busy-ness nor productivity; it is based on what the individual perceives as meaningful.

Purposeful and Meaningful Activity Related to One's Place in the Lifespan

The particular activities and occupation that will be experienced as purposeful and meaningful by an individual and contribute to his or her mental well-being depends in part on the person's age and place in the life span. As people age and mature, the goals that people want to achieve change. Developing throughout our lives, we often find it especially satisfying to try new projects or to hone our skills. The very process of growth and development imposes a structure of physical, psychosocial, and cognitive abilities and expectations that help determine what an individual will choose as personal goals, as well as activities through which he or she can hope to achieve these goals. It also helps determine what others will expect of the person. In this way, **periods of devel-**

opment are part of a larger time frame that gives structure to people's lives and impacts how each will go about achieving a satisfying life (see Appendix C).

Within the discussions of the models for intervention in the text, the reader will consistently be advised to offer activities that fit with the client's/patient's age, interests, and culture, as well as to modify or present therapeutic activities in such a way that they are consistent with the client's age and level of ability and maturity. What makes an activity purposeful and meaningful is often that it makes an optimum match with what the client—child, adult, or older adult—sees as right for him- or herself at the current time in his or her life. For example, the 6-year-old feels especially proud when he or she masters riding a two-wheeler; the middle-aged adult values his or her ability to learn something new or to teach others; the older adult takes pleasure from spending time with grandchildren and telling them stories about their mom or dad. Highly regarded and broadly accepted developmentalists like Erik Erikson (1950, 1959, 1969) propose that during each life stage in the life span there are specific psychological challenges that must be met by the person if he or she is to feel a sense of well-being and readiness to move on to subsequent life challenges (see Appendix C).

Csikszentmihalyi (1990), whom we have previously cited, describes the three types of goals experienced throughout one's life, each of which contributes to a person's development of meaning in life. He identifies these as sensate, ideational, and idealistic goals (see Types of Meaningful Goals).

Bridging from Meaning to Life Theme

Even as an individual's goals and activities will change and evolve throughout his or her life, there typically develops an overarching **life theme** that provides coherence to these changing goals and gives direction and meaning in his or her life. Such themes can come from within the person and his or her experiences; can emanate from messages or directives taken from parents, family, or others; or be a combination of both. One may, for example, have a life theme of trying to help others or consistently putting the family first, or one may have a life theme of avoiding challenges and seeking the easy way out. Themes relate to our beliefs about ourselves and our hopes, aspirations, and fears. They relate to what we know, what we believe, and what we perceive as our reason for being alive. Being able to make choices and engage in activity and occupation that fits with what we perceive as our own life theme is more likely to lead to a feeling of quality of life (Csikszentmihalyi, 1990).

In occupational therapy, we see people whose life themes have been disrupted by accident, trauma, disease, or illness. Thus, it is not just that they can or cannot participate in a specific activity; the bigger issue may be that it appears to the person that he or she can no longer live his or her life in accordance with the theme he or she had embraced. In this way, medical conditions further disrupt quality of life; however, changing health conditions can create what some individuals perceive as a challenge and an opportunity for growth and development. You may know someone who has, in a sense, refused to allow his or her quality of life to be reduced by illness or trauma.

Occupational therapists use activities, tasks, and a person's occupations to help the client meet his or her goals, and in a manner in accordance with his or her style of approaching tasks. We strive to facilitate engagement in activities that are both purposeful and meaningful, that promote growth and development through the life span, and that contribute to quality of life. It is this that enables intervention to be client-centered.

MODELS OF PRACTICE PROVIDE CRITERIA FOR THERAPEUTIC ACTIVITY

As you read about the role of activity and occupation within each of the models presented, you will see one theme repeated: the activity in itself can be something important to the client, or that the activity can help the person meet his or her goals. How the activity can be best used to achieve this end or what activity should be chosen is guided by the theoretical postulates of the model.

If, for example, in the **cognitive-behavioral model**, the belief is that a client's sense of well-being and ability to function successfully increase when the client modifies negative beliefs about him- or herself, then the activity chosen will be one that facilitates the reappraisal of beliefs. To evaluate one's beliefs, perhaps the client will be asked to keep a log or journal. In a **sensorimotor approach**, the premise might be that the client can be more successful in ADLs if his or her CNS is better able to process information; then the activity chosen will be one believed capable of enhancing the person's ability to process sensory information. An activity selected for sensory processing might be that the client engages in a heavy work task that he or she enjoys, such as preparing the ground for a garden. In this way, each framework for practice in the text has postulates about the role of activity in the therapeutic process. The reader is referred to Functions of Activity in a Psychosocial Context (Table 2-1 on p. 41) for a summary of these postulates about activity.

Psychosocial Theory and Client-Centered Activity

Bearing this in mind, the same activity could be used for different purposes. To use our previous example, the person who has negative beliefs about him- or herself might be encouraged to create and nurture a garden as a means to

Types of Meaningful Goals

Sensate goals arise from within us, from our five senses. They identify pursuits that we expect will make us feel good and are realistic for specific circumstances. When we achieve our sensate goals, or when we satisfy our need to see beauty, taste good food, or experience pleasure from physical activity, we can experience pleasure and comfort and can meet our survival needs. For example, our need for rest and relaxation satisfies physical needs and restores energy for daily activity. Our need to see beauty can satisfy several of our senses when we view art and the beauty in nature. The pleasure that can come from sensual or sexual experiences throughout one's life pursues sensate goals and also may satisfy a need for starting a family.

Ideational goals originate in the social and cultural environment and are incorporated as our values and attitudes. They are usually culturally sensitive and provide a direction for meeting role expectations and for a particular lifestyle. These goals help us learn to be a "good neighbor" or a "good Catholic." They can orient us to the values, expectations, and pursuits that result in a "professional" or "academic" lifestyle.

Ideational goals can influence clients' or patients' progress in therapy. For example, in the milieu of rehabilitation programs, experienced clients may reach out to new patients. They introduce themselves, welcome them, and ensure these new patients that they will "get better" just as they themselves improved since being in the program, saying, "This program has really helped me." Over time they share stories and give each other encouragement. Sometimes their challenges help each other move forward to new performance levels. In this way, individuals internalize the goal to be "good patients." This in turn can contribute to a positive therapeutic milieu and to clients' sense of well-being.

With **idealistic goals**, we look inward to establish our values while continuing to monitor cultural expectations. Idealistic goals help us balance internal and external needs and expectations as we build autonomy and work for self-actualization while simultaneously being sensitive to the needs of our family, our community, and society.

For example, a client who was finishing outpatient rehabilitation described his new volunteer role in an intensive care waiting room. He was available to provide coffee or tea or to talk with those persons who wanted to talk with a "survivor." This helped meet his goal, which was to give the family members a sense of hope.

Another outpatient client who owned a video store negotiated a movie night for the patients, staff, and families at an acute rehabilitation setting. He provided complementary movies and enjoyed visiting and sharing time with people who were struggling as he had earlier in his rehabilitation. His goal was to provide comfort and support to clients and families and give them an opportunity for leisure. One day he shared with the occupational therapist, "Before my injury, the goal of my business was to get others to work for me and contribute to my financial well-being. Today, [post injury] I think about how my business helps others. I can bring pleasure for a brief period of time, and I provide additional work for my employees who are raising families."

Note: The goal descriptions are based upon the definitions by Csikszentmihalyi (1990). The examples are based upon experiences of the authors.

---

demonstrate to the person what he or she is capable of accomplishing. Therefore, the postulates about activity are not a cookbook of what activities to use; rather, they are a guide for what the occupational therapist would think about when considering activities.

In reasoning about how activities could be used to carry out client-centered intervention, the occupational therapist must establish what activities are compatible with the client's interests. At the same time, the occupational therapist will provide the kind of sensory, motor, cognitive, and psychosocial information and challenge as needed to build desired skills and contribute to mental health. This often necessitates a careful evaluation or analysis of the activity itself, as the therapist determines its attributes and the performance components needed to do the activity. The analysis also gives the therapist information about the environments and contexts that would be expected to support or to detract from performance.

Activity Analysis for Client-Centered Intervention

According to Crepeau (1998), the choice of activity is usually the result of multiple types of activity analyses. She describes three types of activity analyses that are used by clinicians when making clinical decisions about what activity to use in intervention. First, the clinician analyzes the client's goals to identify the tasks and activities that can contribute to goal achievement. Next, the therapist evaluates the relationship between activities and intervention theories, such as those in models of practice presented in this text. The therapist considers the psychodynamic, behavioral, or cognitive and sensorimotor elements of the activity. During the third analysis, the therapist compares the outcomes of the previous two analyses to the individual needs of the client and his or her activity preferences, performance abilities, occupations,

Table 2-1
FUNCTIONS OF ACTIVITY IN A PSYCHOSOCIAL CONTEXT

Psychodynamic Theory

- Activity is a subjective experience and a catalyst for learning.
- Activity facilitates interactions and understanding among group members.
- Activities are vehicles for increased self-awareness, sense of self, self-expression, and a way to achieve a meaning.
- Activity can connect the person's perception of past, current, and future events.
- The process of the activity (what is learned about the self and others) is as important as the end product.
- Activities provide opportunities for trying out new roles and new ways of relating to people, objects, and environments.
- Structured activities, activities with clear boundaries, and routines can help people who lack internal coherence feel safe and function more effectively.

Behavioral Context

- Activity produces an outcome that reflects client performance.
- Activity is a medium for learning task procedures.
- Activity is a medium for learning simple or complex skills.
- Activity is a medium for learning strategies to achieve a goal.
- Activities can serve as reinforcers for behavior.
- Simulated activities provide a vehicle for practice of real-life skills.

Cognitive Behavioral Context

- Activity increases knowledge of one's self, others, and the environment.
- Activity is a medium for assessing cognitive function.
- Engagement in activity can facilitate cognitive performance.
- Engagement in activity can support or change a person's beliefs and attitudes.
- Activity can increase a person's effective behaviors.
- Activity can increase a person's problem-solving strategies.
- Activities are used in educational modules and homework.

Cognitive Disability Context

- Activities are structured to provide the right cognitive demand.
- Activities can be used to assess the person's cognitive ability.
- Performance within activities can identify a person's level of cognitive function.
- Activities can be graded to match the person's cognitive ability.
- Activities support the person's use of remaining abilities to compensate for loss of cognitive ability.
- Activities are used to monitor the effect of medication on the person's performance.

Dynamic Interactional Cognitive Rehabilitation Context

- Activities are a medium for assessing cognitive performance.
- Activities are the vehicle for learning and re-learning cognitive skills.
- Participation in activities can increase a person's awareness of one's abilities and functional limits.
- Activities provide opportunities for using problem-solving skills.
- Activities are a medium for learning strategies that improve performance.   *(continued)*

Table 2-1 (Continued)

- Participation in activities used in multiple contexts supports generalization of learning.
- Engagement in activities can increase a person's quality of life.

Model of Human Occupation Context

- Activities are components of tasks and occupations.
- Activities may be structured to be simpler or more complex.
- Activities are used to achieve occupational performance goals.
- Activities produce an end product.
- Activity outcomes provide feedback regarding the person's performance.

Sensorimotor Context

- Activities provide sensory input.
- Engagement in activities can normalize movement.
- Participation in activities can facilitate spontaneous movement.
- Activities can facilitate motor planning.
- Activities can increase body awareness.
- Activities are a medium for pleasure and enjoyment.
- Activities can facilitate the person's adaptive response in various contexts.
- Activities provide opportunities for cognitive skill building.

---

and lifestyle (Crepeau, 1998). Each of these three analyses, as described by Crepeau, influences the clinician's reasoning during evaluation and intervention (see Activity Analyses for Clinical Reasoning).

Psychosocial Theory and Client-Centered Practice

While we have been focusing on the role of therapeutic activities and occupation, it becomes clear that when looking at the role of activity in the person-activity-environment triad, it is always with the person as referent. It is the activity's purpose in the eyes of the client and its ability to foster his or her personal goals, it is the meaningfulness of the activity as determined by the client, it is the person's sense of well-being or mental health that we strive to enhance. Activities are analyzed to determine the likelihood that they can be successfully comprehended and mastered by the person, and they are selected in accordance with what the client prefers. Even where some of the models in the text acknowledge that activities and occupation help the person to engage in reciprocal, social relationships or that occupational function of the individual impacts the well-being of others, they never stray from the driving premise that it is the person-at-center in the process of therapy. This, then, can be offered as evidence of person-centered (client-centered) practice, as the term has come to be used by occupational therapists. This will be addressed further in the chapters to follow.

ENVIRONMENT

Therapy, like occupation, never takes place in a vacuum—it occurs within a life space—including a physical space that we can see and touch; an internal, emotional environment (the inner world of thoughts, beliefs, and feelings); and a place composed of other people, their beliefs, and values. To understand whether or not therapeutic goals will be met, the therapist must always pay attention to what exists within the multiple environments in which the activity is being performed. Environments are not like stage scenery that sits at the back of the performance—they are an integral part of the action. An activity or occupation that is taking place in one environment will necessarily be different in some way than it would in another environment. Environments must provide the necessary resources for activities and occupations to be carried out. They can nurture or support activity, or they can impede it. Environments also create expectations for performance, that is, for certain activities to be done, and to be done in a specific manner. For example, eating a meal at home alone might look quite different than it would if one were eating out at a formal banquet. Environments also provide feedback to the person, let-

ACTIVITY ANALYSES FOR CLINICAL REASONING

Task activity analysis identifies the activities that contribute to the tasks related to one's daily living, work, and leisure. This analysis results in a description of:

- The activities that contribute to the task; those required to prepare a meal, write a resumé, or plan a vacation
- The meaning of the task within the context of culture and the typical age of persons who participate in the activity
- The environment in which the task occurs, such as home, school, work, playground
- The safety and possible hazardous conditions for performing the task; the physical and social environments

The therapist also lists the steps of the activity or task and the equipment and supplies needed for doing the activities or task. This analysis helps us understand the demands of the task, its specific activities, and the contextual variables of the activity (Crepeau, 1998).

Performance activity analysis is based upon the performance components described in *Uniform Terminology* (3rd ed.) (AOTA, 1998b) (see Appendix B for this document). The therapist evaluates the need for each of these components to perform an activity. The identified components of performance are sensorimotor, cognitive integrative and cognitive psychosocial skills, and psychological components. Each of these components has multiple variables that are defined (e.g., strength, coordination, memory, sensation, organization, time management, values, interests, etc.). Because of the details of this analysis, the therapist summarizes the essential components of performance for the activity and contrasts this with the client's occupational performance strengths and limits (Crepeau, 1998).

Theory activity analysis is based upon the theoretical beliefs of the therapist, the practice environment, and the occupational therapy profession. These theories may be blended to grade and adapt activities that meet the client's values, interest, motivation, and rehabilitation needs. Theories influence evaluation and intervention approaches and, thus, the choice of activity that can best achieve the goals of occupational therapy (Crepeau, 1998).

Individual activity analysis focuses on the person's current and previous interests, values, goals, performance boundaries, roles, and their relationship to one's activity patterns. This information is used to identify meaningful activities that can be used during intervention. The information can also guide the therapist in adapting activities to achieve client's goals and fit with his or her life theme (adapted from Crepeau, 1998).

---

ting him or her know whether or not his or her behavior is acceptable within that place or setting.

Types of Environments

When we think of "environments," many types come to mind: cultural, physical, social, and economic. Each of these environments can impact in a subtle or very obvious way how easy or difficult it will be for a client or groups of persons to follow through with the activities, occupations, and (ultimately) goals he or she or they have chosen. The significance of the environment in occupational therapy practice has been given increased attention, and the reader is referred to the multiple references in this area, which are provided later in this chapter. Borrowing from the literature (Spencer, 1998) and definitions provided by AOTA (see American Occupational Therapy Association Defines Environments) we begin by identifying terms used to describe environments.

The **cultural environment** refers to the customs, standards, beliefs, and accepted ways of participating in activities shared by the society of which the person is a member. It also includes laws of the society (e.g., it encompasses the legislation that guides health care and community services). Whether or not an individual will value a particular activity or occupation can be closely tied to its acceptance by the people with whom he or she identifies. There are specific cultural beliefs that influence how the person views his or her role in the therapy process as well as the roles of therapists and others. In some cultures, for example, the individual is more likely to perceive the therapist as "expert" and less likely to question recommendations made by the therapist. What is considered "normal behavior" is not the same in all cultures, whether one refers to the carrying out of everyday tasks of living, fulfilling job responsibilities, or raising one's children. While we do not discuss cultural difference in detail in this text, the therapist must always be aware of the cultural environment or climate with which the client is most familiar, the culture in which he or she will be enacting activities, and the internalized culture of values he or she holds.

The **physical environment** refers to non-human components of the environment: physical objects, observable spaces and dwellings, the terrain, and the accoutrements of the physical setting in which one functions, as well as how these accoutrements are arranged in the physical space. Occupational therapists may assess whether or not physical environments are physically accessible and safe, and whether they contain the objects or equipment that the person needs

AMERICAN OCCUPATIONAL THERAPY ASSOCIATION DEFINES ENVIRONMENTS

Environmental Terms

Cultural environment—"Customs, beliefs, activity patterns, behavior standards, and expectations accepted by the society of which the individual is a member. Includes political aspects, such as laws that affect access of resources and affirm personal rights. Also includes opportunities for education, employment, and economic support" (AOTA, 1994, p. 1054).

Physical environment—Non-human aspects of contexts. Includes the accessibility to and performance within environments having natural terrain, plants, animals, buildings, furniture, objects, tools, or devices (AOTA, 1994, p. 1054). "That part of the environment that can be perceived directly through the senses. The physical environment includes observable space, objects and their arrangement, light, noise, and other ambient characteristics that can be objectively determined" (Christiansen & Baum, 1997, p. 601).

Social environment—"Availability and expectations of significant individuals, such as spouse, friends, and caregivers. Also includes larger social groups, which are influential in establishing norms, role expectations, and social routines" (AOTA, 1994, p. 1054). "Those social systems or networks within which a given person operates; the collective human relationships of an individual, whether familial, community, or organization in nature, constitute the social environment of that individual" (Christiansen & Baum, 1997, p. 604).

Virtual environment—An environment in which individuals or objects are not actually present in the immediate physical space but are experienced through the senses by electronic means. Related to the term "virtual reality," which is defined as "a realistic simulation of an environment including three-dimensional graphic by a computer system using interactive software and hardware" (Random House Unabridged Dictionary, 1993).

Note: These definitions are excerpts from Draft IV, OT Practice Framework (AOTA, August 2000). Most recent editions of these terms and other current official documents can be obtained by down loading information and documents from the AOTA network (www.AOTA.org).

ting. One may, for example, be distracted from work in a physical environment that is too cluttered, too warm, too cold, or in which there is a significant amount of noise. While we might tend to pay little attention to an environment in which we are comfortable, we can probably think of instances in which we have been in a setting in which the environment interfered with our being able to accomplish our task.

The **social environment** consists of different groups (e.g., family, friends, co-workers) that influence one's participation in daily life. These groups help to create the expectations for performance and can provide the support that a person needs for learning and participation in one's environment. Social environments also influence a person's quality of life. The occupational therapist considers the social environment during evaluation, treatment, discharge planning, and consultation. Social groups, especially the family, may be impacted by the client's disability. Thus, the clinician may also provide services to families or other social groups in order to help integrate the client into his or her social environment.

Technology has introduced another type of environment. This is referred to as the **virtual environment**, which provides an electronic medium for clients to practice skills that can be transferred to the physical environment. Use of the virtual environment can contribute to the evaluation of safe function in a controlled environment. Safety has a strong relationship with many of the psychosocial issues that arise during occupational therapy interventions in multiple contexts. For example, when individuals have been confused, have a cognitive impairment, or are fearful, driver and work simulations can provide a safe environment for the initial evaluation of the client's ability to drive prior to highway tests or resumption in the job setting.

The **economic environment** also affects performance as well as issues related to mental health throughout the continuum of occupational therapy services. This perspective may or may not be referenced in theory and practice literatures, but it often emerges as a critical variable when talking with clients. Economics can relate to the person's lifestyle and participation in daily activities and one's goals and choices of activity. It is a variable that influences the time available for intervention and the resources available for problem solving.

Environment or Context—Is There a Difference?

Just as the terms "activity" and "occupation" are sometimes used interchangeably, this also occurs with the terms "environment" and "context." Where they are differentiated, some theorists use the term **environment** to describe the broad or general conditions (i.e., physical, social, and cultural) that influence a person's participation in daily life. Some may include the specifics that other theorists describe as "context." **Context** describes the individual conditions that

if he or she is to perform a desired activity. Physical environments have multiple attributes. They include sights, sounds, and odors—all of which may enhance or detract from the individual's comfort and successful performance in the set-

influence the person's performance (e.g., the person's specific place in the life span, the nature of the illness or disability, place, available social support and equipment, and so on). With both environments and personal contexts, the occupational therapist pays attention to the effect that these have on the person's ability to perform activity/occupation in a given life span, and also to the effect that they appear to have on the person's mental health. Keep in mind that the examples in the remainder of this text related to specific frames of reference may or may not influence terminology used.

The Person's Place in the Environment

It is not just the type of environment to be taken into account, there is also the person's relationship to that environment. This idea is discussed by Spencer (1998) and contributes to the understanding of the relationship among person-activity and environment.

Spencer (1998) acknowledges each of the previously identified types of environments (e.g., physical, social, cultural). Within each of these, the person's position in the environment can be immediate, proximal, community, and societal. The person's position in the environment influences his or her occupational performance. It influences the person's control in the environment, which in turn is one of the major psychosocial issues that influences everyday life and the outcome of intervention. One's position in the environment also influences the number of variables that the person manages while participating in tasks, activities, and occupations in daily life.

As identified by Spencer, the **immediate environment** is a person's personal space and objects such as a chair, bed, closet, personal automobile, desk, and personal locker. Clients who cannot get to the second floor of their home may be frustrated by this limitation or depressed by the loss of privacy. The person who must sell his or her car because he or she can no longer drive experiences the psychosocial changes that come with decreased independence, which in turn impacts not only one's quality of life but also limits the range of choices the person has for participating in daily life.

The **proximal environment** consists of the places where a person participates in activities and occupational roles: a person's home, work, school, etc. Clients with impairments and disability must learn to cope with psychosocial stress that can come from the challenges of architectural barriers or new performance challenges at home, work, school, or elsewhere.

The **community environment** has the places that help us meet our basic needs as well as those for quality of life. For example, the supermarket, a museum, movie theater, library, bank, restaurant, shopping mall, place of worship, and park are just a few of the community environments that people frequent. After a disability, clients may need increased time and assistance to use these community resources. Clients

often must re-learn strategies that were once automatic and may become frustrated trying to perform activities that were previously pleasurable or easily accomplished. These changes can produce decreased ability to carry out IADLs and may contribute to feelings of decreased competence, psychosocial stress, or isolation and decreased community participation.

The **societal environment** may not be represented by a concrete place and yet it is a major influence in our daily lives. It represents social policy and laws, such as the American with Disabilities Act (ADA) and mental health legislation. It is the attitude of others toward a person's disability and the emotional and social support from others. The attitudes of others and the support from society are major factors that contribute to a person's psychosocial well-being. The laws as well as the attitudes of society can influence the person's place in society and the opportunities they have for occupational performance.

The Environment in Theoretical Frameworks

We know that people's environments influence whether they will be able to accomplish the activities and occupations that they choose and the very activities and occupations they pursue. The role of the environment is addressed in all of the models in this text, some more explicitly than others. The most comprehensive discussion of the environment is within the model of human occupation (MOHO) (Chapter Seven). Kielhofner (1995), the architect of this model, uses the term **affords** to refer to what the environment makes available as resources and opportunities to enact chosen activities. The term **press** is used to convey the expectations within the environment for certain behaviors (i.e., some activities are expected, sanctioned, and/or encouraged while others are not). It follows that MOHO will pay particular attention to the environment given that one of MOHO's central postulates is that occupational therapists do not change people directly; rather, clinicians "change the relevant environment to support or precipitate a change in the human system" (Kielhofner, 1995, p. 261).

Each of the frameworks for practice in this text emphasizes attributes of the environment in accordance with the overall postulates of the model. The psychodynamic model, for example, pays special attention to how social and emotional environments either support or impede the person's ability to make healthy choices for the self. It emphasizes that if we create an accepting and supportive environment, then people are more likely to risk trying new behaviors within their activity or roles. The same **psychodynamic model** postulates that when people are confused and lack the ability to effectively organize their thoughts and behaviors, an external structure in the environment can increase their feeling of ease and their ability to conduct themselves appropriately. Claudia Allen's **cognitive disabilities model** pays particular attention to the physical setting of home or work, with a special concern for the individual's safety in those settings. Toglia's **dynamic interactional model** and the **sensorimotor models** advise occupational therapists to pay particular attention to the nature and relative amount of sensory information in the environment and to consider the ability of the environment to calm or alert the central nervous system. As we have said, the occupational therapist's goal is to discern the impact of environmental variables in the relationship between the person, activity, and environment and use this information to address psychosocial issues in daily practice.

It is vital that the therapist engaging in clinical intervention or helping to create or support service delivery gives careful thought to the therapeutic environment. It has been a painful lesson for many therapists to observe a client who is doing well leave an inpatient setting, only to go to his or her home and lose therapeutic gains because the home, employment, or community setting did not support therapeutic gains. It may be even more painful for patients and clients whose self-confidence and feelings of personal control seem to rise and fall capriciously because they are tied to things in the environment that are beyond their control.

There is no absolute standard for what constitutes a helpful or nurturing environment, or one that is likely to maintain therapeutic progress. What can be a helpful or supportive environment for one person may be too busy or sterile for another. An activity that fits within one setting may be totally out of place in another. Once again we are reminded that the person-activity and environment are in an ever-changing interrelationship with each other in establishing and maintaining opportunities for participation in daily life. This relationship and its effect on occupational performance is examined in the professional literature, and numerous models have been developed to describe this relationship (Christiansen & Baum, 1997; Clark et al., 1991; Dunn, Brown, McClain, & Westman, 1994; Dunn, McClain, Brown, & Youngstrom, 1998; Fidler & Fidler, 1978; Kielhofner & Burke, 1980; King, 1978; Law et al., 1996; Llorens, 1970; Mathiowetz & Bass Haugen, 1994; Neistadt & Creapeu, 1998; Nelson, 1988; Reilly, 1962; Schkade & Schultz, 1992; Spencer, 1998). Specific occupational therapy models that detail the person-environment-activity/occupation interactions or transactions are identified in Person-Environment-Occupation Practice Models in Occupational Therapy.

Environmental Theory—Contributing Resource to Occupational Therapy

The previously listed person-environment-occupation models have been influenced by environmental theories that were developed in other disciplines. These environmental theories contribute to the occupational therapist's under-

---

PERSON-ENVIRONMENT-OCCUPATION PRACTICE MODELS IN OCCUPATIONAL THERAPY

- Person-Environment-Occupation Model (Law et al., 1996)
- Person-Environment-Occupational Performance Model (Christiansen & Baum, 1997)
- Ecology of Human Performance Model (Dunn et al., 1994)
- Occupational Adaptation Model (Schkade & Schultz, 1992)
- Model of Human Occupation (Kielhofner & Burke, 1980)

---

standing of the roles of the environment in the person-activity-environment relationship (Auerswald, 1971; Baker & Intagliata, 1982; Bandura, 1986; Berlin, 1989; Bronfenbrenner, 1979; Gibson, 1977, 1979; Hancock, 1985; Hart, 1979; Kahana, 1982; Kaplan, 1983; Lawton, 1986; Moos, 1980; Weisman, 1981; Wicker, 1979). These scholars, as well as others, are cited in occupational therapy's professional literature and their concepts contribute to occupational therapy theory and practice. They influence evaluation, intervention, and research methodology in occupational therapy. Key principles or features of these theories that relate to occupational therapy have been outlined by Law et al. (1997). These principles and their influence in occupational therapy are summarized and reproduced in Key Elements of Person-Environment Models (Appendix D). The reader is referred to the original source (Christiansen & Baum, 1997) for related details. When choosing assessments and planning intervention, the occupational therapist can blend some of the theories with some of the psychosocial theories described in the second half of this text.

Evaluation and Research of Person-Environment-Activity/Occupation

To gain insight into the effect of the environment or context on the person and one's activities, occupational therapists may use self-report and ethnographic methods to study the relationship among these variables (Spencer, 1998; Spencer, Krefting, & Mattingly, 1993). These methods also increase one's understanding of psychosocial issues in occupational therapy.

Ethnographic methods, frequently used in anthropology, have been adapted for health care and occupational therapy contexts. For example, occupational therapists have conducted studies to solicit the person's perspective (also called insider perspective) on environments, occupational life, the effects of culture, the meaning and value of activities and occupations, the relationship between the client and the clinician, and the roles of significant others in the life of a person with a disability (Spencer, 1998).

Additionally, the occupational therapist can choose an assessment instrument that evaluates variables in the environment and their relationship to client participation in daily life before or after occupational therapy and his or her quality of life. For example, the Home Observation for Measurement of the Environment (HOME) (Caldwell & Bradley, 1979), the Community Integration Questionnaire (CIQ) (Willer et al., 1993), and the Craig Handicap Assessment and Report Technique (CHART) (Whiteneck et al., 1988, 1992) are just a few of the choices available to clinicians. Environmental Assessment Instruments (see p. 48) identifies tools used in occupational therapy practice. Some are more frequently used in specialty areas of practice; many can provide information relative to psychosocial concerns. The reader is referred to the original sources.

Summary: The Psychosocial Impact of the Environments

Earlier we referred to activities being carried out in physical, sociocultural, and internal environments (i.e., the world of personal perceptions, knowledge, beliefs, attitudes, and motivation). These internal variables interact with the external environments previously described. Internal environments are created by psychological constructs that we already have said can be imagined but have no definitive meaning. Both internal and external environments and their relationships ultimately support or interfere with the person's participation in activities and occupations and influence one's quality of life.

Each of the frames of reference presented in this text places the spotlight on differing attributes of the environment as these impact the person's ability to function optimally. Recognizing that the clients and patients whom we serve are often individuals who have illnesses, disabilities, or limitations—both visible and invisible—the following are some ways in which the environment can directly affect these persons' mental health and sense of well-being:

- The interactions between the person, activity/occupation, and the physical environment can engender stress or beliefs that one can cope, realistic challenge or a sense of defeat, and build or detract from feelings of self-confidence and personal worth.
- Consistency and predictability in the environment can help a person feel safe.
- A structured environment in which rules and expectations are in place and are clear necessitates less decision making by the person than one that is less structured.
- Unpredictability can be unsettling or contribute to curiosity and the pleasure associated with novelty.

- On a sensory level, environments can range on a continuum from arousing to calming.
- Environments can be perceived as physically and emotionally safe and "friendly" places, which makes it easier for people to relax, take risks, and learn. Conversely, they may be perceived as unsafe or unaccepting and should be avoided, which makes it more difficult for people to be themselves, to take risks, and to learn.
- The social interactions within the environment can foster friendship, opportunity for self-expression, and enhancement of esprit de corps or can require the person to cope with silence, misunderstanding, prejudice, or isolation.
- Participation and appreciation of natural and aesthetic environments can contribute to people's quality of life.
- In order to develop feelings of internal control and to establish a realistic basis for understanding one's own abilities and limitations, one needs opportunities to function within a fair and responsive environment.
- The person's perception of being in a fair and responsive environment can contribute to and sustain motivation; an unfair and/or nonresponsive environment can negatively impact motivation.
- The dynamic nature of the person-activity-environment relationship, over time, influences the person's opportunities in daily life, current performance, and one's sense of well-being.

REFERENCES

American Occupational Therapy Association. (1997). Special issue on occupation, spirituality, and life meaning. *Am J Occup Ther, 51*, 167-234.

American Occupational Therapy Association. (1998a). Psychosocial concerns within occupational therapy practice. In *Reference manual of the official documents of the American Occupational Therapy Association, Inc.* (7th ed., pp. 373-379). Bethesda, MD: Author.

American Occupational Therapy Association. (1998b). Uniform terminology for occupational therapy (3rd ed.). In *Reference manual of the official documents of the American Occupational Therapy Association, Inc.* (7th ed., pp. 155-175). Bethesda, MD: Author.

American Occupational Therapy Association. (2000). *Occupational therapy practice framework—Engagement and participation in occupation, draft IV.* Bethesda, MD: Author.

American Psychological Association. (1994). *Diagnostic and statistical manual of mental disorders* (4th ed.). Washington, DC: Author.

American Psychological Association. (2000). *Diagnostic and statistical manual of mental disorders—TR* (4th ed.). Washington, DC: Author.

ENVIRONMENTAL ASSESSMENT INSTRUMENTS

- Work Capacity Evaluation (Velozo, 1993)
- Baltimore Therapeutic Equipment Work Simulator (Neimeyer, Matheson, & Carlton, 1989)
- The Assistive Technology Evaluation Process (Cook & Hussey, 1995)
- The Fine Motor Task Assessment (McHale & Cermak, 1992)
- The Negotiability Rating Process (Bates, 1994)
- The Interview-in-Place (Lifchez, 1987)
- The Readily Achievable Checklist (Cronburg, Barnet, & Goldman, 1991)
- The Accessibility Checklist (Goltsman, Gilbert, & Wohlford, 1992)
- The Neighborhood Environment Survey (Cantor, 1979)
- The Disability Rights Guide (Goldman, 1991)
- The Mother-Child Interaction Checklist (Barrera & Vella, 1987)
- The Cost of Care Index (Kosberg & Cairl, 1986)
- The Family Assessment Device (Epstein, Baldwin, & Bishop, 1983)
- The Ward Atmosphere Scale (Moos, 1974)
- The Environment Assessment Scale (Kannegeiter, 1987)
- The Work Environment Scale (Moos, 1981)
- The Social Support Inventory (Rowles, 1983)
- The Disability Social Distance Scale (Tringo, 1970)
- The Ethnographic Assessment Process (Spencer et al., 1993)
- The Home-Based Intervention for Caregivers of Elders with Dementia (Corcoran & Gitlin, 1992)
- The Classroom Observation Guide (Griswold, 1994)
- The Home Observation for Measurement of the Environment (Caldwell & Bradley, 1979)
- The Craig Handicap Assessment and Report Technique (Whitneck et al., 1988, 1992)
- The Community Integration Questionnaire (Willer et al., 1993)

Note: This list of environmental assessments is selected from Cole Spencer, J. (1998). Evaluation of performance contexts. In M. E. Neistadt & E. B. Crepeau (Eds.), *Willard & Spackman's occupational therapy* (9th ed., pp. 291-310). Philadelphia, PA: Lippincott, Williams & Wilkins.

The reader is referred to Spencer's comprehensive descriptions of environmental assessments and their purpose. Readers should also read the original sources of the assessments. Original sources are cited in this list and in the references at the end of this chapter.

Auerswald, E. H. (1971). Families, change, and the ecological perspective. *Fam Process, 10*, 263-280.

Baker, F., & Intagliata, J. (1982). Quality of life in the evaluation of community support systems. *Evaluation and Program Planning, 5*, 69-79.

Bandura, A. (1986). *Social foundation of thought and action: A social cognitive theory*. Englewood Cliffs, NJ: Prentice-Hall.

Barrera, M., & Vella, D. (1987). Disabled and nondisabled infants' interactions with their mothers. *Am J Occup Ther, 41*, 168-172.

Bates, P. (1994). The self-care environment: Issues of space and furnishing. In C. Christiansen (Ed.), *Ways of living: Self-care strategies for special needs* (pp. 423-451). Rockville, MD: American Occupational Therapy Association.

Berger, M. M. (1977). *Working with people called patients*. New York, NY: Brunner/Mazel.

Berlin, S. (1989). The Canadian healthy community project: Shapes of the reality. *Plan Canada, 29*, 13-15.

Borg, B., & Bruce, M. A. (1991). Assessing psychological performance factors. In C. Christiansen & C. Baum (Eds.), *Occupational therapy: Overcoming human performance deficits*. Thorofare, NJ: SLACK Incorporated.

Borg, B., & Bruce, M. A. (1997). *Occupational therapy stories: Psychosocial interaction in practice*. Thorofare, NJ: SLACK Incorporated.

Breathnach, S. B. (1995). *Simple abundance: A daybook of comfort and joy*. New York, NY: Time Warner.

Bronfenbrenner, U. (1979). *The ecology of human development*. Cambridge, MA: Harvard University Press.

Caldwell, B., & Bradley, R. (1979). *Home Observation for Measurement of the Environment (HOME)*. Little Rock, AR: University of Arkansas.

Canadian National Health and Welfare. (1988). *Mental health for Canadians: Striking a balance*. Ottawa, Canada: Ministry of Supply and Services.

Cantor, M. (1979). Life space and social support. In T. Byerts, S. Howell, & L. Pastalan (Eds.), *Environmental context of aging: Lifestyles, environmental quality, and living arrangements* (pp. 33-61). New York, NY: Garland STPM Press.

Christiansen, C. H. (1997). Person-environment occupational performance: A conceptual model for practice. In C. Christiansen & C. M. Baum (Eds.), *Occupational therapy: Enabling function and well-being* (2nd ed., pp. 46-72). Thorofare, NJ: SLACK Incorporated.

Christiansen, C. H. (1999). Defining lives: Occupation as identity: An essay on competence, coherence, and creation of meaning. *Am J Occup Ther, 53*, 547-557.

Christiansen, C. H., & Baum, C. M. (1997). *Occupational therapy: Enabling function and well-being* (2nd ed.). Thorofare, NJ: SLACK Incorporated.

Christiansen, C. H., Backman, C., Little, B. R., & Nguyen, A. (1999). Occupations and well-being: A study of personal projects. *Am J Occup Ther, 53,* 91-100.

Ciulla, J. B. (2000). *The working life: The promise and the betrayal of modern work.* New York, NY: Random House.

Clark, F., Parham, D., Carlson, M., Frank, G., Jackson, J., Pierce, D., Wolfe, R. J., & Zemke, R. (1991). Occupational science: Academic innovation in the service of occupational therapy's future. *Am J Occup Ther, 45,* 300-310.

Cook, A., & Hussey, S. (1995). *Assistive technologies: Principles and practice.* St. Louis, MO: C. V. Mosby.

Corcoran, M., & Gitlin, L. (1992). Dementia management: An occupation therapy home-base intervention for caregivers. *Am J Occup Ther, 46,* 801-808.

Crepeau, E. B. (1995). Rituals (Module 6). In C. B. Royeen (Ed.), *The practice of the future: Putting occupation back into therapy.* Bethesda, MD: American Occupational Therapy Association.

Crepeau, E. B. (1998). Activity analysis: A way of thinking about occupational performance. In M. E. Neistadt & E. B. Crepeau (Eds.), *Willard & Spackman's occupational therapy* (9th ed., pp. 135-147). Philadelphia, PA: Lippincott, Williams & Wilkins.

Cronburg, J., Barnet, J., & Goldman, N. (1991). *Readily available checklist: A survey for accessibility.* Washington, DC: National Center for Access Unlimited.

Csikszentmihalyi, M. (1990). *Flow—The psychology of optimal experience.* New York, NY: Harper Collins Publishers, Inc.

Csikszentmihalyi, M. (1996). *Creativity—Flow and the psychology of discovery and invention.* New York, NY: Harper Collins Publishers, Inc.

Csikszentmihalyi, M. (1997). *Finding flow—The psychology of engagement with everyday life.* New York, NY: Harper Collins Publishers, Inc.

Cynkin, S., & Robinson, A. M. (1990). *Occupational therapy and activities health: Toward health through activities.* Boston, MA: Little Brown.

Darnell, J. L., & Heater, S. L. (1994). Occupational therapist or activity therapist: Which do you choose to be? *Am J Occup Ther, 48,* 467-468.

Dunn, W., Brown, C., McClain, L., & Westman, K. (1994). The ecology of human performance: A contextual perspective on human occupation. In C. B. Royeen (Ed.), *AOTA self-study series: The practice of the future: Putting occupation back into therapy.* Rockville, MD: American Occupational Therapy Association.

Dunn, W., McClain, L. H., Brown, C., & Youngstrom, M. J. (1998). The ecology of human performance. In M. E. Neistadt & E. B. Crepeau (Eds.), *Willard & Spackman's occupational therapy* (9th ed., pp. 531-535). Philadelphia, PA: Lippincott, Williams & Wilkins.

Emerson, H. (1998). Flow and occupation: A review of the literature. *Can J Occup Ther, 65,* 37-44.

Enquist, D., Short-DeGraff, M., Gliner, J., & Oltjenbruns, K. (1997). Occupational therapists' beliefs and practices with regard to spirituality and therapy. *Am J Occup Ther, 51*(3), 173-180.

Erikson, E. (1950). *Childhood and society.* New York, NY: Norton.

Erikson, E. (1959). Identity and the life cycle. *Psychol Issues, 1,* 1-171.

Erikson, E. (1969). *Identity, youth, and crisis.* New York, NY: W. W. Norton.

Epstein, N., Baldwin, L., & Bishop, D. (1983). The McMaster family assessment device. *J Marital Fam Ther, 9,* 171-180.

Fidler, G. S., & Fidler, F. W. (1978). Doing and becoming: Purposeful action and self-actualization. *Am J Occup Ther, 32,* 305-310.

Gibson, J. (1977). The theory of affordances. In R. Shaw & J. Bransford (Eds.), *Perceiving, acting, and knowing* (pp. 67-82). Hillsdale, NJ: Erlbaum.

Gibson, J. (1979). *The ecological approach to visual perception.* Boston, MA: Houghton-Mifflin.

Goldman, C. (1991). *Disability right guide: Practical solutions to problems affecting people with disabilities.* Lincoln, NE: Media.

Goltsman, S., Gilbert, T., & Wohlford, S. (1992). *The accessibility checklist: An evaluating system for buildings and outdoor settings.* Berkeley, CA: M.I.G. Communications.

Griswold, L. (1994). Ethnographic analysis: A study of classroom environments. *Am J Occup Ther, 48,* 397-402.

Gutterman, L. (1990). A day treatment program for persons with AIDS. *Am J Occup Ther, 44,* 234-237.

Hancock, T. (1985). The mandala of health: A model of the human ecosystem. *Family and Community Health, 8,* 1-10.

Hart, R. (1979). *Children's experience of place.* New York, NY: Irvington.

Hasselkus, B. R., & Rosa, S. A. (1997). Meaning and occupation. In C. Christiansen & C. Baum (Eds.), *Occupational therapy—Enabling function and well-being* (pp. 363-377). Thorofare, NJ: SLACK Incorporated.

Howard, B., & Howard, J. (1997). Occupation as spiritual activity. *Am J Occup Ther, 51*(3), 173-180.

Jackson, J. (1998). The value of occupation as the core of treatment: Sandy's experiences. *Am J Occup Ther, 54,* 466-473.

Jacobs, K. (1994). Flow and occupational therapy practitioner. *Am J Occup Ther, 48,* 989-995.

Jahonda, M. (1958). *Current concepts of positive mental health.* New York, NY: Basic Books.

Kahana, E. (1982). A congruence model of person-environment interaction. In M. P. Lawton, P. G. Windley, & T. D. Byerts (Eds.), *Aging and the environment: Theoretical approaches* (pp. 97-121). New York, NY: Springer.

Kannegeiter, R. (1987). The development of the environmental assessment scale. *Occupational Therapy in Mental Health, 6,* 67-83.

Kaplan, S. (1983). A model of person-environment compatibility. *Environment and Behavior, 15,* 311-332.

Kidner, T. (1924). Work for the tuberculosis patient during and after care: Part II. *Archives of Occupational Therapy, 3,* 169-193.

Kielhofner, G. (Ed.). (1995). *A model of human occupation: Theory and application* (2nd ed.). Baltimore, MD: Williams & Wilkins.

Kielhofner, G., & Burke, J. P. (1980). A model of human occupation, part 1. Conceptual framework and content. *Am J Occup Ther, 34*, 527-581.

King, L. J. (1978). Toward a science of adaptive responses. *Am J Occup Ther, 32*, 429-437.

Kirsch, B. (1996). A narrative approach to addressing spirituality in occupational therapy: Exploring personal meaning and purpose. *Can J Occup Ther, 63*, 55-61.

Kosberg, J., & Cairl, R. (1986). The cost of care index: A case management tool for screening informal care providers. *The Gerontological Society of America, 26*, 273-278.

Law, M., Cooper, B., Strong, S., Stewart, D., Rigby, P., & Letts, L. (1996). The person-environment-occupation model: A transactive approach to occupational performance. *Can J Occup Ther, 63*, 9-23.

Law, M., Cooper, B. A., Strong, S., Stewart, D., Rigby, P., & Letts, L. (1997). Theoretical context for the practice of occupational therapy. In C. Christiansen & C. Baum (Eds.), *Occupational therapy: Enabling function and well-being* (2nd ed.). Thorofare, NJ: SLACK Incorporated.

Lawton, M. P. (1986). *Environment and aging* (2nd ed.). Albany NY: Plenum.

Levey, J., & Levey, M. (1998). *A dynamic approach for creating harmony and wholeness in a chaotic world.* Berkley, CA: Conari Press.

Lifchez, R. (1987). *Rethinking architecture: Design students and physically disabled people.* Berkeley, CA: University of California Press.

Llorens, L. A. (1970). Facilitating growth and development: The promise of occupational therapy. *Am J Occup Ther, 24*, 93-101.

Mathiowetz, V., & Bass Haugen, J. (1994). Motor behavior research: Implications for therapeutic approaches to central nervous system dysfunction. *Am J Occup Ther, 48*, 733-745.

McHale, K., & Cermak, S. (1992). Fine motor activities in elementary school: Preliminary findings and provisional implications for children with fine motor problems. *Am J Occup Ther, 46*, 898-903.

Moore, T. (1992). *Care of the soul.* New York, NY: Harper Perennial.

Moore, T. (1996). *The re-enchantment of everyday life.* New York, NY: Harper Perennial.

Moore, T. (1997). *On meaningful work.* Boulder, CO: Sounds True.

Moos, R. (1974). *Evaluation of treatment environments: A sociological approach.* New York, NY: Wiley.

Moos, R. (1980). Specialized living environments for older people: A conceptual framework for evaluation. *Journal of Social Issues, 36*, 75-94.

Moos, R. (1981). *Work environment scale manual.* Palo Alto, CA: Consulting Psychological Press.

Neidstadt, M. E., & Crepeau, E. B. (Eds.). (1998). *Willard & Spackman's occupational therapy* (9th ed.). Philadelphia, PA: Lippincott, Williams & Wilkins.

Neimeyer, L., Matheson, L., & Carlton, R. (1989). Testing consistency of effort: BTRE work simulator. *Industrial Rehabilitation Quarterly, 2*, 5-32.

Nelson, D. L. (1988). Occupation: Form and performance. *Am J Occup Ther, 42*, 633-641.

Pedretti, L. W. (Ed.). (1996). *Occupational therapy—Practice skills for physical dysfunction* (4th ed.). St. Louis, MO: Mosby.

Ram Dass. (2000). *Still here: Embrace aging, changing, and dying.* New York, NY: Riverhead Books.

Random House unabridged dictionary (2nd ed.). (1993). New York, NY: Random House.

Reilly, M. (1962). Occupational therapy can be one of the great ideas of 20th century medicine. *Am J Occup Ther, 23*, 299-307.

Rowles, G. (1983). Geographical dimensions of social support in rural Appalachia. In G. Rowles & R. Ohta (Eds.), *Aging and milieu: Environmental perspectives on growing old* (pp. 111-130). New York, NY: Academic Press.

Schkade, J. K., & Schultz, S. (1992). Occupational adaptation: Toward a holistic approach for contemporary practice, part 1. *Am J Occup Ther, 46*, 829-837.

Slagle, E. C. (1922). Training aids for mental patients. *Archives of Occupational Therapy, 1*, 11-17.

Spencer, J. C. (1998). Evaluation of performance contexts. In M. E. Neistadt & E. B. Crepeau (Eds.), *Willard & Spackman's occupational therapy* (9th ed., pp. 291-309). Philadelphia, PA: Lippincott, Williams & Wilkins.

Spencer, J., Krefting, L., & Mattingly, C. (1993). Incorporation of ethnographic methods in occupational therapy assessment. *Am J Occup Ther, 47*, 303-309.

Stein, S. K., & Cutler, S. K. (1998). *Psychosocial occupational therapy.* San Diego, CA: Singular Publishing Group, Inc.

Toomey, M. A. (1999). The art of observation: Reflecting on a spiritual moment. *Can J Occup Ther, 66*, 197-199.

Tringo, J. (1970). The hierarchy of preference toward disability groups. *The Journal of Special Education, 4*, 295-306.

Trombly, C. A. (1995). Occupation, purposefulness, and meaningfulness as therapeutic mechanisms—1995 Eleanor Clarke Slagle lecture. *Am J Occup Ther, 49*, 960-972.

Urbanowski, R., & Vargo, J. (1994). Spirituality, daily practice, and the occupational performance model. *Can J Occup Ther, 61*, 88-94.

Velozo, C. (1993). Work evaluations: Critique of the state of the art of functional assessment of work. *Am J Occup Ther, 47*, 203-208.

Weisman, G. D. (1981). Modeling environment-behavior systems. A brief note. *Journal of Man-Environment Relations, 1*, 32-41.

Whiteneck, G., Charlifue, S., Gerhart, K., Overholser, J., & Richardson, G. (1988). *Guide for use of the Craig Handicap Assessment and Report Technique (CHART).* Englewood, CO: Craig Hospital.

Whiteneck, G., Charlifue, S., Gerhart, K., Overholser, J., & Richardson, G. (1992). Qualifying handicap: A new measure of long-term rehabilitation outcomes. *Arch Phys Med Rehabil, 73*, 519-526.

Wicker, A. W. (1979). *An introduction to environmental psychology.* Cambridge, England: Cambridge University Press.

Willer, B., Rosenthal, M., Kreutzer, J., Gordon, W., & Rempel, R. (1993). Assessment of community integration following traumatic brain injury. *J Head Trauma Rehabil, 8*, 73-87.

World Health Organization. (2001). *International classification of impairments, activities, and participation, beta 2 draft, short version.* Geneva: Author, Assessment, Classification, and Epidemiology Group.

Yerxa, E. J. (1998). Health and the human spirit for occupation. *Am J Occup Ther, 52*, 412-418.

Zukav, G. (1980). *The dancing Wuli masters. An overview of the new physics.* New York, NY: Bantam Books.

Zukav, G. (1989). *The seat of the soul.* New York, NY: Simon Schuster.

Zukav, G. (2000). *Soul stories.* New York, NY: Simon Schuster.

CHAPTER THREE

Bases for Best Occupational Therapy Practice

KEY POINTS

✧ Professional Standards
  - Code of Ethics
  - Standards of Practice
  - Guide to Occupational Therapy Practice
✧ Therapeutic Relationship
  - Establishing and Maintaining a Therapeutic Relationship and Context
  - Intervention Relationships
  - Therapy as Change
  - Guides for Establishing a Therapeutic Context
  - Occupation as a Vehicle and as an Outcome
✧ Clinical Reasoning
  - The Application of Theory and Knowledge in Practice
  - Developing Clinical Reasoning
  - Client Ability for Clinical Reasoning in the Collaborative Process
  - The Science and Art of Therapy for Change

FOCUS QUESTIONS

1. Identify several ways the *Code of Ethics, Standards of Practice*, and other official American Occupational Therapy Association (AOTA) documents contribute to best practice.
2. Is there a difference between being client-centered and caring about a client?
3. What are the characteristics of an emotionally safe, therapeutic setting?
4. Think for a moment of yourself with teachers, friends, and people who have had a significant influence in your life. In what type of setting and/or in the context of what kind of interpersonal relationship have you felt most supported to make positive changes? Do you feel that this is different for different people?
5. Describe each type of intervention relationship. Where have you observed these types of relationships?
6. How does reasoning change as the therapist becomes more experienced?
7. In what respect is occupational therapy both an art and a science?

INTRODUCTION

Collectively, the chapters in this book describe multiple ways in which person, activity, environment, and their interrelationship can be framed. The chapters also describe diverse intervention approaches. In some instances readers will find that they are being advised to go in not only different, but contradictory directions if one model is compared to another. Thus, the reader may ask, "Are there some guidelines for intervention that are common across practice settings and that contribute to the best possible practice?" Some have been articulated in our previous chapters: the use of activities or occupation and the focus on the whole person in his or her environment. In this chapter we will discuss three additional types of guides or "common denominators" that act as a basis for best occupational therapy practice in mental health, regardless of theoretical orientation. The first of these are formalized standards for practice as articulated in multiple documents published by the AOTA. These include the *Code of Ethics* (AOTA, 2000) and *Standards of Practice* (AOTA, 1998j). The second of these is much less formalized and describes beliefs shared by many professionals about how best to establish a therapeutic context for intervention. In a way, these less formal guides identify ways that, in everyday practice, the occupational therapist can establish and maintain the ethical, professional, respectful climate mandated in the more formal ethical code. These standards were updated by AOTA and published in 1999. These most recent additions to the foundation of best practice include the *Guide to Practice* (Moyers, 1999) and the Practice Guidelines that are listed later in this chapter. The third of these lies in the use of clinical reasoning, which describes how one uses knowledge to make practice decisions.

ADHERENCE TO STANDARDS OF PRACTICE

During the 1970s, the Representative Assembly of the AOTA became a policy-making body. With its approval, AOTA published and has subsequently revised numerous documents and position papers intended to standardize and ensure the quality of occupational therapy service. Among these are the *Occupational Therapy Code of Ethics* (AOTA, 2000), the *Standards of Practice* (AOTA, 1998j), and the *Guide to Occupational Therapy Practice* (Moyers, 1999).

Code of Ethics

The *Occupational Therapy Code of Ethics* (AOTA, 2000) applies to occupational therapy personnel at all levels and in any service capacity. It is intended to promote the highest standards of ethical behavior. The Code of Ethics is based upon seven principles:

1. **Beneficence**, which states that OT personnel must be concerned with the well-being of recipients of service, appreciate cultural contexts, set reasonable fees, and advocate for persons in need of service.
2. **Non-maleficence** speaks of maintaining relationships that are non-exploitative.
3. **Autonomy/privacy/confidentiality** mandates collaborating with recipients of service or their surrogates, informing recipients regarding the nature and expected outcome of service, respecting the rights of recipients to refuse service, and maintaining confidentiality.
4. **Duties** addresses being properly credentialed, staying abreast of current knowledge, and not treating problems beyond one's area of expertise.
5. **Justice** mandates complying with laws and regulations, including local, state, federal, institutional, and those of AOTA, and taking steps to ensure that those one supervises adhere to the Code of Ethics.
6. **Veracity** calls for providing accurate information regarding occupational therapy services, disclosing any potential conflict of interest, and making no false or deceptive claims.
7. **Fidelity** mandates treating colleagues and other professionals with fairness, discretion, and integrity; accurately representing their qualifications and views; and supporting adherence to the Code of Ethics by others (see Appendix E for the Code of Ethics).

Standards of Practice

The *Standards of Practice* (AOTA, 1998j) provides recommended guidelines to assist occupational therapy practitioners in the provision of occupational therapy services. These standards apply to both registered occupational therapists and certified occupational therapy assistants. The *Standards of Practice* articulates clear expectations for the occupational therapist to be certified and to behave in an ethical manner (in accordance with the *Code of Ethics*) when providing services. The guide also expects the clinician to understand and use current research to guide practice. The standards identify the components of occupational therapy intervention planning and implementation. It recommends screening to determine the need for service, assessment of occupational performance components and environments, client strengths and limitation, intervention planning, intervention and the discontinuation of services, and provisions for **continuous quality review**. As mandated by the document, the intervention plan should include the following:

- Short- and long-term observable and measurable goals
- Content based upon the theories of the profession
- A time frame that is compatible with the system in which occupational therapy services are housed
- An individualized plan that integrates purposeful activity
- A system that monitors and updates the initial plan
- Resource and educational components for the person in occupational therapy and his or her significant others
- A system of documentation

These standards were recently revised. Currently, they are used in multiple contexts of occupational therapy. The profession also has official documents that identify the roles for occupational therapists with specific populations or for roles outside of direct service provider. For example, refer to the *Official Documents of the American Occupational Therapy Association* (1998a-k) and you will find papers, guidelines, and statements that discuss occupational therapy service in a neonatal intensive care unit, in early intervention, and with clients who have human immunodeficiency virus (HIV). The profession also publishes statements regarding services for persons with Alzheimer's disease, with cognitive impairment, and with learning disabilities. There are also statements that suggest the roles for occupational therapists in independent living centers, in hospice, and as case managers (AOTA, 1998a-k). The roles of consultants are broadly defined and comprehensively discussed in Jaffee and Epstein (1992).

Guide to Occupational Therapy Practice

Another document that provides shared guidelines for practice is the *Guide to Occupational Therapy Practice* (Moyers, 1999). It was initiated to educate persons who refer clients to occupational therapy. It also influences clinicians' daily problem solving and reasoning with clients and communication with third parties. The purpose of this document is to communicate to those clients who refer to occupational therapy and to third-party payers the roles and values of occupational therapy and the multiple and potential outcomes of occupational therapy in rehabilitation contexts. The practice guide gives general information about occupational therapy. It is not a refereed document; however, it was carefully reviewed by experts in the profession and by members of the Commission on Practice of the AOTA.

The guide describes the scope of occupational therapy practice for persons who have problems that interfere with their participation in daily life and compromise their general health and well-being or their quality of life. The general information in the document contributes parameters for occupational therapy practice. The guide does the following:

- Defines occupational therapy and the populations who are served
- Outlines intervention principles and the terminology used by the profession
- Identifies the multiple outcomes of occupational therapy function and occupational performance to promote health, well-being, and quality of life
- Outlines the language for communicating with third-party payers
- Establishes a reference list of the significant studies that specifically relate to occupational therapy
- Describes the two stages of the occupational therapy process: Stage one—referral, screening, and evaluation, and Stage two—the clinician develops an intervention plan, implements and monitors it, and revises the plan as needed
- States that clients may be referred by health care professionals, family members, community agencies, and organizations in business and industry or those at state and local levels
- Recommends discharge planning and, when needed, a follow-up program

This document, available from the AOTA and updated online, provides many examples that illustrate the processes it describes and is a helpful resource for therapists (Appendix F).

Occupational Therapy Practice Guidelines (AOTA)

Because of the general nature of the previous documents, additional and more specific information may be needed to ensure the maintenance of high standards in practice with particular clients. Thus, the AOTA has developed and continues to develop more detailed guides for intervention that are specific to an identified client population or a person's condition or problem (see Sample Practice Guidelines for a sample of the guidelines published by the AOTA).

The reader is encouraged to refer to the AOTA web page (*www.AOTA.org*) for additional guidelines as they become available. As you can see from their titles in the box on the next page, these brief guides are specific to a population, disease, injury, diagnosis, or disabling condition. They follow a format that:

SAMPLE PRACTICE GUIDELINES

AOTA's Practice Guidelines Series

- Adults with Alzheimer's Disease (Corcoran, 2001)
- Adults with Carpal Tunnel Syndrome (Rossman, 2001)
- Adults with Hip Fracture/Replacement (Verner Platt, 2001)
- Adults with Low Back Pain (Larson, 2001)
- Adults with Low Vision (Warren, 2001)
- Adults with Mood Disorders (Denton & Skinner, 2001)
- Adults with Neurodegenerative Diseases (Balsdon Richer & Bhasin, 2001)
- Adults with Rheumatoid Arthritis (Yasuda, 2001)
- Adults with Schizophrenia (Kannenberg & Dufresne, 2001)
- Adults with Spinal Cord Injury (Dolhi, 2001)
- Adults with Stroke (Acquaviva, 2001)
- Adults with Traumatic Brain Injury (Radomski, 2001)
- Attention-Deficit/Hyperactivity Disorders (Hanft, 2001a)
- Cerebral Palsy (Colangelo & Gorga, 2001)
- Chronic Pain (Engel, 2001)
- Substance Use Disorders (Stoffel & Moyers, 2001)
- Tendon Injuries (Rivet, 2001)
- Young Children with Delayed Development (Hanft, 2001b)

- Outlines construct definitions (e.g., etiology, incidence, DSM-IV diagnostic criteria)
- Integrates occupational therapy uniform terminology (e.g., performance areas, performance components, and performance contexts) related to the functional outcome of a diagnosis
- Provides referral guidelines (e.g., who can refer and the basis for referral—change in activities of daily living, work, and leisure performances)
- Is a general guide to the occupational therapy intervention process (e.g., sample frequency and duration, general evaluation guide, general intervention process [acute, partial hospitalization, in home, etc.] and discharge planning and case follow-up suggestions)

They also identify resources that contribute to the knowledge a clinician uses during problem solving and clinical reasoning. The guides do not give specific theoretical descriptions for planning and implementing interventions; nor do they describe the specific assessment instruments suggested.

They provide:

- Case studies that demonstrate the application of the guidelines; cases give the context for the disability and identify an area of occupational performance that is the focus of intervention with sample goals and objectives
- A list of general intervention strategies but not a list of details for their purpose and use
- A sample of possible outcomes of occupational therapy intervention
- A list of references that clinicians can explore for more information

While these practice guides provide a framework for occupational therapy services, they are not prescriptive. They are based upon the general guidelines for occupational therapy practice. They tell the clinician to consider the focus of occupations, their components, and contexts. They give sample goals that integrate components of occupational performance with occupation outcomes. They are not specific to a model of practice or a specific frame of reference. They are intended as a guide that can accommodate individual client needs. The fear that these guides compromise the individualization of practice is unfounded; however, the expertise of the clinician in being able to effectively integrate these guides with occupational therapy theories is the key to intervention in a client-centered context (see Appendix G).

In summary, the AOTA, through its published documents, has established and continues to modify guides that help to ensure the provision of quality, ethical, and professional service by occupational therapists.

ESTABLISHING AND MAINTAINING A THERAPEUTIC RELATIONSHIP AND CONTEXT

We have already spoken several times about the critical place of humanistic philosophy within occupational therapy and have indicated that humanistic philosophy is enacted through the creation of a client-centered (client/practitioner) relationship. Humanistic philosophy and the idea of a client-centered relationship have strong theoretical roots. We have chosen to discuss these concepts in more detail in Chapter Four, Psychodynamic Frame of Reference—Person Perspective and Meaning, in which their tie to other theoretical constructs can be more fully developed.

A **client-centered relationship** is one in which the therapist tries to determine what is important to the client and tries to involve the client in the decision-making process. The therapist respects the client and what he or she brings into the therapeutic context and recognizes that it is ultimately the client's vision as to whether or not therapeutic goals have been met. At its heart it is a collaborative relationship.

There are specific types of intervention relationships, however, including those in which the client is unable or minimally able to collaborate. The practice setting will influence the manner in which the practitioner and patient/client interact, the abilities of the client, and the expectations of the person or persons seeking a service. Additionally, as suggested by Peloquin (1998), the person's and the clinician's perceptions of each other influence their interactions. Some of the different types of intervention relationships often (but not necessarily) seen in contemporary practice settings are identified by McColl and Bickenbach (1998).

Intervention Relationships

In a **medical model** of care, it may occur that the therapeutic relationship is one in which the therapist determines and prescribes treatment to a person who is unable to participate in the problem-solving process. This model is usually identified with hospital and health care environments.

In a **client-centered** relationship, the therapist facilitates change by actively recruiting the ideas, skills, and needs of the person. The client comes into the relationship with specific goals and expects the therapist to assist him or her in achieving the desired outcome. Together they use each of their expertise to negotiate the problem-solving plan in occupational therapy. The therapist monitors the process, ensuring that the humanistic philosophies of the profession's founders and of contemporary mental health practice are integrated. The preference for this model grew out of the community mental health movement and endures today.

In the **community-based rehabilitation** and **independent living models** of practice, other types of collaboration evolve. Relationships focus on the community, not the individual person. The occupational therapist is a "catalyst" who facilitates community development intended to increase the opportunity for a person with a disability to find and use resources and participate in the environment. Occupational therapists in community-based environments educate the community about disability and rehabilitation as well as the person's right to adequate resources for participation in the community. The therapist is an advocate and consultant.

The person in the **community relationships model** may be identified as a consumer, member of a community, and/or resource to the community. In this model, therapists help persons with a disability contribute to society, not just use resources. Therefore, the therapist helps the person with a disability to collaborate with community leaders to bring the change needed at the community level. Fountain House is an example of the community model that is familiar to many mental health clinicians. See Fountain House Model for a brief description.

To facilitate community change, the therapist uses research and advocacy approaches and self-help, support, and educational models. The desired outcome is for occupational therapy to be a resource to individuals, populations,

FOUNTAIN HOUSE MODEL

The Fountain House Program is a community model that serves persons who have chronic mental health problems, and many must cope with being homeless. The program provides individualized flexible programming through a case management process of rehabilitation. Members (clients) may be "lifetime members" and participate in the Fountain House programs as needed. They collaborate with peers and staff teams to choose the resources that they feel meet their needs. Resources may include: emergency funds for food, shelter and clothing, temporary shelter, and connections to state and federal social and health care services. Clients also can select from a continuum of employment programs, (volunteer, transitional, independent, or individual or group work placements). The goals of Fountain House and similar programs are to empower the client/members, and to produce customer/client satisfaction through a case management process where "client choice" is central and criteria for entering programs is flexible (Asmussen, Romano, Beatty, Gasarch, & Shaughnessey, 2000).

and community agencies. In addition to providing direct care services, occupational therapists are a resource for community problem solving. Clinicians work to increase available resources for people with disabilities, resources for increased opportunity for employment, and accessible housing and transportation. Clinicians educate the general public to the role that persons with disabilities can play in the community. A disability does not prevent a person from contributing to society, and a person with a disability is not only capable of assisting his or her peers but can be a key resource for problem solving (McColl & Bickenbach, 1998).

Therapy as Change

In real practice, any of these types of relationships may emerge in any setting and can be consistent with written standards for ethical, professional practice. What is common to all of these relationships, and we propose common to all therapy, is that they are intended to bring about change. Often, the change process is one in which the person becomes a learner, and he or she will learn new information and new skills. Other times, adaptations will be made to the environment or to the occupations/activities in which the person is engaged so that the client does not need to change or needs to change only minimally. Sometimes, many, many things change. We know that life constantly changes—we get older, our physical body changes, people come and go from our lives, circumstances around us change. When people seek or are referred to the services of an occupational therapist, they need assistance in bringing about specific kinds of change or adjusting to change. Keeping this in mind, we turn to some practical, less formal guides for establishing and maintaining a helpful or "therapeutic" relationship and context for therapy. By helpful we mean that both the therapist/client relationship and the manner in which therapy is structured makes it easier for a person or persons to learn and accommodate to change, regardless of the therapist's theoretical orientation or intervention strategies applied. If you read carefully, you will see that what is discussed is consistent with those recommendations in the formalized standards for occupational therapy practice. Therapeutic relationships and the creation of a therapeutic context do not happen immediately, and there are no absolutes as to how they are established or maintained; without them, little therapy occurs.

GUIDES FOR ESTABLISHING A THERAPEUTIC CONTEXT

Occupation as a Vehicle and an Outcome

In occupational therapy, we recognize that characteristics of the person, physical and social environments, and the task all enter into and can help or hinder the change process. In occupational therapy, meaningful and purposeful activities, tasks, and occupations are seen as essential change agents.

Through involvement with activities and occupations, many persons can learn new skills, gain knowledge, mobilize physical energy, and learn more about themselves and others. Although reflecting upon personal experiences may enhance the ability to learn from them, clients do not just talk about what they would like to experience or change. They set priorities for change, and they also try out and practice new behaviors. After practice, they are often given the opportunity to use feedback from the therapist, others, and the experience itself to reflect on their goals and progress. Other persons who find themselves in the client or patient role are not as able to learn new skills but need help to better use the skills and abilities they have. For them, therapy may mean adjusting to new environments, adaptive equipment, or modified activities. Therapy may mean learning to allow others to assist them in order that they can engage in activities or occupation in a more satisfying way. However activities or occupation are used, they have a critical place in the therapeutic context.

Risking Change

Many of the activities in occupational therapy are not unusual or new; they are often the stuff of life. In both mental health and physical medicine, however, we sometimes see people who cannot imagine themselves trying, much less succeeding at, the tasks and activities they see around them. For these people, activity and participation in the environment remain inaccessible until they are able to picture themselves in a new role or are willing to risk changing, or a combination of both. The therapeutic relationship opens windows and widens pathways when risks are taken within its support, encouragement, caring, and guidance. When people risk change, they risk failure as well as success. They may face upheaval and uncertainty; they move to unfamiliar ground. Often, they risk letting go of old, perhaps comfortable, ways of viewing themselves and relating to others with no assurance regarding what will come next. To let go of the old and familiar, a person must first feel safe, and it is an essential role of the therapist to ensure safety.

Safety—Choice, Knowledge, and Consistency

Think for a moment about the situations in which you were willing to test a new idea or experiment with an activity that was quite foreign to you. We suspect that you needed to feel emotionally safe first. Few of us have so much self-assurance that we will easily risk ridicule or tempt criticism. Perhaps someone assured you that if you faltered, he or she would be there to offer support.

Choice

Patients, clients, learners, residents all need to know that they will not be humiliated. Beyond that, they need to know that they will not be forced into going further than they wish, that their limitations will be respected. This means therapists must respect that people have different paces at which they can learn, change ideas, and accommodate to external changes. There may be just so much change people can cope with at a given time. Individuals must also feel physically safe. If they fear loss of control or physical harm, they need to know that they will not be allowed to harm themselves or others.

Knowledge

Coming from and providing a firm knowledge base enables the clinician to establish a safe environment. The therapist needs to be knowledgeable about the person's physical, emotional, and cognitive abilities and limitations, and also about the demands and limitations of a broad range of human activities and as imposed by physical and social environments. Providing patients/clients with information helps them gain power and control in relation to their own safety or well-being and is an important part of the continuing effort to enhance the person's ability to be and feel effective and appropriately self-reliant.

Consistency

While no one can predict the outcome of therapy, when we as therapists behave in a manner that is consistent and predictable, others tend to feel more safe with us, for they know what they can expect from us and what is expected of them. Similarly, people tend to feel safest in a setting that is organized and consistent.

We all hear about professionalism and may mistake it for being stiff or acting aloof. In fact, as professionals, therapists strive to be consistent, ethical, dependable, and knowledgeable, and they make a statement of their commitment to the best of care. Such a commitment helps establish the context in which the person feels safe and is able to entrust the therapist with his or her efforts to change.

Trust

An essential part of creating a therapeutic climate depends on the ability of the occupational therapist to foster trust, which is integral to the sense of safety just addressed. Three kinds of trust between two persons are emphasized here: respecting confidences, congruency, and valuing ourselves. These same principles apply when three or more persons are involved in the therapeutic process.

Respecting Confidences

Trusting someone with confidential information means trusting that they will care for something that is important—one's privacy. Maintaining confidentiality is addressed in the profession's Code of Ethics and is so essential in a professional practitioner/client relationship that law protects it. It may be helpful for therapists to be very explicit and let clients know that what they relate during their intervention will be kept in confidence. At the same time, it is important for clients to know what cannot be kept in confidence, or what "confidentiality" means within the intervention setting. For example, they need to know that information related to their therapy is shared with other intervention team members. We have probably all been in situations in which we were not certain if our confidences would be kept. In such situations, we tend to close up rather than open up, feeling a need to protect our thoughts, our concerns, and ourselves. Such an environment does not make it easier for us to take the risk needed for change. Consider some of the variables in the environment that compromise confidentiality and your response to these possible dilemmas (see Increasing Your Understanding: Maintaining Confidentiality).

Being Congruent

There is also trust based on finding the other person to be authentic or "real." That is, there are certain values and characteristics that emerge consistently in a person's behavior; the person is not a chameleon. Patients and clients are more likely to experience therapists as genuine when they are, as described by Rogers (1972), congruent. **Congruent** in this usage means that a person's words, affect, and actions go together to give a clear and consistent message.

Being congruent requires that we, as therapists, be aware of our beliefs and values. As stated by Rogers (1972), "...if I

INCREASE YOUR UNDERSTANDING: MAINTAINING CONFIDENTIALITY

The following are examples from clinical experiences that can compromise confidentiality. Discuss with peers possible strategies for managing these environmental circumstances:

- Your client is in a "double" room. The focus of occupational therapy treatment is basic self-care. How do you provide a confidential environment that allows physical privacy and also confidential discussion of the person's concerns and clinician feedback to the client regarding occupational performance?

- You enter a client's room in an acute rehab setting and the client's family is present. Before you begin your occupational therapy intervention, what do you say to your client and his or her family? Do you ask the client if he or she wishes the family to stay and observe or participate?

- You are in the cafeteria or on an elevator in a health care environment and one of your colleagues initiates a conversation about a client. How do you respond?

- You are working in a client's home and have been working with the client for approximately 2 weeks when the client shares with you that he or she is being abused by his or her spouse or caregiver. What is your professional responsibility? Legal responsibility? Response to the client?

- A client shares with you in confidence a concern about a family situation and requests that it not be discussed with the family. What is your response? Does it differ for an adult or minor client?

- Share some situations you have seen or anticipate that present confidentiality dilemmas. Consider your own code or guide for confidentiality as well as that of the profession and the environment of the situation.

can form a helping relationship to myself—if I can be sensitively aware and acceptant toward my own feelings—then the likelihood is great that I can form a helping relationship toward another" (p. 14). Knowing what we think, feel, and believe helps us to keep our needs separate from those of others, helps us to be clear about our own boundaries and limitations, and allows us to behave in a manner that is consistent and establishes trust.

Valuing Ourselves

Trust is also nurtured when therapists behave openly, as if they trust themselves and believe in the worth of their therapy and in themselves. This behavior includes acknowledging that they do not have all the answers and showing that they are willing to learn. When patients and clients can see that therapists are willing to be vulnerable and open to learning, they find that they do not have to be perfect to be trustworthy and they have a model of self-acceptance from which they can learn.

Caring

Another important contributor to trust is making our clients' well-being the highest priority. When we do this, they can trust that we care about them. Devereaux (1984) describes caring as the heart of the therapeutic relationship and notes "...its presence enriches all other aspects of the relationship." As she states, being cared about is the opposite of anonymity within and being disconnected from the rest of the world. If you ask prospective or practicing therapists about their desire to be therapists, they will very often cite their wish to help or care about others. Brammer (1979) refers to the need to care as a valuing of altruism. He reminds us that in our reaching out to others we fulfill our own need to feel valuable and connected to others. In recognizing that as therapists each of us gains something important for ourselves, we are better able to distinguish our own needs from those of our clients.

Valuing the Person

Each person has his or her own ideas about how caring can best be expressed. Indeed, each human relationship will bring special circumstances and unique opportunities for caring. At its core, **caring** means that we believe that our patient or client is valuable, that we desire to know each person in a real way, and that the individual's needs, feelings, and aspirations direct our service. Mothering or infantilizing a person should not be confused with caring. Rather, in caring for their clients, occupational therapists try to help persons become empowered, more independent, and better able to meet the challenges of life. Most would agree that people are more likely to be committed to the goal that they have established or helped to establish and to a therapeutic process that they understand.

It may happen that patients or clients who seek or come reluctantly to occupational therapy will state that they have no need to learn or change because, as they say, "No one cares about what I do." When therapists show they care, they do not act as a substitute for friends, parents, spouses, or others, but they do provide a person-to-person relationship in which someone does care. At times, this creates an evocative challenge to long-held suppositions as the individual may confront the possibility, "Perhaps someone does care. Perhaps I am worthy of being cared about."

Open Communication

Safety, trust, and the confirmation of caring all depend in their vitality on open communication within the therapeutic relationship. Where there is open communication, all persons (client/patient[s] and therapist) can express themselves, bring up their concerns, clarify areas of doubt or ambiguity, and move toward the common goals of intervention.

Much has been written about specific skills and clinician attitudes believed to enhance communication (Avilla, Combs, & Purkey, 1972; Carkhuff, 1969; Combs, Avilla, & Purkey, 1971; Egan, 1975; Rogers, 1951). For example, when therapists maintain good eye contact, indicate verbally and nonverbally that they are listening, and avoid a judgmental stance, it is believed to increase the likelihood that the person will share his or her thoughts and actively participate in the change process. More fundamentally, clients need to believe it is all right to be honest.

Permission to be Genuine

Open communication implies something deeper than encouragement to talk. It depends on an attitude of true permission for our patients and clients to be genuine with us. Can you recall any instances in which a parent, teacher, friend, or other said, "Tell me what you really feel" or "Be yourself"; yet, when your response was received as challenging, the permission to be honest was rescinded? An essential part of open communication is allowing the person to experience negative as well as positive feelings about what he or she is experiencing in therapy and to share those that he or she wishes to share with us. That is not always as easy as it sounds.

Patients and clients may be angry with us when we feel they have no cause. They may express romantic feelings. They may behave unpredictably and threaten our personal need for order and control. They may disagree with us, state that what they are being expected to do is "too hard" or "useless," or they may refuse our services. While not making themselves targets of abuse, when clinicians listen to those feelings that may make them uncomfortable, they let the person know that their commitment to the process of therapy does not come and go with the client's ability to please them. In the process, therapists grow professionally. They learn how therapy looks from the other side of the client/practitioner relationship. Therapists do not have to agree with or feel the same way that their patients and clients do.

In fact, communication is a reciprocal process, and it often includes us stating when and how things look different from our perspective. Open communication depends on both the person and the therapist having respect for the right of the other to think and feel as each does, and it provides an opportunity for each to gain insight into the perceptions of the other.

Understanding

Open communication is necessary if clients and patients are to believe that they are understood and that the therapist really knows the person. Depending on the conceptual model, therapists may seek specific kinds of information from the person. It is important that they gain not only information that they believe is necessary from their viewpoint, but also that the person knows that the therapist understands what he or she thinks is important.

Often a client who is going through a particularly difficult time may feel isolated. For example, a woman newly divorced might say, "No one can know how I feel." An amputee being encouraged to put pressure on a painful stump might say, "It's easy for you to tell me to bear down; you don't feel the pain I do." In a way, both persons are correct. We cannot know exactly how each feels. But, if we can draw on our own experiences and attempt to look and listen for the purpose of understanding, we can go a long way toward appreciating the frustration and pain each experiences. In doing so, we increase our ability to communicate caring and to serve the best interests of the persons we serve. Further, our encouragement to patients and clients to take risks does not become an insensitive demand.

Valuing Change

In any therapeutic context, it is vital that patients and clients see the therapist as someone who values change and believes in the person's ability and potential for positive change. While each individual is ultimately responsible for taking risks, each of us is encouraged when someone we trust says, in essence, "I really believe you can do this."

The psychology literature emphasizes the devastating effects of parenting in which a child is told over and over again, "You are inept. You'll never amount to anything." As therapists, we are unlikely to imagine ourselves making such statements. Yet, in our efforts to care or help we may give our own undermining messages. When, for example, a therapist overprotects the person to prevent them from failing, or because their reliance on the therapist makes him or her feel important, the therapist communicates, "I don't believe in your ability to take care of yourself or to be successful."

At times we must use careful clinical judgment to determine the presence of an actual risk of physical harm and to assess how it can best be managed; however, much of the changing and risk taking in a psychosocial context relates to emotional risk taking. Therapists may find themselves wishing to protect the person from disappointment, failure, or rebuffs. The clinical judgments therapists make in these instances are some of the most difficult. If, however, there is a sound therapeutic relationship, it enhances the person's ability to manage. When we let patients and clients know that we value them regardless of what they have accomplished, we facilitate their attempts to change.

Accepting Tentativeness

Within the course of therapy both the client and the practitioner must accept some tentativeness in therapy. A person may understandably try to limit ambiguity and perhaps ask for assurances that everything will go according to plan. This desire is not unlike the wish that many people have had at some time for life to go according to plan. Learning to cope with the everyday vicissitudes depends on the confidence that each of us—patient/client and therapist—has in ourselves, our knowledge and skills, and on the degree to which we are aware of the uncompromising values that help us maintain our equilibrium.

As occupational therapists, we need to realize that while intervention plans give us direction, some of the most memorable learning occurs when we and our clients can respond spontaneously to unscheduled events or unexpected feelings. If we remember our initial premise that therapy facilitates change, we can better realize the essential need to accept tentativeness as part of the client-centered process.

Boundaries

Finally, the process of therapy has boundaries, as does the therapeutic relationship. Some of the boundaries in therapy relate directly to the characteristics of the person, the therapeutic goals, and the availability of resources. It is important that both therapist and client share an understanding of these boundaries. The following are some additional boundaries that bear upon therapy and the therapeutic relationship.

Time Limits

Occupational therapy is a temporally bounded process; it cannot and will not go on endlessly. Helping the person to be aware of the probable duration of intervention enables patients/clients and therapists to establish reasonable expectations for what can be accomplished. If therapy facilitates change, one might speak metaphorically of therapy serving as a bridge into unfamiliar terrain. The therapist is the guide. Once the bridge is crossed, however, there is a point at which the guide departs, and the person continues independently. Therefore, the client or patient and therapist must always consider ways in which, as Devereaux (1984) states, they can "create opportunities for reconnecting the patient with other human beings and the environment."

Other limitations relate to the structure of the intervention: mutually agreed upon boundaries regarding the length of each therapy session, the therapist's availability at times other than those scheduled, and the responsibilities specific to the person and to the therapist as they work together in therapy. Whether the structure of therapy is negotiated informally or formally (e.g., through verbal or written contract), it is important to recognize the purpose of such a structure. In part, the creation of this structure enhances predictability in therapy and increases the level of safety, as discussed earlier. It also provides expectations by which therapists and the client can judge if the goals of intervention are being met.

Dependency

Just as important, such a structure provides a mechanism that helps keep therapists from slipping into patterns of relating that could keep the person perpetually and increasingly dependent on them or their service. In special instances, dependency will appropriately be fostered especially, for example, when a patient or client has had extreme difficulty in asking for or accepting help from anyone. What we caution against are those times in therapy when a clinician becomes so involved in helping that he or she loses sight of the others in the person's world who could effectively and better relate to the person around given needs.

Friendship

Beyond the obvious ethical boundaries prohibiting the clinician from compromising the emotional or physical well-being of the patient/client, the therapist must also understand that he or she is not a friend. Although our patients and clients may understandably feel friendly toward us and we may feel friendly toward them, a friendship is not created for the purpose of therapy, or therapy for the purpose of friendship. Therapists will like many of their patients and clients very much, but when therapy ends so does the therapeutic relationship. If the people served by occupational therapy can be helped to recognize all they have accomplished as an outcome of therapy and the personal qualities that they bring to an interpersonal relationship, they begin to see in themselves the potential to build other meaningful relationships.

Summary—Establishing a Therapeutic Context

Thus far, we have identified both written and unwritten guides that are designed to maintain an ethical, respectful, and professional therapeutic experience, regardless of any other theoretical orientation the therapist might have.

As you were reading, we hope that you recognized in the described values and behaviors reminiscences of helpful relationships and contexts you have known in your life. From your own experience you bring both intuitive and well-informed ideas about the conditions that facilitate your making positive changes, and those that do not. See Increase Your Understanding: Occupational Therapy Relationship and answer the questions posed.

CLINICAL REASONING

Given the therapist's desire to adhere to the standards of practice and commitment to maintaining an ethical, therapeutic relationship and climate, the occupational therapist nevertheless has many questions to answer or "problems" to solve. With each new referral or request for service, the therapist must consider:

- Why has this client sought or been referred to therapy?

INCREASE YOUR UNDERSTANDING: OCCUPATIONAL THERAPY RELATIONSHIP

The next time you observe or participate in a therapeutic interaction between clinician and client/patient, try to identify comments made, nonverbal behaviors, or other behaviors by the clinician and client that would help you answer the following:

- Does the client feel he or she is liked in this relationship?
- Does the client like him- or herself?
- Does the client feel accepted?
- Can he or she accept him- or herself?
- Does the clinician respect the client and treat him or her with dignity?
- Does the client have a sense of dignity?
- Does the client appear to feel capable or able?
- Has the client been given an opportunity to succeed?
- Does the clinician convey a belief in the person's ability to succeed?
- Does the client understand the purpose of therapy?
- Does the client understand the purpose of specific therapeutic strategies or procedures?

Combs (1971) suggests that the answers to these questions contain the guidelines to the "...encouragement of growth and development everywhere" and "[are] the bases for the conditions of therapy."

- What are the biggest challenges that must be addressed?
- What additional information do I need before we proceed, and how can I best obtain that information?
- What does it mean for this person that I act in his or her best interest (what is best for this person)?
- What is important to this person? What motivates him or her? What does his or her affect, behavior, and verbalization tell me about his or her psychological health?
- What model(s) of practice seems to make the best fit with the client's problems, strengths, preferences, and style of relating to people and activities?

Having selected one or more theoretical models as a basis for proceeding, the therapist might then ask:

- Where should we begin?
- What specific strategies are most appropriate in this situation?
- How do I implement these strategies with this particular client?
- (And later) How are these strategies working?

In helping clients respond to and manage psychosocial issues as well as their physical and cognitive symptoms or disabilities, occupational therapists may draw from multiple theoretical principles during occupational therapy intervention. These principles come from occupational science and environmental, physical, sensorimotor, cognitive, and psychosocial theories.

Each client and therapeutic situation represents a new challenge for the therapist. Establishing and following through with a service plan requires one to draw upon available knowledge and think through these plus multiple other questions and problems. The process by which this occurs is that of clinical reasoning.

The Application of Theory and Knowledge in Practice

In occupational therapy, **clinical reasoning** has been broadly defined as the application of theory in practice (Neistadt et al., 1998). Schell (1998) describes it as an interactive process "...used by practitioners to plan, direct, perform, and reflect on client care" (p. 99).

Clinical reasoning requires and enables occupational therapists to make judgments about what is most important to pay attention to, what actions to take, and the likely outcomes of taking specific actions in the context of therapy (see Reflective Reasoning Process). It is also a way to learn from therapy once it is has been completed. It entails reasoning about not only the outcome of intervention decisions in the present context, but also what these outcomes could be expected to mean to the client in the future.

REFLECTIVE REASONING PROCESS

The "judgment in action" process of clinical reasoning is derived from the views of Schön (1983), who recommends that a clinician use a reflective reasoning process to identify and define problems within the context of the client's situation and the personal meaning of the problems to the client. When the occupational therapist is a reflective practitioner, he or she uses tacit knowledge, which comes from the clinician's experience in practice. The source of this information may be difficult to pinpoint, but the clinician can use it automatically to respond in the present situation and build the client's performance for the future.

The literature indicates that when we say that occupational therapists use what they know in clinical reasoning, we actually refer to many types of "knowing" (Mattingly & Fleming, 1994; Schell, 1998). Types of knowledge may include information from many sources:

- There is the information that one learns in books or was taught in school; for example, the principles and theories related to each of the models described in this text.
- There is the information that the therapist "knows" based on his or her life experiences and clinical experiences as an occupational therapist, even intuitive information (**tacit knowledge**).
- There is the information that one "knows" because one has been told this by the client, other persons, or professionals involved with the client, or because events are unfolding in the moment within the therapeutic experience.

Because there is such diverse information that is brought together in the clinical reasoning process, it is not possible for one to say ahead of time exactly what will be the best thing to do at the moment a therapeutic decision is made and carried out. But bringing this information together (often using many types of "knowing" simultaneously) in the process of clinical reasoning enables the therapist to respond flexibly throughout the therapy to the changing conditions encountered in daily practice.

Developing Clinical Reasoning

The literature also suggests how clinical questions are posed and how problems are thought through and solved changes as one becomes more experienced as a therapist. For example, a new practitioner might rely more heavily on theoretical knowledge (e.g., refer back to one's textbooks), while the experienced practitioner has more professional experiences to draw from during the clinical reasoning process. Developing Expertise in Clinical Reasoning outlines the stages of development. It is not that one type of reasoning necessarily brings about a superior outcome, but there is a qualitative difference in the process used.

Client Ability for Clinical Reasoning in the Collaborative Process

Just as client-centered practice is, to the extent possible, a collaborative process, so is the process of clinical reasoning. That is, when possible, it will not be the therapist pondering, "What should I do next?" it will be the therapist involving the client in the process of solving problems and making decisions.

Client-centered reasoning strives for a balance of responsibility between clinician and client. Thus, there is a coming together of scientific knowledge, knowledge based on evidence for practice, the therapist's knowledge based on his or her personal and previous clinical experiences, and the client's perspective or his or her experiencing of the illness or disability (Ersser & Atkins, 1999). In order to enhance the clients' ability to engage in the clinical reasoning process, therapists need to take into account the clients' level of understanding, their preferences (whether they wish to be

DEVELOPING EXPERTISE IN CLINICAL REASONING

Integrating the work of multiple theorists (Dreyfus & Dreyfus, 1986; Benner, 1984; Clark, Ennevor, & Richardson, 1996; Creighton et al., 1995; Mattingly and Fleming, 1994; Slater & Cohn, 1991; Strong et al., 1995), Schell (1998) characterizes the differences in expert and novice reasoning. Schell's synthesis identifies five levels of expertise that span from no experience to 10 years of practice experience. Reasoning moves from:

- **Novice reasoning** that relies on theory practice decisions

- **Advanced beginner reasoning** that uses theory in context and can identify the differences between the classical problem and the presenting problems

- **Competent reasoning** that supports managing multiple clinical issues and automatic use of skills

- **Proficient reasoning** that supports flexible use of clinical experiences and repertoire of resources

- **Expert reasoning** that uses intuition and knowledge organized around cases

Each level relies on different reasoning processes and has some variance in the problem-solving outcome (Schell, 1998, p. 97). The reader is referred to the original source for details.

involved in this process and to what extent), and the time frame and practical constraints that may exist. If therapists are going to include clients in this process, they need to provide information that clients can understand. Some things that the therapist should consider include the following:

- The client's age, education, and knowledge regarding his or her present condition

- The client's interest in and ability to contribute to the process

- The client's understanding of his or her role in decision making

- The purpose of the intervention (e.g., to increase quality of life versus extending life) and the severity of the client's problems

- The types of condition (Emergency? Long-term? Chronic?)

- The client's potential benefit from therapy

- The health status of the client

- The client's culture and its perspective of health care and rehabilitation

- The time frame for intervention and any organizational constraints on therapy (e.g., the possible length of stay and the level of professional expertise available for interventions) (Ersser & Atkins, 1999)

Frames of Reference—The Scientific Foundation for Change

There has been a great deal written about clinical reasoning, which we have only touched upon (Creighton et al., 1995; Ersser & Atkins, 1999; Mattingly, 1991a, 1991b, 1994; Mattingly & Fleming, 1994; Neistadt, Wight, & Mulligan, 1998; Rogers, 1983; Rogers & Holm, 1991; Schell, 1998; Schell & Cervero, 1993; Schön, 1983), and it is beyond the scope of this text to describe the reasoning process in detail. We do propose that the frameworks for psychosocial practice that are described in this text assist occupational therapists in the reasoning process. Therapists use models of practice to define the constructs of concern, frame the client's problems, and form hypotheses for change. These models help therapists determine what problems need to be addressed first and when problems are beyond the scope of concern. These models and frames of reference identify evaluation and intervention strategies that can be expected to best respond to the client's needs in the context of occupational therapy, and they provide parameters by which therapists can evaluate the outcomes of therapeutic intervention. In these ways, frames of reference or models of practice contribute to the science of therapy and the core of occupation-based practice.

THE ART OF THERAPY— FACILITATION OF CHANGE

Given all that the therapist might know about a specific clinical problem and all the treatment strategies he or she might be aware of, there is no cookbook for the actual implementation of therapy. Some therapists can consistently think on their feet and seem to know intuitively what actions are best at a given time. It might be said that they are expert clinicians, or effectively use clinical reasoning, or that they are experts in the art of therapy. The art of therapy is that elusive yet powerful ability to bring knowledge, caring, and skills together in a way that fosters positive growth and change. The frameworks for practice represent a vital starting place for the cultivation of both science and an art that continue to develop throughout one's professional life.

REFERENCES

Acquaviva, J. (2001). *Occupational therapy practice guidelines for adults with stroke.* Bethesda, MD: American Occupational Therapy Association.

American Occupational Therapy Association. (1998a). Knowledge and skills for occupational therapy practice in the neonatal intensive care unit. In American Occupational Therapy Association, *The reference manual of the official documents of the American Occupational Therapy Association* (pp. 179-191). Bethesda, MD: Author.

American Occupational Therapy Association. (1998b). Occupational therapist as case manager. In American Occupational Therapy Association, *The reference manual of the official documents of the American Occupational Therapy Association* (pp. 333-336). Bethesda, MD: Author.

American Occupational Therapy Association. (1998c). Occupational therapy for individuals with learning disabilities. In American Occupational Therapy Association, *The reference manual of the official documents of the American Occupational Therapy Association* (pp. 357-370). Bethesda, MD: Author.

American Occupational Therapy Association. (1998d). Occupational therapy roles. In American Occupational Therapy Association, *The reference manual of the official documents of the American Occupational Therapy Association* (pp. 271-298). Bethesda, MD: Author.

American Occupational Therapy Association. (1998e). Occupational therapy services for persons with Alzheimer's disease and other dementias. In American Occupational Therapy Association, *The reference manual of the official documents of the American Occupational Therapy Association* (pp. 327-332). Bethesda, MD: Author.

American Occupational Therapy Association. (1998f). Occupational therapy services in early intervention and preschool services. In American Occupational Therapy Association, *The reference manual of the official documents of the American Occupational Therapy Association* (pp. 231-232). Bethesda, MD: Author.

American Occupational Therapy Association. (1998g). Occupation therapy services in work practice. In American Occupational Therapy Association, *The reference manual of the official documents of the American Occupational Therapy Association* (pp. 383-388). Bethesda, MD: Author.

American Occupational Therapy Association. (1998h). Providing services for person with HIV, AIDS and their caregivers. In American Occupational Therapy Association, *The reference manual of the official documents of the American Occupational Therapy Association* (pp. 237-242). Bethesda, MD: Author.

American Occupational Therapy Association. (1998i). Sensory integration evaluation and intervention in school-based occupational therapy. In American Occupational Therapy Association, *The reference manual of the official documents of the American Occupational Therapy Association* (pp. 389-394). Bethesda, MD: Author.

American Occupational Therapy Association. (1998j). Standards of practice for occupational therapy. In American Occupational Therapy Association, *The reference manual of the official documents of the American Occupational Therapy Association* (pp. 317-324). Bethesda, MD: Author.

American Occupational Therapy Association. (1998k). The role of occupational therapy in the independent living movement. In American Occupational Therapy Association, *The reference manual of the official documents of the American Occupational Therapy Association* (pp. 353-356). Bethesda, MD: Author.

American Occupational Therapy Association. (2000). Occupational therapy code of ethics (2000). *Am J Occup Ther, 54,* 614-616.

Asmussen, S. M., Romano, J., Beatty, P., Gasarch, L., & Shaughnessey, S. (2000). Old answers for today's problems: Integrating individuals who are homeless with mental illness into existing community-based programs: A case study of Fountain House. In Cottrell, R. P. (Ed.), *Proactive approaches in psychosocial occupational therapy.* Thorofare, NJ: SLACK Incorporated.

Avilla, D., Combs, A., & Purkey, W. (Eds.). (1972). *The helping relationship sourcebook.* Boston, MA: Allyn & Bacon.

Balsdon Richer, C. B., & Bhasin, C. A. (1999). *Occupational therapy practice guidelines for adults with neurodegenerative diseases.* Bethesda, MD: American Occupational Therapy Association.

Benner, P. (1984). *From novice to expert.* Menlo Park, CA: Addison-Wesley.

Brammer, L. (1979). *The helping relationship: Process and skills.* Englewood Cliffs, NJ: Prentice Hall.

Carkhuff, R. (1969). *Helping and human relations.* New York, NY: Holt, Rinehart & Winston.

Clark, F., Ennevor, B. I., & Richardson, P. L. (1996). A grounded theory of techniques for occupational storytelling and occupational story making. In R. Zemke & F. Clark (Eds.), *Occupational science: The evolving discipline* (pp. 373-392). Philadelphia, PA: F. A. Davis.

Colangelo, C., & Gorga, D. (2001). *Occupational therapy practice guidelines for adults with cerebral palsy.* Bethesda, MD: American Occupational Therapy Association.

Combs, A. (1971). Some basic concepts in perceptual psychology. In A. Combs, D. Avilla, & W. Purkey (Eds.), *Helping relationships: Basic concepts for the helping professions.* Boston, MA: Allyn & Bacon.

Combs, A., Avilla, D., & Purkey, W. (Eds.). (1971). *Helping relationships: Basic concepts for the helping professions.* Boston, MA: Allyn & Bacon.

Corcoran, M. (2001). *Occupational therapy practice guidelines for adults with Alzheimer's disease.* Bethesda, MD: American Occupational Therapy Association.

Creighton, C., Dijkers, M., Bennett, N., & Brown, K. (1995). Reasoning and the art of therapy for spinal cord injury. *Am J Occup Ther, 49,* 311-317.

Denton, P. L., & Skinner, S. R. (2001). *Occupational therapy practice guidelines for adults with mood disorders.* Bethesda, MD: American Occupational Therapy Association.

Devereaux, E. (1984). Occupational therapy's challenge: The caring relationship. *Am J Occup Ther, 38*(12), 791-798.

Dolhi, C. D. (2001). *Occupational therapy practice guidelines for adults with spinal cord injury.* Bethesda, MD: American Occupational Therapy Association.

Dreyfus, H. L., & Dreyfus, S. E. (1986). *Mind over machine: The power of human intuition and expertise in the era of the computer.* New York, NY: Free Press.

Egan, G. (1975). *The skilled helper.* Monterey, CA: Brooks/Cole.

Engel, J. M. (2001). *Occupational therapy practice guidelines for chronic pain.* Bethesda, MD: American Occupational Therapy Association.

Ersser, S. J., & Atkins, S. (1999). Clinical reasoning and patient-centred care. In J. Higgs & M. Jones (Eds.), *Clinical reasoning in the health professions* (2nd ed., pp. 68-77). Oxford, England: Butterworth Heinemann.

Hanft, B. E. (2001a). *Occupational therapy practice guidelines for attention-deficit hyperactivity disorders.* Bethesda, MD: American Occupational Therapy Association.

Hanft, B. E. (2001b). *Occupational therapy practice guidelines for young children with delayed development.* Bethesda, MD: American Occupational Therapy Association.

Jaffee, E. G., & Epstein, C. F. (1992). *Occupational therapy consultation—Theory, principles, and practice.* St. Louis, MO: Mosby Year Book.

Kannenberg, K. R. (2001). *Occupational therapy practice guidelines for adults with schizophrenia.* Bethesda, MD: American Occupational Therapy Association.

Larson, B. A. (2001). *Occupational therapy practice guidelines for adults with low back pain.* Bethesda, MD: American Occupational Therapy Association.

Mattingly, C. (1991a). What is clinical reasoning? *Am J Occup Ther, 45,* 979-986.

Mattingly, C. (1991b). The narrative nature of clinical reasoning. *Am J Occup Ther, 45,* 998-1005.

Mattingly, C. (1994). The narrative nature of clinical reasoning. In C. Mattingly & M. H. Fleming (Eds.), *Clinical reasoning: Forms of inquiry in a therapeutic practice* (pp. 239-269). Philadelphia, PA: F. A. Davis.

Mattingly, C., & Fleming, M. H. (Eds.). (1994). *Clinical reasoning: Forms of inquiry in a therapeutic practice.* Philadelphia, PA: F. A. Davis.

McColl, M. A., & Bickenbach, J. E. (1998). *Introduction to disability.* Philadelphia, PA: W. B. Saunders Co Ltd.

Moyers, P. (1999). *Guide to occupational therapy practice.* Bethesda, MD: American Occupational Therapy Association.

Neistadt, M. E., Wight, J., & Mulligan, S. E. (1998). Clinical reasoning case studies as teaching tools. *Am J Occup Ther, 52,* 125-132.

Peloquin, S. (1998). The therapeutic relationship. In M. E. Neistadt & E. B. Crepeau (Eds.), *Willard & Spackman's occupational therapy* (9th ed., pp. 105-119). Philadelphia, PA: Lippincott, Williams & Wilkins.

Radomski, M. V. (2001). *Occupational therapy practice guidelines for adults with traumatic brain injury.* Bethesda, MD: American Occupational Therapy Association.

Rivet, L. B. (2001). *Occupational therapy practice guidelines for tendon injuries.* Bethesda, MD: American Occupational Therapy Association.

Rogers, C. (1951). *Client-centered counseling.* Boston, MA: Houghton Mifflin.

Rogers, C. (1972). The characteristics of a helping relationship. In D. Avilla, A. Combs, & W. Purkey (Eds.), *The helping relationship sourcebook.* Boston, MA: Allyn & Bacon.

Rogers, J. C. (1983). Clinical reasoning: The ethics, science, and art. *Am J Occup Ther, 37,* 601-616.

Rogers, J. C., & Holm, M. B. (1991). Occupational therapy diagnostic reasoning: A component of clinical reasoning. *Am J Occup Ther, 45,* 1045-1053.

Rossman, D. L. (2001). *Occupational therapy practice guidelines for adults with carpal tunnel syndrome.* Bethesda, MD: American Occupational Therapy Association.

Schell, B. A., & Cervero, R. M. (1993). Clinical reasoning in occupational therapy: An integrative review. *Am J Occup Ther, 47,* 605-610.

Schell, B. B. (1998). Clinical reasoning: The basis of practice. In M. E. Neistadt & E. B. Crepeau (Eds.), *Willard & Spackman's occupational therapy* (9th ed., pp. 90-99). Philadelphia, PA: Lippincott, Williams & Wilkins.

Schön, D. (1983). *The reflective practitioner—How professionals think in action.* New York, NY: Basic Books.

Slater, D. Y., & Cohn, E. S. (1991). Staff development through analysis of practice. *Am J Occup Ther, 45,* 1038-1044.

Stoffel, V., & Moyers, P. (2001). *Occupational therapy practice guidelines for substance use disorders.* Bethesda, MD: American Occupational Therapy Association.

Strong, J., Gilbert, J., Cassidy, S., & Bennett, S. (1995). Expert clinicians and student view on clinical reasoning in occupational therapy. *British Journal of Occupational Therapy, 58,* 119-123.

Verner Platt, J. V. (2001). *Occupational therapy practice guidelines for adults with hip fracture/replacement.* Bethesda, MD: American Occupational Therapy Association.

Warren, M. (2001). *Occupational therapy practice guidelines for adults with low vision.* Bethesda, MD: American Occupational Therapy Association.

Yasuda, L. (2001). *Occupational therapy guidelines for adults with rheumatoid arthritis.* Bethesda, MD: American Occupational Therapy Association.

CHAPTER FOUR

Psychodynamic Frame of Reference— Person Perspective and Meaning

KEY POINTS

◇ History and Current Theory
- Theoretical Basis—Freud, Jung, Hartmann, White, Rogers, Maslow, Goldstein
- Feelings Influence Motivation and Decision Making
- Development of Personality and Adaptation
- Awareness, Motivation, Defenses, Adaptation, and the Therapy Process
- Sign of Personality in Occupational Therapy Assessment and Intervention
- Learning by Doing—The Therapeutic Activity and Fidler's Task Oriented Group
- Evolution of an Existential-Humanistic Psychodynamic Model
- Client-Centered Occupational Therapy—Individualized Intervention

◇ Theory in the Context of Occupational Therapy Practice
- Person—Dynamic Energy System Motivated for Competence and Meaning
- Collaborative Relationship—Therapist and Client/Patient Contribute
- Activity—Medium for Expression, Creativity, Improved Coping, and Confidence
- Activity Provides Necessary Boundaries

◇ Theoretical Assumptions Guide Evaluation and Intervention
- Evaluation
  —The Subjective and Objective Perspectives Through Interview, Drawings, and Tasks
  —Client-Centered Methods—Interview, Observation, Dialogue, Feedback, and Tasks/Activities
- Intervention
  —Collaboration to Identify Client-Centered Objectives and Plans
  —Occupational Therapy Groups Today—Sample Groups Across the Life Span
  —Group Treatment—Process, Social Microcosm, Activity Processing, Member Feedback
  —Regard for Subjective Experience

◇ Contributions and Limitations of a Psychodynamic Framework

FOCUS QUESTIONS

1. What themes do existential humanism and occupational therapy have in common? Describe them.

2. What have psychodynamic models contributed to occupational therapy's understanding of the whole person?

3. What does it mean that clients are the "experts" on their own lives? Do you think that this view of expertise is always true?

4. Given that people are believed to seek challenge, suggest several reasons why a patient/client might avoid a challenge in occupational therapy.

5. What does it mean that an assessment is "subjective?" What place should subjective assessment have in OT?

6. What is the sign of personality approach in assessment? Discuss what you perceive as the legitimacy of this approach in OT.

7. How does having an understanding of a client's ego function guide the therapist in creating a therapeutic environment?

8. How does a structured environment contribute to the well-being of persons who are confused or lack internal control?

9. What guidelines does this framework provide for giving feedback to individuals about their behavior and activity performance?

10. How does a therapeutic milieu contribute to a person's enhanced self-awareness?

11. What is the purpose of processing an activity experience?

12. What is the role of expressive activities in OT today?

13. What have psychodynamic models contributed to practice with persons having mental illness?

14. What have psychodynamic models contributed to practice outside of the mental health arena?

HISTORICAL UPDATE

In the previous two editions of this text (Bruce & Borg, 1987, 1993), the psychodynamic framework was referred to as the "object-relations" frame of reference. The basis for this choice of terms was in its use by occupational therapist and educator Dr. Anne Mosey in her groundbreaking text, *Three Frames of Reference for Mental Health* (1970). In the denotation of an object-relations framework, Mosey created an umbrella for diverse theories, which were drawn from outside of occupational therapy but used to guide OT practice. These theories generally fell within the rubric of either Freudian/neo-Freudian psychodynamic theory or humanistic/existential theory in psychology and philosophy. The object-relations framework described by Mosey in 1970 was a model for occupational therapy practice closely linked to the psychodynamic orientation prevalent in psychiatry at that time. In her text, Mosey states that the application of an object relations framework is not specific to age, diagnosis, or socioeconomic status (Mosey, 1970, p. vi).

Psychological Constructs

A psychodynamic framework for OT is one in which psychological **constructs** are believed to account for one's occupational and social behavior. Psychological constructs describe mental states, abstract or metaphorical in nature, which have a shared colloquial meaning but because they are abstract, no definitive meaning. For example, one can talk about "anxiety," "satisfaction," or a person's "sense of self-esteem" and recognize that it is probably not possible for everyone to come to full agreement about the meaning of these terms. Few would disagree, however, that any of these constructs could impact an individual's occupational choices or perseverance in a task. The term "psychodynamic" reminds us that, although diverse in origin, the theories contributing to Mosey's model as well as those that will contribute to this current chapter are concerned with the persons' "inner life" as these impact their engagement in meaningful occupation.

Height of Use—Emphasis 1950-1970

Psychodynamically based occupational therapy in mental health was at its height during the 1950s through the early 1970s. It was used to guide intervention with children, adolescents, and adults. During that period it was quite common for persons with identified mental illness to be treated as inpatients in private or public psychiatric hospitals. It was not unusual for intervention to last 2 or 3 months, or even longer. Typically, patients were administered psychotropic medication and participated in a variety of therapies, including OT. The purpose of these lengthy intervention periods was often to provide initial protection, if patients were believed unable to control their own behavior, and facilitate behavior change. The goal was that patients gain insight into their ways of behaving, experience and work through troubling feelings, achieve self-control, and/or try out and practice new ways of behaving. Such lengthy hospitalizations still exist for children/adolescents and adults, but they are most often reserved for persons exhibiting highly disturbed behavior.

Today, individuals with acute psychiatric illness or acute exacerbation of chronic illness may be hospitalized for very brief periods (3 to 5 days), and once stabilized medically, they may be discharged or transferred to outpatient or supported living settings. Thus, as we consider the viability of a psychodynamic model, we do so thinking both within but also beyond the medical system in which it was originally conceived.

Two Different Applications

As we take another look at the application of psychodynamic principles in occupational therapy, it appears most clear to distinguish between two different but related applications of a psychodynamic model. The first is the application of a psychodynamic model based on Freudian and neo-Freudian (newer adaptations of Freudian) ideology. Such a model can be used with children, adolescents, and adults and is more likely to be used in a medical setting. A somewhat different set of psychodynamic beliefs come together in humanistic/existential theory and are evident in occupational therapy practice within mental health settings but also more broadly in practice.

Collectively, a psychodynamic orientation to understanding and responding to behavior in occupational therapy appears to be most applicable in six key areas:

1. Such an orientation helps therapists intervene with persons of all ages having mental disorders in which a psychodynamic explanation for behavior is especially compelling. These disorders include (but are not limited to) those resulting from trauma and abuse (e.g., post-traumatic stress disorder, dissociative disorder), some depressive reactions, eating disorders, and borderline personality disorder.

2. A psychodynamic model provides a useful means by which the occupational therapist can evaluate and respond to the often-confused behavior exhibited by persons with mental illness.

3. It provides a means for understanding and supporting the feelings, thoughts, and emotions (or "inner life") of persons of all ages who may not have mental illness but are coping with physical illness, injury, or adversity, including those who are grieving.

4. It alerts the therapist to the styles of relating within occupation that individuals come to prefer and for responding accordingly.

5. It provides a framework for understanding how occupation becomes meaningful to all persons—underscoring that it is the person's **experience** of illness or physical limitations and their perceptions of occupational choices that must concern us.

6. It speaks to the significance of the therapeutic relationship and provides guidelines for creating and sustaining this relationship.

The Influence of a Person's Feelings

An enduring contribution of a psychodynamic framework has been that it alerts occupational therapists to attend to the emotional or affective part of the person. It reminds us as occupational therapists that sometimes what our client thinks or knows may be quite different from what he or she feels, and that feelings exert a powerful influence on peoples' choices, motivation, and continued engagement in occupation.

Occupational therapy's concern with meaningful occupation and function is "based on the belief that performance is influenced by biological, psychological, and social factors," writes occupational therapist and educator Susan Fine (1993, p. 9). Yet, she continues, "...we continue to ignore these principles where they count most: in many of our educational and clinical programs" (p. 10). As we turn our attention to the "inner life" or psychological domain to which Fine refers, we echo her challenge:

> The psychosocial domain is everybody's business. It must not be disregarded as something irrelevant to your practice, disposed of because you think you won't be reimbursed, or dismissed because someone else on your team is expected to deal with it. The fact is, you can't discard it, because it won't go away. It's omnipresent—to help or hinder you in your work with each individual. (p. 10)

DEFINITION

A psychodynamic frame of reference is one that provides an explanation for how mental processes, including perceptions, thoughts, and feelings that are in conscious awareness as well as those that are not, influence one's selection of, participation in, and satisfaction with occupation. Beginning at birth and through occupation, the person creates a relationship with his or her human and nonhuman environment, thereby satisfying both basic needs and the need to use one's unique talents, skills, and interests; engage socially with others; and ultimately find a purpose in life.

Therapeutic activity is selected in accordance with its utility in enhancing interpersonal communication, facilitating healthy emotional experiences, enhancing self-awareness and self-acceptance, and enabling the client to identify and pursue his or her skills and interests. A psychodynamic framework can serve as a restorative model in which some aspect of the person is expected to change as a consequence of intervention. It may also be used to identify compensatory strategies that can be used to assist persons of all ages to achieve and function optimally within their environment, and to identify caregiver adaptations in those instances in which individuals are limited in their ability to change.

THEORETICAL DEVELOPMENT

The psychodynamic frame of reference in occupational therapy is an outgrowth of the early psychoanalytic and communication approaches in occupational therapy. In 1963, occupational therapist Gail Fidler and her husband, psychiatrist Jay Fidler, collaborated to write *Occupational Therapy—A Communication Process in Psychiatry* (1963), a book that described the implementation of psychodynamic principles in a therapeutic group context. Occupational therapist Lela

Llorens (1966; Llorens & Rubin, 1967) described the application of these psychodynamic principles with disturbed children. In 1970, occupational therapist Ann Mosey took a Freudian term, **object-relations**, and used it to describe an eclectic approach in occupational therapy that applied Jungian, neo-Freudian, humanistic-existential, as well as classical Freudian influences that originated in medicine and psychology.

In an **eclectic approach**, several theories are integrated to formulate a new and disciplined approach. Eclecticism provides a rationale for evaluation and intervention based on identified theoretical concepts and clinical techniques. It is not a license of total freedom for the therapist to do as he or she pleases, nor is it a simple common sense approach.

In the Beginning: Freud

Because the mental health field as a whole and psychodynamic theory in particular have their roots in ideas professed by Sigmund Freud, a brief summary of several of these beliefs is provided in order that we might highlight critical components that have influenced early psychodynamically oriented occupational therapy and that continue to bear on practice. We recognize, as will the reader, that this review does not substitute for more complete accounts of Freud's work, nor do we wish to diminish the important contributions made by all of those who have followed since Freud. Our goal in this cursory theoretical review is to assist the reader in placing psychodynamic occupational therapy into the context of psychodynamic practice in the greater mental health community. Freud lived and wrote nearly a century ago, and his ideas have been subject to immense scrutiny and change. That they have been modified along the way may be less remarkable than the extent to which they have endured.

Society and mental health treatment have come a long way since Freud first elaborated his beliefs in *The Interpretation of Dreams* (Freud, 1950). If his peers and eventually the public were outraged then by his emphasis on the role of sexual feeling in unconscious thought and conscious behavior, they nonetheless were given a new way to conceptualize human thought, feeling, and behavior.

Today people talk about their feelings as if they have a life of their own. They describe thoughts as being **conscious**, **unconscious**, or **subconscious** and expect others to understand what they mean by these terms. They may substitute our term **hang-up** for Freud's **complex**, but they discuss their hang-ups and feelings and those of people around us with the expectation that these influence behavior and one's overall sense of well-being.

From early psychodynamic theory we have been given a vocabulary and the license to talk about and understand ourselves in a way that we now take for granted. Not only do we have words to describe our "inner life," we have a better understanding of how this inner life develops and differentiates into the "self" we take for granted.

Life's Energy: Libido

Freud saw the person as a closed energy system and labeled the energy **libido**. The term libido means "vital energy." He viewed this energy or libido as limited and directed either inward (to self) or outward (to other persons or things), both of which were referred to by Freud as **objects**. Investing their energy in objects is how people satisfy their needs. In everyday terms, we may hear someone say, "This project is important to me; I've put all my energy into it," or, "I'm so worried about my children's problems, I have no energy left for anything else." The person was believed born with libido but, in and of itself, having libido did not meet the person's needs. To use an analogy suggested by Hall (1954) we might think of a newborn infant, exemplifying ourselves, as being born with 16 ounces of libido.

The newborn infant experiences hunger, thirst, and pain and will cry vigorously when uncomfortable. Our rather typical infant will have caring parents who act to meet the child's needs, and the infant can picture the people and non-human objects that provide comfort and satisfaction. Soon, the child is able to imaginatively long for mother, bottle, soft toys, and any other objects experienced as enjoyable. Unfortunately, at this stage, the 16 ounces of libido can only be used for reflexive physical activity and for wishing or picturing. The infant wants what it wants now but can't create a plan to get it.

Ego Emerges from Id

That portion of the mind or psyche that was unable to differentiate between reality and fantasy and that wanted immediate gratification was said to reside in a portion of the self Freud called the **id**. The id is present at birth and houses the instincts, including those related to survival. The id experiences intolerable tension when biological needs are not satisfied and pleasure when needs are met and tension is released; however, the id is not capable of logical thinking. Out of necessity, some of the 16 ounces of energy develops into a second intrapsychic area that could relate functionally with the outside world. This area Freud termed the **ego**.

The ego also strives to satisfy, or bring pleasure, but unlike the id, it is able to realistically assess the outside world. As Freud said, ego functions help the individual perform a task by "becoming aware of stimuli, by storing up experiences about them (in memory), by avoiding excessively strong stimuli (through flight), and... by learning to bring about expedient changes in the external world to its own advantage (through activity)" (Stafford-Clark, 1966, p. 134). There are no actual boundaries in the brain or elsewhere between the id, ego, and superego. Rather, these terms are a shorthand way of conceptualizing and identifying psychological processes within the personality.

Other Ego Functions

The ego is considered to be the organizer of the personality. It houses those mental processes that recognize "I am myself," "I am real," and "I am not part of anyone else." It is the part of us that can identify a problem and solve it. It can distinguish between a wish and a mental image, and what exists in the physical world. The mental processes housed by the ego can focus attention on one part of experience (the foreground) while putting the rest into the background. The ego is aware of time and sequence and is given the job of postponing gratification. The ego can also use energy to plan actions capable of removing obstacles to satisfaction in a function Freud called **aggression**. When the ego collects data, establishes priorities for the self, and puts a plan of action into effect to see if it works, the ego is said to be doing **reality testing** (Hall, 1954). Stated another way, the ego does not randomly invest energy to meet needs. It orchestrates a plan that ultimately becomes meaningful occupation.

Freud in his later writing proposed aggression as an innate human drive in addition to the drive for pleasure. It was, according to Menninger (1963) and Stafford-Clark (1966), viewed as neither more nor less important than other drives, described rather matter-of-factly as influencing human behavior.

Back to our analogy: Our developing child, now 2 years old, has some sense of self as separate, calls that self by a name, knows what he or she wants, possesses a functioning ego, and does not need to cry on the hopes that a bottle will magically appear. With determined ego direction, the child can use 1/4 ounce of libido to crawl up to his mother with an empty bottle, pull the family cat out of the mother's lap (aggression), and ask for the bottle to be filled (using a primitive form of sign language or insistent whines typical of the young child). Because energy is limited and the child has only 16 ounces to invest, should he or she direct too much effort to satisfying daily needs, such as those for the bottle, there might be too little left to meet new challenges. As the child matures, his or her ability to take in and use information will increase, as will his or her experiences in problem solving. What begins as a primitive ego becomes more and more complex and capable of adapting to the world.

The premise that everything the person does takes energy and that energy can be tied up by mental/emotional tasks and problem solving as well as physical activity is an idea helpful for occupational therapists to imagine why clients sometimes seem to have little energy available for the tasks in therapy.

Psychological Influence in Occupational Therapy

Applying an understanding of the function of ego processes, the occupational therapist working within a setting (often medically based) in which Freudian or neo-Freudian psychodynamic principles were used had several concerns. Was the client able to invest his or her energy in meaningful activities that met his or her needs? Did the individual have energy invested in a wide enough variety of objects and interests so that a full range of needs was being met? When an "object" (thing, event, or person) was no longer need-satisfying, could this person pull back energy from it and reinvest the energy in other productive, socially acceptable relationships or activities? When the patient/client was involved in tasks, was the ego in control or was the primitive need for immediate gratification leading to impulsive, chaotic behavior? Because the ego was believed to house all those mental functions that enabled a realistic appraisal of the external world and functional performance, assessing and enhancing ego function by means of functional activity became a primary goal in occupational therapy in mental health, especially in those settings in which individuals had identified mental illness. This is articulated clearly in the following passage taken from a text by occupational therapist Gail Fidler, along with her physician husband, Jay Fidler, a book that served as one of the most influential within in the field during the 1960s:

> Building and reconstructing a more healthy ego is the purpose of all psychotherapeutic endeavors. Thus all formulations presented here are, hopefully, directed ultimately toward helping the patient develop a more complete and realistic concept of himself as a person separate from others, understand the nature and potential of this, and increase his capacities to realize his potential. (Fidler & Fidler, 1963, p. 83)

Relation Between Ego Function and Task Choice

An important function of the psychiatric diagnostic categories used in the past and currently in mental health is that they give information about the relative strength or limitation of ego function. Those mental disorders in which the ability of the ego to do its job is severely impaired are identified as **psychoses**. Knowing that a client exhibits psychotic behavior is a signal for the therapist to pay special attention to safety issues, structure the task environment, and reduce the demands for decision-making by the individual. In principle, the more impaired the ego, the less able the individual is to make sound judgments and control his or her own behavior; therefore, the more the therapist will structure and organize the external environment. Mental illness is not the only factor that bears on ego function, however. Stress, physical illness, fatigue, and the use of alcohol or other intoxicants can all be expected to influence ego function. To increase your understanding of the use of this term by occupational therapists, the reader is referred to Functions of the Ego in Daily Life Tasks. It becomes clear when looking at this list that the occupational therapist has been concerned about the person's ego function because the ego enables adaptation and participation in purposeful occupation.

FUNCTIONS OF THE EGO IN DAILY LIFE TASKS

The ego is that part of the person that oversees adaptive function in the everyday environment. As identified in this model, the following are key functions of the ego that impact one's ability to engage successfully in daily life tasks.

- To distinguish between reality and fantasy
- To postpone gratification until such time as satisfaction of needs is appropriate to the situation
- To control impulses
- To oversee selective memory
- To weigh options and make judgments based on real information
- To create and maintain an accurate self-image
- To be aware of one's strengths and limitations
- To be able to integrate changes in body image as the body changes
- To be able to devise a plan to meet needs, including the need to establish relationships with people and nonhuman objects in the environment
- To oversee one's occupational being-in-the-world
- To manage feelings
- To restore and maintain internal equilibrium
- To feel a sense of mastery upon accomplishment
- To intervene between wants/desires and what one believes is correct to do (conscience)

Superego and Performance Expectations

Logic, not moral imperatives, guide the ego. Because the child's survival depends initially on the love and approval of parents/caregivers, some energy is used in assessing which courses of action will be approved of and which actions his or her parents will think are "bad." The child develops what is commonly called a conscience, an inner voice that influences actions by evoking guilt, when he or she has displeased others, and pride when he or she does what is perceived as right or approved of. This occurs in the area of the psyche that Freud called the **superego**.

The ego's job became one of steering a course that satisfied what the person wanted in a way that would be socially acceptable. Sometimes occupational therapists treat children and adults who have a **punitive** or overly critical superego. In this instance, the person's expectations for him- or herself are too demanding or inflexible. Conversely, the therapist might work with individuals who seem to have too little superego; they tend to be unconcerned about hurtful, immoral, or amoral behavior. In either instance, the therapist might try to engage these individuals in therapeutic groups in which the person can be given realistic feedback about the impact of his or her behavior.

The Unconscious and Making Choices

The id, ego, and superego must share that "16 ounces" of original libido. All three portions of the psyche want success and satisfaction for the person and must find a way to work together in relative balance and harmony so that each part can do its necessary work. For what one might call efficiency of operation, some knowledge that our infant has gained—knowledge that might be interesting but of no practical value—may be pushed out of current awareness or consciousness into the area Freud termed the **unconscious**.

LATERALITY OF BRAIN FUNCTION

It is interesting to compare Freud's constructs of id-ego and conscious-unconscious to what is known about the laterality of brain function. For the right-handed person, the left hemisphere is considered primarily (but not solely) responsible for the ability to verbalize, do mathematics, think logically (i.e., in terms of cause preceding an effect), and to deal in ordinary time-space constructs; these describe "ego" functions. The right, or nondominant, hemisphere has more responsibility for the ability to intuit, visualize, and deal with affect. The right hemisphere lives in timelessness, does not see events proceeding logically one before another, and is, therefore, acausal; this describes "id" (Gazzangia, 1988, 1989; Ornstein, 1973; Springer & Deutsch, 1981).

Likewise, knowledge or thoughts that the child's evolving superego judges as shameful may be pushed from consciousness into the unconscious or may never have been allowed into conscious awareness at all. Much material held in the area of the unconscious includes thoughts one would be ashamed of, were he or she conscious of them. Also pushed or kept from consciousness are perceptions that are too much for the ego to handle, meaning the ego can't create a logical way to explain or to accept these thoughts. A child or adult who has been abused, for example, or experienced other trauma might not be able to recall details surrounding this experience or might be able to recall only fragments. Nevertheless, the person might experience overwhelming feelings of fear or anxiety that he or she cannot explain or control. Although it represents an area of non-awareness, the unconscious continues to exert a powerful influence over behavior. Freud believed that only a small portion of perceptions and thoughts are conscious. Many perceptions and thoughts reside in either the unconscious, where they are generally inaccessible, or in the **preconscious**, where they are not in current awareness but are able to be recalled (Freud, 1950).

It is this notion— behavior being influenced by perceptions, thoughts, memories, or feelings that are outside awareness—that can assist occupational therapists trying to make sense of and/or help clients make sense of feelings or behavior that seem illogical or difficult to understand. Stated another way, sometimes our clients have feelings, experience anxiety, or do things that they don't understand and feel helpless to change. This can make it difficult for them to freely pursue choices, including occupational choices, that would appear to be healthy for them.

Development of the Personality and Skill Development

Complementary to his theories about id-ego-superego and conscious-unconscious, Freud conceptualized that while a person is pleasure-seeking by nature, the objects and activities that would be experienced as especially satisfying would change as the individual matured. Freud began with the newborn and outlined progressive stages of what was termed **psychosexual** or **psychosocial development**. He attributed special importance to the first three developmental stages, which span the first 5 years of life, citing preferred object choices and preferred ways of relating to significant others as well as to non-human objects/media. These Freud related directly to changes in the physical development of the child. During each of these developmental stages, the child also has emotional tasks he or she must accomplish, including those related to learning to trust others, establishing a sense of internal control and autonomy, establishing a moral code, establishing gender identity, and learning and gaining confidence in one's own social and occupational skills (Table 4-1). Developmental, cognitive, and social learning theorists who

followed Freud have elaborated upon these skills, describing in much greater detail the manner in which these skills are developed (see Bowlby, 1969; Colby & Kohlberg, 1987; Erikson, 1950, 1959, 1969; Gilligan, 1982; Havighurst, 1974; Kohlberg, 1969, 1971, 1976; Levinson, 1974; Piaget, 1962, 1965, 1973; Piaget & Inhelder, 1969; Selman, 1971, 1976; Sheehy, 1978). Especially pertinent to occupational therapists who work with children has been the work done in the area of play (Axline, 1969; Bundy, 1997; Ellis, 1973; Florey & Greene, 1997; Perry & Bussey, 1984; Piaget, 1962; Pronin Fromberg & Bergen, 1998; Reilly, 1974; Takata, 1974). Play has been shown to be a primary vehicle by which the child establishes myriad intrapsychic, cognitive, social, physiomotor skills that enable satisfying daily function. Knowing the developmental stages and related skills is especially important to the therapist applying a psychodynamic model in work with children, and the interested reader is encouraged to pursue the literature in this area. Adult behavior, however, may also reflect difficulties with progressing through and meeting developmental challenges.

It was in *Three Essays on Sexuality* (Freud, 1953) that Freud fully described how he viewed the development of object preferences. Freud noted that as the child develops, specific regions of the body become especially sensitive to touch or stimulation and that touch to that area is very pleasurable. Freud termed all bodily pleasure as sexual pleasure and did not limit his use of the term sexuality to genital sexuality, as we tend to do today. Along with favored objects, the child progressed through "stages" in the manner in which he or she related to significant people. Stage theory describes a sequential progression by which the person moves from the protection of infancy out into his or her world, learns about this world, and achieves satisfaction and mastery within it. The following summary provides an encapsulated review only.

Psychodynamic Stage Theory

The descriptions of the five stages of dynamic theory give insight into the variables in the relationships between the person and his or her environment and the possible outcomes of each developmental period.

Oral Stage and Bonding

For the newborn infant to about the age of 2, the oral region is the focus of pleasure, and the child is in the **oral stage**. For these children, activities that stimulate the mouth, such as those involved in sucking at their mother's breast or one's own fingers, or biting are favored. According to Freud, mother is the most important person-object at this stage. Subsequent developmentalists and social learning theorists (Perry & Bussey, 1984) have recognized that other consistent caregivers (father, siblings, and grandparents) may be equally important. It is imperative that caregivers be responsive to the infant's biological as well as emotional needs for consistent nurture. The child also needs a safe and nurturing envi-

Table 4-1

NORMAL PSYCHOSOCIAL DEVELOPMENT

Age	Region, special sensitivity	Pleasurable activities	Object choice	Potential problems
Birth to 2	Oral stage (a) early oral (b) late oral	(a) Sucking, incorporating, swallowing (b) Biting, destroying	Self; oral object Maternal figure	Person fixated at this stage may be clingy, over-dependent, or have trouble trusting others; enjoys talking; finds comfort in food, smoking, etc.; unable to form close relationships
1 to 3	Anal stage (a) early anal (b) late anal	(a) Excreting, touching excrement, being messy (b) Controlling, retaining, holding on to excrement; being very neat	Parent figure; anal object	Early: Might be overly messy Late: Finds being messy repugnant; enjoys being the organizer, the collector; generates conflicts over who is in charge
3 to 5	Early genital stage (phallic)	Touching or exploring genitals; learning about own and genitals of opposite sex	Parent; superparent (hero)	May have difficulty accepting appropriate roles, manner of dressing, etc., or may have exaggerated sex role behavior May be most comfortable with same sex relationships or fear them due to homosexual concerns May appear to be without conscience or remorse for antisocial-behavior

Table 4-1 (Continued)

Age	Region, special sensitivity	Pleasurable activities	Object choice	Potential problems
5 to 12	Latency (no new zone)	Sublimation of energy into learning new skills	Companion of same sex	May be unable to engage with peers in reciprocal relationship; lacks confidence in skills and abilities
12 to 18	Late genital stage (adolescence)	Touching, investigating, fantasizing about own genitals and genitals of opposite sex	Self; emergence of love for companion of opposite sex	Struggles with issues of independence versus dependence May appear especially concerned regarding own physical appearance; may be preoccupied with matters of genital sexuality May experiment with homosexual and heterosexual activity

Adapted from Hall, C. S. (1954). *Primer of Freudian psychology.* New York, NY: New American Library and Stafford-Clark, D. (1966). *What Freud really said.* New York, NY: Schocken Books.

ronment: one that provides stimulation and opportunities for physical interaction. Through rudimentary play, also called sensorimotor play, the child in this stage gains an awareness of his or her body as well as the physical environment. The abilities to receive nurture, to learn to trust that needs will be satisfied, and to **attach** or **bond** emotionally with parents/caregivers are critical social developmental tasks for the child at this stage.

Anal Stage and Control

For the child about age 1 to 3 years, the anal region is especially sensitive. Activities associated with excreting, particularly in terms of mastering control over excrement, will be satisfying. At this **anal stage**, mother and father continue their important roles as nurturers, but the child's relationship with them is changing. He or she has learned to say "No!" and tries to gain a sense of autonomy and control over the environment, while not alienating parents. The child is more mobile and able to scoot or amble about his or her environment, and the nurturing environment is one that provides materials and a safe setting in which the child can venture

out and explore; develop motor, cognitive, and social skills; and develop feelings of mastery.

Phallic Stage and Identity

When the child is 3 to 5 years of age, he or she is in the third stage of development—the **early genital** or **phallic stage**. Freud viewed the early genital stage as the key period for appropriate gender identity (Eichenbaum & Orbach, 1983, p. 71). Boys see themselves like dad (or other significant males) and girls see themselves like mom and begin to imitate their behaviors in a process termed **identification**. (Again, social theorists have emphasized that the child may identify with adults or other role models in addition to parents.) Freud considered the male and female child as essentially **bisexual** (demonstrating traits of both sexes) until this stage. Children in this stage also take large strides in a process known as **separation-individuation**, in which the child begins emotional separation from the parents. The child, who is practicing being separate and independent, needs to know that the parents will be there, emotionally as well as physically, when he or she returns. It requires that parents allow the child to have needs and opinions of his or her own. Play often includes the use of imagination or "pretend," which is another way the child can venture off and practice independence. In addition, during the early genital phase, the child actively incorporates parental ideas about good and bad. Parents remain a primary object choice, but this is the period in which the child seeks a superparent or hero.

Latency Stage and Social Relationships

From about age 5 to puberty, the child is in the **latency stage**. Later developmentalists would divide this period into two stages, that of early and later childhood. No new body area assumes special significance, and energy is channeled into developing or enhancing performance skills and forming peer friendships. Latency is a key time for the child to develop life skills such as those involved in helping his or her family or community, achieving academically, and socializing comfortably. During this time the child has the ability to establish truly reciprocal friendships with peers. Play now includes games with rules as well as organized, cooperative play (e.g., going off with friends to catch crawdads, building a sledding run that all can enjoy, and so on).

Late Genital Stage and Independence

From puberty though adolescence, referred to as the **late genital stage**, the genital area is again experienced as especially pleasure-related, and there is movement toward adult heterosexuality. The heterosexual love object takes on special significance.

The adolescent is in many ways caught between childhood and adulthood, still financially and legally dependent on parents and emotionally attached, but very concerned about peer approval and becoming increasingly independent in multiple areas.

Fixation

It must be stressed that the age boundaries given for each developmental stage are not really boundaries, but flexible conceptual divisions that allow for the overlapping of stage-related behaviors. Sometimes, however, the individual, child, or adult gets stuck or **fixated** at a certain level of psychosexual development. His or her behavior, including object preferences and interpersonal relationships reflect this fixation. In this case, an excess of energy will be directed toward trying to meet needs at a specific level, and the individual will not successfully move on to the next stage. The result can be an immature and/or restricted manner of dealing with self, others, and things.

For example, a child who does not successfully attach with a parent in infancy may in later years have difficulty trusting any adults. The child may not feel secure to go off and explore his or her environment; he or she may cling, or conversely, reject adult contact, and may fail to interact with peers (Lieberman, 1977).

Similarly, an adult fixated at the oral stage may select objects and activities (perhaps symbolic) that reflect an over-reliance on oral pleasure (e.g., eating). In relationships the person may want to be parented, rather than engage in a mature adult relationship.

Psychosexual Development and Children

Frequently, children seen within the mental health community have behavior and emotional problems that disrupt their ability to meet the expected stage requirements for their ages. Psychological problems and skill deficits demonstrated by these children may include those related to:

- An inability to establish a close, trusting relationship with parents or care providers
- A lack of confidence in venturing off to play and learn new skills; difficulty establishing appropriate peer relationships
- Disruptive and/or amoral behavior including aggression, impulsivity, and other problems with self-control; depression/sadness
- Failure to engage in expected skills in self-maintenance and self-care

Additionally, psychologically healthy children coping with and managing physical or cognitive disabilities, children from impoverished or chaotic environments, or children experiencing illness may have a more difficult time transitioning through the various stages. In occupational therapy with children, Freudian and neo-Freudian postulates are used within a context that provides the child opportunities to engage in normal activities and master age-appropriate skills, often using play but also activities that emphasize cooperation and task accomplishment (Olson, 1993).

Reflection in Adult Behavior

There are probably few adult readers who have not heard or shared comments about one's self or another being too "oral" or "anal," so common is that vernacular. Perhaps more useful is the recognition that often, and at a young age, individuals settle into a favored style of relating to their environments. For example, one person may have a strong preference for order, keeping his or her workspace organized and schedules routine; others may be more inspired by a playful environment and a schedule that invites spontaneity. On the one hand, being "fixated" at any given psychosexual stage of development tends to limit the range of need-satisfying objects and ways of dealing with the environment. The person may be less flexible. On the other hand, and without needing to judge or label behavior, recognizing the differences people have in their preferred way of approaching tasks and relating to the environment enables therapists to accommodate to their clients' preferences. Occupational therapists can't typically change people's styles and make them match their own. Often, they can help individuals cope with changes in their lives by helping them maintain the styles with which they are most comfortable.

Example: Frances was 79 years old and had had Parkinson's disease for more than 20 years. For the past 10 years she had required a wheelchair for mobility. Despite this, she had been able to work part-time as a realtor until the age of 70. She had been a widow for 5 years and took pride in the fact that she was able to live alone; to independently groom, bathe, and dress herself; prepare her own meals; and manage her finances. All this she accomplished by being very organized. Recently, however, Frances had become increasingly quiet, and her family felt she was becoming depressed. A home care nurse called in the occupational therapist to assist in an evaluation of Frances' living situation. Dialogue revealed that it was becoming increasingly difficult for Frances to organize her physical environment. Trying to be helpful, various family members had been moving things in Frances' house to make them easier for her to access. The result was clutter on the counter, and a clothes closet with items half-falling out through the doors. If Frances would complain, family members suggested that she be more relaxed. "After all," they asked, "Who's going to see your closet?" Once the therapist talked with Frances and determined that Frances had a strong need for order and a feeling of being able to control her own living environment, the therapist was able to work with Frances to re-create an accessible and highly ordered environment and use her home management skills. Frances' affect soon brightened.

Freud's View of Motivation

The person wants to satisfy him- or herself on the one hand (the so-called **pleasure principle**), whereas reality often requires that gratification be postponed or even abandoned. The pull of pleasurable activities versus the reality of a situation in which it is difficult to reach desired goals creates a tension that motivates the person to act.

At times this tension is felt as anxiety, especially when needs cannot be met or when the individual fears that he or she will engage in behavior that would be harmful or guilt-inducing. This anxiety would be likely to result when ego strength was diminished or when demands on the ego were increased. The ego might try to manage anxiety by trying to "deny, falsify, or distort reality" via special constellations Freud termed **defense mechanisms** (Hall, 1954).

Defense Mechanisms and Adaptation

Defense mechanisms enable a "very special kind of coping" that occurs mostly unconsciously and involuntarily (Vaillant, 1993, p. 9). **Defenses** are ways in which the ego can alter the perception of both inner reality (feelings or thoughts) and external reality. They are likened to the body's immune system. The immune system goes to work when

bacteria invades the physical body. Defense mechanisms go to work when sudden change or conflict threatens to overwhelm the ego's sense of what it can manage. If the immune system has done its job "wisely" (neither too much nor too little), the person doesn't show signs of illness; if the defense system does its job "wisely," the person will be judged to be "healthy, conscientious, funny, creative, (and/or) altruistic." If defenses are used badly, society may view him or her as mentally ill, "unpleasant," or "immoral" (Vaillant, 1993, p. 11). Defense mechanisms are summarized in Appendix H, although the reader is advised that there is not unanimous agreement regarding what constitutes the full spectrum of defenses. Freud and writers who followed (Freud, 1937; Vaillant, 1993) agreed that use of some defenses is more adaptive than is use of others, and their relative utility may depend in part on how long the defense is used and in what situation.

Occupational therapists often work with persons who are faced with challenges that are unexpected and highly stressful. Defenses, unlike other coping strategies (e.g., cognitive stress management techniques, going for a walk to clear one's head, or seeking emotional support from friends and family) are not used consciously. One of the healthy uses of a defense is that it can help clients meter pain and anxiety (i.e., make it more manageable). A familiar example is the initial use of denial upon learning that one has a potentially fatal illness. Sometimes individuals faced with overwhelming stress due to illness or trauma may **regress**, which means that they revert to more childlike behavior. Overall, people tend to have preferred defenses that, along with their typical manner of approaching tasks, evolve over time and characterize their way of meeting needs. Combined, these are reflected as **personality**.

The Therapy Process

Believing that the unconscious portion of the person's mental activity exerted a powerful influence over behavior, Freud attempted to determine thoughts that were held in the unconscious. One approach he took was to look in depth at the individual's symbol production through free word association, "slips of the tongue," and by exploring with a person his or her dreams. The belief was that it took energy to keep thoughts out of consciousness (or **repressed**) and that if unconscious thoughts and conflicts could be brought into conscious awareness, they could be worked through by the individual, thereby freeing up energy to be invested in other, more satisfying activity.

Freud saw his role as neutral in which he could allow the patient to play out on the "therapist screen" the unresolved conflicts and unconscious dramas that needed to be remedied. The major activity in this process, which he called **psychoanalysis**, was interpretation, especially interpretation of the patient's behavior and affect during therapy sessions with the analyst, plus interpretation of dreams recounted by the patient. This interpretation was designed to increase insight and understanding. Although the past was inevitably recounted in the psychoanalytic process, it was the patient's memory of the past, "the world of reconstructed subjective experiences," that was considered important. The accuracy of such memory was not a primary concern (Michels, 1983, p. 61). The idea that it is the individual's perception of events and not the event itself that is important is a belief that was adapted by humanistic theorists who followed.

It is interesting to note that Freud viewed the personality as tending to become more fixed (inflexible) as the individual reaches maturity. As a result, the adult aged 50 or older was not believed to be a good candidate for change nor for psychoanalytic intervention (Sadler, 1978).

Because Freud believed that old conflicts left unresolved would dictate current behavior, he emphasized the significance of understanding the patient's history, especially those events that were being held by the unconscious and tying up too much energy. In accounting for behavior by looking at past events, Freud's theories are referred to as **causality**.

THE EARLY MODEL: OCCUPATIONAL THERAPY AND "PROJECTIVE" ACTIVITIES

Early occupational therapists applied a model similar to Freud's using art media such as clay, paints, and collage as a tool for encouraging expression and potentially accessing this unconscious material. This was reflected in the use of what were termed "projective" assessment batteries in occupational therapy. Therapists lacked clear guidelines for interpreting the meaning of this artwork, however, and the appropriateness of such interpretation as an occupational therapy function came into question (Allen, 1985; Drake, 1999). However, occupational therapists continue to use art as an expressive outlet. Some of these uses are described in this chapter.

Sign of Personality in Occupational Therapy Assessment

Judgment in occupational therapy based on Freudian and neo-Freudian principles often employed and may continue to employ a **sign of personality** approach. In such an approach, the therapist looks at the client's or patient's performance in an assessment or with various materials as representative of the personality and the person's general way of handling specific media or engaging in tasks (Borg & Bruce, 1991). For example, the person who dislikes handling "messy" materials within occupational therapy would be presumed to be a person who overall dislikes handling messy materials. The person who approaches a particular task with precision and organization would be believed to be someone who will approach other tasks in life with precision and

organization. Many occupational therapy assessment batteries developed during the height of neo-Freudian OT intervention included tasks that were **structured** (having inherent guides as to how they were to be executed) and **unstructured** (lacking external guides and encouraging creative problem solving), thereby allowing the client to exhibit his or her preferred style through a variety of means (Azima & Azima, 1959; O'Kane, 1968; Williams & Bloomer, 1987).

The person's performance in occupational therapy tasks may also be viewed as representative of his or her ability to organize, problem-solve, and in other ways successfully perform occupationally, which are all functions of the ego. For instance, people who manage their frustration during a task by throwing up their hands and giving up might be expected to respond similarly to other frustrating situations.

Another focus in psychodynamic occupational therapy assessment and intervention has been self-image and body image. Many occupational therapy assessment batteries included a request for a human figure drawing, often for an image of the self (Azima & Azima, 1959; Hemphill, 1982; O'Kane, 1968; Shoemyen, 1970; Williams & Bloomer, 1987). Dialogue was sometimes used to assist the drawer to describe his or her feelings about the drawing, but the therapist might also interpret or make inference about the drawer based on what was depicted in the drawing and/or how the task was approached.

Learning By Doing: The Therapeutic Activity or "Task" Group

In the 1960s through mid-1980s, psychodynamic OT in mental health settings often occurred in the context of either inpatient or outpatient settings in which individuals, typically identified as patients, lived together and/or engaged within the context of what was called the **therapeutic community** or **therapeutic milieu** (Jones, 1953). Typically, patients participated together in a treatment program that extended throughout the day, often into the evening. The environment was designed to emulate one's everyday environment, and participants engaged together throughout the day in meetings and activities, as well as during mealtime and unstructured time. Therapeutic groups might include occupational therapy, recreation therapy, verbal group therapy, psychodrama, medication group, and/or patient government. Free or unstructured time allowed participants the opportunity to talk, reflect, and learn to manage their own unscheduled time, similar to that needed at home. With staff support, clients were expected to take responsibility for getting along, resolving differences, and planning leisure activities. Within such a context, there were many opportunities for participants to give each other feedback, to learn from and support each other, and to practice social skills and other functional living skills. In this respect, the work of therapy was believed to be done within the milieu.

Task-Oriented Group

During the 1960s, Gail Fidler published her article "The Task-Oriented Group as Context for Treatment" (1969). Task groups in occupational therapy (also referred to as **therapeutic activity groups**) provided an opportunity for clients to learn about themselves while working together. Occupational therapy groups were described as a "microcosm of life—work situations," which could be "seen and explored" as they occurred rather than in retrospect (Fidler, 1969). These groups were structured in accordance with the relative abilities (ego function) of participants. As clients worked together in group tasks, the emphasis was not just on the outcome or **product** (what they accomplished) but equally on the **process** or dynamics of the activity group (how they worked together to accomplish their goals). Thus, the therapeutic activity group was a good philosophical match with therapeutic milieu.

Group Model for Young Clients

Occupational therapist Lela Llorens and Rubin (1967) described a similar group model for intervention with older children and adolescents; however, reflecting on the outcome as well as process in a task was not restricted to group work. The occupational therapist might also talk with young clients about tasks or projects they work on independently. When looking at the **dynamics** of an activity, the individual and the therapist together look at the end product, form, content, and process that occurred. Patients or clients might be encouraged to talk about the significance of a particular activity and answer the following questions:

- How did it feel to have so many others compliment you on your work?
- Is this (product) for you or a gift for someone else?
- What did you learn about yourself while engaged in this task?
- How did you feel?
- How did you respond to your frustrations?
- What part(s) of the activity process did you most enjoy? Or not enjoy?

Activity to Increase Awareness

In their book, Fidler and Fidler (1963) provided a substantive discussion on the use of activities as a means to increase self-awareness. As they wrote, the "extent to which (an individual or group) is encouraged to talk about feelings associated with the activity process will depend partially on" (their) readiness or ability to communicate certain associations verbally (1963, p. 81).

What characterized clinical reasoning in this neo-Freudian approach in occupational therapy was that while the therapist was interested in what the client felt or perceived, the final judgment about what was significant in occupational behavior was often made by the therapist.

INFLUENCE OF JUNG

In her description of an "object-relations" (psychodynamic) framework, Mosey (1970) included ideas attributable to psychotherapist Carl Jung. It is difficult to assess how this man, who was a contemporary of Freud's and a groundbreaker in the field of psychology, influenced beginning psychodynamic occupational therapy practice. It is not within the scope of this text to discuss Jung's constructs in depth, and the reader is referred again to the reference list; however, several influences in current practice are credited to Jung and are discussed here. In some respects, Jung's work acts as a link to that of humanistic theorists, as we shall see.

Jung was a psychoanalyst who, like Freud, believed in the existence of an unconscious. He too identified tensions within the individual. Jung saw behavior as motivated by past events (**causality**) as well as future aims (**teology**). That is, Jung saw in the person a constant, internal striving for creativity, a search for wholeness, and a yearning for the development of the self (Jourard, 1971; Jung, 1966, 1979).

Polarities in the Self

Jung was himself well versed in and influenced by Eastern philosophy. The image of the individual as struggling to balance many opposing forces, as is conceptualized in the Eastern image of the yin and yang, is key in Jungian thinking. Agreeing with Freud that much memory and thought is unconscious, Jung thought that the predominant tension in the unconscious was created by the pull of opposite forces that exist in the self (Campbell, 1971).

Some opposing forces identified by him include:

- The tendency of the self to be **introverted** (focused on the self) versus **extroverted** (focused on others)
- The tendency of the individual to gain information through tangible seeing versus the tendency to favor gaining information through intuition
- A striving in the self for material comfort versus a striving for spirituality
- The existence in males of latent or unexpressed feminine qualities and in females of latent masculine qualities

Jung thought that all these polarities in the inner-self needed to be developed and given expression in a person's life. He called this process **individuation**. Further, he conceived of a governing structure that would strive to bring all these polarities into balance and work toward the goal of wholeness. This force he called the **transcendent function**; and the process, the ultimate goal of personhood, he termed **transcendence**.

Jung introduced concepts that have found significant contemporary acceptance among a generation that is concerned about achieving personal balance, inner harmony, and spiritual wellness (see Occupational Dualities).

OCCUPATIONAL DUALITIES

The dualities discussed by Jung also correspond to the dualities suggested by split-brain studies. In the right-handed person, the left or dominant hemisphere corresponds to feelings of "light" and to a sense of masculinity, as well as the verbal-intellectual function, as was mentioned earlier. The right, non-dominant hemisphere corresponds to a sense of "dark" or night, to feelings of femininity, as well as the acausal-intuitive function of perceiving and problem-solving. Ornstein (1973) makes the observation that various occupations tend to depend more on the function of one or the other hemisphere: "Many different occupations and disciplines involve one of the major modes of consciousness. Science and law are highly involved in linearity, duration, and verbal logic. Crafts, the 'mystical' disciplines, and music are more present-centered, aconceptual, and intuitive" (p. 83).

Changes in the Second Half of Life

Whereas Freud's discussion of psychosocial development stops with the advent of a person's adulthood and sexual maturity, Jung addressed the changes that occurred in self-perception, values, and social roles throughout the life process until death. In accordance with his belief that both men and women carry within themselves latent qualities of the opposite gender, Jung felt that in middle age, after relative success in meeting societal role expectations, both men and women could allow themselves to express some of these qualities.

For example, a rather passive mother of 40 years of age might become more assertive in her relationships and seek a significant role in the business community. In contrast, the 40-year-old man who perhaps has been very focused in his business pursuits may start to feel that business is not so important and may want to spend more time nurturing his children. Both men and women at middle age would, according to Jung, tend to turn from materialistic concerns to spiritual concerns.

As indicated by Hall and Nordby (1973), Jung was one of the first psychologists until recently who had tried to understand the psychology of the middle years. In an evocative passage Jung states, "A human being would certainly not grow to be 70 or 80 years old if this longevity had no meaning for the species. The afternoon of human life must also have significance of its own and cannot be merely a pitiful appendage to life's morning" (Jung, 1971, p. 17).

Jung felt that "middle age" extended well into the 50s, 60s, and even 70s—old age implying senility or a return to the unconscious. He predicted that it was the older person who could achieve real wisdom and wholeness. Implicit is the premise that Jung valued the roles and accomplishments of the older person, in contrast to Freud's inference that older age brings rigidity and little growth.

With much of our current population aged in the middle to older years, it is understandable that much popular lay psychology literature reflects Jungian theory (Moore, 1992, 1996; Pinkola-Estes, 1992).

Collective Unconscious and Culture

Perhaps the greatest stir in the analytical community was raised by Jung's conception of a **collective unconscious**. Jung conceived of the psyche as being conscious and unconscious in content, as did Freud. He went further, however, in suggesting that the unconscious held not only thoughts and reflections of personal experience, but images, ideas, and a predisposition to seek certain experiences in a way that our ancestors had experienced them. These universal images and predispositions, thought to be genetically inherited, were called collective and said to be stored in the **collective unconscious**. Pointing to similar themes and content in mythology, religion, and cross-cultural art and finding these same themes in the symbolic expression of his patients, he looked at symbols in a much broader vein than Freud. *Man and His Symbols* (Jung, 1979), the writings of Joseph Campbell (1968, 1976, 1981, 1990), and the more recent work of Thomas Moore (1992, 1996) are among the well-received publications that explore cross-cultural themes in art, literature, and myth.

Jung and the Use of Art

As his ideas about the unconscious developed, Jung began to encourage his patients to make drawings of their dreams and daydreams (or fantasy material). Although the drawings were not usually made during a therapy session, they were shared between patient and therapist (Edwards, 1987). The purpose of such drawings appeared to be to help the individual understand and integrate what was depicted therein; just executing the drawings was not enough.

Jung does not specify in his writing techniques for involving patients in drawing; however, many contemporary therapists who specialize in the use of art as an expressive and integrative medium refer to Jungian theory as their base (Edwards, 1987; Uecker, 1986). The occupational therapist that is well-acquainted with cross-cultural themes in mythology, art, and religion has the opportunity to help the individual reflect on his or her own life and struggles in terms of broad themes common to humanity.

EGO PSYCHOLOGY AND MOTIVATION

Although Freud regarded the ego as the decision-maker in the personality, he continued to view it as subservient to the whims of the id, trying to reduce tensions and resolve conflicts. Many of those who followed in psychiatry (a medical discipline) and psychology (non-medical) thought that the ego had a broader, more autonomous role. Writing mainly in the 1950s and 1960s, these persons came to be referred to as **ego psychologists**. Heinz Hartmann and R. W. White are two ego psychologists often referred to in the occupational therapy literature. Hartmann wrote that the ego does not develop out of the id but upon the birth of the individual. He said that although the ego uses some energy to meet instinctual needs and reduce tension, the rest is used to help the person adapt and prosper within the environment in ways that are not conflict-ridden. The person not only adapts to his or her environment but helps to create that environment (Hartmann, 1958, p. 31). This belief is echoed in the writing of White, who stressed that the ego (the person) gains great satisfaction from exploring and accomplishing within his or her world (White, 1959, 1971).

Hartmann refers to his own ideas as differing in emphasis from Freud's ideas, not as a major break from them. The difference in emphasis, however, was one that occupational therapists would increasingly point to in the literature because it helped explain why "doing" (occupational therapy's key tool) is a natural part of a healthy state of being and is satisfying in and of itself.

FREUDIAN PSYCHODYNAMICS AND IDEOLOGY TODAY

Mental health treatment and psychodynamic practice continue to be affected by Freudian ideology, albeit with modification. Whether or not it is accurate to refer to most contemporary psychodynamic treatment as "Freudian" at all is probably a valid question, as it has moved far from Freud's original model, which is why we have preferred the term "neo-Freudian" in describing this model.

Another term for the application of this model in occupational therapy has been **ego-adaptive** (Llorens, 1966; Cole, 1993). Today's psychosocial occupational therapist will likely be directly or indirectly influenced by this neo-Freudian ideology in contemporary practice, especially when this practice occurs within a medical or medical-model setting.

Current trends in psychotherapy are not duplicated in psychodynamic occupational therapy, but intervention within medically based settings is likely to reflect some of the following changes.

Altered View of the Role of Past History

Whereas Freud stood firmly by his belief that events in the past (through their retention in conscious and unconscious memory) caused events in the present and that therapy should attempt to understand these causes, current neo-Freudian thinking operates under a newer model. Today, childhood experiences are not conceived as necessarily causing events to occur in adult life, and therapy is believed to be most productive when it focuses on the here-and-now interactions between the therapist and the patient (Gruenbaum & Glick, 1983; Malone, 1983).

New Conceptualization of the Development of Gender Identity

Altered View of Femininity

Freud's perspective on women has been especially criticized as patriarchal, biased, and totally inadequate (Bernstein, 1983; Blum, 1976; Eichenbaum & Orbach, 1983; Lerner, 1983; Money & Ehrhardt, 1972; Notman & Nadelson, 1982). It was a view based on the belief that psychology was rooted in biology; that women wished (unconsciously) to be men; that appropriate female behavior was dependent, passive, and masochistic; and that the proper feminine role was associated with nurturing and child-bearing. It was an interpretation that was based on the belief that female and male gender was not established until about 4 years of age, with the advent of the early genital phase. Undoubtedly, it represents Freud's own observations of the women of his times and, as such, represents his incorporation of the cultural bias and values of his day.

Gender Identity

Today's psychodynamically oriented therapist is knowledgeable about the information gained in the area of child development and regards the importance of cultural shaping in gender identity. **Gender identity** is "the knowledge and awareness, conscious or unconscious, that one belongs to one sex and not the other" (Notman & Nadelson, 1982, p. 5). The child is now understood to be establishing gender identity upon birth (and quite possibly before birth). Countless studies and simple observation have shown that males and females begin to diverge in interests, mannerisms, and conduct by 12 to 16 months of age (Grinspoon, 1984; Hales & Frances, 1985; McFarlane, 1983; Money & Ehrhardt, 1972; Stoller, 1968).

The understanding of gender identity is one of many areas in which contemporary theory views Freud's original premises as too rooted in biology and as placing too much emphasis in the phallic period. Differences in gender role are now attributed to many antecedents including biological differences, social learning, scripting, and cultural myths.

Changing Roles of Men and Women

Western society has challenged the Freudian bias that women need to be passive and dependent to be "feminine" and psychologically healthy. Cultural changes, the emerging role of women in positions of power and authority, and the increasingly diversified models for child-rearing and family role-taking have all affected the societal norms regarding appropriate female and male conduct. Contemporary therapists have a much broader view of masculinity and femininity (Fausto-Sterling, 2000; Gruenbaum & Glick, 1983; Kimmel, 1998).

Gender Stereotypes

Gender stereotypes have special implication for the occupational therapist working to facilitate meaningful occupation for patients/clients, both male and female. Even if the therapist has incorporated a liberalized perspective on appropriate gender activity, he or she may encounter in practice individuals who still hold sexual stereotypes about themselves and others. The occupational therapist needs to be aware that both in terms of the activities and media made available to patients/clients and in terms of his or her role of therapist (possibly a female in a position of authority), the therapist may precipitate individuals' conflicting feelings about gender role.

Challenging the Supremacy of Biological Determination

The change in views regarding appropriate male and female behavior reflects a contemporary ability to see behavior as determined by more than anatomy. Freud is described as never having been able to adequately resolve the conflict between cultural injunction and individual psychology (Person, 1983).

Today, psychodynamic theory attempts to understand the significance of all aspects of the external world (environment and culture) as experienced by the individual and giving unique meaning to his or her existence. Even sexual objects (e.g., those related to genital sexuality) are considered in light of their cultural-societal association, not merely as appendages to an instinctive, biological drive.

Child-Parent Relationship

For a long time, the Freudian and neo-Freudian therapist thought the therapist-patient relationship was, at an affective level, a re-experiencing of the child-parent relationship of the early genital period; in other words, the therapist was the longed-for Oedipal parent (Eichenbaum & Orbach, 1983).

Today, we are aware of the special relationship of infant to parents, which is critical in terms of parents' physical and emotional nurture. As the ego develops, the child is increasingly able to go off alone, thus beginning the process of separation-individuation. Successful separation-individuation depends on the ability of the child to experience mother/father as consistent and nurturing, to retain them in memory, and to trust that they will be there when he or she returns.

With much more emphasis placed on early (pre-phallic) development, it is not surprising that current psychotherapists also perceive the development of superego as beginning much earlier than conceived by Freud (Brickman, 1983).

This view would be more consistent with the work of such developmentalists as Piaget and Kohlberg.

Geriatric Psychiatry

With the increased longevity of the average American, public priorities about the elderly are changing. Whereas Freud thought that change was not likely to occur in the older individual, psychiatrists have become increasingly involved (within their professional organizations and as reflected in their practice) in better understanding the special problems of the elderly and making treatment available to them. In the mid-1990s geriatric psychiatry was identified as the "fastest growing field in psychiatry" (Kaplan, Sadock, & Grebb, 1996, p. 1155; 1998).

By presidential proclamation, 1900 to 1999 was declared the "decade of the brain." In an associated shift in priorities, those individuals with known cognitive impairment (e.g., individuals with senile and presenile dementia, traumatic head injury, autism, and schizophrenia) have been the focus of many studies conducted by the National Institutes of Health and the National Institute of Mental Health (Kaplan, Sadock, & Grebb, 1996, p. vii). The medical community's renewed interest in the function and chemistry of the brain is reflected in its extensive coverage in recent literature. As more and more is being learned about the physiology of the brain, much hope is being placed in the direction of better management of psychiatric symptoms through the use of medication. Yet, the belief continues to be expressed that medications alone do not ameliorate the functional problems of living encountered by persons with mental illness (Kaplan, Sadock, & Grebb, 1996, p. vii-ix; 1998; Wallis & Willworth, 1992).

Supportive Treatment

The final trend that has emerged in practice is the acknowledgment of a need for shortened psychotherapeutic treatment. Shortened treatment duration is, in some cases, a reflection of changing therapeutic priorities, including that for cost containment. Intervention that is not expected to bring about personality change or change in ego function but is designed to bolster existing ego strengths is referred to as **supportive**.

EVOLUTION OF AN EXISTENTIAL-HUMANISTIC PSYCHODYNAMIC MODEL

With its roots in the writing of such articulate philosophers as Sartre, Camus, Tillich, Kafka, and Heidegger and in the neo-Freudian therapies of Karen Horney, Robert White, Hartmann, Sullivan, Klein, Adler, Rank, Fromm, and Erikson, existential-humanism has evolved over the past 40 years into a significant influence in philosophy, psychology, and education.

Generally included as part of the existential-humanistic movement are those theories or therapies referred to as Gestalt or field theory, perceptual psychology, organismic theory, phenomenology, Rogers' client-centered therapy, Frankl's logotherapy, plus others. We focus here on the elements common to or shared by these existential-humanistic philosophies and those in particular that have contributed to the humanistic psychodynamic model for occupational therapy.

Although proclaiming themselves as separate from Freud and as a "third force" in psychology (the Freudian psychodynamic model and the behavioral model served as the other two "forces"), existential humanism is also a psychodynamic model. It too offers an explanation for the development of the psychological self and describes how psychological constructs impact behavior, engagement in occupation, and one's sense of well-being.

While existential-humanistic approach within the field of psychology was vigorously elaborated in the literature in the 1960s and early 1970s (see especially Rogers [1951, 1961], May [1950, 1953, 1969], Maslow [1968, 1971], Jourard [1971], Perls [1969], and Moustakas [1956, 1961]), one can discern the continued influence of existential-humanism across a broad range of theoretical frameworks and across many disciplines today.

Existential-humanism has focused on the essence of the human condition and how one individual might best help another. With science now able to extend or maintain life, questions of life, death, and quality of life push us to reexamine our beliefs in this regard.

Challenging Freud

Believing as Freud that the therapist must understand and appreciate the subjective experiencing of the individual, the existential-humanist professes a much different view of what constitutes an optimum therapeutic relationship. In this unique conceptualization of the therapeutic relationship, existential-humanism has been and continues to be evident in the field of occupational therapy. Existential-humanism also conceives of a much different human nature than that identified by Freud, a view consistent with the generally positive posture taken by occupational therapy.

Existential-humanism became part of the movement across Western society encouraging the individual to be "true to yourself" and to act in accordance with one's own values and cultural traditions. One result, evident in the practice and literature of contemporary occupational therapy, is the importance given to respecting diversity among all persons (Law, Baptiste, & Mills, 1995; Rochon & Baptiste, 1998) and the emphasis given to respecting and maximizing client choice (Law & Mills, 1998).

Subjective Nature of Experience

Like Freud, existential-humanistic writers proposed that one's life be experienced from an internal or subjective base.

If you (as a therapist) want to understand my life experiences, you must do so by trying to imagine how they are for me. That is to say, each of us personally selects what we will pay attention to in our experiences and will make sense of those events according to the personal meaning they have for us. To offer a simple illustration: Imagine that you and four friends go to a concert and sit together to listen and enjoy the evening. What each of you pays special attention to, feels, and recalls as a result of your shared experience will be different. In that sense, you each experienced a different concert.

In the same way, life changes will be experienced differently by each individual. Assume two men, Mitchell and Jim, have both had an accident that resulted in an arm being amputated. Mitchell, age 27, is married and the father of three young children; he makes his living as a stunt rider in professional rodeo. Jim, age 43, is also married, but his children are in their early 20s; he is a high school math teacher. While Mitchell's and Jim's injuries might appear identical, their losses may be very different. Based on this model, occupational therapists will strive to understand both men's unique needs, concerns, and priorities as each copes with his loss.

Nature of Motivation

Humanistic theorists echoed the sentiments of writers like White, Hartmann, Maslow, and Jung, who proposed that the individual is innately motivated to explore and master his or her environment. All believed that people gained satisfaction from challenging themselves, developing skills, and meeting goals. Whereas Freud conceptualized a tension-reduction model of behavior, and ego psychologists and Jung saw both tension-reduction and fulfillment as motivating behavior, existential-humanists conceived one driving force: the innate striving in each individual to be all he or she can be. They termed the life-long striving toward this ultimate goal as a striving for **self-actualization**.

As described by humanistic psychologist Carl Rogers (1961), self-actualization is "…the urge which is evident in all organic and human life to expand, extend, become autonomous, develop, mature. It is the tendency to express and activate all the capacities of the organism…" (p. 35). One is reminded of Jung's conceptualization of transcendence—a state perhaps achieved by only a few—in which all dimensions of the individual find expression during the course of his or her lifetime.

If there appears to be loftiness to this goal of self-actualization, a humility and integrity inherent in existential-humanism should not go unnoticed. This ideology holds the basic belief that all individuals have wisdom and worth, that one person's path to knowledge and purpose is no more or less valuable than another's provided that each is using his or her abilities as best each can and living according to one's personal values and beliefs. Therefore, a simple task or basic skill has as much essential worth as an endeavor requiring what one might view as exceptional intellect or skill.

Implicit is the belief that the occupational therapist adopting this philosophy does not need to externally motivate the client (as through offering "rewards" or recognition for compliance); rather, the therapist needs to provide opportunities for developing skills and potentialities, and achieving mastery within one's occupational choices.

Self-Approval

Humanists like Rogers recognized, however, that the process sometimes breaks down. Believing with Freud that past experiences influence present awareness and functioning, Rogers, for example, saw in early childhood experiences the basis for many distortions in the individual's self-awareness. The youngster, seeking parental approval, may behave according to parent wishes and mimic the feelings that parents communicate are valid. If this behavior continues into maturity, the individual loses touch with personal values and perceptions. Parental hopes for the individual become the person's hopes for him- or herself. Frequently, adult life is spent seeking external approval or validation, and the person may make choices, sometimes unknowingly, that reflect only what others want. One outcome might be that the individual would experience anxiety.

Existential Anxiety

Anxiety is viewed by existential-humanists as deriving from one or more of the following:
- The individual recognizes the need for a significant change in life or is in the midst of change
- The individual recognizes his or her failure to live authentically (i.e., consistently and in accordance with personal beliefs and values)
- The individual can find no real meaning or purpose in his or her life
- The individual recognizes that he or she has not developed unique skills and has failed to be "all he or she can be" (Corey, 1982)

Bearing this in mind, the occupational therapist using this framework encourages the person to give one's self approval, rather than seeking it from outside sources, and provides opportunities to explore his or her own values, beliefs, and preferences.

Pressing Needs and Closure

From the field of perceptual psychology came another principle that could help explain how persons make choices to act. It is that in any situation or experience, whatever is most important will come to the forefront, and what is less important will recede to or stay in the background. Stated simply, people will naturally be inclined to attend to what they experience as their most pressing needs.

The writings of Abraham Maslow (1968, 1970, 1978) have been cited in the occupational therapy literature in regard to his work in which he identified a hierarchy by which personal needs would necessarily be addressed. According to Maslow, people will first and foremost need to have their basic safety and physiological needs met before they can turn to meeting their needs for social affiliation or mastery within occupations, or at the highest level, the striving for self-actualization. This premise has served as an enduring guide for occupational therapists as they collaborate with clients to prioritize intervention goals and strategies.

Perceptual psychologists also demonstrated that obtaining **closure** will be important; that having tasks or issues unfinished is not satisfying, while seeing a task finished or an issue resolved is. Further, when persons leave a task or issue unfinished or unresolved, it is difficult for them to turn their attention to anything else. Think, for example, of yourself: You are in the midst of a quarrel with a significant other or perhaps having a disagreement with an instructor about a grade you've received on an assignment. You look up at the clock and realize that it's time to go to class; the disagreement is not resolved. As you sit in class, you may find yourself having an internal dialogue in which you practice all the things you want to say to resolve this disagreement. It is difficult to pay full attention to class and what the instructor is presenting because your mind is still on the quarrel. Think of yourself deeply engrossed in a task at home; perhaps you are re-organizing your drawers or balancing your checkbook. Your goal is to finish the job, but the phone rings and you are needed elsewhere. Often it is difficult to put the job aside. Thus, the person experiences less satisfaction in a job half-done than one completed.

The implication for occupational therapists is that they need to help clients identify what they experience as most pressing and help each to resolve that first. Another implication is that therapists should enable clients to complete meaningful "chunks" of activity. A simple strategy the therapist might use, for example, would be to have the client help set the agenda for a therapy session. Another strategy would be to inform clients before therapy sessions are over in order that they could find a way to meaningfully wrap-up their activity for that session.

People Can be Trusted to Make Good Decisions

Existential-humanists stressed that the individual has the ability for self-awareness and, with it, freedom to choose his or her actions and determine a personal destiny (Baptiste & Rochon, 1999, p. 43; Corey, 1982). With this freedom of choice comes the responsibility for one's own behavior, a responsibility that includes a need to acknowledge one's effect on and relatedness to others.

Existential-humanistic thinkers proposed that people are basically positive and can be trusted to make good choices, although they may learn to behave in ways that are unacceptable to themselves and/or others. In order to make healthy choices, people need to believe they are in a setting that is safe both physically and emotionally. People need to have information about what choices they have, what resources are available, and often guidance in regards to how they can go about following through with a decision. Providing this is an important piece of **empowerment** or **enablement**.

When The Process of Engagement Breaks Down

The work of Kurt Goldstein suggests one reason why a person might withdraw from or avoid challenges. Goldstein's work was done many years ago and was largely with soldiers with brain injury. His work is especially pertinent to occupational therapists because he studied persons with cognitive impairment and physical disabilities and not healthy individuals, who are more often cited in support of humanistic ideology. He observed in these injured soldiers' behavior a natural tendency toward "balance" and self-healing (Goldstein, 1939, 1942), including the tendency to withdraw from situations they believed they could not master. Goldstein believed that this helped them maintain a sense of well being.

This same principle can be applied when working with mentally ill individuals. Many of the currently classified mental disorders (e.g., schizophrenia, depression, and bipolar disorder) are known to have a physiological substrate. That is, there are identified changes in the brain's structure and/or chemistry that account for changed feelings and altered behavior. Persons with mental disorders can also be viewed as striving to achieve balance and make sense of their experiences and may withdraw from situations they perceive as more than they can respond to or manage.

To illustrate: A woman describes her feelings and behavior at the beginning of her mental illness:

> I felt as though there was a huge gap between the rest of the world and me... I watched dispassionately as my two younger sisters matured, dated, shopped, and shaped their lives, while I seemed stuck in a totally different dimension. (Leete, 1993, p. 277)

Nature of the Therapist-Client Relationship

Originally schooled in Freudian ideology, existential-humanists challenged Freud's premise that a therapist must be passive and impersonal and that he or she must facilitate a re-enactment of the parent-child relationship or the doctor-patient relationship. As Rogers stated, "I was asking the question, 'How can I treat, or cure, or change this person?' Now I would phrase the question in this way: 'How can I provide a relationship that this person may use for his own

personal growth?'" (Rogers, 1961, p. 32). The humanists suggested that the therapist and individual are each responsible for their own behavior and the ultimate outcome of therapy. Using a term originally coined by humanist therapist Carl Rogers, the enactment of humanistic philosophy in helping intervention was termed **client-centered** practice.

KEYS TO CLIENT-CENTERED OCCUPATIONAL THERAPY

Client-centered practice in occupational therapy has evolved over a 30- to 40-year period. The integration of humanistic theory into occupational therapy reminds us of the individual differences that influence the process and outcomes of intervention. Responding to these differences is challenging for clinicians and requires knowledge and understanding of the key variables that are described next.

Choice

The reader will discern many themes in the philosophical basis for existential-humanism that are parallel to basic tenets of occupational therapy. Beginning in the professional literature of the 1960s through today, occupational therapists have identified the philosophical beliefs shared in common by occupational therapy and existential-humanism (Baum, 1980; Canadian Association of Occupational Therapists, 1997; Gilfoyle, 1980; Law & Mills, 1998; Law, Baptiste, & Mills, 1995; Yerxa, 1967, 1978). Key among these has been the importance of client choice.

In her 1966 Slagle lecture, entitled "Authentic Occupational Therapy," occupational therapist Dr. Elizabeth Yerxa stated, "Choice is so fundamental to our thinking that we have questioned whether procedures that are done to the person, over which he has no control, should be called occupational therapy. ...since self-initiated activity is our 'stock in trade' and since it is impossible to force any human being to initiate without his choosing to do so, choice is one of the keys to our unique therapeutic process" (Yerxa, 1967, p. 3). Thirty-eight years later, Mary Law, a leading advocate of client-centered occupational therapy, writes, "A fundamental concept of client-centered occupational therapy is that therapists show respect for the choices that clients have made, choices that they will make, and their personal methods of coping" (Law & Mills, 1998, p. 9).

The Authentic Relationship

Client-centered occupational therapists, like client-centered psychotherapists, also believe that to assist the individual in meeting personal goals, the therapist needs to understand the subjective-experiencing or **phenomenal world** of the individual. They proposed that the individual is most able to be honest with the therapist and honest with one's self in the context of an **authentic** relationship. In her 1966

Slagle lecture, Dr. Yerxa also described authentic occupational therapy as based "upon a commitment to the client's realization of his own particular meaning... the therapeutic experience is primarily an opportunity for self-actualization. Therefore, the occupational therapist does not force his value system upon the client..." (Yerxa, 1967, p. 8). In such a relationship, the therapist openly expresses concern for the individual, shares his or her attitudes and feelings, and conveys a message (verbal or nonverbal) of acceptance. The therapist communicates that he or she would not reject the person upon really "knowing" the person (Rogers, 1951, 1961). Rogers had coined the term **unconditional positive regard** to describe the therapist's attitude (1951, 1961). Unconditional positive regard does not mean that the therapist necessarily agrees with or likes everything the individual does, but he or she continues to value the individual and respect his or her right to feel differently from the therapist and to make choices that were different from what the therapist might choose.

The occupational therapist does not see the individual as there to make the therapist feel important, to follow his or her advice, or to model the therapist's expectations.

In the 1980s, Canadian occupational therapists as a professional group adopted client-centeredness as an "ongoing paradigm" for the practice of occupational therapy in Canada (Baptiste & Rochon, 1999, p. 41). The literature has reiterated the goals of client-centered occupational therapy as assisting the individual to become more aware of personal needs, feelings, options/resources, and goals; to understand realistically the needs and feelings of others; and to facilitate the acceptance of personal responsibility for one's own life.

Giving Information at the Client's Level

Toward these goals the client-centered occupational therapist collaborates with the client, gives information to the client at his or her level of understanding, and provides opportunity for the client to make choices about the direction of his or her own therapy (Law & Mills, 1998).

Given that some persons are more or less cognitively able to understand and choose, the therapist strives to maximize choices at the level of the client's ability. That includes breaking larger goals into smaller steps that enable the client to meet or accomplish personal goals, using a vocabulary that clients can comprehend, and engaging clients in the decision-making process whenever possible. With persons who experience periods of psychosis, it may mean informing the primary caregiver (e.g., the family) at a level he or she can understand. Once the client becomes lucid, the therapist can review with him or her what intervention has gone on and then include him or her in the decision-making process. Working with the family-as-client may often occur when working with children or persons with developmental delay. As Pollock and McColl (1998) remind us, it does not pre-sume that children or persons with cognitive limitations cannot be asked to express their concerns or preferences. It means a commitment by the therapist to helping clients communicate their wishes if possible (p. 93). It also means respecting the decisions clients make.

Client as Expert: Respecting Client Decisions

In the client-centered model, it is believed that clients are the experts on their own lives and have the ultimate responsibility for making the decision about what they wish to achieve through occupational performance and as an outcome of occupational therapy.

Especially with individuals who have chronic mental illness, there has too often been a tendency in mental health to discount what clients/patients have expressed because they often have periods of impaired judgment or ability for reality testing. Nevertheless, many individuals with chronic mental illness have periods of lucidity, and they too are presumed to be the experts on what they experience and what they need to function optimally.

Sometimes occupational therapists are in the difficult position of making recommendations and having them not followed. It is difficult because therapists are typically recommending what they believe will enhance the well-being of their client. If therapists have informed the person to the best of their ability, then in accordance with the model, they must respect his or her choices (Law, Baptiste, Carswell, McColl, Polataijko, & Pollock 1994).

Individualization of Intervention

> All client-centered occupational therapy frameworks begin by emphasizing the need for respect for clients and their families. Clients of occupational therapy come from many different backgrounds, have encountered different life experiences, and have made choices regarding occupation that are unique to them and the situations in which they live. (Law & Mills, 1998, p. 9)

It follows then that the intervention plan for each client needs to match his or her unique needs and experiences. What "works" for one client may not meet the needs of another. The assessment information considered vital with one person may be vastly different than that for another.

It is not that intervention principles are useless, but they are only guides that help therapists direct their attention. How intervention principles are applied in real practice will be different for each situation.

Spirituality and Meaning

The occupational therapy literature of the 1990s expressed a renewed interest in spiritual issues as they related to practice (Egan & DeLaat, 1994; Enquist, Short-DeGraff,

Gliner, & Oltjenbruns, 1997; Gutterman, 1990; Howard & Howard, 1997; Kirsch, 1996; Schkade & Schultz, 1992; Urbanowski & Vargo, 1994). Differentiating spirituality from religiosity, **spirituality** refers to the person's subjective perception of something greater than one's self, or a connection to a greater life force; religion refers to the more formalized aspects of spirituality, including worship (Howard & Howard, 1997, p. 181). Spirituality has been described in the occupational therapy literature as the "impetus and motivation to discover purpose and meaning in life" (Enquist et al., 1997, p. 174; Gutterman, 1990), and as "the experience of meaning in everyday activities" (Urbanowski & Vargo, 1994, p. 91). Viewed in this light, spirituality influences quality of life and fits with the essential feature of client-centered occupational therapy, which is to help facilitate activities that are meaningful to the client. Further, spirituality is viewed as a part of the whole person and as such should be important to occupational therapists (Short-DeGraff, 1988). Practitioners' beliefs in the importance of spirituality was affirmed in a survey of 500 registered occupational therapists, but this survey also indicated that therapists were unclear as to how or if they should address "spiritual" issues with their clients (Enquist et al., 1997).

The Canadian Association of Occupational Therapists formally recognized spirituality as one of five fundamental elements of client-centered intervention (Canadian Association of Occupational Therapists, 1991; Townsend, 1998, p. 52). Yet, as Hammell writes, occupational therapists have had a "traditional and predominant preoccupation with self-care activities" even when self-care and the severity of disability have not been shown to be directly related to life satisfaction (Hammell, 1998, p. 127). Given the common themes of purpose and meaning in both spirituality and occupational therapy, and the critical reference to spiritual issues that often occur when people face serious illness or trauma, the suggestion made by Trieschmann (1988) and reiterated by Hammell (p. 127) that best fits the client-centered model might be that "rehabilitation... should not only focus on the acquisition of skills to enable clients to get out of bed in the morning, but should assist them in finding their own reasons for doing so" (Hammell, 1998, p. 127).

Finding Meaning Through Narratives

Existential-humanists focused on the wholeness of the individual. This "whole" person, wrote Yerxa (1967), is one in whom not only "reason and intellect" but also "emotion and will" must be aroused in his or her discovery of personal potential through occupation (p. 7). That meant that the occupational therapist applying this model would recognize that physical limitations would have a psychological impact, and likewise that psychological concerns could be expressed through physical symptoms. It meant always trying to appreciate the meaning of a person's experiences in terms of how they affected his or her entire life, and not just a piece of his

or her life. Sometimes having that fuller appreciation helps occupational therapists perceive how a piece of behavior that seemed random or senseless is meaningful.

In concert with the interest in the area of spirituality and the wish to help clients identify meaningful activity, the profession has increasingly emphasized the use of narratives or stories. **Narrative** here refers to the recounting or creation of stories or "biographical reconstruction" (Hammell, 1998, p. 125) by clients or families in which they look at the clients illness, loss, or injury as part of the client's larger life story. Clients/families might be encouraged in an interview, for example, to talk about the direction their life has taken in the past and how they see that direction as changing. The use of narrative helps clients recognize and reaffirm priorities and values, and enables therapists to place a specific illness, trauma, or impairment into a person's larger life story and thereby better understand its meaning to the person (Fleming, 1991; Helfrich & Kielhofner, 1994; Helfrich, Kielhofner, & Mattingly, 1994; Kirsch, 1996; Mattingly, 1991; Mattingly & Fleming, 1994; Peloquin, 1990, 1995).

Therapeutic Occupation and the Present Challenge to Client-Centered Practice

Activities used in mental health settings that have their origin in existential-humanistic ideology include values clarification activities, body awareness experiences, gestalt art experiences, and non-competitive games (Fluegelman, 1976; Rhyne, 1973). The therapist realizes, however, that all activities have the potential to be both purposeful and meaningful and to facilitate change.

Appreciating that each client is unique, the therapist operating from a client-centered model understands that what works for one client may not be best suited for the next. Through the evolution of a client-centered model comes the mandate that assessment and intervention be individualized so that a plan and process can evolve that truly fit the concerns, strengths, limitations, and special circumstances of each client, family, and group with whom the therapist interacts.

Nevertheless, maintaining client-centeredness is not always easy in the climate of health care in which standardization of practice and mandates to curtail cost may press therapists to move quickly, fall back on familiar routines, or to not fully engage the client in the process of goal setting.

CURRENT PRACTICE IN OCCUPATIONAL THERAPY

Person and Behavior

When applying the psychodynamic frame of reference in occupational therapy practice, the clinician considers the relationships between the dynamic person system and the environment. These relationships influence the person's motivation and object choices throughout the life span.

Dynamic Energy System

A person is a dynamic energy system whose nature it is to create relationships with people and non-human objects through the process of active "doing" or engagement within the environment. In addition to the physical self, the person is composed of psychological parts known to the self and parts of which one is unaware. One such set of psychological constructs identified within neo-Freudian psychodynamic theory is that of id, ego, and superego; other constructs are those labeled as defense mechanisms (see Appendix H). These plus such other psychological constructs as "self-awareness" and "self-actualization" describe inner "workings" that describe something of how the individual adapts to the real world and why he or she engages in occupation that will be meaningful to the self. Occupational therapists view these parts of the person and dimensions of personhood as reflecting pieces of a meaningful whole, each part striving for personal fulfillment.

Object Choices and Relationships

There is a developmental progression by which persons engage with human and non-human objects, establish self-identity, and build increasingly complex social and occupational skills. Early experiences influence object preferences and preferred ways of relating to human and non-human objects, but objects and occupations have no meaning in and of themselves. Individuals give meaning to them through their unique perceptions and experiences. Occupational therapists respect that people have preferred ways of interacting in their environments but recognize that not all styles are equally adaptive for all situations. Further, changes in health or abilities may make it difficult to use one's familiar style. Understanding his or her own behavior (becoming more self-aware) and/or being given the opportunity to develop new styles, a person may change the manner in which he or she relates to human and non-human objects and participates in occupation.

Motivation

The person may fear change or resist trying something new, especially if he or she does not expect to succeed; however, each person is believed to have an innate striving to grow, mature, be competent, and relate in a meaningful way to the people and world around them. When mature, the individual accepts responsibility for his or her own actions, his or her behavior is consistent with personal values, and he or she changes personal perceptions according to real data and values of self and of others (Rogers, 1961).

Both neo-Freudians (like White) and client-centered practitioners (like Rogers and Yerxa) use the term **self-actualization** to describe the process by which a person strives to meet and master personal challenges. A person moves toward self-actualization when he or she uses thoughts, feelings, senses, and perceptions to increase self-awareness, pursue interests, and develop personal talents, while respecting one's limitations and the rights and boundaries of others. In using this term, occupational therapists have emphasized the importance of maximizing choices given to the client within the context of therapy.

Function and Dysfunction

The continuum of function and dysfunction represents the effects of a person's ego functions during tasks and occupations to adapt to the environment, participate in daily life, and support optimal health.

Function

Within neo-Freudian applications of this model, function suggests that the person has a sound, functioning ego. He or she can make realistic assessments about what is going on in the environment; adapts to environmental expectations, which include exerting self-control and deferring gratification; and uses intellect, insight, and judgment to solve problems and satisfy personal needs in a socially acceptable way. These **ego functions** are often very evident when the individual is engaged in task behavior. Other related ego functions include having an accurate image of one's self as separate from others, and having a realistic self-image and body image, including knowledge of one's strengths and limitations. These too may be developed within the context of occupational engagement in which the person can see the outcome of his or her own efforts and be given feedback about how he or she is viewed by others.

Quite similarly, but without necessarily applying the term "ego," existential-humanistic theory suggests that the **optimally healthy person** is one who is self-aware and can alter his or her self-image according to real information. The person uses skills/talents to meet needs in a manner that respects the rights of others, and he or she takes responsibility for his or her own behavior and occupational choices. Further, in the pursuit of spiritual health, the person participates in activities that are meaningful to him or her and feels that he or she has a quality of life.

Dysfunction

Freudian ideology contributed to a system of labeling a person's behavior according to psychodynamics (psychiatric diagnoses), and dysfunction in the neo-Freudian application is frequently identified as mental illness.

Humanistic-existential proponents have challenged this system of labeling, often seeing it as presumptive, unnecessary, and even demeaning (Scheff, 1975, 1984). Whether or not the occupational therapist will refer to these diagnostic labels will likely be determined, in part, by the setting in which he or she is employed.

Overall, within this framework, from an occupational therapy perspective, **dysfunction** suggests that the person views him- or herself or situations outside of the self in ways that are very different from how others see these. The person is unaware of feelings that are shaping decisions. He or she is not developing talents or skills or is making choices that are not in accordance with personal values. The person is unable to function satisfactorily and meaningfully in either activities of daily life, in pursuit of personal interests, at work, and/or in social relationships. Dysfunction may also be evident as a breakdown in self-motivation. Often, dysfunction is characterized by feelings of helplessness, hopelessness, and/or anxiety.

Role of the Occupational Therapist

The occupational therapist serves as a knowledgeable, empathetic guide who believes that the client has strength and wisdom about his or her needs. The therapist endeavors to establish a collaborative relationship with the individual and maintains the framework of intervention.

Mutual Responsibility

In this **collaborative relationship**, the occupational therapist acknowledges that the individual has a will and responsibility for making decisions and choices. The aim is for the individual and therapist to mutually assume responsibility for assessment, identification of intervention goals and development of an intervention plan, and to work together cooperatively during the intervention process. Both therapist and client pool their knowledge to enable the development of an intervention plan that reflects what is important to the client.

Since individuals will vary in their abilities to be self-reflective and make or follow through with sound judgments, the occupational therapist strives to maximize the person's ability to make healthy choices and moderates the degree of structure and direction given in accordance with what the individual needs to succeed. In a mental health setting, clients may initially be seen in treatment in an acute state of distress or confusion that may necessitate waiting until their thinking has cleared. In the instance of clients who are confused and not expected to be able to make healthy choices (as with dementia), the family or other caregivers may become the identified "client."

Establishing a Safe Context

One of the therapist's first jobs is to ensure the clients' safety. When individuals are disoriented, confused, or frightened as a consequence of their mental disorders, the therapist's ability to provide necessary structure and to moderate the environment can help establish a safe context for intervention.

When the occupational therapist has an attitude of unconditional positive regard, he or she sees the person as a worthwhile human being and accepts the person's thoughts, feelings, and behavior without attaching a value to them. This too can enhance a feeling of safety and engender the belief that it is safe to "be one's self." When therapy occurs in a group context, the occupational therapist has a similar role

as group **facilitator**, establishing group norms that create an emotionally and physically safe setting and acceptance, and that provide information and feedback at the clients' level of understanding. This role as a group leader is discussed later in the chapter.

Function of Activities

As each therapist looks at activities or occupation in relation to each individual or group of people, the following will be at the very core: What activity (occupation) can best provide this individual or these persons with an opportunity to learn more about the self and/or successfully perform occupation that he or she or they choose? Closely akin to this question: What is this person's most pressing need? Therapeutic activities provide an opportunity for increased self-awareness, the ability to learn one's effect on and within the world around them, accepting and coping with feelings, an opportunity for positive change and increasing one's own efficacy, and a means to connect in a satisfying way with people and the world. Each of these can be examined more closely.

Meaningful Expression of Feeling through Art

When we think about activities as a means for self-expression, we often think of art. Art (e.g., drawing, painting, poetry, music, photography, and expressive movement) has diverse uses. These uses may be included as a means of self-expression, as a vocational or avocational pursuit, as a vehicle to increase self-awareness and self-acceptance, and to facilitate transition.

In discussing the use of art as a medium for working with persons who have been abused, Frye and Gannon (1990) describe it as a "way to tell," a "way to structure time," and as a "safe alternative to violence." Unchanneled anger, for example, can be released acceptably through expressive media. Then, when some of the energy behind the anger has been released, the person can identify the source of this anger. No matter what feelings are expressed, the process depends on the individual knowing that he or she will not be criticized nor punished for his or her feelings, nor will he or she be permitted to get out of control and hurt him- or herself or anyone else.

This use of art may occur in the context of group or individual intervention with children, adolescents, and adults. Use of art media for expression is based in part on the belief that repressed feelings or perceptions may emerge first through visual symbols, before the person can put them into words, and that such expression is health promoting. In persons who have experienced traumatic events, for example, unmanageable feelings may be preventing them from moving forward in their lives. In describing the use of art experiences with a group of men who have combat-related post-traumatic stress disorder, Short-DeGraff and Englemann (1992) describe self-expression as a way to "let go of past trauma" and make a "positive transition to healthful and productive living" (p. 27). With children, art media is a familiar form of play and self-expression. Occupational therapists who encourage expression through art or use art to meet other therapeutic goals need to clearly articulate the therapeutic goal in the use of art.

Though Frye and Gannon discuss the use of art with persons having dissociative disorder, their recommendations are generally suited to the use of expressive media in multiple contexts and are summarized here:

- Introduce the idea of art as a possible therapeutic task; do not push.
- Establish a verbal or written contract or agreement for safety in which participants clearly commit to not harming themselves, the physical space, or anyone else, if that is a concern.
- Acknowledge the work.
- Accept all work nonjudgmentally.
- Invite participants to tell you about their work.
- Avoid analyzing or interpreting the artwork; be aware of your own prejudices, biases, and opinions.
- The artwork belongs to the client. Let him or her decide what to do with it (i.e., display it, hide it, keep it, or destroy it).
- Consider encouraging clients to use art in an ongoing way, like a written journal, in which case they may wish to sign and date each piece; this enables the artist to reflect on changes over time (Frye & Gannon, 1990, p. 6).

In a similar vein, Short-DeGraff and Englemann describe multiple uses of expressive media for the treatment of combat-related post-traumatic stress disorder (1992). In their discussion they provide guidelines for using popular music, movies, and videotapes as well as art and written media. For example, one activity that they suggest, which can be done either individually or within a group context, has the participant write a letter or letters to "home" expressing "feelings of survivor guilt, shame, anger, either directed at themselves or directed toward others for leaving/deserting them or not showing them support" (p. 40). Short-DeGraff and Englemann echo the sentiments of Frye and Gannon and point out that self-expression by persons who have strong feelings can be an intense emotional experience, and clients need support and encouragement during and following the process (see Increase Your Understanding: Writing Confrontation Letters).

Regaining Self-Control

When an individual does not seem able to manage feelings, is confused or overwhelmed by them, or has a tenuous ego, the exploration of feelings may not be appropriate. In those instances, it may be that the therapist will help the person become involved in activities that are much less affect-driven and that have a strong task-focus. Being able to engage in a familiar, structured task (e.g., organizing supplies by type or color, re-potting plants) that is less emotionally

charged is something the person may be able to succeed at and be less emotionally stimulated by. It is not just that the person is diverted from troublesome feelings (though he or she may be), it is also that the task itself may be organizing or calming. In summarizing her findings about the internal or subjective experiences of persons having schizophrenia, Hatfield says, "Structure and predictability in the external world help compensate for the unpredictability of (their) inner world. Daily routines give pattern and a sense of order to life" (1993, p. 286). In this way, engagement in occupation is a means of establishing or maintaining a safe context for the individual. Remembering Maslow's hierarchy, the therapist respects the need for clients to be and feel safe, both physically and emotionally, in the environment.

As one individual with recurring episodes of schizophrenia writes,

> Because new experiences and environments create enormous pressures, I need the security of a predictable environment. I also know I must go slow when confronted with anything new, avoiding stressful situations... I know now that at times I may need to spend some time alone, and I take "time out," but not too much. (Leete, 1993, p. 281)

Establishing or Regaining a Sense of Self-Confidence and Coping Ability

In some persons, the most urgent need may be to regain or strengthen confidence and coping ability. Hence, the occupational therapist is equally concerned about ego function as it is reflected in an individual's ability to comprehend and use information for problem-solving, to manage frustration, to persevere and accomplish a task, to feel confidence in one's ability, and to integrate new insight into awareness and put it into action. The following example illustrates this.

A woman in her early 30s came into the occupational therapy facility during her brief hospitalization following an episode of alcohol abuse. She was attractive, articulate, and very pleasant as she assured the therapist that there was "nothing" that occupational therapy could do for her. When asked what she might do for herself, the woman laughed and said, "Are you kidding? Everything I touch, I mess up. I'm a walking disaster area." The pressing need in this situation was for this woman to experience herself as successful, and it became clear, as she gradually did try some activities, that she was determined to fulfill her prophecies. Through her interaction with several occupational therapy activities of her choice and by her willingness to pause and reflect on her behaviors, she was able to see that she often gave up or "messed up" just short of success, as if to prove her own beliefs about herself. Determined to change this pattern, she and the therapist worked together to help her try out some new, more successful ways of participating.

INCREASE YOUR UNDERSTANDING: WRITING CONFRONTATION LETTERS

Confrontation letters are letters, often not mailed, written by a person to another, typically to express powerful feelings that they have been previously unable to verbalize to someone who has hurt them (emotionally and/or physically). The intent is that the writer of the letter is able to freely express thoughts and emotions that have remained unexpressed. The writer is advised that the letter need not be mailed and that the point of writing such a letter is in the freedom of expression and catharsis that it permits. The ultimate outcome is that the individual has the ability to identify these painful feelings in order that he or she might be able to get emotional closure and move on (Forward, 1989; Short-DeGraff & Englemann, 1992, p. 41). Persons who have been traumatized by abuse or abandonment (Bass & Davis, 1994; Davis, 1990) may, for instance, write confrontation letters. Short-DeGraff and Englemann (1992) recommend their use in occupational therapy intervention with Vietnam War veterans who are dealing with unresolved feelings of rejection by loved ones at home. The person to whom the letter is directed need not be living, and such letters can also be a vehicle for helping a person cope with the grief process.

The following serve as very general guides for writing confrontation letters and can be used by occupational therapists wishing to facilitate this process:

- The writer needs to consider how long he or she will spend writing this letter. Some authors recommend that writers take as long as needed (Forward, 1989); others recommend that the writer set a time of 20 to 30 minutes in which he or she writes without stopping (Bass & Davis, 1994; Davis, 1990).
- Writers should choose a time and place where they won't be interrupted.

- Such letters are typically composed in private, but they could be composed within a group; ultimately, the decision may be made to share or not share with others in a group. Writers need to know that the letter's contents can be kept totally private; the decision regarding what to do with the letter is always the writer's.
- The goal is free expression and catharsis; therefore, the writer should not censor his or her writing. The writer doesn't need to use correct vocabulary, complete sentences, or proper spelling. Davis (1990) suggests writers not erase or cross out because, in her estimation, they probably meant what they initially wrote.
- Writers don't have to be "reasonable."
- Letters don't have to be mailed, but writers may choose to mail them.
- A letter can be written more than once.
- Forward (1989) suggests that though similar content may be covered with several people, it is important to write a separate version of the letter to each person.

Forward (1989, p. 239) proposes a structure that helps focus the letter:

1. This is what you did to me.
2. This is how I felt about it at the time.
3. This is how it affected my life.
4. This is what I want from you now.

Writing these letters is often an intense emotional experience; the writer needs to give him- or herself time afterward to readjust. Some persons may need emotional support, consolation, or a place to express rage; if carried out in a clinical setting, professional staff should be apprised that this activity has taken place and be available to provide support and follow-up.

In this example, therapeutic activities served as a vehicle for learning as this woman became more consciously aware of how she went about doing things. In this case, the activity process (and not just the outcome) was explored.

Persons with mental illness frequently have an impaired ability to perform functional activity. For some persons, this is a life-long impairment, and they have what can be termed persistent or recurring impairment of ego-function. That does not mean that they cannot be assisted to identify conditions in their own environments or things that they can do which support their optimal function.

For individuals with chronic mental illness, **increasing insight** means helping them to use information to manage their own lives. By becoming more knowledgeable about the nature of their own disability and about the psychotropic medications that can help them alleviate or lessen troubling symptoms, clients learn to establish sleeping and eating routines that optimize their health, and they get help to participate at a level at which they can succeed. This insight may enable them to have a quality of life. In this regard, mental illness is approached as is any chronic illness (e.g., diabetes or arthritis) in which one learns to best manage one's own limitations.

Relapse and Coping

As this woman writes of her own persistent mental illness,

> Those of us with mental illness must... learn what we can from the unfortunate experience of relapse and remember what helped us to recover and what did not... Like those with other chronic illness, I know to expect good and bad times... (Leete, 1993, p. 282).

The woman in Leete's book also goes on to say about her mental illness,

> I have come to understand that life may be more difficult for me than it is for others... Yet every individual... must develop skills in general coping, interpersonal relations, and management of work and leisure time. (Leete, 1993, p. 282)

As the hope increases that medications will enable persons with chronic mental illnesses like schizophrenia and major depression to participate more fully in everyday life activities, we recognize that these persons often need to learn the basic life skills that many of us take for granted. Describing a group for patients in rehabilitation at Case Western Reserves Psychosocial Rehabilitation Clinic, one reads:

> ...participants are asked to make a pie chart of a typical day. How big a slice does sleep get? Work? Television? Many schizophrenics are accustomed to sleeping 16 hours a day... They help one another... cook breakfast, buy Mom a birthday card, look for a job. (Wallis & Willworth, 1992, p. 56)

One woman says, "I can't drive a car. I can't follow a map. I have no idea what a computer is. It's really embarrassing. Just about everybody with an I.Q. over 70 can do things I can't do (Wallis & Willworth, 1992, p. 56)."

Other Means of Enhancing Performance: External Boundaries

Supporting ego function often means that the therapist will adapt the environment or task so that the client can succeed or will teach caregivers to make these adaptations. When persons are disorganized or have chaotic problem-solving, the occupational therapist might create boundaries for the client, lessening the number of choices to be made, making expectations explicit, or providing activities that have steps, a plan, or a design to follow. The therapist imposes external control to compensate where the person lacks internal control. Gradually, the client can recognize that he or she can do this for him- or herself.

Sometimes, for example, adolescents who have behavior problems are quite impulsive. In their impulsivity, they may unwittingly sabotage their own success because they don't take the time and devote the attention needed to complete a task or job successfully. In their frustration, they may blame themselves, their peers, or adults, or they may insist that "it doesn't matter anyway." If able to establish trust with this young man or woman, the therapist may be able to help the person look at their own behavior more realistically and identify alternatives to rushing through. Using the activity experience as a vehicle for learning, they can be encouraged to take a time-out when they get frustrated or feel hurried, or they can be taught to develop a blue-print for a task before they jump into a job. In addition to learning about their own task behavior in one situation, they can be encouraged to consider other situations in which they may find themselves in a similar jam. Overall, in increasing their repertoire for problem-solving, they strengthen future ego-function.

Reaffirming Priorities or Seeing One's Self in a New Way

For others, occupational therapy activities may be a vehicle to explore untapped skills and see themselves in new roles. When we ask our clients, "What would you like to learn?" or "What would be most important for you to accomplish right now?" it may raise questions that they haven't thought about in a long time. What are my priorities now? What do I enjoy? Illness and life changes may necessitate reappraisal; they also provide an opportunity for reappraisal of values, career, and lifestyle. One occupational therapist who treats persons managing rheumatoid arthritis makes it a point to always ask a new client, "What are you doing for yourself, that you enjoy, each day?" Depending on the therapeutic setting, the client may have the opportunity to explore new interests, hobbies, or ways of relating to others that would have been outside the routine he or she had previously maintained. The process may begin with a clarification of one's values and beliefs. We might think for a moment of what has probably happened in occupational therapy many times. An older man comes to the occupational therapy setting for the first time. He looks around and sees what appears to be a great deal of art and craft material, or perhaps a greenhouse, or even a woodshop. Red flags figuratively flash before him, and he announces in his own fashion something like, "Get me out of here!" Appreciating the roles and values this individual brings into the occupational therapy setting, he can be encouraged to look at the ideas he has about himself and the kind of tolerance he has for others. Perhaps he has never allowed himself to enjoy play, a hobby, or time for quiet thinking. The choices may be reaffirmed or disavowed. It will always be up to him to decide.

When occupational therapy offers group activities, clients may learn about themselves and their concerns in a group. They have an opportunity to learn more about how others view them and may have a chance to test out their ideas about others. These individuals have a vehicle for developing trust and for trying out dependence or independence. They may have the chance to compete or to try non-competitive play. They may learn more about their feelings toward sharing, losing, and winning. They may try out a new role as a leader, as a follower, or as a person who no longer identifies him- or herself as a "patient." In this model, the therapist appreciates that making external changes must often begin with seeing one's self in a new way.

In this reflection, the person ultimately asks him- or herself, "Who am I? What is important to me? What have I done today or do I have planned for tomorrow that makes my life meaningful?" For persons who have chronic mental illness, this question can raise painful realization of what has been missed as they see their peers marry, raise children, and celebrate life accomplishments that they have not been able to achieve. The occupational therapist that makes available learning experiences recognizes the critical importance of providing support and encouragement to the person.

Summary of Function of Activities

In summary, occupational therapy activities in the psychodynamic framework are seen as serving one or more of the following functions:

- They provide an avenue for increasing self-awareness and the appropriate expression of feeling.
- The structure in activities can assist persons with tenuous self-control or who are confused to feel safer and help them to increase their internal organization and to strengthen or re-establish self-control.
- They are an opportunity to enhance performance and improve functional skills.
- They provide an opportunity for examining priorities and trying out new roles or gaining confidence within already established roles.
- They provide a vehicle for learning more about one's relationship to others and enhancing social skills.
- They provide a means toward increased self-acceptance.
- They provide an avenue for improving one's quality of life—experiencing enjoyment, feeling competent, and connecting to something greater than the self.

Theoretical Assumptions—Guide to Evaluation and Intervention

The theoretical assumptions (see Psychodynamic Theoretical Assumptions on p. 96) are a summary of basic beliefs about the person, activities or occupations, and the environment or context. These beliefs are adapted from the psychodynamic theories previously described in this chapter. The assumptions about the person-environment-occupation variables and their possible relationships guide evaluation and intervention in occupational therapy.

Evaluation

The evaluation process in the psychodynamic framework uses subjective and objective assessments to gather data for planning interventions. The data increases our understanding of the relationship between psychological constructs and function and gives insight into client-centered variables.

Neo-Freudian Assessment

Assessment in occupational therapy has been described as the process of collecting information for the purpose of making informed decisions about the intervention process (Christiansen & Baum, 1991, p. 137; Opacich, 1992, p. 356). Psychological assessment in occupational therapy is the process of gathering information about the person's mind or mental function (including thoughts, perception, conscious and unconscious processes) and how it impacts the ability to engage in satisfying occupation.

As we have indicated, assessment within a neo-Freudian psychodynamic application is concerned with identifying the relative strengths and limitations and sometimes "style" of the ego in enabling functional performance and in assessing the effect that emotions or unconscious influences have on performance. This in turn is used to increase the mutual understanding of the individual's specific concerns, to identify the occupational performance areas in which the person wishes to make changes, or to identify adaptations and resources that will enhance the person's ability for functional performance.

Data Gathering in the Psychodynamic Model

To gather data, the occupational therapist uses assessment tools that may elicit information from both the subjective and objective perspective (i.e., the therapist will typically ask clients about their perception of personal needs and concerns, and their perception of their abilities). Additionally, the therapist may observe the clients engaged in task behavior and make judgments about the clients' effectiveness in approaching and following through with task behavior.

Projective or "Expressive" Assessment Today

Early occupational therapy assessments were identified as **projective** because the person was believed to project his or her personality into task performance. These early batteries typically incorporated art media (drawing materials, paints, collage, and clay), and as such, they encouraged the free expression by the client of feelings and emotions, as well as providing opportunity for creativity. For that reason they are also referred to as **expressive assessments.** The occupational therapist would observe the client's performance with a variety of these media in order to note favored object choices, symbolic representations, the manner in which materials were handled, and the use of defenses. This **sign of personality** approach is in contrast to a **sample of behavior** approach in assessment, which assumes that task behavior is situation specific (Goldfried & Kent, 1972). While projective batteries are seldom used today in mental health, the use of expressive media continues. These early assessments brought attention to the manner in which the ego enabled functional performance within a task and to the preference in styles in client performance. These assessments also brought attention to attributes/characteristics of various media and activities.

PSYCHODYNAMIC THEORETICAL ASSUMPTIONS

The psychodynamic theoretical assumptions listed below are adapted from the theories that contribute to the psychodynamic frame of reference. These assumptions contribute to the framework for evaluation and intervention in occupational therapy practice. Details of their application are described below.

The Person/Unique Individual

1. A patient/client is a valuable, unique individual.
2. He or she is the expert on his or her life, including his or her feelings, emotions, and what he or she needs to change in order to function more successfully in the environment.
3. He or she is capable of developing increased understanding of self and others, cause and effect, and to learn from experience in a process referred to as insight.
4. Each person has an internal drive to love and be loved, to use unique skills, and to feel that life has meaning.
5. Human behavior is influenced by what is conscious and by what is not conscious in the individual.
6. Increased self-awareness contributes to one's ability to make satisfying choices.
7. The person who is more self-accepting and has less need to keep "secrets" from personal awareness has more energy to put toward establishing an abundance of satisfying object relationships.
8. The person has an innate tendency to restore internal equilibrium.
9. An individual needs to feel both physically and emotionally safe in order to be open to new perceptions and to make changes.
10. A person's most pressing needs will naturally emerge and need to be dealt with first.
11. The person can be described via psychological constructs that refer to components and attributes of the psychological self. When the wholeness and integrity of the self is lost in focusing on these components and attributes, these have ceased to be useful constructs.

Activity/Occupation

12. Activities provide an avenue for appropriate self-exploration and expression of feelings.
13. When increased learning, self-awareness, and self-satisfaction are goals, the process of doing an activity is as important as its outcome.
14. The structure in activities can contribute to improved functional performance by people who have tenuous self-control.
15. The structure in activities can contribute to enhanced feelings of safety in confused persons.
16. Activities provide an avenue to connect to and find meaning in the world.
17. Activities and objects have no meaning in and of themselves—people give them meaning.
18. Being able to actually "do" an activity rather than just talk about doing it is a powerful learning tool that allows the person to integrate what they think, what they know, and what they believe. It can also change one's very identity in a way that introspection or "talk" alone cannot achieve.

Environment/Context

19. What is most important in the person's physical and internal environment will come to the forefront.
20. The patient/client-therapist relationship significantly impacts therapeutic process and outcomes.
21. Structure, predictability, and boundaries in the external (physical) environment help compensate for feelings of unpredictability, confusion, or tenuous internal boundaries within the person.
22. The creation and maintenance of an atmosphere of mutual respect/regard contributes to the members' sense of safety and helps members function optimally in a group milieu.

The occupational therapists who initially used these projective batteries made many inferences about clients' personality and the relative strength of their ego-function and the influence of these on performance. Today the occupational therapist can use expressive assessment in other ways. When expressive activities elicit emotions or feelings that a client has about him- or herself, he or she is viewed as the expert in terms of what these emotions may be. It is not the therapist analyzing the creative product. Clients can be encouraged to keep the products they have created and use creative expression in an ongoing way, as was described earlier in the chapter. In this way, assessment is the first step of the ongoing intervention process.

Expressive Assessment Instruments

The literature gives an extensive list and description of projective instruments, and includes the following:

- The Azima Battery
- The Shoemyen Battery
- The Goodman Battery
- The Lerner Magazine Picture Collage
- The Barbara Hemphill (BH) Battery
- The Ehrenberg Comprehensive Assessment Process
- Human figure drawing (including the kinetic person drawing and kinetic family drawing)
- Build A City

Table 4-2
EARLY OCCUPATIONAL THERAPY PROJECTIVE ASSESSMENTS

Name of Assessment	Tasks	Behavior and Constructs Assessed
Azima Battery (Azima & Azima, 1959)	Paper and pencil drawing of man or woman Make an object out of clay Finger painting	Mood Drives Ego organization Object relations
Shoemyen Battery (Shoemyen, 1970, pp. 276-279)	Tile mosaic trivet Finger painting Carve object from 4-inch vermiculite cube Model human figure from clay	Responses to tasks
Goodman Battery (Drake, 1999, p. 132)	Mosaic tile trivet Spontaneous drawing Human figure drawing Make an object out of clay	Organization Discrimination Sequencing Problem solving Ability for independence Ego boundaries Preferences Emotional tone Object and style preferences Need for control Use of tools
Lerner Magazine Picture Collage (Lerner, 1977, pp. 156-161)	Given colored construction paper and magazines; told to construct a collage	Cognitive-perceptual skills Nature and quality of defenses Affect Sense of self Quality of object relations

The first four of these are summarized in Early Occupational Therapy Projective Assessments (Table 4-2).

Barbara Hemphill (BH) Battery

The BH Battery (Hemphill-Pearson, 1999) consists of a mosaic tile trivet and finger painting. The therapist evaluates the patient's approach to the media in regard to ability to follow directions and problem solve; frustration tolerance; ability to perceive parts as belonging to a whole; ability to abstract, make decisions, and follow through in logical sequence; internal organization; intrinsic gratification; body concept; use of structure and flexibility; ability to handle limits and boundaries; and feeling tone. Observations made include those related to the manner in which the tasks are performed, statements made about the tasks, as well as observations of the outcome or "content" of what has been created. Preliminary studies have demonstrated inter-rater reliability in scoring during the performance of the two tasks include those related to posture, characteristics of verbalizations, the manner in which he or she uses space, and the patient's verbal responses.

Ehrenberg Comprehensive Assessment Process: A Group Evaluation (Drake, 1999)

During three 1-hour group sessions, patients are asked to complete a tile trivet, then to choose one of three projects (a collage, group drawing, or a problem-solving task) and complete it. The therapist is guided to look at interaction skills. The therapist also includes an interview about general education, employment and recreation history, and activities of daily living, and participants are asked to complete a daily schedule.

Draw-a-Person and Other Human Figure Drawing Assessments

Occupational therapists have used several versions of a draw-a-person test to assess body image in children and adults. Many of these came out of psychology and were designed as assessment tools for children, including the Draw-a-Man Test (Goodenough, 1926), later revised to the Draw-a-Person (DAP) (Naglieri, 1988); the House-Tree-Person (Buck, 1966); and Kinetic Family Drawings (Burns & Kaufman, 1970, 1972). Guidelines for the understanding and use of these assessments are in the citations provided.

Children and Human Figure Drawings as Maturational Indicators: Draw-a-Person (DAP)

Cross-cultural studies have demonstrated that there is a universal sequence by which children draw increasingly accurate human figures (Harris, 1963; Livesley & Bromley, 1973). In the DAP (Naglieri, 1988) a child is given an 8 inch x 11 inch response form and a pencil with eraser and is asked to complete, in order, three person drawings: one of a man, one of a woman, and one of the self. The DAP is a standardized assessment tool that has been normed on thousands of children from a broad spectrum of race, socioeconomic status, age, and ability. It can be scored according to a qualitative scoring, which attempts to identify atypical characteristics of the drawing (so-called **emotional indicators**), or a quantitative scoring system, which determines the developmental or maturational level (age-norm) of the drawings based upon the presence of key body parts, the extent of detail in the drawing, accurate placement of body parts, and the relative accuracy of proportion. Professionals outside of psychology, including educators and occupational therapists, may purchase the test. Practice drawings are provided in the test manual for the prospective assessor to gain the skills needed for scoring the assessment.

Human Figure Drawing With Adults

A request for one or more human figure drawings (or person drawings) when working with adults is also part of other OT batteries, including the Bay Area Functional Performance Evaluation, the Schroeder Block Campbell Adult Psychiatric Sensory Integrative Evaluation (discussed in Chapter Ten of this text), and the Azima and Goodman Batteries (see Table 4-2).

Human figure drawings and family drawings are considered useful as assessments not only because they permit the expression of issues related to self, body concept, and family relationships, but they also represent very graphically the ability to present one's self in an integrated fashion. There are classical indicators of neuropathology that are evident in human figure drawings. These include gross distortions in the placement of body parts, hemi-neglect, simplification and fragmentation within the drawing, and perseveration. As such, human figure drawings can act as a quick screen for central nervous impairment that suggests the need for further assessment and referral (King, 1982; Schroeder et al., 1978).

Build A City

The Build A City (Clark, 1999) projective task was developed in 1975 and presented in 1977 at the American Occupational Therapy Association national conference by occupational therapists Clark and Downey. It is based in part on the work of Erik Erikson in the area of play with children (Erikson, 1941), Lowenfield's Build A World technique (Bowyer, 1970), and Mucchielli's Le Jeu Monde et le Test du Village Imaginaire (Mucchielli, 1960). In all of these previous studies children and adults were given toys (representing people, cars, and buildings) and asked to create a scene, city, or village. Children and adults who had behavior problems displayed this in scenes that were chaotic or disordered.

In Clark and Downey's Build A City task, a group of adult clients are given a standardized number and size styrofoam blocks, construction paper, string, brads, clay, pipe cleaners, scissors, wooden clay tools, and a blunt knife and asked to work together to "build your ideal city." The time limit for this shared task is 30 minutes. The purpose of the task is not only to assess the task and social skills of individual participants but also the ability of the group as a whole to work together (see Working Through Grief). The task is believed to help stimulate a sense of community among group participants. A rating scale is provided to enable easy and consistent recording of observations.

WORKING THROUGH GRIEF

A similar task group has been used as a treatment tool with children who are grieving the loss of a family member. As described in the video, "Children Die, Too" (Films for the Humanities, 1990), children worked through feelings of loss and lack of control by creating a city for themselves in which all would be safe.

While Clark describes no studies of validity or reliability, the author cites instances from his 20-year experience with the tool in support of its utility.

Assessing the Impact of Psychological Constructs on Performance

Bay Area Functional Performance Evaluation (2nd ed.)

The BaFPE (Klyczek, 1999; Williams & Bloomer, 1987) is an assessment also summarized in this text with the discussion of behavioral assessments. Williams and Bloomer describe it as a functional performance evaluation. As cited by Klyczek (1999, p. 88), Williams and Bloomer define function as "the employing of useful activity" to satisfy "physiological and psychological needs through interaction with both people and objects." What makes the BaFPE particularly suited to the psychodynamic model is that it attempts in its scoring to rate how psychological constructs (e.g., self-esteem, self-confidence, motivation, and frustration tolerance) impact the person's performance.

The BaFPE consists of two sections: the Task Oriented Assessment (TOA) and the Social Interaction Scale (SIS). In the TOA, the client is asked to complete five different tasks: sort shells by like kind, complete a simulated money and marketing task, draw a home floor plan, duplicate a block design from memory or with the use of a cue card if needed, and complete a kinetic person drawing.

For the SIS, the client's social behavior in five different social settings is observed. These settings are a one-to-one interview, at mealtime, an unstructured group situation, a structured activity group, and a structured verbal group. As with the TOA, behaviors are ranked that include those related to psychological constructs.

Research: A number of studies have been conducted to establish the reliability and validity of the original and revised BaFPE (Curtin & Klyczek, 1992; Klyczek, 1999; Mann & Klyczek, 1991; Mann, Klyczek, & Fiedler, 1989). Included among these are studies in support of the tool's ability to discriminate among psychiatric and nonpsychiatric populations (Curtin & Klyczek, 1992), concurrent validity with the Functional Needs Assessment (Tardiff, 1993), Allen's ACL (Newman, 1987), subtests of the Wechsler Adult Intelligence Scale (Thibeault & Blackmer, 1987), and Part 1 of the American Association on Mental Deficiency Adaptive Behavior Scale (Klyczek & Mann, 1990), and predictive validity in regard to post-treatment functional performance (Accardi, 1985; Olson & Jamal, 1987). Studies in the use of the BaFPE with special populations include persons having eating disorders (Stanton, Mann, & Klyczek, 1991), nursing home residents (Mann & Small Russ, 1991), and adolescents (Wener-Altman, Wolfe, & Staley, 1991). Inter-rater reliability has been established for the original and revised BaFPE (Bloomer & Williams, 1982; Williams & Bloomer, 1987).

With the exception of money management and grocery market tasks, the nature of these assessment tasks are not likely to be tasks that are necessary for the client to function in his or her everyday environment. We would define the BaFPE as an assessment that incorporates the sign of personality approach in assessment. It also evaluates components of function.

Client-Centered Assessment

The preceding assessments have in common the rating by the therapist of client/patient behaviors. It is the assessor who has structured the assessment process and is making judgments about the influence of psychological constructs on behavior and the relative success of functional performance. In that respect these assessments represent the **outsider** or **objective perspective**.

When assessment data is gathered from the client's perspective, one can refer to it as **subjective** or from the **insider perspective**. Client-centered assessment strives to be subjective. Assessment can be subjective according to one or more of three criteria:

1. The client determines the feelings, behaviors, performance, and/or environment to be assessed.
2. The client reports on the feelings, behaviors/skills, and environment being addressed.
3. The client judges the adequacy of behaviors, skills, and conditions (Margolin & Jacobson, 1981).

Clearly, a subjective approach in assessment believes that the person is a reliable reporter and is the "expert" on his or her own life.

Another attribute of client-centered assessment is that it is individualized for each client; therefore, in a client-centered application of a psychodynamic model not every client is administered the same assessments. Rather, specific tools or procedures are selected after the occupational therapist has ascertained strengths, limitations, and concerns that are specific to this individual.

Because client-centered assessment has as its goal to determine what is important to the client, one often-used tool is the **unstructured interview**, punctuated by the open-ended request to please, "Tell me about your concerns," or "What would you like to accomplish?" Another often used tool is the **semistructured interview**, as exemplified by the Occupational Performance History Interview (OPHI-II) (Kielhofner et al., 1998) in which the therapist has specific areas that he or she covers within the interview but provides ample opportunity for the client to elaborate his or her specific concerns within that structure. A third format is the **self-report inventory**.

An assessment that has been designed with the intent of being client-centered and uses the format of a loosely structured interview and self-report is the Canadian Occupational Performance Measure.

Canadian Occupational Performance Measure (2nd ed.)

The COPM (Law et al., 1994) resulted from a collaboration between the Department of National Health and Welfare and the Canadian Association of Occupational Therapists to develop a client-centered outcome measure of occupational performance.

The COPM is described as an individualized measure designed for use by occupational therapists "to detect change in a client's self-perception of occupational performance over time" (Law et al., 1994, p. 1). It identifies problems in areas of occupational performance, evaluates performance and satisfaction relative to those problems, and measures change in the client's perception of his or her performance. It is designed to be used as an initial measure to determine client concerns, as an ongoing tool to help with goal reappraisal, and as a follow-up measure to assess client satisfaction. Occupational performance is addressed in the three areas of self-care, productivity, and leisure. The COPM is an outgrowth of the mandate within Canada to create a client-centered assessment of occupational performance that could be employed across specialty areas and with persons across the life span and from all cultures.

The COPM asks clients to report on occupational performance concerns and does not seek to externally validate or substantiate these self-reports.

Research: As of the 1994 second edition, the COPM had been tested with more than 500 persons. Surveys indicated that the COPM was useful to clinicians for identifying assessment issues (Law et al., 1994; Toomey, Nicholson, & Carswell, 1995). Preliminary studies supported test-retest reliability (Law et al., 1994). Validity has been explored in regard to the COPM's responsiveness to changes in client performance. Initial studies of validity were promising (Law et al., 1994; Rudman, Tooke, Eimantas, Hall, & Maloney, 1997; Sanford et al., 1994).

Guides for the Assessment Process

There are some general guides for psychodynamic assessment that reflect the desire shared by neo-Freudian and humanistic/client-centered therapists—that both therapist and client better understand the impact of psychological constructs on occupational performance.

Interview

If there is an initial interview, the therapist allows time to establish **rapport** with the patient. Rapport is enhanced by the therapist's attitude of warmth, openness, and regard, as discussed previously. In addition, the therapist may use the initial interview as a time to discuss confidentiality and to orient the client to the goals of occupational therapy and the purpose of the interview, as well as other assessment tasks. The therapist communicates his or her interest in understanding what is important and meaningful to the client.

Instructions

When there are specific instructions for an assessment, the therapist gives clear, specific instructions but does not offer suggestions for methods of task accomplishment. As the individual works, the therapist observes and notes verbal and nonverbal behaviors. These can be shared with the client when he or she is done. Typically, the therapist allows the client to complete the task before initiating discussion because discussion during the activity may be too distracting for the person and can affect his or her performance.

Atmosphere

The atmosphere during the evaluation should be one of mutual sharing and learning, not interrogation. The goal is for the client to gain personal awareness of his or her thoughts/feelings, skills, limitations, and/or concerns and have an opportunity to communicate these to the therapist. In the psychodynamic frame of reference, the therapist is often open in sharing his or her views with the patient, not as a form of judgment but as another perspective or as part of the information-sharing process.

The Figure Drawing as an Evaluation Task

Because the person drawing is used in several of the aforementioned batteries, as well as in assessments to be discussed in other frames of reference that follow in this text, we will illustrate how a person drawing might be presented and followed up as part of the psychodynamic intervention process. It is important to realize that use of a human figure drawing does not need to be part of a formal assessment but rather as a tool for enhanced awareness. For example, in a group described later in the chapter, women with eating disorders are asked to draw a figure of themselves as a vehicle for exploring their perceptions and beliefs around having an ideal body.

Adapted Person Drawings

The request for a human figure drawing might be part of an assessment battery, presented singly with an interview, or used as therapeutic activity. The drawing requested might be of a person, the self, or the self engaged in an activity; of the self doing something with the family; of the self in the future; or of the idealized self.

Person Drawing Protocol

The therapist has available several pieces of white, unlined paper (at least 8-1/2 x 11 inches; larger pieces can produce more expressive results) and two or more pencils with erasers. Crayons or colored marking pens or pencils are available if the therapist wishes to allow color to be an aspect of the drawing and increase the opportunity for expression.

The activity may be done individually or within a group. The client is typically seated with the therapist and asked, "Please draw a picture of yourself" (or "yourself with your family"). Patients/clients may express the concern that they "can't draw" or "can't do this." The therapist will communicate his or her understanding and give assurance that artistic ability is not the concern and that he or she would like the patient/client to try and draw a "whole person" and may add, "please don't draw a stick figure." The therapist can also assure the individual that when the drawing is finished, they will look at it together. This approach lets the patient/client know that the drawing will not be interpreted, but rather, the person will have the opportunity to look and see what he or she thinks. This attitude of valuing the individual's opinion frequently lessens the resistance to what can be a very anxiety-laden task. If possible, there is no limitation on the time allowed for the drawing. Individuals frequently feel a strong need to get the drawing right. When there is a time limit, however, the patient/client is told about it in advance.

Guide for Activity Processing and Feedback

The occupational therapist may help the person pay attention to the following:

- The manner in which the person selects and uses the media
- Comments made while engaged in the task
- The parts or aspects of the body or drawing that are given special time or care or that are ignored or glossed over
- The individual's general affect while doing the drawing
- Peripheral drawings or scribbles on the page and when, in the process, they were made
- The person figure itself

After the drawing is completed, one might ask the person or group members to pause, look at the drawing, and give it a title.

In this example, when the drawing is done as part of a battery of evaluation tasks, the drawing is often the last task presented in the sequence. This task sequence also allows time for the therapist to establish rapport with the patient/client and for the person to become comfortable with the evaluation process while completing the other tasks. As a consequence, there is usually less discomfort when it comes time to draw.

After completing the drawing, the therapist communicates a wish to look at the drawing with the patient/client (or group) with the goal of helping the person become more self-aware. The process might be started with a statement such as, "I am hoping that together we can look at this drawing and learn more about you and get a better understanding of what you want to accomplish for yourself while you are in treatment. What can you tell me about the person in this drawing?" or "Please tell me about the person in this drawing."

When an individual is reluctant or unable to respond to an initial request to tell about the drawing, the therapist might facilitate the process by making an observation about the drawing, or the manner in which it was approached. The therapist should always do this with a note of tentativeness in his or her voice, so that the patient/client feels invited to expand on or correct the therapist's observation. For example, the therapist might say, "I noticed that you drew a very light figure, almost as if it wasn't supposed to be seen. What are your thoughts now, as you look at it?" or, "I noticed that you erased your drawing several times, and I wondered how you felt while doing the drawing?"

Using Observation and Discussion Questions

Some individuals are unable to talk about their figure drawing even with support and assistance, and their limitations must be respected. Occasionally, these patients/clients are able to structure their thoughts in writing, and the therapist might ask them to respond to one or more issues this way.

Some questions that might be posed about the figure drawing include the following:

- What is the figure doing?
- Is the figure male or female? (if that is not evident)
- What does the figure in the drawing like about him- or herself?
- What would he or she like to change?
- What are his or her roles? To whom is he or she responsible?
- If engaged in a task, why was this task chosen?
- If the patient makes a family drawing, who is he or she placed near?
- Who is close to whom in the family? Who is isolated?
- What is the significance of the title (if one was requested)?
- What is the person in the drawing thinking?
- What is the person in the drawing feeling?
- What does the patient feel while looking at the drawing?
- What has he or she learned about him- or herself from doing the drawing?
- If a physical change or disability is reflected, what does the person feel about it? Are physical changes accurately depicted?

Human figure drawings and especially self-drawings are viewed as a communication about the self. In a way, it is as if the "self" is standing before the viewer and communicates non-verbally, much as one's body language communicates in any setting. Some things to consider are as follows:

- Small, lightly drawn and frequently erased drawings tend to appear apologetic; they do not communicate confidence or comfort.
- Large, bright drawings may exude confidence and a sense of importance; however, only the drawer knows.
- Body parts may be omitted or covered, scribbled, and erased when there is discomfort with their function.
- Drawings tend to appear masculine, feminine, asexual, or bisexual. What does the drawing communicate about the individual's comfort with his or her sexuality?
- A figure's expression, posture, and use of color communicate an affect or feeling-tone. Is it sorrow, confusion, "flatness" (lack of affect), joy, anger, other?

- A loss of integration in the figure (e.g., body parts disconnected, distorted, or missing) or the use of excessive symbolism often reflects a loss of integration in the individual.
- Inability to complete the task or a highly symbolic rendering may reflect an inability to deal with the self as a real and meaningful entity.
- Background objects placed with the figure in the drawing may provide emotional support or help define the individual's roles or what is important to the drawer.
- Drawings may be internally congruent or incongruent. For example, the title of the drawing is "I'm Me and I'm OK," but the figure in the drawing is frowning. The drawing may also be congruent or incongruent in relation to the drawer. For example, the person doing the drawing may appear sad and state that he or she is in treatment due to "depression," but the figure in the drawing is smiling.
- The amount of time and energy spent on the figure and on specific figure parts may relate to their importance to the individual.

Figures I-1 through I-18 in Appendix I are self-drawings completed by patients with whom we have worked. Some pertinent biographical data are included. They illustrate the manner in which figure drawings can vividly reflect an individual's sense of self and related concerns.

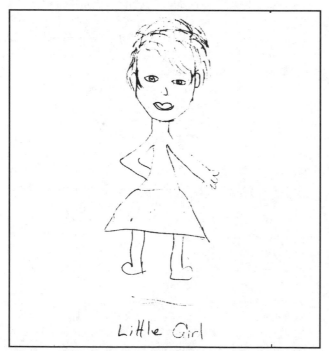

Figure 4-1. Self-drawing of a 19-year-old female (reprinted with permission from Bruce, M., & Borg, B. [1993]. *Psychosocial occupational therapy: Frames of reference for intervention* [2nd ed.]. Thorofare, NJ: SLACK Incorporated).

Sample Interview Dialogue

For Figure 4-1, we have included the beginning patient-therapist dialogue to further illustrate how communication around a task can be developed. A 19-year-old caucasian woman drew this figure. She sought outpatient treatment because of feelings of depression but was then hospitalized because of her physician's concern about her suicide potential. Her parents are recently divorced. In the interview she appears mildly overweight, wears a very short dress, and is well groomed. When asked to "please draw a picture of yourself," she uses the pencil to draw a figure about 6.5 inches tall in the middle of a 12 x 16-inch piece of paper and titles it "Little Girl." When the task is completed, the therapist initiates the following interview:

Therapist: What can you tell me about this drawing?

Patient: I like my eyes; I think they're my best feature.

Therapist: And the rest of your body?

Patient: I'm too fat. (pause) I don't like my body.

Therapist: Can you say more about what you don't like?

Patient: I don't like my legs and thighs. (pause) I just don't like any of it really.

Therapist: I'm struck by the title that you gave this picture. Can you tell me how you came to this title?

Patient: Sometimes I feel like a little girl. (pause) I wish I were a little girl again. It was so much easier.

Therapist: Easier than being a woman?

Patient: I know my parents don't approve of me, especially my father. They don't like the way I dress or the guys I date. I'm dating a guy right now, "R." Sometimes he calls me at 11 o'clock and wants me to come over. (pause, looking down) You know what I mean. He doesn't even ask me out on regular dates. When I come home, I feel really crummy.

Therapist: It sounds like you disapprove of yourself as much as your parents do.

Patient: That's right—I really hate myself. I wish I could be little again; then my parents would love me, and they'd be together and I wouldn't have to feel so crummy. I don't even know what I want to be and I have a crummy job as a... I'm a big flop. Do you know what I mean?

Therapist: Well, I think I'm starting to understand why being little again could seem so appealing.

Summary of Evaluation Process

The assessment process is designed to help clarify both the problem and pressing need(s) as perceived by the patient/client and to help identify the individual's strengths and available resources. The person drawing was discussed to illustrate the development of an evaluation task in the assessment process. Both structured and unstructured evaluation tasks as well as patient-therapist dialogue are used to help identify the patient's/client's personal perceptions, goals for therapy, and the ways in which these goals might be accomplished. During the assessment, the person is taught to focus on and identify specific goals for treatment and for occupational therapy. A person unfamiliar with occupational therapy may need assistance from the therapist in understanding what resources are available and how these can be used. Once the initial assessment has been completed, the therapist turns the process to goal setting and intervention. The assessment process is an ongoing one in which the patient's/client's progress continues to be evaluated and modifications in intervention are made as warranted.

Intervention

In the early history of psychiatric occupational therapy, an analytically oriented approach was used under the close supervision of the physician who prescribed treatment. Knowledge of psychodynamics and activities were used to identify personality structures, object relationships, defenses, and conscious and unconscious meanings of behavior. The occupational therapist used projective activities to develop object relationships, ego function, and defenses, and to increase the conscious awareness of the dynamic reason for symptoms (Fidler & Fidler, 1963).

Collaborating to Set Goals

Currently, in psychodynamic mental health intervention, the physician or primary therapist refers the client to occupational therapy and expects the occupational therapist to meet with the client and conduct an assessment to determine his or her needs/strengths and limitations as pertaining to occupational function. Often, the occupational therapist functions as part of an intervention team, (in a medical setting, this would most likely be referred to as the treatment team) and may collaborate with family members as well. Establishing intervention goals encompasses the following:

- Determining with the individual (or family) what the patient/client would like to accomplish as an outcome of therapy
- Planning a program that will provide the patient/client a means to this goal

The therapist strives to increase the patient's/client's ability to identify and satisfy personal needs, achieve greater insight, and to use this insight to interact more effectively within the environment. Within the broad goals of increasing self-awareness, developing insight, and improving problem solving, the occupational therapist sets specific individualized treatment goals for the person.

Specifying Intervention Objectives

The contemporary occupational therapist writes specific objectives that are easily understood and are stated in terms of patient/client outcome. Usually the goals are behaviorally identified and agreed on by the patient/client and intervention team. Third-party payers may use this when making reimbursement decisions.

While goals will be driven by client wishes and priorities in treatment, the client cannot necessarily identify his or her goal in the way that therapists write them. Clients may know, for example, that they are uncomfortable or want to be happier, want to be less depressed, want to be able to hold down a job, or want to get rid of the voices in their head. They may need considerable assistance identifying steps toward these larger objectives or goals. In talking to the client and/or his or her family and helping the client to set achievable goals, the therapist does an important piece of client education.

If the intervention duration warrants, treatment goals may be re-evaluated periodically, typically weekly or bimonthly, and modified as needed.

We have referred throughout this chapter to the general goals of intervention in this model. These include enhanced performance ability, including taking responsibility for one's own life, exhibiting improved functional problem solving, and being able to adapt to one's own circumstances; increased knowledge of what one needs to function optimally, self-awareness, and self-acceptance; recognition, expression and acceptance of one's thoughts and feelings; improved social skills (including communication skills and being able to cooperate with others in task performance); and increased ability for impulse control. How these goals will be articulated will depend in part on the length of intervention. When intervention is for a longer period (e.g., 2 to 6 weeks), both long-term and short-term goals may be written. For example, a long-term goal might be that the client exhibits improved impulse control in order that he or she be able to hold down a job; a short-term goal (or enabling objective) might be that during a given week, the client maintains self-control during the duration of an OT task group. When the intervention duration is short, then distinguishing between long- and short-term goals may be less clear. Nevertheless, one can look at the client's functional history and his or her (or family) concerns and determine appropriate goals given the person's concerns and probable discharge plans. For example, as described by Mary Conrad, MBA, OTR/L, a senior therapist working with severely disturbed children at Ohio State University Hospital, most of the children have extreme difficulty with managing feelings. They either express them inappropriately in an out-of-control manner, or they ignore them, as if feelings didn't exist. Since recognizing, appropriately managing, and expressing feelings are important components in one's being comfortable with one's self, being welcome to play with peers, and being able to succeed at school, an individual goal for many of the children is that they "learn/use one effective strategy to express feelings during their hospitalization." According to this same therapist, a child might be discharged to outpatient treatment or be discharged to home, only to be re-admitted at a later time. Often the children demonstrate skills learned in a previous hospitalization, and these can be built upon in subsequent treatment. This model is similar to that used for goal setting with adult patients who often begin as inpatients and then move to the outpatient setting.

Neo-Freudian Implementation

From the theoretical assumptions there are four guiding principles particularly evident in application of psychodynamic principles in the neo-Freudian (typically medical model) setting:

1. Adjust the degree of external structure and expectations for problem solving and internal control according to the patient's/client's ego strength
2. Safety first
3. Generally, persons do the best they can to maintain internal equilibrium and cope
4. Persons with a range of ability for "insight" can be taught to be more self-aware and thereby better cope if information is given in a manner that they can understand

OT Groups Today

The idea of a therapeutic group as described by Fidler (1969) embodies OT's commitment to learning by doing. One of the big changes in mental health care has been the shortened length of inpatient treatment. As we have indicated, those individuals who are hospitalized are often very confused or agitated. That being the case, these persons initially may be unable to participate in a treatment program. Then, when first entering OT groups, the groups in which they can succeed have a high degree of structure. Psychodynamic principles can also guide intervention in residential or community outpatient settings. In many instances, task groups similar to those envisioned by Fidler are part of extended community programming provided to assist those individuals who continue to need support in order to manage in the community. Residential living settings and halfway houses may incorporate similar principles in helping residents learn to get along and function in their daily lives.

Impact of Group Process in Treatment

According to this model, there are several things the therapist will need to consider when planning intervention for a population of persons having special mental health needs.

Patient/Client Expectations

Patients/clients who are new to treatment are often quite uncertain about what is expected of them in a patient or resident group. They may be frightened that the patient group will see them as sick or a "mental case," and they may be equally concerned about the pathology they see in other patients. The therapist needs to respect these concerns while setting a tone of mutual regard. The therapist also needs to be certain that the members or residents are introduced to each other and that they are given a chance to become more comfortable before numerous demands for interaction are made of them.

Varied Forms of Interaction

Depending on the format within a clinical or residential setting and on the therapist's goals, the following degrees of interaction may be evident and suggest the degree of social cooperation that best matches participants' abilities. These are listed in order of increasing demand:

- Individuals are working by themselves on their own projects or tasks, with little interaction but in the same work space as other patients.
- Several participants are sitting together, sharing materials, and talking, but each is working on an individual activity.
- Several participants or the entire group are working together, cooperating on accomplishing an agreed upon task; interaction and sharing, which are high as well as personal feelings, occur around the task.

Therapist as Group Participant

Within group sessions the occupational therapist may be a facilitator, observer, or participant-observer. Therapist participation can help ease patient/client anxiety or the initial reluctance to participate. For example, in this excerpt from a student therapist's journal, the OT student describes how she encouraged residents in a homeless shelter to paint newsprint to help decorate a dumpster for a Christmas food drive:

> I wasn't sure how this whole evening was going to go... I carried a pile of newspapers into the dining room and got someone to carry in the newsprint. Right on schedule, two people jumped up to see what I was doing. (Heubner & Tryssenaar, 1996, p. 29)

This is one way of **role modeling** and acts as an invitation to join in. If the group resists this permission, however, the therapist should be sensitive to this resistance and not try to force anyone to go beyond his or her present need or capacity. The process of change may be both inviting and threatening and, thus, tends to occur slowly.

Therapist as Gatekeeper

Within the therapy group, the occupational therapist has a **gatekeeping** responsibility. In this role he or she sees that safety needs (physical and emotional) are met, disruptions (subgrouping, scapegoating, abusive behavior) are responded to, materials and equipment are shared and used appropriately, and individual client and clinic or residence scheduling needs are met.

When the therapist wants individuals to function cooperatively as a group, materials and seating can be arranged to facilitate sharing and interaction, as in the preceding example. Group tasks, activities, or games may be introduced that will have their vitality depend on patient interaction.

Establishing Behavior Norms

To ensure that the group is one in which patients/clients feel accepted and safe and one in which feedback is given constructively, the therapist must be cognizant of the important role he or she has in helping set the norms of behavior. These norms would typically include free interaction among members; nonjudgmental acceptance; respect for individual boundaries; honest expression of affection, discomfort, and other feelings; and confidentiality (Yalom, 1975).

One way for a therapist to help establish norms is to be a model-setting participant, as we have discussed. Another is to clearly articulate expectations at the beginning of a group session. Often members who are familiar with the group's norms can be asked to re-state these to newer participants.

Increasing Participant's Self-Knowledge/ Processing the Activity Group

As an observer during the group process, the occupational therapist notes significant task and social behaviors, as well as the affect of members during the activity process. These behaviors and their possible significance to the person, to the groups' accomplishments, and to the emotional climate of the group can be discussed when the activity is completed. During the discussion, the occupational therapist may do the following:

- Highlight themes or concerns that the group may have in common in order to enhance the means by which participants can feel mutual support and learn from each other.
- Help patients/clients explore the thoughts, feelings, and memories aroused by the activity, including their satisfaction with the process and outcome of the activity.
- Help participants make a conscious association between the activity experience and past, present, and future experiences and difficulties.
- Using conscious associations, help the patients/clients increase their self-understanding and broaden their perspective on current social and task behavior, problems, and possible solutions (Mosey, 1970, pp. 71-81).
- Validate the clients' accomplishments and encourage them to validate themselves in the process.
- Assist members in looking at their task behaviors including:
  - —The choice of the activity and how this choice was made
  - —Individual skills demonstrated when engaged in the task (e.g., motor coordination, workmanship, ability to follow instruction)
  - —How members managed frustration and other feelings
  - —The type, quality, and system of communication that occurred during the group
  - —How decisions were made
  - —The extent to which members cooperated, including roles taken by each member
  - —The attitude displayed by group members toward each other and toward the therapist (Fidler, 1969; Fidler & Fidler, 1963)

Group as a Social Microcosm

It has been suggested that whenever people get together in this way, a **social microcosm** is formed. An individual tends to replicate in each group of which he or she is a member the patterns or behaviors that typify everyday social interactions. Thus, the occupational therapy group experience is a vehicle for learning about and possibly enhancing task and social skills that can be used in one's everyday environment. When the group provides a chance for intimacy and mature interaction, which may be lacking or minimal in everyday life, the patient in the group has an opportunity for what Alexander (1963) called a **corrective emotional experience**.

Member Feedback

If the group has been open in its verbal sharing, the participant can be given **feedback** about behavior not just from the therapist, but the entire group. Yalom (1975) suggests that in a group context, the participant may gain insight at several levels. Those most applicable to an occupational therapy group are the following:

- Insight as to how I am perceived by others: Am I tense? Warm? Aloof?
- Insight as to how I interact with others: Do I tend to exploit them? Reject them? Overdepend? Do I behave differently toward men than toward women?
- Insight about why I behave the way I do: How does my behavior make me feel? (Yalom, 1975, pp. 32-33)

By receiving this kind of feedback, the patient/client can engage in **consensual validation** (i.e., he or she can compare thoughts and viewpoints with the statements made by others and can reassess these views when he or she becomes aware of discrepancies). Studies suggest that whether the patient receives so-called "superficial" or "deep" insight appears to not influence the degree to which the patient finds feedback to be helpful. Any accurate feedback is considered helpful (Yalom, 1975).

The ultimate aim is to assist group participants in better understanding their social and task behavior, thereby enabling them to make conscious efforts to change or expand the manner in which each relates interpersonally and approaches activities. Further, when patients/clients have the chance to try out new, more successful behaviors within the group, they may have the added advantage of having the group express its approval and appreciation of this new manner of relating. Participants may increase self-esteem, and this confidence is hopefully carried into future situations.

We'll look next at a group that exemplifies the first two intervention principles: structure the occupational therapy group in accordance with ego strength, and consider safety first. After reading the description of the group, please see Sample Group Format: A Re-Entry Group for Adults with Chronic Mental Illness for details related to the group format.

Sample Group Format: A Re-Entry Group for Adults with Chronic Mental Illness

Orientation

Members are welcomed by name, including the therapist who introduces him- or herself and introduces new participants. The group will be identified (e.g., occupational therapy "Re-entry Group") and the purpose of the group reviewed. If the group meets each day at a given time, that information may also be shared. The general goals of the group are restated (e.g., "Our purpose in getting together is to help prepare you to get back to a healthy routine at home."). Goals specific for a particular session may be stated also (e.g., "Today our goal will be to learn ways to identify stress," or "We're going to practice paying attention," or to "practice sharing."). As leader, the occupational therapist will be responsible for establishing an emotionally safe climate in which members feel accepted and welcome. If there are any house "rules" they will be reviewed as well. Old members may be able to restate these for new members or the therapist may review them. The purpose is to not intimidate members with many rules, and rules may be as simple as "please stay and participate if you can; if you need to leave, we'd appreciate it if you'd quietly excuse yourself." Or, "It helps us all feel comfortable if we listen and try to respect the wishes of each other. Several of our members have said they'd prefer not to be touched, so we'll respect that wish."

Warm-Up

To help participants feel comfortable and to help engage them in the group, the therapist may lead one or more brief "warm-up" activities, which will be selected by the therapist to suit the mood and needs of the participants. For example, people who have been sitting much of the day may be encouraged to stand and stretch and "shake out the kinks," or if members have been involved in a hectic day they can be asked to identify something new they saw or learned today. The expectation will not be for lengthy discussion but rather for an appropriate comment. To enhance familiarity and comfort when participants are frightened by change, the therapist may use a similar warm-up each session in a series of therapeutic group meetings.

Group Task

Next, the group is introduced to the central task for the day. The task or activity will be brief, typically completed within 10 to 20 minutes, and will be selected in accordance with the needs and abilities of the participants. For example, the task could be around baking or decorating some cookies in which the dough has been pre-made. Each participant may be given a different colored icing to share, and all participants are instructed to get every color icing on the cookies that they decorate. Where participants are anticipating going home soon or moving to a different residential setting, members are anticipating discharge to home or prevocational setting, the task could be to make and exchange greeting cards that express one's feelings toward group members.

As described by Yalom (1983), the task could be a meaningful game in which members take turns leaving the room; while one member is gone, another member alters his or her appearance in some way; when the person is called back into the room, he or she has to identify who has altered their appearance and how (p. 302). Because the behavior of group participants may be erratic and the mood of the group changes, it helps if the therapist has several alternative activities that could be used if the one planned no longer seems suited to what the group needs.

Wrap Up

Typically, the therapist will wrap up the session, though he or she may elicit help from the members in doing this. The therapist can summarize what the group did that day, including restating the purpose of the activity. This helps emphasize what the purpose was in the tasks, as well as to highlight for members what they have accomplished. If certain themes emerged during the group activities, these can be stated. This serves to enhance the sense of "universality" that Yalom (1975) describes—the feeling that "I am not alone in what I am going through."

There is an opportunity provided for participants to give each other feedback. Since members can be quite fragile, this could be done in the form of "appreciations" in which members are encouraged to tell one or more persons in the group something that they did that they appreciated. The therapist can serve as a model for how this is done, especially in recognizing the smallest contribution or measure of appropriate behavior.

Example 1: A Re-Entry Group for Adults with Chronic Mental Illness

Persons with severely compromised function are often hospitalized for short periods, longer if necessary. They may have thought disorder, be markedly impaired in their ability to care for themselves and to relate meaningfully to others; some may be given a diagnosis that includes periods of psychosis (e.g., schizophrenia, psychotic depression, or bipolar disorder); others may not have a thought disorder but may be very unmotivated, or depressed, and therefore minimally functioning.

The task and social expectations in any type of group can easily overwhelm these people. The size of a group is kept small—usually four to eight clients. Applying the "safety first" principle, the role of the therapist is to structure a safe, supportive environment in which expectations will be kept low. Persons will be invited to stay the full length of the group (30 to 45 minutes), but if they cannot tolerate the full stay they know that they may leave. They may not be able to actively participate at first so just coming and watching may be an initial goal. The larger goal of the group will be for participants to be successful in brief social or task accomplishments.

Intervention with Younger Clients: Guidelines

The same general principles are applied when working with children and adolescents. The younger the child, the more rudimentary the ego skills and the less sophisticated the verbal and reasoning skills. The aim will be the same for the child as the adult: to increase his or her self-awareness, to experience success, to be comfortable with one's self, to be able to cope with feelings, and to feel competent to meet daily challenges. Children can have severe emotional disturbances that interfere with age-appropriate ego-function. In the instance of psychotic disorders, children may receive the same medications as adults. Therapists expecting to engage with severely disordered children are encouraged to go more deeply into the literature and gain experience in that specialty area. The following serves only to highlight the application of psychodynamic principles with children:

- Children are not miniature adults. The therapist needs to be cognizant of their place in the developmental scheme described previously.
- Children are people with thoughts and feelings who need to accept these feelings and find an appropriate way to express them.
- Children too have a sense of who they are, what they look like, and what they are capable of. Engagement in purposeful and meaningful activity can enrich that understanding, helping it to become more differentiated and more accurate.
- Children need a safe, trusting relationship with the occupational therapist to participate optimally in therapeutic experiences.

- Children have preferences and can usually be included in making decisions about activity choices; the younger child typically does best with limited choices. The parents/caregiver of very young children or non-communicative children may be able to identify the child's preferences, temperament, and special concerns.
- The younger the child or the more disturbed the child, generally the less his or her ability for impulse control, sustained attention, and the ability to postpone gratification; activities need to be graded accordingly.
- Like adults, children may avoid experiences or challenges in which they expect to fail.
- Play is the vehicle through which younger and mid-aged children can enjoy themselves; learn social, physical, cognitive, and occupational skills; learn coping strategies; and express and accept unfamiliar or uncomfortable feelings. Older children can also participate in playful experiences, but are developmentally ready for other forms of creative expression, group projects, and more work-oriented activities.
- Children can generally learn to understand the effect of their behavior on others and gain skills in self-control if adults use vocabulary that is at their level of understanding.
- Activity groups with peers provide a potent tool for helping children to learn social/emotional skills and practice problem solving. The extent to which the therapist as adult leader needs to impose a structure and control the group will vary according to the age and skills of the participants. It will be important to consider not only the children's cognitive level, but also their level of moral development (their manner of making decisions about right and wrong), their skills in problems solving, and the extent to which they are familiar with the games and tasks being used in the group.

As with adult groups, the therapist has a role in creating and enhancing an atmosphere of safety and acceptance in the group.

Example 2: A Group for Highly Disturbed Children (as described to the authors by Mary Conrad, MBA, OTR/L, Ohio State University Hospital)

The children in this group have a variety of psychiatric diagnoses including schizophrenia, psychotic depression, and conduct disorder. The children average in age from 5 to 12; most are between 6 or 7 and 12. If a 12-year-old seems to have more in common with older clients, he or she may be treated in the adolescent group, which typically is for young people age 13 to 17. These children come into treatment very disturbed, and the first order of business is often to get them stabilized on one or more psychotropic medications. Medication is not expected to solve all their problems. Most have a history of poor social and task skills, few friends, often a history of bizarre or inappropriate behavior, and many have been abused.

Because of the variety of their ages and developmental needs and because many are initially unable to cooperate in a task group, the therapist most often sees the children in a group context in which all are working on a craft project and sharing materials, but doing the project at their own levels. The use of crafts in this instance makes a good fit with the interest that children in the 7 to 11 age group often have in doing craft projects. The goal is for each child to create an end product in which he or she feels successful. Task goals can include better sharing, being able to ask for what one needs, learning strategies for impulse control, being able to express needs and feelings in an appropriate and effective manner, and having and expressing feelings of pride in what one has accomplished.

While cognizant of behavior management principles (discussed in our next chapter), the therapist is especially interested in helping the child learn some effective strategies for internal control, which include increasing his or her awareness of his or her needs and feelings and finding a way to express these. Many of these children have seldom, if ever, had an opportunity to engage successfully in age-appropriate play or tasks, so creating an environment in which they can succeed at "being normal" is another goal. In observing the children select and work on their "project" the therapist gains important information about the children's strengths and limitations that help him or her make recommendations related to post-discharge planning.

Example 3: A Cooking Group for Persons with Substance Abuse Disorders and Dual Diagnoses

One outpatient group at a community health center experienced frequent change in patient population, with the average length of patient treatment being 1 month. A criterion for this group was that the participant had either a substance abuse disorder or a dual diagnosis of substance abuse and a second diagnosis (e.g., bipolar disorder, depressive disorder). Common problems for the individuals in this group were poor eating habits, inconsistent work skills, lack of enjoyable leisure activities, and difficulty getting along with peers. Most in the patient group had been inpatients for a brief stay during which they withdrew from alcohol and medications were regulated.

To encourage interaction and build specific skills, the occupational therapist had the patient group, which varied in size from 5 to 10, plan and carry out the preparation of a noon or evening meal. Patients purchased all supplies, prepared food, and cleaned up. The occupational therapist was a resource person only. On some occasions, the patient group would vote to invite one guest each to share their meal. It was useful for the group to consider their own feelings about having guests. When the group had achieved a strong sense of unity and each patient felt accepted by the group, the issue of having guests was not volatile. When there were less ease and cohesion, the prospect of having guests made many patients anxious. When potential guests included persons not in psychiatric treatment, many patients had to confront the personal struggle they were experiencing about being in treatment.

This group had many tasks and subtasks that required good organization and problem solving. Equally significant, patients had the opportunity to experience themselves in a social setting that was quite similar to an everyday social situation.

This cooking group was a popular patient activity. Food and sharing food with others play important symbolic functions in our culture. In breaking bread together, patients could give to themselves and to each other in a meaningful and enjoyable way.

Example 4: A Group for Women with Eating Disorders (conducted by Leanna Noonan, MA, OTR)

This group is composed of 5 to 10 women, all of whom have an eating disorder and are inpatients on the psychiatric unit of a rehabilitation hospital. The duration of inpatient treatment is typically 1 to 2 weeks, during which time an important goal is to medically stabilize the women. Once this has been accomplished, many of the women will be discharged to become outpatients in a follow-up group.

The larger goal of the OT group is for the women to confront the feelings they have about themselves and their personal effectiveness, including their perceptions and feelings about their bodies. More immediate goals might include those related to articulating/expressing values and beliefs related to self-image, body image, effectiveness in one's life, and control. The women are neither necessarily underweight nor overweight; however, all have a preoccupation with and/or aversion to normal eating. Some, who may appear of average weight, are preoccupied with not only their weight but their overall physical appearance. Art media and drawing in particular are often used in therapeutic activity.

For example, in one group session each participant is asked to draw a picture of herself as she currently appears. The therapist pays attention not only to what each participant draws, but also the relative amount of time and attention given to various parts of the body in each drawing. Participants are then encouraged to look at their own drawings and notice how they depicted themselves, as well as those areas of the body in which they spent the most time or energy drawing. Group dialogue might be around the drawings and one's own feelings, as well as societal values/expectations and what the participant has learned in her own family about food, eating, or the importance of physical appearance. Ultimately, the group members support each other's efforts toward enhanced self-awareness, self-acceptance, and healthier lifestyles.

Combining Neo-Freudian and Client-Centered Principles in Helping Individuals Cope with Loss and Grief

A premise throughout the chapter is that psychodynamic principles apply not only to mental health settings, but any therapeutic encounter with the "whole" person. One instance in which this is especially evident is when therapists engage with clients who are coping with loss. Such loss may be around loss of independence, loss of physical prowess, loss of abilities, loss of a significant other, and loss of wage-earning ability. For family members of persons with chronic mental illness and for the chronically mentally ill individual, loss may be protracted around hopes for "'normalcy, as the mentally ill person may have episodes of health or being his or her 'former self'" (Miller, 1999, p. 417). Whatever the loss, grief is viewed as a normal response that ultimately allows the person to move forward and re-engage in life.

While the work of Elisabeth Kubler-Ross (1969) focused on the stages of grief people go through when they learn they have a terminal illness, similar models have described the typical stages of grieving any loss (Burnell & Burnell, 1989; Worden, 1982). To review, **grief** can be defined as an intense feeling of emotional suffering associated with physical and behavioral change, which is a normal response to loss. Grief is believed to be a universal experience that, to be resolved, requires that the griever accept the reality of the loss, accept the grieving as painful, adjust to changed circumstances, and re-invest or redirect energy from what is not to what is possible/available (Burnell & Burnell, 1989).

Grief begins with shock and denial, which can be understood psychodynamically as defenses against overwhelming information. The next phase of grief involves confronting the loss, which typically includes strong emotional responses—anguish, anger, and sorrow—as the reality of the loss sinks in. A normal part of this confrontation is preoccupation with thoughts about what has been lost and trying to make sense of the loss. Finally, in the last or resolution phase, the individual becomes increasingly able to withdraw energy from thinking about the loss and re-invests that energy in new activities or new roles. Resolution involves acceptance of the loss and that something has been irrevocably changed in the griever's life.

Guided by their understanding of the progression of grief, occupational therapists can intervene in a manner that makes use of psychodynamic principles and that equally respects the need to respond to what the client/griever experiences as his or her most pressing need.

Example 5: Groups for Children Dealing with Serious Illnesses or Loss of a Family Member

The video *Children Die, Too* (Films for the Humanities, 1990) depicts a group for children who have experienced the death of a family member. As depicted in the video, one group session began with members drawing whatever they would like. One participant drew a city, and soon other members followed his lead, and together the entire group, over the span of several meetings, created a mock city in which each member took on a special role. This was done not only through drawing but also through the children's enactment in play and with props. The outcome of the activity was the creation of a city in which everyone would be safe. As described in the video, the group facilitator believed that through this experience the children dealt with their need to feel safe and to feel a sense of control.

It is similar to other groups for children who are themselves dealing with serious illness. Carolyn Porter, MS, OTR describes one such group: The children meet one or more times per week in a room rich in art supplies, toys, stuffed animals, puppets, and other enticing supplies. One "rule" of the group and of the environment itself is that no hospital staff member may enter uninvited. Thus, the room in which the children gather represents a safe haven from the tests and treatments so often associated with a hospital setting. Sometimes group participants engage in free play and structured games that represent the normal play of children. Because these are psychologically healthy children, it is not necessary for the therapist to be as structured; often she takes on the role of encourager and resource, and the children have the primary responsibility for determining what they would like to play or do on a particular day. Other times, the group may be encouraged to draw and paint and, in doing so, has an opportunity to express feelings and emotions that may be hard to put into words.

Example 6: Using Psychodynamic/Client-Centered Principles in Therapeutic Interaction with One Client Who Has Experienced Loss (Note: the following example is based on actual therapeutic sessions).

Shock

When Maggie, a home-care therapist, walked through Mr. E's front door, she sensed immediately that something was wrong. Mr. E had a hip fracture 5 weeks ago and still needed assistance in the home to take care of himself. She found him sitting in his favorite chair looking dazed. Usually he was smiling and appeared eager to begin "working" as he called it, so Maggie immediately asked, "What's wrong?" He told her that his wife had "passed away" yesterday. His wife, herself quite ill, lived in a skilled nursing facility across town, and Mr. E was only able to see her on weekends when their children would come to town and drive him. Maggie looked around and saw indications that the certified nursing assistant (CNA), who came early each day, had been there; there were breakfast dishes in the sink, and Mr. E was clean-shaven. She wondered why no one from the agency had notified her. She knew that he was in no place to be practicing meal preparation, as was her plan for today. Concerned for his safety and well-being, she asked Mr. E what he needed to do today and how she could be helpful. He indicated that his children were coming later and that he didn't know what to do other than wait. His eyes were teary-looking, but he was not actively crying. Maggie sat down and took his hand into hers and said nothing.

Before she left, she made a call to the agency to make sure that all staff realized what had happened. It had been arranged that the case manager, a registered nurse (RN), would come by later that day to check on Mr. E and would call his family.

Confrontation

The next time Maggie saw Mr. E. in therapy was about a week later. She had dropped by one time before then just to make sure he was "okay" and had brought him a dish of lasagna. The funeral had been held, and his family was back to their own homes, and he was again alone. This time Mr. E was much more talkative. He spoke about his wife, how they had met, their courtship, and what a wonderful mother she had been to their two boys. Maggie listened attentively, while able to suggest that Mr. E could practice making bacon and eggs standing at the stove, as they had planned. With a bit of extra attention on Maggie's part, she was able to let Mr. E practice at the stove and was still able to let him talk. She stayed longer than usual so that she could be there when he ate his breakfast but nevertheless made it to her next appointment on time.

Moving On

Maggie's last intervention session with Mr. E was about 6 weeks after his wife had died. In each of her preceding visits he had talked about her, but he talked about other things too. He had known she was very ill and, as he said, every time he had said "goodbye" to her, he knew this might be the last time he would see her. It was hard to not be able to visit her any more, yet somewhat a relief because it made him "feel bad" that she was "failing" physically. He and Maggie used the last two treatment sessions to talk about what Mr. E would like to do now that his wife was gone. Did he still want to live in this house, or might he wish to move in with one of his boys? He indicated that he had thought about it, and this was still his home. As long as he was able, he wanted to live here on his own. Maggie was concerned that without his weekly visits to his wife, he had very little to look forward to each week. She inquired about his interest in joining the Senior Center, or at least getting on their mailing list so that he'd know about any outings they might be planning. He said he wasn't interested in "hanging around a bunch of old people." He then shared with Maggie that one of his neighbors down the street had begun visiting with him and invited him to go along with him and some of his cronies to a gambling town not far away. He said they met for breakfast on Friday mornings, then spent the day at the casinos. He "reckoned" that he'd like to join them.

Accountability: Demonstrating the Efficacy of Psychodynamic and Client-Centered Approaches

Does Client-Centered Practice Make a Difference?

According to Hammell (1998), occupational therapists frequently state that their primary goal is to enhance a client's quality of life, but most outcome measures have sought to assess functional achievements (p. 138): Can the client dress himself? Can she write a resume? The attention is not usually on, "Does he or she desire to do so?" or "Will he or she do so once therapy has concluded?" The push in quality assurance is for measurable, functional outcomes, as third-party payers ask in particular, "Is this person capable of being more independent?"

In the edited text, *Client-Centered Occupational Therapy* (Law, 1998), in her chapter entitled, "Does Client-Centered Practice Make a Difference?" Law summarizes her review of the literature for evidence in support of client-centered practice. The three areas she focuses on are the relationship of client-centered principles with:

1. Adherence by clients to intervention recommendations
2. Client satisfaction with intervention outcomes
3. Positive functional outcomes

Her search is not exclusive to the field of occupational therapy service and includes studies that employ both quantitative and qualitative research designs. Law (1998) cites numerous studies that demonstrate a significant relationship between giving of information and shared decision-making, supportive and respectful care, and patient/family satisfaction (Caro & Derevensky, 1991; Doyle & Ware, 1977; Dunst, Trivette, Boyd, & Brookfield, 1994; Henbest & Stewart, 1990; King, Rosenbaum, & King, 1996; Stein & Jessop, 1984); a positive relationship between supportive/respectful care, client-therapist partnership, and client adherence to intervention recommendations (Avis, 1994; King, King, & Rosenbaum, 1996); and a positive relationship with improved family/client functional outcomes (Dunst, Trivette, & Deal, 1988; Greenfield, Kaplan, & Ware, 1985; Landefeld, Palmer, Kresevic, Fortinsky, & Kowal, 1995; Moxley-Haegert & Serbin, 1983; Starfield et al., 1981). The reader is referred to Law (1998) and Law and Mills (1998) for further citations in this area.

The evidence in support of client-centered practice, while compelling, raises other questions and is evocative of similar research studies in the 1960s and 1970s. During that time, as mental health practice expanded well beyond that of the traditional Freudian model, there was a plethora of literature and research in the quest to demonstrate which psychiatric and psychological approach (e.g., Freudian, Rogerian, behavioral) was the most efficacious. While stated very simply here, three conclusions that seemed to come from this and that could reasonably apply to occupational therapy were:

1. One should not be asking which is the best approach, but instead, "What treatment, by whom, is most effective for the individual with a specific problem, and under what circumstances?" (Patterson, 1974, p. 539)

2. Regardless of clinical orientation, there needs to be a "good" relationship between the therapist and the client.

3. What was meant by "good" resided largely in the client's perceptions but most likely included respectful, empathic concern for the client (Patterson, 1974, pp. 528-531).

Individualized intervention, which respects the client and seeks to establish a good therapeutic relationship, is not exclusive to what has been labeled "client-centered" within this model, but the conclusions drawn are that regardless of any other model or orientation embraced, "client-centeredness" has a powerful impact on therapy.

This research in support of client-centered practice within occupational therapy leads one back to a very old question asked when Carl Rogers and other humanists were writing in the 1960s. This question was, "Is client-centered intervention both *necessary* and *sufficient* to account for change?" As occupational therapists apply the client-centered model in their intervention, it continues to be a provocative question.

The Utility of Psychodynamic Constructs

What then of the efficacy of a neo-Freudian, psychodynamic application? As described in this chapter, such an application is, in large part, conceived of as a "paying attention" to things internal—feelings, emotions, and thoughts not held in conscious awareness but believed to have a powerful impact on behavior and occupational performance. Within a medical model, particularly a psychiatric setting, it may be easier to recognize when a psychodynamic model is the predominant orientation. The early descriptions by Fidler (1963, 1969) of patient groups and individual patients engaged in what is clearly a psychodynamic program allude to the effectiveness of task groups in occupational therapy that emphasize insight and self-awareness, much as do the case examples provided to us by contemporary therapists. But, such a "paying attention" to psychological constructs may be much subtler yet just as significant in a non-psychiatric context. The narratives described in the occupational therapy literature by Mattingly, Fleming, Peloquin, Kielhofner, and Helfrich, to name just a few, suggest that to not pay attention

to these internal constructs is a failure to consider what is meaningful to the client and may ultimately sabotage therapy. One possible avenue for further study would be meta-analyses of such narratives to better identify what factors contribute to client satisfaction and improvement.

Whether or how psychodynamic language is introduced and perpetuated within the psychodynamic community is helpful in broadening not only therapists' but also clients' understanding of what people and their families need, and how it may or may not help in our framing of intervention remains to be clearly demonstrated not only within OT but psychiatry at large.

Summary

Physical concepts are free creations of the human mind and not, however it may seem, uniquely determined by the external world. In our endeavor to understand reality we are somewhat like a man trying to understand the mechanism of a closed watch. He sees the face and the moving hands, even hears its ticking, but has no way of opening the case. If he is ingenious he may form some picture of the mechanism that could be responsible for all the things he observes, but he may never be quite sure his picture is the only one which could explain his observations. He will never be able to compare his picture with the real mechanism and he cannot even imagine the possibility of the meaning of such a comparison.—Albert Einstein (Zukav, 1980)

Regard for Subjectivity

Collectively, the psychodynamic framework for understanding a person and his or her endeavors depends on the therapist's belief in the integrity of subjective experiencing. Although the framework draws its philosophical base from a diversity of sources both within and outside of occupational therapy, the following beliefs are key:

• As a person sees his or her world, so is the world.

• A person's feelings and perceptions about personal endeavors have a significant impact on his or her actions.

• People can make better decisions when they are informed.

• The more a person is aware of personal needs, beliefs, values, and feelings, the more real freedom he or she has in making choices.

• Understanding an individual's history of experiences can assist the therapist in understanding what is important to the person and his or her current approach to life.

- The patient-therapist or client/therapist relationship significantly affects the therapeutic process and its outcome.
- Each individual has an internal drive to love and be loved, to use unique skills, and to feel purposeful and significant, and this is achieved through active engagement with people, things, and occupations.
- Human endeavor is influenced by what is conscious and unconscious in the person.
- The person who is more self-accepting has more means available to interact positively with others and to develop his or her potential.

Although consideration is given to the social context and the quality and function of activity, the locus for looking at occupational performance is from the view of the individual. While not specifically addressed in this text as a developmental theory, the psychodynamic model is, in fact, developmental in its ascribing to the person a sequential development in self-perception, relatedness to others, relatedness to objects, and ability to successfully engage in activity and participate in one's community.

CONTRIBUTIONS AND LIMITATIONS OF A PSYCHODYNAMIC FRAMEWORK

Contributions

Understanding Meaning

As has been stated, the psychodynamic framework provides a vocabulary and hypothetical constructs for talking about and understanding feelings or the subjective self and what lies at the very heart of the human condition. Proponents of this framework emphasize that subjective experience is a valid and integral part of being a person and is the only way that "meaningfulness" of engagement in occupation can be truly determined. It is the psychodynamic model that directly addresses "meaningfulness" of activities and quality of life. Further, based in this framework, the occupational therapist acknowledges that what one "feels" and what one "knows" may be quite different and that feelings are not always logical or easy to understand. Yet, they are so important in determining whether or not the patient/client will profit from occupational therapy. Preliminary studies suggest that persons who have the opportunity to express their feelings and trust that they are understood and accepted can focus more easily on tasks that are meaningful to them, are more satisfied with therapy, and are more successful in meeting functional outcomes. Further, viewing the individual patient or client as capable of insight, even if limited, helps direct therapy toward a goal of enablement and empowerment rather than caretaking by the therapist.

Connections to One's Life History

The psychodynamic framework provides a context for approaching and understanding an individual's history or previous experience. This characteristic has been considered by many to be a detriment rather than a contribution to the extent that traditional Freudian ideology was judged by many as having placed too much emphasis on patient history. However, when individuals are given an opportunity to reflect on and better understand their past experience as it relates to their goals for the present and the future, it helps provide continuity and, again, helps secure the meaningfulness of therapeutic engagement.

Positive Emphasis

We might each pause to reflect on our own feelings about our personal past. How often do we, upon making new friends, wish to share with them information about where we come from, our family upbringing, and meaningful events and relationships in our lives? How often do our children ask us to tell them about ourselves when we were children? In occupational therapy, this interest in clients' life histories has recently been pursued through the use of narratives. Given what has been learned about the physiologic basis for many mental illnesses and the importance of experience and learning, neither the neo-Freudian nor client-centered applications view behavior as predetermined. Both engender a positive set in regard to the person and his or her potential for change. It is an optimistic posture that emphasizes the possibilities, not fallibilities of the individual.

Humanism Supports Client-Centered Model

Existential-humanistic input and the re-embracing of the client-centered model in particular have focused attention on the significance of the therapeutic relationship in intervention. It encourages the occupational therapist to be more conscious of his or her role and responsibilities in the therapeutic relationship, calling for active participation and not passivity nor inappropriate care-taking. For those new therapists who may be especially concerned that they will harm a patient/client by saying or doing the wrong thing, the emphasis on listening to the individual/family and respecting his or her pace and choices provides a good starting place.

In encouraging patients/clients to be independent and emphasizing their responsibility for their welfare, the psychodynamic framework strives to facilitate carryover of gains made through intervention to home or post-discharge. In addition, by looking to internal, naturally evolving rewards rather than rewards designed by staff members, changes made by the person are viewed as more enduring.

An important contribution of existential-humanistic and neo-Freudian applications of this theory is that they encourage the therapist to consider each person as unique, in terms of personal style, preferences, and life history. In accordance, the therapist is encouraged to approach each person/family as special and unlike any other. Intervention is individualized, and diversity is respected.

Increase Understanding of Behavior

At the same time, the psychodynamic model when applied by occupational therapists provides a way to put behavior by individuals who may be confused, frightened, chaotic, aggressive, or defensive into perspective. Psychodynamic principles provide a means by which to determine when structure and boundaries in the therapeutic setting are necessary and helpful. Therapists who understand the principles behind defensive behavior by clients/patients, for example, can appreciate that individuals might reject information that they are given, or refuse to try something new, when they are not ready to change their self-perceptions.

The examples of intervention provided in this chapter were instances in which psychodynamic principles appear to be especially useful for understanding what is not adequately explained by any other models. These instances included applications with persons experiencing grief and loss, persons who have been abused, persons with post-traumatic stress disorder, and persons with eating disorders.

Limitations

Psychiatry's methods and outcomes have long been criticized. The bottom line for these critics is that many persons who have mental illness do not improve or, if they do improve, may relapse. Mental health treatment has historically been expensive, and in the eye of critics, taken too long. The treatment of mental illness through pharmacological means has become increasingly popular and, at times, has appeared to border on the medicalization-away of any uncomfortable feelings.

As they write in the introduction to their textbook on psychiatry, Kaplan, Sadock, and Grebb (1994) observe that we are in the midst of "seismic changes in the delivery of health care in this country... Drugs, rather than psychotherapy, will become the treatment of choice, in spite of the fact that many studies have found the superior efficacy of drugs when used in conjunction with psychotherapy in the treatment of most mental disorders" (p. ix). They conclude their comments with their belief that "prejudice toward psychiatry and fear of mental illness are largely responsible" for the limitations being imposed in psychiatric treatment (Kaplan et al., 1994, p. ix).

Research Needed to Evaluate Outcomes

To the extent that occupational therapy is a part of that mental health system and that the psychodynamic approach depends on a reference to something unseen, psychodynamic OT is in the same position as psychodynamic mental health intervention overall—if it works, prove it. Even proponents of a psychodynamic approach suggest that shortened intervention doesn't allow for the implementation of a true psychodynamic intervention, especially if increased insight and self-awareness are among the goals. Further, as with the examples given in this chapter, a psychodynamic approach seems to imply direct service. One could ask, is it viable where the therapist is increasingly assuming the role of consultant?

The group programs described in this chapter are actual programs provided within the last 3 years. They seem to have validity in regard to the intervention methods used, but without more scrutiny and research in support of the efficacy of programs like these, their utility remains in question.

Limited Understanding by Clinicians

Eventually, the theorist and practitioner within this framework must ask, "Does feeling-oriented, psychologically based occupational therapy improve the quality of individuals' lives? If so, how can this improvement be demonstrated?" It would appear that both qualitative and quantitative research must continue and become more rigorous to demonstrate the viability of this model.

As with any body of knowledge, there is a danger in knowing just enough to be conversant and believing that one knows all that he or she needs. We have been acquainted with students and long-time therapists who became quite fascinated with their encounter with elements of the unconscious. However, haphazard dabbling with unconscious constructs and misguided efforts to analyze behavior lend themselves to a great deal of useless interpretation, much misinterpretation, and little in the way of helpful intervention. Further, therapists may think that they somehow know more about patients or clients than they know about themselves.

When humanistic client-centered principles are applied, there can be a tendency to view therapy as overly simplistic. Being warm and concerned about patients/clients is important but does not mean that therapy has occurred. Unconditional positive regard is not viewed as desirable by all therapists and may be one of the most difficult postures to achieve; yet, it may appear simple. Finding one's own place within this construct depends on experience and a maturing into the therapist role. Phony acceptance by the occupational therapist of behaviors that he or she finds unacceptable confuses the patient and confounds the relationship. Carl Rogers believed that client-centered therapy contained a methodology that stood on its own and led to change in the person. It is often difficult for the occupational therapist to trust that, given information, the client will make healthy choices. We all know people—children and adults—who do not make healthy choices, and one can ask, "What then?"

Client Needs Capacity for Insight

The psychodynamic striving to increase clients' insight is most successful with persons who have a good functioning ego and capacity for realistic thinking. One must remember, however, that even individuals who are confused some of the time are lucid at other times, and they may have more ability for insight than treatment staff acknowledges. Further, when insight is not the goal, the therapist's ability to conceptually understand the behavior may make the behavior more meaningful and manageable and thereby facilitate a constructive response. Attempts at empathic understanding and the communication of positive regard are believed to be important with all persons.

Eclectic Framework

The psychodynamic framework as presented is a highly eclectic framework. Therefore, it is open to criticism on a variety of grounds. As Patterson (1974) writes, eclecticism has been viewed as undesirable for its lack of direction, the inevitable inconsistencies in practice, and the difficulties in its examination through research. If one accepts that no one current theory or technique best fits each individual treated or each situation, however, then one can try to synthesize common, compatible, and workable constructs from a range of therapy approaches. Patterson cites the definition of **eclecticism** given by English and English (1958) in *A Comprehensive Dictionary of Psychological and Psychoanalytic Terms:*

> **Eclecticism** in theoretical system building, the selection and orderly combination of compatible feature from diverse sources, sometimes from incompatible theories and systems; the effort to find valid elements in all doctrines or theories and to combine them into a harmonious whole. The resulting system is open to constant revision even in its major outlines. Eclecticism is to be distinguished from unsystematic and uncritical combination, for which the name is syncretism. The eclectic seeks as much consistency as is currently possible but he is unwilling to sacrifice conceptualizations that put meaning into a wide range of facts for the sake of what he is apt to think of as an unworkable overall systematization. The formalist finds the eclectic's position too loose and uncritical. For his part the eclectic finds formalism and schools too dogmatic and rigid, too much inclined to reject if not facts, at least helpful conceptualizations of facts. (Patterson, 1974)

The psychodynamic framework for understanding a person and his or her engagement in daily life occupation is an attempt at the kind of integration of which English and English speak. As we leave this model and move to the next, we will be confronted again with trends toward eclecticism in other theoretical frameworks. The reader is encouraged to be open-minded and journey with us.

REFERENCES

Accardi, M. (1985). *The Bay Area Functional Performance Evaluation: A validity study.* Unpublished master's thesis, Boston School of Occupational Therapy, Tufts University, Medford, MA.

Alexander, F. (1963). *Fundamentals of psychoanalysis.* New York, NY: Norton.

Allen, C. K. (1985). *Occupational therapy for psychiatric diseases: Measurement and management of cognitive disabilities.* Boston, MA: Little, Brown & Co.

Avis, M. (1994). Choice cuts: An exploratory study of patients' views about participation and decision making in a day surgery unit. *Int J Nurs Stud, 31*, 289-298.

Axline, V. (1969). *Play therapy* (Rev. ed.). New York, NY: Ballantine.

Azima, H., & Azima, F. (1959). Outline of a dynamic theory of occupational therapy. *Am J Occup Ther, 8*(5), 215.

Baptiste, S., & Rochon, S. (1999). Client-centered assessment: The Canadian Occupational Performance Measure. In B. Hemphill (Ed.), *Assessments in occupational therapy mental health.* Thorofare, NJ: SLACK Incorporated.

Bass, E., & Davis, L. (1994). *The courage to heal: A guide for women survivors of child sexual abuse* (3rd ed.). New York, NY: Harper Perennial.

Baum, C. (1980). Occupational therapists put care in the health system. *Am J Occup Ther, 34*(8), 505-516.

Bernstein, D. (1983). The female superego. *Int J Psychoanal, 64*(2), 187-201.

Bloomer, J., & Williams, S. (1982). The Bay Area Functional Performance Evaluation. In B. Hemphill (Ed.), *The evaluative process in psychiatric occupational therapy.* Thorofare, NJ: SLACK Incorporated.

Blum, H. (1976). Masochism, the ego ideal, and the psychoanalysis of women. *J Am Psychoanal Assoc, 24*, 157-191.

Borg, B., & Bruce, M. A. (1991). Assessing psychological performance factors. In C. Christiansen & C. Baum (Eds.), *Occupational therapy: Overcoming human performance deficits.* Thorofare, NJ: SLACK Incorporated.

Bowlby, J. (1969). *Attachment and loss.* New York, NY: Basic Books.

Bowyer, L. (1970). *The Lowenfield world techniques.* New York, NY: Pergamon Press.

Brickman, A. (1983). Pre-oedipal development of the superego. *Int J Psychoanal, 64*, 83-91.

Bruce, M. A., & Borg, B. (1987). *Psychosocial occupational therapy: Frames of reference for intervention.* Thorofare, NJ: SLACK Incorporated.

Bruce, M. A., & Borg, B. (1993). *Psychosocial occupational therapy: Frames of reference for intervention* (2nd ed.). Thorofare, NJ: SLACK Incorporated.

Buck, J. (1966). *The House-Tree-Person technique* (Rev.). Beverly Hills, CA: Western Psychological Services.

Bundy, A. C. (1997). Play and playfulness: What to look for. In L. D. Parham & L. S. Fazio (Eds.), *Play in occupational therapy for children* (pp. 52-66). St. Louis, MO: Mosby.

Burnell, G., & Burnell, A. (1989). *Clinical management of bereavement.* New York, NY: Human Science Press.

Burns, R., & Kaufman, S. (1970). *Kinetic family drawings.* New York, NY: Brunner/Mazel.

Burns, R., & Kaufman, S. (1972). *Actions, styles, and symbols in kinetic family drawings: An interpretive manual.* New York, NY: Brunner/Mazel.

Campbell, J. (1968). *Creative mythology.* New York, NY: Viking Press.

Campbell, J. (Ed.). (1971). *The portable Jung.* New York, NY: Viking Press.

Campbell, J. (1976). *The masks of God.* Harmondsworth, England: Penguin Books.

Campbell, J. (1981). *The mythic image.* Princeton, NJ: Princeton University Press.

Campbell, J. (1990). *Transformations of myth through time.* New York, NY: Harper and Row Perennial Library.

Canadian Association of Occupational Therapists. (1991). *Occupational therapy guidelines for client-centred practice.* Toronto, Canada: Author.

Canadian Association of Occupational Therapists. (1997). *Enabling occupation: An occupational therapy perspective.* Ottawa, Canada: CAOT Publications ACE.

Caro, P., & Derevensky, J. L. (1991). Family-focused intervention model: Implementation and research findings. *Topics in Early Childhood Special Education, 11*(3), 66-80.

Christiansen, C., & Baum, C. (1991). *Occupational therapy: Overcoming human performance deficits.* Thorofare, NJ: SLACK Incorporated.

Clark, E. N. (1999). Build A City: A projective test concept. In B. Hemphill-Pearson (Ed.), *Assessments in occupational therapy mental health: An integrative approach.* Thorofare, NJ: SLACK Incorporated.

Colby, A., & Kohlberg, L. (1987). *The measurement of moral judgment.* Cambridge, MA: Cambridge University Press.

Cole, M. (1993). *Group dynamics in occupational therapy.* Thorofare, NJ: SLACK Incorporated.

Corey, G. (1982). *Theory and practice of counseling and psychotherapy* (2nd ed., pp. 30, 34). Monterey, CA: Brooks/Cole.

Curtin, M., & Klyczek, J. (1992). Comparison of BaFPE-TOA scores for inpatients and outpatients. *Occupational Therapy in Mental Health, 12*(1), 61-75.

Davis, L. (1990). *The courage to heal workbook: For women and men survivors of child sexual abuse.* New York, NY: Author.

Doyle, B. J., & Ware, J. E. (1977). Physician conduct and other factors that affect consumer satisfaction with medical care. *Journal of Medical Education, 52*(10), 793-801.

Drake, M. (1999). The use of expressive media as an assessment tool in mental health. In B. Hemphill-Pearson (Ed.), *Assessments in occupational therapy mental health: An integrative approach.* Thorofare, NJ: SLACK Incorporated.

Dunst, C. J., Trivette, C. M., Boyd, K., & Brookfield, J. (1994). Help-giving practices and the self-efficacy appraisals of parents. In C. J. Dunst, C. M. Trivette, K. Boyd, & J. Brookfield (Eds.), *Supporting and strengthening families: Methods, strategies, and practices* (Vol. 1). Cambridge, MA: Brookline Books.

Dunst, C. J., Trivette, C. M., & Deal, A. (1988). *Enabling and empowering families: Principles and guidelines for practice.* Cambridge, MA: Brookline Books.

Edwards, M. (1987). Jungian analytic art therapy. In J. Rubin (Ed.), *Approaches to art therapy* (pp. 92-113). New York, NY: Brunner/Mazel.

Egan, M., & DeLaat, D. (1994). Considering spirituality in occupational therapy practice. *Can J Occup Ther, 61*, 95-101.

Eichenbaum, L., & Orbach, S. (1983). *Understanding women—A feminine psychoanalytic approach* (p. 71). New York, NY: Basic Books.

Ellis, M. (1973). *Why people play.* Englewood Cliffs, NJ: Prentice-Hall.

English, H. B., & English, A. C. (1958). *A comprehensive dictionary of psychological and psychiatric terms.* New York, NY: Longmans, Green.

Enquist, D., Short-DeGraff, M., Gliner, J., & Oltjenbruns, K. (1997). Occupational therapists' beliefs and practices with regard to spirituality and therapy. *Am J Occup Ther, 51*(3), 173-180.

Erikson, E. (1941). Sex differences in play configuration of pre-adolescents. *Am J Orthopsychiatry, 21*, 667-692.

Erikson, E. (1950). *Childhood and society.* New York, NY: Norton.

Erikson, E. (1959). Identity and the life cycle. *Psychol Issues, 1*, 1-171.

Erikson, E. (1969). *Identity, youth, and crisis.* New York, NY: W. W. Norton.

Fausto-Sterling, A. (2000). *Sexing the body: Gender politics and the construction of sexuality.* New York, NY: Basic Books.

Fidler, G. (1969). The task-oriented group as a context for treatment. *Am J Occup Ther, 23*(1), 43-48.

Fidler, G., & Fidler, J. (1963). *Occupational therapy—A communication process in psychiatry* (p. 82). New York, NY: MacMillan.

Films for the Humanities. (1990). *Children die, too.* Princeton, NJ: Author.

Fine, S. (1993). Interaction between psychological variables and cognitive function. In C. Royeen (Ed.), *AOTA self-study series: Cognitive rehabilitation* (pp. 6-25). Rockville, MD: American Occupational Therapy Association.

Fleming, M. H. (1991). Clinical reasoning in medicine compared with clinical reasoning in occupational therapy. *Am J Occup Ther, 45*, 988-996.

Florcy, L. L., & Greene, S. (1997). Play in middle childhood: A focus on children with behavior and emotional disorders. In L. D. Parham & L. S. Fazio (Eds.), *Play in occupational therapy for children* (pp. 126-143). St. Louis, MO: Mosby.

Fluegelman, A. (Ed.). (1976). *The new games book.* New York, NY: Dolphin Books/Doubleday and Co.

Forward, S. (1989). *Toxic parents: Overcoming their hurtful legacy and reclaiming your life.* New York, NY: Bantam Books.

Freud, S. (1937). *The ego and the mechanisms of defense.* London: Hogarth Press.

Freud, S. (1950). *Interpretation of dreams* (pp. 242-243, 465). (A. A. Brill., Trans.). New York: Random House. (Original work published 1900)

Freud, S. (1953). Three essays on sexuality. In J. Strachey (Ed. and Trans., in collaboration with Anna Freud, assisted by A. Starchey and A. Tyson), *The standard edition of the complete psychological works of Sigmund Freud* (Vol. XII, pp. 135-243). London: The Hogart Press. (Original work published 1923)

Frye, B., & Gannon, L. (1990). The use, misuse, and abuse of art with dissociative/multiple personality disorder patients. *Occupational Therapy Forum, 5*(24), 3.

Gazzangia, M. S. (1988). *Mind matters.* Boston, MA: Houghton Mifflin.

Gazzangia, M. S. (1989). Organization of the human brain. *Science, 245,* 947-952.

Gilfoyle, E. (1980). Caring: A philosophy for practice. *Am J Occup Ther, 34*(8), 517-521.

Gilligan, C. (1982). *In a different voice: Psychological theory and women's development.* Cambridge, MA: Harvard University Press.

Goldfried, M. E., & Kent, R. N. (1972). Traditional versus behavioral personality assessment: A comparison of methodological and theoretical assumptions. *Psychol Bull, 77,* 409-420.

Goldstein, K. (1939). *The organism.* New York, NY: American Book Co.

Goldstein, K. (1942). *After-effects of brain injuries in war.* New York, NY: Grune & Stratton.

Goodenough, F. (1926). *Measurement of intelligence by drawings.* New York, NY: Harcourt, Brace.

Greenfield, S., Kaplan, S. H., & Ware, J. E. (1985). Expanding patient involvement in care: Effects on patient outcomes. *Ann Intern Med, 102,* 520-528.

Grinspoon, L. (Ed.). (1984). *Psychiatry update: The American Psychiatric Association annual review* (Vol. III). Washington, DC: American Psychiatric Press.

Gruenbaum, H., & Glick, I. (1983). The basics of family treatment. In L. Grinspoon (Ed.), *Psychiatry update: The American Psychiatric Association annual review* (Vol. II, pp. 185-203). Washington, DC: American Psychiatric Press.

Gutterman, L. (1990). A day treatment program for persons with AIDS. *Am J Occup Ther, 44,* 234-237.

Hales, R., & Frances, A. (Eds.). (1985). *Psychiatry update: The American Psychiatric Association annual review* (Vol. IV). Washington, DC: American Psychiatric Press.

Hall, C. S. (1954). *Primer of Freudian psychology* (pp. 29, 35, 85). New York, NY: New American Library.

Hall, C. S., & Nordby, V. (1973). *Primer of Jungian psychology* (p. 93). New York, NY: New American Library.

Hammell, K. W. (1998). Client-centred occupational therapy: Collaborative planning, accountable intervention. In M. Law (Ed.), *Client-centered occupational therapy.* Thorofare, NJ: SLACK Incorporated.

Harris, D. (1963). *Children's drawings as measures of intellectual maturity.* New York, NY: Harcourt/Brace.

Hartmann, H. (1958). *Ego psychology and the problem of adaptation* (p. 31). New York, NY: International Universities Press.

Hatfield, A. (1993). Patient's accounts of stress and coping in schizophrenia. In R. F. Cottrell (Ed.), *Proactive approaches in psychosocial occupational therapy.* Rockville, MD: American Occupational Therapy Association.

Havighurst, R. J. (1974). *Developmental tasks and education.* New York, NY: David McKay.

Helfrich, C., & Kielhofner, G. (1994). Volitional narratives and the meaning of therapy. *Am J Occup Ther, 48,* 318-326.

Helfrich, C., Kielhofner, G., & Mattingly, C. (1994). Volition as narrative: Understanding motivation in chronic illness. *Am J Occup Ther, 48,* 311-317.

Hemphill, B. J. (1982). *Training manual for the BH battery.* Thorofare, NJ: SLACK Incorporated.

Hemphill-Pearson, B. (1999). How to use the BH battery. In B. Hemphill-Pearson (Ed.), *Assessment in occupational therapy: An integrative approach.* Thorofare, NJ: SLACK Incorporated.

Henbest, R. J., & Stewart, M. (1990). Patient-centeredness in the consultation. 2: Does it really make a difference? *Fam Pract, 9,* 311-317.

Heubner, J., & Tryssenaar, J. (1996). Development of an occupational therapy practice perspective in a homeless shelter: A fieldwork experience. *Can J Occup Ther, 63*(1), 24-32.

Howard, B., & Howard, J. (1997). Occupation as spiritual activity. *Am J Occup Ther, 51*(3), 173-180.

Jones, M. (1953). *The therapeutic community: A new treatment method in psychiatry.* New York, NY: Basic Books.

Jourard, S. (1971). *The transparent self* (Rev. ed.). New York, NY: Van Nostrand Reinhold.

Jung, C. (1966). *The practice of psychotherapy: Collected works* (Vol. 16). Princeton, NJ: Princeton University Press.

Jung, C. (1971). In J. Campbell (Ed.), *The portable Jung* (p. 17). New York, NY: Penguin Books.

Jung, C. (Ed.). (1979). *Man and his symbols.* Garden City, NY: Doubleday and Co.

Kaplan, H., Sadock, B., & Grebb, J. (1994). *Synopsis of psychiatry* (7th ed.). Baltimore, MD: Williams & Wilkins.

Kaplan, H., Sadock, B., & Grebb, J. (1996). *Pocket handbook of clinical psychiatry.* Baltimore, MD: Williams & Wilkins.

Kaplan, H., Sadock, B., & Grebb, J. (1998). *Synopsis of psychiatry* (8th ed.). Baltimore, MD: Williams & Wilkins.

Kielhofner, G., Mallinson, T., Crawford, C., Nowack, M., Rigby, M., Henry, A., & Walens, D. (1998). *Occupational Performance History Interview (II).* Chicago, IL: Model of Human Occupation Clearinghouse, Department of Occupational Therapy, University of Illinois.

Kimmel, M. S. (1998). *The gendered society.* Oxford, England: Oxford University Press.

King, G., King, S., & Rosenbaum, P. (1996). Interpersonal aspects of care-giving and client outcomes: A review of the literature. *Ambulatory Child Health, 2,* 151-160.

King, L. J. (1982). The person symbol as an assessment tool. In B. J. Hemphill (Ed.), *The evaluative process in psychiatric occupational therapy.* Thorofare, NJ: SLACK Incorporated.

King, S., Rosenbaum, P., & King, G. (1996). Parents' perceptions of caregiving: Development and validation of a measure of processes. *Dev Med Child Neurol, 38*, 757-772.

Kirsch, B. (1996). A narrative approach to addressing spirituality in occupational therapy: Exploring personal meaning and purpose. *Can J Occup Ther, 63*, 55-61.

Klyczek, J. (1999). The Bay Area Functional Performance Evaluation. In B. Hemphill-Pearson (Ed.), *Assessments in occupational therapy mental health: An integrative approach*. Thorofare, NJ: SLACK Incorporated.

Klyczek, J., & Mann, W. (1990). Concurrent validity of the task-oriented component of the Bay Area Functional Performance Evaluation with the American Association on Mental Deficiency Adaptive Behavior Scale. *Am J Occup Ther, 44*, 907-912.

Kohlberg, L. (1969). Stage and sequence: The cognitive-developmental approach to socialization. In D. Goslin (Ed.), *Handbook of socialization: Theory and research*. Chicago, IL: Rand McNally.

Kohlberg, L. (1971). Stages of moral development as a basis for moral education. In C. M. Beck, B. S. Critlenden, & E. V. Sullivan (Eds.), *Moral education*. Toronto, Ontario: University of Toronto Press.

Kohlberg, L. (1976). Moral stages and moralization. In T. Lickona (Ed.), *Moral development and behavior: Theory, research, and social issues*. New York, NY: Holt, Rinehart & Winston.

Kubler-Ross, E. (1969). *On death and dying*. New York, NY: Macmillan.

Landefeld, C. S., Palmer, R. M., Kresevic, D. M., Fortinsky, R. H., & Kowal, J. (1995). A randomized trial of care and hospital medical unit especially designed to improve the functional outcomes of acutely ill older patients. *New England Journal of Medicine, 332*, 1338-1344.

Law, M. (1998). Does client-centred practice make a difference? In M. Law (Ed.), *Client-centred occupational therapy* (pp. 19-27). Thorofare, NJ: SLACK Incorporated.

Law, M., Baptiste, S., Carswell, A., McColl, M. A., Polatajko, H., & Pollock, N. (1994). *Canadian Occupational Performance Measure* (2nd ed.). Toronto, Ontario: CAOT Publications.

Law, M., Baptiste, S., & Mills, J. (1995). Client-centred practice: What does it mean and does it make a difference? *Can J Occup Ther, 62*(5), 250-257.

Law, M., & Mills, J. (1998). Client-centered occupational therapy. In M. Law (Ed.), *Client-centered occupational therapy*. Thorofare, NJ: SLACK Incorporated.

Leete, E. (1993). The treatment of schizophrenia: A patient's perspective. In R. F. Cottrell (Ed.), *Proactive approaches in psychosocial occupational therapy*. Rockville, MD: American Occupational Therapy Association.

Lerner, C. (1977). The magazine picture collage: The development of a scoring system. *Am J Occup Ther, 31*(3), 156-161.

Lerner, H. (1983). Female dependency in context. *Am J Orthopsychiatry, 53*(4), 697-705.

Levinson, D. (1974). *The seasons of a man's life*. New York, NY: Ballantine.

Lieberman, A. F. (1977). Preschoolers' competence with a peer: Influence of attachment and social experience. *Child Dev, 48*, 1277-1287.

Livesley, W., & Bromley, D. B. (1973). *Person perception in childhood and adolescence*. London: John Wiley and Sons, Ltd.

Llorens, L. (1966). Occupational therapy in an ego-oriented milieu. *Am J Occup Ther, XX*(4), 178-181.

Llorens, L., & Rubin, E. (1967). *Developing ego functions in disturbed children*. Detroit, MI: Wayne State University Press.

Malone, C. (1983). Family therapy and childhood disorders. In L. Grinspoon (Ed.), *Psychiatry update: The American Psychiatric Association annual review* (Vol. II, pp. 228-241). Washington, DC: American Psychiatric Press.

Mann, W., & Klyczek, J. (1991). Standard scores for the Bay Area Functional Performance Evaluation Task Oriented Assessment. *Occupational Therapy Journal of Mental Health, 11*(1), 13-24.

Mann, W., Klyczek, J., & Fiedler, R. (1989). Bay Area Functional Performance Evaluation (BaFPE): Standard scores. *Occupational Therapy Journal of Mental Health, 9*, 1-7.

Mann, W., & Small Russ, L. (1991). Measuring the functional performance of nursing home patients with the Bay Area Functional Performance Evaluation. *Physical and Occupational Therapy in Geriatrics, 9*(3), 113-129.

Margolin, G., & Jacobson, N. S. (1981). Assessment of marital dysfunction. In M. Herson & A. Bellack (Eds.), *Behavioral assessment*. New York, NY: Pergamon Press, Inc.

Maslow, A. (1968). *Toward a psychology of being* (Rev. ed.). New York, NY: Van Nostrand.

Maslow, A. H. (1970). *Motivation and personality*. New York, NY: Harper & Row.

Maslow, A. H. (1971). *The farther reaches of human nature*. New York, NY: Viking Press.

Maslow, A. H. (1978). *Dominance, self-esteem, self-actualization—Seminal papers of A. H. Maslow* (R. J. Lowry, Ed.). Monterey, CA: Monterey Books/Cole Publishing.

Mattingly, C. (1991). The narrative nature of clinical reasoning. *Am J Occup Ther, 45*, 998-1005.

Mattingly, C., & Fleming, M. H. (1994). *Clinical reasoning: Forms of inquiry in a therapeutic practice*. Philadelphia, PA: F. A. Davis.

May, R. (1950). *The meaning of anxiety*. New York, NY: Ronald Press.

May, R. (1953). *Man's search for himself*. New York, NY: Norton.

May, R. (1969). *Love and will*. New York, NY: Norton.

McFarlane, W. (1983). New developments in the family treatment of psychotic disorders. In L. Grinspoon (Ed.), *Psychiatry update: The American Psychiatric Association annual review* (Vol. II, pp. 242-256). Washington, DC: American Psychiatric Press.

Menninger, K. (1963). *The vital balance: The life process in mental health and illness*. New York, NY: Viking Press.

Michels, R. (1983). Contemporary psychoanalytic views of interpretation. In L. Grinspoon (Ed.), *Psychiatry update: The American Psychiatric Association annual review* (Vol. II, pp. 61, 69). Washington, DC: American Psychiatric Press.

Miller, F. (1999). Grief therapy for relatives of persons with serious mental illness. In R. F. Cottrell (Ed.), *Psychosocial occupational therapy: Proactive approaches* (2nd ed., pp. 417-420). Rockville, MD: American Occupational Therapy Association.

Money, J., & Ehrhardt, A. (1972). *Man and woman, boy and girl.* Baltimore, MD: Johns Hopkins University Press.

Moore, T. (1992). *Care of the soul.* New York, NY: Harper Perennial.

Moore, T. (1996). *The re-enchantment of everyday life.* New York, NY: Harper Perennial.

Mosey, A. C. (1970). *Three frames of reference for mental health.* Thorofare, NJ: SLACK Incorporated.

Moustakos, C. (1956). *The self: Exploration in personal growth.* New York, NY: Harper.

Moustakos, C. (1961). *Loneliness.* Englewood Cliffs, NJ: Prentice-Hall.

Moxley-Haegert, L., & Serbin, L. A. (1983). Developmental education for parents of delayed infants: Effects on parental motivation and children's development. *Child Dev, 54,* 1324-1331.

Mucchielli, R. (1960). *Le jeu monde et le test du village imaginaire.* Paris, France: Presses Universitaires de France.

Naglieri, J. (1988). *Draw-a-Person manual: A quantitative scoring system.* New York, NY: Psychological Corp.

Newman, M. (1987). *Cognitive disability and functional performance of individuals with chronic schizophrenic disorders.* Unpublished master's thesis, University of Southern California, Los Angeles.

Notman, M., & Nadelson, C. (Eds.). (1982). *The woman patient: Aggression, adaptations, and psychotherapy* (Vol. 3, p. 5). New York, NY: Plenum Press.

O'Kane, C. (1968). *The development of a projective technique for use in psychiatric occupational therapy.* Buffalo, NY: State University of New York at Buffalo.

Olson, B., & Jamal, J. (1987). *The BaFPE: Standardization and clinical application in acute adult psychiatry.* Irvine, CA: University of California Irvine Medical Center.

Olson, L. (1993). Psychosocial frame of reference. In P. Kramer & J. Hinajosa (Eds.), *Frames of reference for pediatric occupational therapy.* Baltimore, MD: Williams & Wilkins.

Opacich, K. J. (1992). Assessment and informed decision-making. In C. Christiansen & C. Baum (Eds.), *Occupational therapy: Overcoming human performance deficits.* Thorofare, NJ: SLACK Incorporated.

Ornstein, R. (1973). *Psychology of consciousness* (p. 83). New York, NY: Penguin Books.

Patterson, C. H. (1974). *Relationship counseling and psychotherapy* (pp. 270-271). New York, NY: Harper and Row Publishers.

Peloquin, S. M. (1990). The patient-therapist relationship in occupational therapy: Understanding visions and images. *Am J Occup Ther, 44,* 13-21.

Peloquin, S. M. (1995). The fullness of empathy: Reflection and illustrations. *Am J Occup Ther, 49,* 24-31.

Perls, F. (1969). *Gestalt therapy verbatum.* Moab, UT: Real People Press.

Perry, D., & Bussey, K. (1984). *Social development.* Englewood Cliffs, NJ: Prentice-Hall.

Person, E. (1983). The influence of values in psychoanalysis: The case of female psychology. In L. Grinspoon (Ed.), *Psychiatry update: The American Psychiatric Association annual review* (Vol. II, pp. 36-50). Washington, DC: American Psychiatric Press.

Piaget, J. (1962). *Play, dreams, and imitation in childhood.* (C. Gattegno & F. Hodgsen, Trans.). New York, NY: Norton & Co.

Piaget, J. (1965). *The child's conception of the world.* Totowa, NJ: Littlefield, Adams, & Co.

Piaget, J. (1973). *The child and reality.* (A. Rosin, Trans.). New York, NY: Grossman Publishers.

Piaget, J., & Inhelder, B. (1969). *The psychology of the child.* New York, NY: Basic Books.

Pinkola-Estes, C. (1992). *Women who run with wolves.* New York, NY: Ballantine Books.

Pollock, N., & McColl, M. A. (1998). Assessment in client-centered occupational therapy. In M. Law (Ed.), *Client-centered occupational therapy.* Thorofare, NJ: SLACK Incorporated.

Pronin Fromberg, D., & Bergen, D. (Eds.). (1998). *Play from birth to twelve and beyond: Contexts, perspectives, and meanings.* New York, NY: Garland Publishers.

Reilly, M. (1974). *Play as exploratory learning.* Beverly Hills, CA: Sage Publications.

Rhyne, J. (1973). *The Gestalt art experience.* Monterey, CA: Brooks/Cole.

Rochon, S., & Baptiste, S. (1998). Client-centered occupational therapy: Ethics and identity. In M. Law (Ed.), *Client-centered occupational therapy.* Thorofare, NJ: SLACK Incorporated.

Rogers, C. (1951). *Client-centered therapy.* Boston, MA: Houghton-Mifflin.

Rogers, C. (1961). *On becoming a person* (pp. 32, 35-36). Boston, MA: Houghton-Mifflin.

Rudman, D. L., Tooke, J., Eimantas, T. G., Hall, M., & Maloney, K. B. (1997). Preliminary investigation of the content validity and clinical utility of the predischarge assessment tool. *Can J Occup Ther, 65,* 3-11.

Sadler, A. (1978). Psychoanalysis in later life: Problems in the psychoanalysis of an aging narcissistic patient. *J Geriatr Psychiatry Neurol, 11*(1), 5.

Sanford, J., Law, M., Swanson, L., & Guyatt, G. (1994). *Assessing clinically important change as an outcome of rehabilitation in older adults.* Paper presented at the conference of the American Society on Aging, San Francisco, CA.

Scheff, T. (Ed.). (1975). *Labeling madness.* Englewood Cliffs, NJ: Prentice Hall.

Scheff, T. (1984). *Being mentally ill.* New York, NY: Aldine Publishing.

Schkade, J. K., & Schultz, S. (1992). Occupational adaptation: Toward a holistic approach for contemporary practice, part 1. *Am J Occup Ther, 46,* 829-832.

Schroeder, C. V., Block, M. P., Campbell, I., Trottier, E., & Stowell, M. S. (1978). *Schroeder-Block-Campbell adult psychiatric sensory integration evaluation* (2nd ed.). LaJolla, CA: SBC Research Associates.

Selman, R. L. (1971). Taking another's perspective: Role-taking development in early childhood. *Child Dev, 42*, 1721-1734.

Selman, R. L. (1976). Social-cognitive understanding: A guide to educational and clinical practice. In T. Lickona (Ed.), *Moral development and behavior: Theory, research, and social issues*. New York, NY: Holt, Rinehart & Winston.

Sheehy, G. (1978). *Passages: Predictable crises of adult life*. New York, NY: E. P. Dutton & Co.

Shoemyen, C. (1970). Occupational therapy orientation and evaluation. *Am J Occup Ther, 24*, 276-279.

Short-DeGraff, M. A. (1988). *Human development for occupational and physical therapists*. Baltimore, MD: Williams & Wilkins.

Short-DeGraff, M. A., & Englemann, T. (1992). Activities for the treatment of combat-related post-traumatic stress disorder. *Occupational Therapy and Health Care, 8*(2/3), 27-47.

Springer, S., & Deutsch, D. (1981). *Left brain, right brain*. San Francisco, CA: W. H. Freeman and Co.

Stafford-Clark, D. (1966). What Freud really said. In S. Freud, *An outline of psychoanalysis* (Vol. 23, p. 134). New York, NY: Schocken Books. (Original work published 1939)

Stanton, E., Mann, W., & Klyczek, J. (1991). Use of the Bay Area Functional Performance Evaluation with eating disordered patients. *Occupational Therapy Journal of Research, 11*(4), 227-237.

Starfield, B., Wray, C., Hess, K., Gross, R., Birk, P. S., & D'Lugoff, B. C. (1981). The influence of patient-practitioner agreement on outcome of care. *American Journal of Public Health, 71*, 127-132.

Stein, R. E., & Jessop, D. J. (1984). Does pediatric home care make a difference for children with chronic illness? Findings from the pediatric ambulatory case study. *Pediatrics, 73*, 845-853.

Stoller, R. (1968). *Sex and gender*. New York, NY: Science House.

Takata, N. (1974). Play as prescription. In M. Reilly (Ed.), *Play as exploratory learning*. Beverly Hills, CA: Sage Publishers.

Tardiff, M. (1993). *Concurrent validity of the Functional Needs Assessment with the Task-Oriented Assessment of the Bay Area Functional Performance Evaluation*. Buffalo, NY: D'Youville College. Thesis.

Thiebeault, R., & Blackmer, E. (1987). Validating a test of functional performance with psychiatric patients. *Am J Occup Ther, 41*, 515-521.

Toomey, M., Nicholson, D., & Carswell, A. (1995). The clinical utility of the Canadian Occupational Performance Measure. *Can J Occup Ther, 62*(5), 242-249.

Townsend, E. (1998). Client-centered occupational therapy: The Canadian experience. In M. Law (Ed.), *Client-centered occupational therapy*. Thorofare, NJ: SLACK Incorporated.

Trieschmann, R. B. (1988). *Spinal cord injuries: Psychological, social and vocational rehabilitation* (2nd ed.). New York, NY: Demos Publications.

Uecker, E. (1986). Tarot thematic projective technique: A structured exercise for facilitation of self-awareness and problem solving. *Occupational Therapy Forum, 1*(14), 1.

Urbanowski, R., & Vargo, J. (1994). Spirituality, daily practice, and the occupational performance model. *Can J Occup Ther, 61*, 88-94.

Vaillant, G. E. (1993). *The wisdom of the ego*. Cambridge, MA: Harvard University Press.

Wallis, C., & Willworth, J. (1992). Schizophrenia: A new drug brings patients back to life. *Time, July 6*, 53-57.

Wener-Altman, P., Wolfe, A., & Staley, D. (1991). Utilization of the Bay Area Functional Performance Evaluation with an adolescent psychiatric population. *Can J Occup Ther, 58*, 129-136.

White, R. W. (1959). Motivation reconsidered: The concept of competence. *Psychol Rev, 66*, 297-333.

White, R. W. (1971). The urge toward competence. *Am J Occup Ther, 25*, 271-274.

Williams, S., & Bloomer, J. (1987). *Bay Area Functional Performance Evaluation* (2nd ed.). Palo Alto, CA: Consulting Psychologists Press.

Worden, J. W. (1982). *Grief counseling and grief therapy: A handbook for the mental health practitioner*. New York, NY: Springer.

Yalom, I. (1975). *The theory and practice of group psychotherapy* (2nd ed.). New York, NY: Basic Books.

Yalom, I. (1983). *Inpatient group psychotherapy*. New York, NY: Harper.

Yerxa, E. (1967). Authentic occupational therapy. *Am J Occup Ther, 21*(1), 1-9.

Yerxa, E. (1978). The philosophical base of occupational therapy. In *Occupational therapy: 2001 AD*. Rockville, MD: American Occupational Therapy Association.

Zukav, G. (1980). *The dancing WuLi masters: An overview of the new physics* (p. 8). New York, NY: Bantam Books.

CHAPTER FIVE

Behavioral Frame of Reference— Objective Perspective

KEY POINTS

✧ History and Current Theory
- Behavior is Learned—Conditioning, Discrimination, Reinforcement
- Eliminate, Shape, or Model Behavior
- Biofeedback in Physical Medicine and Mental Health Contexts

✧ Theory in Context of Occupational Therapy Practice
- Motivation and the Person's Behavior
- Adaptive Performance and Skills
- Performance Deficits and Behavior Excess
- Client-Centered Learning Experiences
- Activities Build Skills and Improve Occupational Performance
- Activities as Reinforcers and for Simulated Learning Experiences
- Therapist Roles: Model, Coach, Consultant, Designer

✧ Theoretical Assumptions Guide Evaluation and Intervention

✧ Evaluation
- Establishing a Performance Baseline—Behavior Data Base
- Assessment Context: Naturalistic, Simulated, Unobtrusive versus Obtrusive
- Temporal Conditions—Evaluation Over Time

✧ Intervention
- The Goal-Setting Process—General Statements to Observable Goals
- Writing Behavior Contracts
- Behavior Programs in Multiple Contexts and Environments
- Behavior Management and Constructive Feedback
- Behavior Occupational Therapy Groups

✧ Contributions and Limitations of the Behavior Frame of Reference

FOCUS QUESTIONS

1. How are function and dysfunction identified in this framework?

2. What is the difference between internal and external reinforcement? Which is more likely to sustain behavior in a variety of settings and why?

3. How is behavior extinguished? Why is it difficult to extinguish most behaviors?

4. What is the difference between a **skill deficit** and a **performance deficit**?

5. Why might a person who is capable of an identified skill or behavior choose to not exhibit that behavior?

6. Why is it so important to be specific when targeting behavior for change?

7. What characterizes the behavioral assessment?

8. Describe three or more means by which new behaviors can be learned.

9. What are the benefits and drawbacks of a token economy?

10. What is meant by the term **behavior management** and for whom is it used?

11. What are the characteristics of a well-written learning/behavioral contract?

12. Support the view that behavioral treatment is a humanizing influence in mental health treatment. Support the opposite view.

HISTORICAL UPDATE

Ann Mosey identified the behavioral frame of reference or model in occupational therapy in 1970 as one of three "frames of reference" for OT in mental health. In her text, Mosey identified principles for using operant conditioning, referring to these collectively not as the "behavioral" framework but rather as an "action-consequence" model. Subsequent literature described the use of a behavioral model in a variety of occupational therapy contexts, frequently to address psychosocial issues but not necessarily in mental health settings. Over time, however, leaders in the field reacted strongly to the implicit suggestions (made explicit by Skinner [1971]) that in the application of behavioral principles, the persons controlling reinforcement were ultimately controlling human behavior. Understanding motivation as an internal phenomenon and wishing to be client-centered, occupational therapists expressed discomfort with practices that would aim to control client behavior. The authors of the occupational literature of the 1980s and 1990s (Kielhofner & Burke, 1985, p. 14; Rogers, 1982; Yerxa, 1991, 1992) spoke out against a behavioral therapy that was viewed as reductionistic and mechanistic and that failed to take into account the wholeness of human experience and the ability of persons to generate creative solutions.

On the flip side, occupational therapists have in behavioral principles clear guides for teaching skills and for identifying and documenting behavior change. In occupational therapy literature, Giles' and Clark-Wilson's (1999) neurofunctional approach is an example of applying behavioral theory to clients who are relearning basic activity of living skills after an acquired brain injury. When considering daily practice, occupational therapists on occasion or with great regularity either use rewards to encourage behavior, use timeouts, negotiate verbal or written contracts with a client, or write behavioral goal statements; all of these intervention approaches originate as behavioral strategies.

Taking the stance that behavioral theories help us as professionals identify and understand the transactions that occur between the person and his or her environment and that behavioral techniques are used extensively in the current practice of occupational therapy in multiple contexts and across the life span, we will describe the behavioral model as it is presently applied in practice and summarize its strengths and limitations.

Definition

T. E. Clayton (as cited in Mosey, 1970, p. 83) says, "Learning results from experience... Learning depends on what the learner does... the end result of the learning process is some change in the learner... (and) tends to be fixed by the consequences of his behavior..."

The behavioral frame of reference is built on experimental inquiry and principles of cognitive, social, and conditioned learning theories. Within the context of a therapeutic relationship, these principles are systematically applied through behavioral techniques and procedures that bring about behavior change within the individual and build performance skills necessary for that individual to function successfully in his or her environment. The behavioral model is a restorative model for therapy.

Where possible, occupational therapists strive to build skills that will enhance occupational performance, regardless of frame of reference (Fine, 1988; Palmer, 1988). Now identifying psychiatric illness in terms of the person's ability to function, the mental health community has placed increasing emphasis on behaviorally identified outcomes in intervention (Anthony, 1979; Lang & Mattson, 1993; Watts & Bennett, 1983). Even in those intervention contexts that are not identified primarily as "behavioral," the occupational therapist is often a teacher, trying to assist the individual to learn new skills. In so doing, the therapist frequently employs learning strategies that originated with the behavioral learning model. Viewed in this light, the behavioral frame of reference can be described as both a theoretical base and an intervention approach that stands on its own, but one that also affects much, if not most, contemporary occupational therapy.

Important Terms

Therapy within the behavioral frame of reference is concerned with identifying and eliminating problem behaviors and building desired functional skills. **Performance skills** consist of overt behaviors that can be observed and measured in occupational therapy and in the patient's or client's expected environment. Those behaviors and skills that contribute to function in one's living environment are referred to as **adaptive behaviors**; those behaviors that create obstacles to function are often referred to as **maladaptive**. Maladaption is viewed as the result of faulty learning, not disease.

The skills that one has learned and therefore has available in a given situation constitute his or her **behavioral repertoire** or **skill repertoire**. The behavioral model is not primarily concerned with feelings, past history, or the development of insight except where understanding these enables one to effect change in current behavior. The therapist and client/patient actively collaborate in identifying skills expected to enhance meaningful occupation and in creating opportunities in which these skills can be taught, practiced, and ultimately become a part of one's skill repertoire.

It is the rigorous application of learning principles that distinguishes a behaviorally oriented occupational therapy intervention program from those programs based on other models.

THEORETICAL DEVELOPMENT

Since the 1960s, occupational therapists have documented the efficacy of the behavioral approach to intervene with persons exhibiting psychosocial behavior problems (Burgess, Mitchelmore, & Giles, 1987; Drouet, 1986; Durham, 1982; Giles, 1987; Gorman, 1991; Jodrell & Sanson-Fisher, 1975; Ogburn, Fast, & Tiffany, 1972; Stein & Nikolic, 1989; Stein & Tallant, 1988; Watts, 1976; Wilberding, 1993). Professionals have also described behavioral intervention within occupational therapy in areas other than mental health (Borg & Bruce, 1997; Diasio, 1968; Giles & Clark-Wilson, 1999; Mosey, 1970, 1986; Norman, 1976; Sieg, 1981; Stein, 1982; Trombley & Scott, 1984; Wanderer, 1974).

Originally, the approaches used in occupational therapy were derived from principles of conditioned learning (Mosey, 1970). Today the behavioral approach in occupational therapy incorporates cognitive, social, and operant learning theory, although cognitive behaviorists tend to view themselves as being in a different camp from traditional behaviorists and are discussed in Chapter Six in this text.

Additionally, many psychologists, counselors, and behavioral scientists have contributed to the theory and development of behavior therapy. Those most often cited in the occupational therapy literature include Hilgard, Bower, Clayton, Tolman, Bandura, Skinner, Wolpe, Dollard and Miller, Goldfried and Davidson, Liberman and Spiegler, Azigan, Bakker, and Armstrong. Although each behaviorist may describe learning differently, the reader should view these differences as being mainly in emphasis.

HOW BEHAVIOR IS LEARNED

To understand how new behavior is learned, we begin by posing the question, "What is a behavior, and what are its characteristics?" Speaking broadly, **behavior** encompasses everything a person does (Murdoch & Barker, 1991, p. 20). Occupational therapists are more specifically concerned with building the skilled behavior that comprises or enables the occupational performance desired by the client. In order to enhance this skilled behavior, therapists may also strive to lessen or eliminate undesirable behavior. Behavior can be **overt** (riding a bike) or **covert** (thinking about what one wants for dinner). All behavior is measurable and, as such, is measurable in one or more of three dimensions: **intensity**, the force with which something is done; **frequency**, the rate of behavior or units of behavior per units of time; and **duration**, the length of time the behavior occurs (Murdoch & Barker, 1991, p. 22). If, for example, we take the behavior of hammering a nail into a piece of wood, we could measure how hard one hits the nail (intensity), how many times in the day one engaged in hammering nails into wood (frequency), or how long a given interval in which one was engaged in driving a nail into wood (duration).

All behavior—adaptive and maladaptive—not attributable to physical maturation or accident is presumed to be learned, and behavioral therapy rests on the assumptions of learning theory. When a person learns, multiple factors come into play:

- The person's physical capacity, intelligence, and bodily functions
- The drive or motives that impel the person to act
- The thoughts, perceptions, and feelings of the person
- The situation or context in which he or she is functioning
- The response or behavior that is present, as well as behavior that is desired

Of these factors, much is internal and is often inferred (e.g., intelligence, motives, feelings, thoughts, and tolerance of change); even when they can be described or verbalized, they are not easily measured.

Characteristics of the physical setting, the person's current behavior, and desired behavior or response(s) can be identified in measurable terms, and these factors define learning in this frame of reference. Although a setting is typically shaped by multiple physical stimuli, we can briefly speak here of "setting" in its most basic unit, as a single **stimulus**. Similarly, most behavior is very complex but is described here as the simplest unit of behavior, a single **response**. When a new stimulus brings about or elicits an already demonstrated response or when a given stimulus brings about a new response, **learning** is said to occur.

For example, yesterday a child could climb only the stairs from the family basement. Today the toddler is able to climb the stairs to the attic. When confronted yesterday with any of the stairs in his or her home, the child could only crawl up them. Today, confronted with these stairs, he or she walks up them for the first time. In both cases, learning has been demonstrated. When an identified stimulus consistently brings about a specific response, one says that an association has been made between them. In everyday behavior, this consistent association may also be termed a habit.

COGNITIVE MAP

Beginning with Tolman's pioneer work in the 1930s, behaviorists began to grapple with the possibility that internal processes, as mediated by the central nervous system, also need to be considered when looking at behavior. Tolman conceived of a "cognitive map" or internal integration of data by the organism (person). He suggested that the individual, rather than responding in an automatic stimulus-response habit, is capable of holding a cognitive awareness of several means to achieve a desired goal. Tolman theorized that in the development of these cognitive maps, the person is learning not just movement patterns but also meaning (Hilgard & Bower, 1975; Tolman, 1951). The attention given to cognitive processes was to be especially significant in the work of behaviorists who were interested in the development of language and has ultimately led to a division between traditional behaviorists and cognitive behaviorists.

Classical Conditioning

According to behavioral inquiry, learning occurs in several ways. In **classical conditioning** (also called respondent conditioning), a new stimulus becomes capable of evoking a given response because the new stimulus is presented together with a stimulus that already evokes the response. For example, eating a piece of lemon will cause a person's mouth to pucker. This puckering is a natural autonomic bodily response and does not need to be learned. Most often, a person tasting a lemon will also be seeing the lemon, and in very short time, just the sight of a lemon, without any necessity for tasting, will elicit the puckering response. For this kind of learning to occur, the two stimuli (taste of lemon, sight of lemon) need to be presented at virtually the same time or in what is termed **close temporal contiguity**. If the lemon was shown over an extended time frame but not tasted, the tendency of the sight of the lemon to elicit puckering would diminish until it had become eliminated or extinguished.

Stimulus Generalization

Classical conditioning has often been carried out in relationship to autonomic functions. As such, its application to therapy might seem limited; however, classical conditioning is very significant in learning. Learning occurs in classical conditioning and in operant conditioning, which will be discussed, in part because of stimulus and response generalization. For example, if the sight of an actual lemon makes your mouth pucker, a photograph of a lemon or perhaps a plastic facsimile evokes the same response as a result of **stimulus generalization**.

Stimuli that seem alike become capable of eliciting the same response. For instance, most newborn and young infants attach emotionally to their mothers and experience a positive response such as body relaxation when their mother holds them. It is not unusual for young infants to relax more quickly when held by another woman than they do when held by a man because women are more like the mother. This response is due to a series of stimulus generalizations. Similarly, a client may respond to a female therapist or a very nurturing man much as he or she does to his or her mother because of stimulus generalization.

In **response generalization**, two or more responses are evoked by the same stimulus because these responses occur in close temporal contiguity, or because the two responses are perceived as similar. For example, we may learn to say "thank you" upon being given a present, or we may, upon receiving a gift, shorten our response to "thanks." As may occur in treatment, when an individual builds certain social skills in the clinic setting (learning to say "please," waiting to take his or her turn), frequently other nontargeted social skills also improve. Response generalization is often complex and therefore difficult to specify; yet it plays a significant role in everyday learning (Martin, 1978).

Facilitating Generalization in Learning

Stimulus and response generalizations are most likely to occur when the stimuli look or act similarly and when the responses are similar or occur in close temporal contiguity. Through an infinite number of response and stimulus generalizations, the stimuli that become capable of bringing about a particular response may become very different, and the repertoire of responses that may be elicited by a given stimulus may become vast. Because of this generalization in learning, we do not need to relearn how to drive a car every time we purchase a new automobile. Nor do we have to relearn how to button our clothes every time we change our shirts.

The ability to generalize learning depends on the ability of the person to recognize and respond to the similarities in a variety of situations and behaviors. The occupational therapist uses this principle when he or she plans learning experiences. The more similarities between two or more environments or the more vivid these similarities, the greater the likelihood of generalization. Therefore, the therapist wishing to increase generalization will point out to the learner how two or more situations are alike. For instance, if the therapist has taught a client how to use a stove in the clinic kitchen, he or she may then have the client practice on other stoves, each time bringing to the client's attention the similarities among all stoves. Practice in multiple and varied contexts increases the opportunities for generalization of learning.

Operant Conditioning

B. F. Skinner focused his attention on the role of reward or **reinforcement** in learning and described the process known as **operant** (also called **instrumental**) **conditioning** (Skinner, 1938, 1953, 1968, 1971). Skinner looked first at the behavior or response that was occurring. When the response was desirable, it was rewarded or reinforced.

Discriminating Stimulus

When the response was reinforced in the presence of one stimulus but not in the presence of another, the response tended to occur in the presence of the former and not the latter. The former stimulus, called a **discriminating stimulus**, was said to act as a **cue**, telling the person when to generate the response. If the stimulus and response were paired repeatedly but without the reward, the response ceased, or was eliminated, and **extinction** was said to have occurred.

To illustrate, a client or patient might have difficulty in asking for help and making his or her needs known to others. As part of his or her personal goal, the individual might agree to come to your desk and ask for assistance when needed. You would wait for the client to come and ask for help; when he or she succeeded, you might smile and say, "I'll be glad to help you" (reinforcement). If this person approached you while you were away from your desk helping someone else in the clinic, you would ignore his or her evocation (no reinforcement). Seeing you at your desk is the cue that he or she should come and ask for help.

Discriminatory Behavior

In the preceding example, the cue has two parts—you are alone and you are at your desk—and two responses are desired—approaching you and asking for help. Being able to perceive the difference between your being at your desk and your being elsewhere in the clinic is the basis for **discrimination**. Discriminatory behavior is the opposite of generalization. It depends on being able to see the differences between situations or settings, thereby enabling the individual to determine when a behavior is appropriate and when it is not. It is because of much stimulus and response discrimination that we know to act differently in a movie theater than during a church prayer.

It is easier to discriminate between gross or obvious differences in stimuli than between subtle differences. For example, the junctions of most busy streets use discriminating stimuli intended to be noticed; these are the red and green traffic signals that cue our traffic behaviors. However, discriminating among subtle differences in stimuli makes possible the execution of more skilled motor and social acts. For instance, if an individual is adept at perceiving slight changes in the voices or nonverbal behaviors of his or her peers and can respond accordingly, one might say this individual is "sensitive" or "gracious." If he or she fails to take notice of such changes, he or she might be considered to be insensitive or crude. One might say that the individual would need to be "hit over the head before getting the message."

In the psychodynamic framework, the ability for discrimination is considered an ego function. In order for effective and adaptive discriminatory behavior to be learned, there must be appropriate giving and withholding of reinforcement according to the situation, and the individual must be able to perceive differences in stimuli and cues.

Facilitating Discrimination in Therapy

The occupational therapist wanting to enhance discriminatory learning within a therapeutic milieu would take care to do the following:

1. Make sure that the individual perceives the differences between specific situations
2. Reinforce only properly discriminated behavior

In regard to this first aim, the therapist might direct the person's attention to the discriminating features of a setting or point out the differences between two settings. In another text (Borg & Bruce, 1997), the authors describe an instance in which the occupational therapist is instructing a young man, "Nathan," who is indiscriminate in asking personal questions of the therapist during therapy sessions. In this instance, the therapist could ignore (not answer) all questions that are of a personal nature (withhold reinforcement), could help Nathan discern the difference between personal and therapy-related questions (enhance discrimination), or could use both learning strategies (pp. 89-92).

REINFORCEMENT

Skinner defined reinforcement as anything that increased the likelihood that a behavior would recur. For our discussion in this chapter, we speak primarily of positive reinforcement, although some behavioral occupational therapists also use what they refer to as negative reinforcement. A significant role for the therapist planning to use operant conditioning is to identify what in the environment serves to reinforce, and therefore maintain, specific client behaviors, both adaptive and maladaptive (see Reinforcement).

Types of Reinforcement

From the time we are very young, we are encouraged to behave through the use of such well-known reinforcers as

REINFORCEMENT

A **reinforcer** is anything that, when it follows a behavior, increases the likelihood that the behavior will be repeated. Whether positive or negative, reinforcement builds or maintains targeted behavior. In **positive reinforcement**, something is presented to the person that is seen as desirable; the targeted behavior is repeated to gain the desired reinforcement. In **negative reinforcement**, the targeted behavior is done to get away from the reinforcement, which may be viewed as aversive. The desired behavior acts on the environment so as to remove the adverse stimuli or to remove or keep the individual from the situation. For instance, in the winter we put on a coat to avoid getting cold. The cold weather outside negatively reinforces the behavior of putting on a coat. A group of children who find the quiet, inactive therapy session to be boring may initiate activity to avoid continued quiet. Allowing them to experience this "boring" environment may provide negative reinforcement for their appropriate initiation of play and engagement in the group.

hugs, attention, praise, sweets, and material goods. Martin (1978) categorizes reinforcers that have been used frequently in therapeutic settings. Combined into three broad categories these are consumable reinforcers, social reinforcers, and activity reinforcers.

Consumable reinforcers are those such as candy, cigarettes, fruit, snacks, and coffee. **Social reinforcers** include any signs of attention, hugs, smiles, pats on the back, verbal praise, recognition, etc. **Activity reinforcers** cover a broad range and may require some diligence on the part of the therapist and client to identify. These include the opportunity to engage in a favored activity (e.g., tinker with one's car, ride a bike, read a book, spend time alone, watch television, play video games, work with arts or crafts, or shopping). Activity reinforcers may also include the opportunity to wear one's favorite shirt, hold a favored toy, or sit in one's favorite chair.

Schedules of Reinforcement

In day-to-day living, material goods and opportunities to engage are reinforcing to the individual, in part, because they are not constantly available. For instance, food is rewarding because we do not eat constantly and we get hungry. Reading a book may be reinforcing because it represents a diversion from a more exacting or job-related task. We function in a world where, although we are not flooded with reinforcement, we are reinforced often enough to encourage desired behaviors.

Continuous versus Fixed Reinforcement

In therapy, reinforcement is supplied according to what is termed a **schedule of reinforcement**. If behavior is reinforced every time it occurs, **continuous reinforcement** occurs. If reinforcement follows a given number of correct responses (e.g., every third or fourth time the behavior is exhibited), a **fixed ratio** of reinforcement occurs. If behavior is reinforced at a consistent interval of time (every 10 minutes), a **fixed interval** of reinforcement occurs. There are also variable or unpredictable ratios and intervals of reinforcement and complex combinations of ratio and intervals. When a new behavior is being learned, the individual may need continuous or very consistent reinforcement. This situation occurs in occupational therapy when the therapist acknowledges the individual's or group's achievement by giving verbal praise or attention, candy, or tokens every time a desired behavior is exhibited.

Intermittent Reinforcement

Over a period of time in therapy, the client or patient is usually weaned to less frequent reinforcement. In **intermittent reinforcement**, behavior is reinforced occasionally. Behavior that is maintained by both intermittent and unpredictable reinforcement is the most difficult to extinguish and, therefore, most stable. This effect is illustrated, for example, by the behavior some may exhibit when hoping for a phone call from a new romantic interest who says, "I'll call you." Initially, we might keep a phone nearby or keep our calendars open, hoping for a call. If he or she calls only once during the week, that may be enough to keep us encouraged for more days because there is the chance that this person will call again. If no such call is ever received (no reinforcement), however, we would typically stop expecting the call within a relatively short period of time. With no reinforcement, the waiting behavior ceases.

Determining Reinforcement

It is difficult to predict how often an individual will need to be rewarded in order to maintain a specified desired behavior. For instance, one employee may require a great deal of recognition and many pats on the back from his or her employer to maintain a high level of productivity; another might find only a yearly brief, "Thanks for a good job," adequate reinforcement. The extent to which each of us needs external and predictable reinforcement from outside sources is related in part to the extent that we get self-satisfaction from our own behavior.

Guide for Using Selective Reinforcement

When an individual who had not previously done so consistently demonstrates a behavior as a consequence of its being reinforced, regardless of whether it is behavior the person has consciously thought about, learning is said to have occurred.

A key strategy used within the behavioral model is that of **selective reinforcement**. Selective reinforcement simply means that the therapist will be careful to reinforce only those behaviors that are desired and can be expected to lead to skill development. Equal care will be taken to not reinforce any behaviors that impede skill development. See Principles of Reinforcement, which summarizes principles for effectively using reinforcement.

Reducing or Suppressing Behavior

Whereas selective reinforcement is used to enhance or maintain a desired behavior, sometimes a goal when responding to problem behaviors is to decrease or suppress behavior. If, for example, an undesirable behavior can be minimized or suppressed, it may create an opportunity for a more positive behavior to take its place.

When behavior is followed by a negative consequence that decreases the incidence of this targeted behavior, this consequence is referred to as punishment. **Punishment**

PRINCIPLES OF REINFORCEMENT

The following summarizes principles for effectively using reinforcement:

1. An agent or event will be particularly reinforcing if one has been deprived of it at least briefly. Therefore, food will be more rewarding in the clinic or home setting to an individual who has not finished lunch; being able to work on a fine-motor craft will be more satisfying if the person had not been working on a similar task before occupational therapy. Even smiles and praise when given in excess tend to lose their capacity to be rewarding. When an agent or activity is no longer experienced as reinforcing because the patient or client has had enough, **satiation** occurs and an alternative reinforcement must be used.

2. An individual should be reinforced immediately after a desired behavior so that he or she will associate the response with the reinforcement.

3. At first, reinforce often, then gradually less often. One may need to reinforce every response to initiate a new behavior but should be able to reward it progressively less frequently to keep it going.

4. Don't reward a person for "something that a dead man can do." This is a picturesque way of stating that it is better to reinforce active behavior, or steps taken toward one's goals, rather than passivity, or the absence of behavior. If applied with children, for example, instead of rewarding an aggressive child for sitting silently for 10 minutes, consider rewarding him or her for appropriate involvement in a group activity.

5. Ask for and reward a specific accomplishment rather than general obedience or good intentions. This requires that a desired behavior be clearly spelled out.

6. By providing verbalization along with the reinforcement, one can, through the principle of stimulus generalization, make the verbalization alone reinforcement. For instance, when a client is on time for therapy 5 days in succession, he or she may earn the right to go to a local shopping mall unaccompanied by a staff member. If, when informing the person of the reward, the therapist adds enthusiastically, "I'm really proud of you, and I'll bet you feel good too!" then therapist's praise has been coupled with the earned walk. If this association is repeated many times, therapist praise alone may eventually be adequate reinforcement for the patient or client to maintain promptness or, even better, the person's self-talk ("I feel good about me") may maintain the behavior.

7. The thoughts or internal statements that an individual tells him- or herself may act as stimuli for action, as cues telling him or her when to act, as drives impelling actions, as responses, and as reinforcement.

8. Behavior that depends solely on an external reward for its maintenance is precarious behavior because reinforcement may be removed by others without recourse by the individual. The most stable behavior is often that in which personal satisfaction (e.g., living up to one's standards) is the primary reinforcement.

occurs when a given behavior is followed by an adverse stimulus that cannot be escaped or avoided. Punishment has been shown to decrease or suppress behavior but not to extinguish it; there is no change in learning.

Let's use an example that often occurs with children. A young child is given a toy (e.g., building blocks) that he or she doesn't know how to use appropriately. Rather than build with the blocks, the child plays with them by tossing them around the room. The upset parent or therapist punishes the child by taking the blocks away and states that one "must not throw toys." Next time the child has the blocks he or she may not throw them, but unless someone has taught the child how the blocks are to be used, he or she still hasn't learned the "proper way" to organize and build for play. Sooner or later, the temptation to throw the blocks may become too strong, and again the child tosses them about. In itself, punishment does not lead to new behavior, but if paired with reinforcement of more appropriate behavior (the child is shown how to assemble the blocks and praised for his or her efforts), it can be used as part of a learning strategy.

There are dangers in the use of punishment. One danger is that behavior stopped through punishment is likely to recur. Further, the therapist who has punished the client (child or adult) has to deal with the possibility that he or she has fostered negative feelings toward the therapy setting or the therapist. Another undesirable consequence is that punishment may lead to passive behavior or withdrawal. Finally, if the use of punishment jeopardizes the client-therapist relationship, it may make it more difficult for the therapist to effectively reinforce desired behaviors (Murdoch & Barker, 1991, pp. 44-48).

Eliminating Behavior

How then can one hope to eliminate undesirable behaviors? Behavioral therapists state very clearly that the way to eliminate a problem behavior is to make sure that it is not reinforced (Murdoch & Barker, 1991). This requires the therapist or therapy team to identify what in the environment is reinforcing and thereby maintaining the behavior. It can be very difficult to identify what acts as reinforcement for behavior. At times, depending on the clients with whom we work, they may get reinforced by responses that one wouldn't expect to be rewarding (e.g., negative attention for misconduct) or for behavior that is not desirable (e.g., sympathy for helpless-appearing behavior).

One strategy intended to eliminate rewards for undesirable behavior is the use of time-outs. The term **time-out** stands for "time out from reinforcement." If an undesirable response is ignored and positive reinforcement is withheld until the desired behavior occurs, the desired behavior is more likely to be learned.

To cite an example from the literature, time-out-on-the-spot (**TOOTS**) is used as a way to neither reward nor punish inappropriate behavior. The therapist responds to a behavior (e.g., a client demanding a third or fourth dessert at lunch) either by walking away for a brief period (20 seconds or so) or by continuing to pay attention to the person but ignoring the behavior and talking with the person about something else (Giles, 1987).

More commonly, the person with misconduct is removed from the situation, typically for a brief time period (Murdoch & Barker, 1991, p. 46). Most of us have seen situations in which a child is sent to his or her room or out of a classroom for the purpose of taking a time-out. Time-outs can also be self-imposed. For example, a person who is experiencing difficulty controlling his or her angry outbursts might be encouraged to remove him- or herself from provocative situations. In some community intervention programs, clients are taught the TOOTS strategy to meet program rules that expect participants to have control of their behavior to avoid physical and verbal altercations. In this situation a time-out can give a person time to regain emotional control and gives staff the ability to problem-solve with one client at a time. Both with children and adults, the use of time-out can be part of a more encompassing set of strategies known as **behavior management**.

Behavior management is used with persons of all ages who have difficulty controlling their behavior. Behavior management emphasizes the use of clearly articulated expectations and an externally structured learning environment designed to optimize order and boundaries. Clinicians use these strategies, and they teach clients and family members to use these strategies for managing emotional outbursts and stressful environments. (Note: Behavior management as a strategy used with children is discussed later in this chapter.)

A therapist using time-out (e.g., removing an individual from the therapy setting) has to be cautious that the time-out from therapy is not viewed by the client as more desirable than participating in therapy, in which case time-out would become a reward for undesirable behavior.

Neither reinforcement nor punishment can be expected to teach a person a behavior that is not in his or her repertoire. When a desired, adaptive response appears not to be in the individual's behavior repertoire, other behavioral techniques may be used. These techniques include shaping, building chains of behavior, and modeling.

Shaping

In an earlier discussion of discriminatory learning, we cited an example of reinforcing a client who asks for assistance from the therapist when the therapist is at his or her desk. If, in this example, the desired behavior of asking for the therapist's assistance is not demonstrated, then shaping techniques could be used. In **shaping**, any action that is similar to or preliminary to the desired behavior is reinforced, as are successive actions that more closely approximate or lead to the desired response. For example, if the client in the earlier example did not succeed initially in approaching the therapist's desk and asking for help, the therapist might watch to see if he or she arose from his or her seat, or even just looked in the therapist's direction. The therapist might then choose to reinforce this anticipatory behavior and continue to reinforce subsequent behavior (e.g., with smiles) that brought the person closer to the therapist's desk. While using the principle of shaping, the therapist would also be careful to not reinforce any maladaptive responses.

Identifying Approximate Steps

When using shaping as part of a behavior program, the therapist must begin with a behavior that the individual can complete and must be prepared to reinforce small steps toward the final, desired goal. Martin (1978) suggests that the therapist begin by making a list of the approximate steps that will lead from the beginning to the final behavior. Be aware that each step in the sequence might have to be repeated and reinforced many times before the therapist can expect the next step in the sequence to be exhibited. In other instances, however, several steps might follow in quick succession.

Building Chains of Behavior

Skinner believed that most complex behavior can be understood as chains of stimulus-response connections; links in which a completed response acts as a stimulus signaling that it is time for the next in the series of responses. Occupational therapists often assist clients who wish to learn complex sequences of skills. One might consider the steps in planting a flower garden. We see the seedlings at the store, which signals to us that it is time for a planting, which cues us to collect our tools and other paraphernalia, which leads us to select a potential site for planting, which when chosen cues us to begin digging a hole, and so on. In fact, each of these major steps by itself consists of even smaller, discrete stimulus-response links.

Backward Chaining

When we think about learning, we tend to conceive of developing learning chains in a forward order; however, **backward chaining** is used frequently in therapy. The term backward chaining might suggest that the individual is taught to do a procedure backward but that is not the case. The example of planting a seedling allows us to illustrate backward chaining and its advantage.

Suppose for a moment that you are teaching a young child or adult who has a short attention span the procedures just indicated. By the time you help the child or adult select the tools, choose a planting site, and dig a hole, he or she may have lost interest in completing the process. For most people, the most rewarding part of planting is seeing the young plant standing upright firmly in the ground. If the therapist prepares the ground and calls the client over to put the plant in the hole or asks him or her to cover the roots of the plant with dirt, the person begins with the final step and immediately gains the reward of seeing the plant in the ground.

After helping the therapist with several plants in this manner, the individual may express the wish to help dig the holes. In that case, one might start the hole for the client so that not too much digging is needed, then let him or her finish the digging, insert the plant, and cover its roots with soil. As the child or adult becomes more interested and better able to persevere, we continue to add steps in a backward chain, always allowing him or her to move from the chosen step through the subsequent steps he or she has already learned to the last step and the reinforcement. In this way, the final reward comes to sustain a long series of stimulus-response links. Very often therapists teaching rehabilitative techniques to clients will set up the therapeutic environment with the same principles in mind, in order that the client can complete the last few steps in a process and achieve the satisfaction of bringing a task to successful completion.

As with shaping, the therapist may find it useful to make a list of the approximate steps taken from start to finish in a given process. The therapist then starts with the last step and, upon its completion, provides a suitable reinforcement. The therapist then proceeds backward down the chain, giving the patient or client ample opportunity to practice each step or series of steps, as needed, before adding a new behavior link.

Forward and backward chaining methods are also used in many intervention environments for relearning basic ADL and IADL skills. The choice of method for learning is influenced by the client's previous level of function and the person's current ability to attend to and follow the activity sequence, as well as the treatment goal.

Modeling

Modeling has been described as a "rapid method of learning" (Murdoch & Barker, 1991, p. 32). In the evolution of learning theory, modeling has been better understood largely due to the investigation of Albert Bandura (1963, 1971a, 1971b). Along with such others as Mischel (1968, 1973) and Rotter (1954), Bandura has proposed a social learning theory that attempts to not only incorporate the traditional reinforcement and contiguity elements of behavioral theory, but also to add to these the role of imitation in learning. Bandura and his associates believe that when a person observes the actions of another, he or she can vicariously learn a new behavior that later can be replicated through imitation.

Some skills appear to be learned more easily by imitation than through the development of stimulus response chains or the shaping of behavior.

For example, when an individual wishes to learn how to swing a golf club correctly, he or she often imitates his or her teacher. Learning new words, learning to drive a car, or learning to play baseball can all be viewed as highly imitative forms of learning. Nothing in this concept is new to most occupational therapists who have long known the value of demonstration and imitation when trying to teach new skills.

However, modeling is recognized as being quite different conceptually from other methods of learning because the **modeled behavior** is conceived as having been learned internally and vicariously before any actual response has been demonstrated or rewarded. This becomes important in the area of social learning, in which one learns how to act based on one's observations of various models whom he or she admires.

For example, learning from modeling occurs in many rehabilitation environments. Clients learn from observing and interacting with each other. On multiple occasions we have heard clients comment that they learned an activity by watching another client or staff member. Families comment that they learned from watching and listening to other families who were participating in the intervention environment.

Guides for Using Modeling

Behavioral literature highlights what has been learned about modeling. The guides can be used by the occupational therapist who wishes to increase imitative learning (see Guides for Using Modeling).

Bandura and other social learning proponents differ from traditional behaviorists with their inclusion of concepts such as vicarious learning, symbolic representation, imagery, and cognitive problem-solving. Social learning has become an increasingly significant part of behavioral theory and, along with cognitive behaviorism, appears to represent the direction of much recent behavioral inquiry. More of Bandura's theory and cognitive behavioral approaches are discussed in Chapter Six.

Token Economies

Token economies are systems of operant conditioning designed to alter behavior with several or more individuals, especially when internal or intangible reinforcements (e.g., social approval or self-satisfaction) have not proven effective. Tokens, which can be metal washers, plastic discs, credit cards that can be punched, and the like, are tangible rewards given for appropriate behavior. They can be exchanged for privileges, cigarettes, candy, involvement in desired activities, and other desired goods or opportunities.

For example, if a person in residential care makes his or her bed, he or she might receive three tokens; if the individual completes an occupational therapy work project, the reward is five tokens. A candy bar might cost three tokens; a pass home might cost 20 tokens. Whereas some token economies use only positive reinforcement, others use negative procedures as well (e.g., fines [tokens given back] are assessed when a patient fails to meet a requirement). The previous example of token use demonstrates a form of punishment known as **response cost**. As noted by Corey (1982), tokens can have several advantages:

- Tokens reduce the delay between appropriate behavior and its reward.

GUIDES FOR USING MODELING

- A person is more likely to be imitated if he or she is perceived as having high status; consequently, a therapist viewed by patients and clients as having status has a potentially significant impact as a social model.

- A person is more likely to be imitated if the observer can see the similarities between self and the model. Such similarities could relate to age, gender, nationality, socioeconomic position, similar disability, or skill level.

- An individual will more likely imitate behavior perceived as leading to reward (e.g., when the person sees the model receiving a reward). In addition, he or she is more likely to inhibit a response perceived as leading to punishment, as when the model is observed being punished.

- A model's relative physical attractiveness will increase the likelihood of his or her being copied (Murdoch & Barker, 1991, p. 34).

- A model that is perceived as warm and caring and has a history of meeting an individual's emotional needs is more likely to be imitated (Murdoch & Barker, 1991, p. 34).

- Hostility, aggression, and moral behavior have all been shown to be highly accessible to learning through modeling.

- To be successfully imitated, the model behavior must be well attended to. Distraction in the learning setting can be expected to decrease imitative learning.

- Many skilled acts, especially those involving fine motor coordination, can be learned only in part through modeling; participation and practice are necessary adjuncts to learning.

- When the individual can give verbal labels or descriptions to the behavior observed, that behavior is more successfully remembered and imitated (Hilgard & Bower, 1974, 1975).

- Tokens can be used as a concrete measure of motivation.
- Tokens involve an element of choice in that the person has an opportunity to decide how he or she wishes to spend them.

Concern for Patients' Rights

During the 1960s and 1970s, there was a proliferation of token economies, especially in programs for individuals with long-term or chronic psychiatric problems, persons with developmental delay, and those in forensic settings. Some major and positive outcomes were seen in the ability to affect behavior, teach new skills to those who up until then had seemed unteachable, and to manage large populations more effectively. As journals cited cases in which bizarre behavior improved dramatically, token economies and the concomitant strict observance of operant behaviorism were touted as breakthroughs in mental health care (Ogburn et al., 1972; Overbaugh, Bradley, & Bucher, 1970).

Subsequently, however, token economies were criticized. Overbaugh et al. (1970) describe a male patient who had been in treatment for 45 years, yet continued to respond with little in the way of appropriate behavior. The decision was made by the treatment team to apply a rigorous token system. As the authors state:

> Throughout the therapy, the patient was on a deprivation schedule. He received no breakfast at any time during the study... Receipt of tokens redeemable for the noon and evening meals was contingent on meeting each day's global performance criterion...

The authors go on to say that in a short time the patient exhibited markedly improved behavior and was more manageable within the institution.

The ethics of depriving an individual of such a basic need as food is at issue—even for what is described as a "short period" and for positive intent.

In 1962, President Kennedy outlined a Consumer's Bill of Rights, which provided for the consumer's right to safety, right to be informed, right to choose, and right to be heard. Since then, patients and clients have been viewed increasingly as consumers, and these rights also extend to them. However, persons in institutions, especially those involuntarily committed, historically did not always receive treatment sensitive to patients' rights.

The 1972 court decision of Wyatt vs. Stickney represented a significant move toward increased specificity regarding patient rights. As part of the resolution of this case, the court, assisted by the American Civil Liberties Union, the American Orthopsychiatric Association, the American Psychological Association, and the American Association of Mental Deficiency specified in detail rights for those individuals who were under involuntary commitment. These rights include the right to privacy, the right to wear one's own clothes, the right to have personal possessions, the right to regular physical exercise, the right to be outdoors from time to time, the right to nutritionally adequate meals, and the right to the "least restrictive conditions necessary to achieve the purposes of treatment" (Geiser, 1976). These are absolute rights and cannot be made contingent on a token economy or other intervention systems.

Effectiveness of Token Economies

Contemporary therapists are sensitive to these legal rights and take care to use tokens as part of programs designed to foster human dignity. Finding effective reinforcements for very regressed and uncommunicative or uncooperative patients or clients can be difficult, as many do not desire customary social and tangible rewards (Liberman, Massel, Mosk, & Wong, 1993). Occupational therapist Lorna Jean King (1974) reframed this problem and noted that many institutionalized patients exhibit **anhedonia**, or the inability to experience pleasure.

Other questions have been raised by token economies. There is no clear evidence that the gains made within a token system are sustained once the individual returns home or to a non-treatment setting. To sustain behavior, internal or other external reward must reinforce behavior that had been maintained by tokens. For instance, self-satisfaction or a spouse's approval must be sufficiently rewarding at home, but this is not always the case. Although token economies do seem capable of managing behavior within a closed treatment community, they are not the panacea for behavior change that they were once believed to be (Martin, 1972).

Desensitization

Since the late 1950s, **systematic desensitization** has been used as a behavioral strategy to reduce anxiety. Although the reasons for the success of this technique are not entirely understood, persons with test anxiety, speech anxiety, interpersonal-social anxiety, stuttering, and phobias have been successfully treated by desensitization (Cormier & Cormier, 1979). After identifying the source of fear or anxiety, the patient or client participates in experiences that help him or her to gradually get comfortable with the situation. The anxiety-provoking stimuli are presented in a series of graded experiences that proceed from low to high intensity. The graded experience may incorporate imagery, role playing, simulated activities, homework, or real situations inside or outside the intervention setting that stimulates fear and anxiety (Cormier & Cormier, 1979). The principle of desensitization is frequently used informally by therapists in a variety of intervention contexts. The child or adolescent who is painfully shy with his or her peers might be encouraged to attend a group activity session and observe, perhaps for only 10 or 15 minutes, before being encouraged to attend for longer periods or to actually participate in a task group. The person who is sensitive to tactile stimulation might be touched or brushed for initial periods of seconds only, as his or her tolerance to touch is gradually increased.

Biofeedback and Stress Management

Biofeedback is "a process of using equipment... to reveal to human beings some of their internal physiological events, normal and abnormal, in the form of visual and auditory signals to teach them to influence these otherwise involuntary or unfelt events by manipulating the displayed signals" (Abildness, 1982). The signals that the individual receives may act as stimuli or cues to act and as reinforcement.

Biofeedback in Physical Medicine and Mental Health Settings

Occupational therapists and other professionals in physical medicine and mental health treatment settings have applied biofeedback. In rehabilitation settings, biofeedback can be used for physical reconditioning, muscle re-education, increasing motor control and coordination, and strengthening muscles. It is also used in physical medicine settings to monitor heart rate, visceral activities, blood pressure, and skin temperature. It has been used in pain management programs and with psychosomatic conditions such as tension, migraine headaches, and fecal incontinence (Abildness, 1982; Engel & Rapoff, 1990).

In mental health, biofeedback is more frequently applied to promote relaxation and manage stress. It has also been successful in helping patients manage symptoms that are an outcome of a variety of disorders including phobic reactions, depression, substance abuse, schizophrenia, and character disorder (Abildness, 1982; Stein & Nikolic, 1989).

Biofeedback in Occupational Therapy

In occupational therapy, biofeedback is used in conjunction with functional activities and is integrated with the application of other major theoretical treatment approaches such as biomechanical, neurodevelopmental, rehabilitation, psychodynamic, or sensory integrative approaches. During evaluation and intervention, biofeedback is used to identify the effects of the occupational therapy task on the individual. Clients have been monitored during group projects, home activities, social experiences, work projects, and community outings. This feedback is used to teach the client or patient self-control, to facilitate the adjustment of intervention strategies, and to document progress (Abildness, 1982).

CURRENT PRACTICE IN OCCUPATIONAL THERAPY

Person and Behavior

From 1940 through the 1960s, the deterministic view of behavior predominated. This view was judged to be "radical" because it saw people as limited in the ability to actively choose and learn (Corey, 1982). The early behaviorists, oper-ating on Skinner's behavioral theory, believed that virtually all behavior was determined, and therefore controlled, by the introduction and maintenance of reinforcement (Skinner, 1971). Persons who controlled reinforcement were identified as those in charge, and the concept of free will was challenged. Since the late 1960s, the behavior position has incorporated cognitive and social learning theories, which consider the individual to be both the product and producer of the environment.

People are viewed as neither innately good nor bad. Whether behavior is considered adaptive or maladaptive depends on the degree to which it meets social expectations.

Motivation

Motivation refers to the process in which goal-directed activity is instigated and sustained (Pintrich & Schunk, 1996, p. 21). It is an internal process that one cannot see directly; rather, one observes its outcome in behavior. Early behaviorists defined motivation in terms of forces beyond the person's control such as the basic biological drives (the need for food, sex, and the avoidance of pain) as well as the secondary needs for love, approval, and other social needs (Pintrich & Schunk, 1996). More recent literature views motivation as something both externally and internally influenced and as a necessary condition for change (Murdoch & Barker, 1991; Pintrich & Schunk, 1996). To elaborate, we do not motivate a person to behave appropriately by enticing him with a reward (e.g., successful achievement of his goal). He must have an internal desire to obtain the reward for it to be rewarding. That is one reason why even stringent behavioral approaches may be ineffective when a client lacks motivation. The client who is extremely depressed, for example, may lack internal motivation, as may the person with long-standing schizophrenia, and behavioral techniques are not necessarily going to "motivate" these persons. That does not mean that behavioral strategies cannot influence motivation.

Literature in the area of goal-setting and motivation suggests that clients will be more motivated to reach therapeutic goals that are specific, moderately challenging, and set by them (Hoppes, 1997; Locke & Latham, 1990). Thus, a client who has an internal drive (motivation) to get healthier would be expected to more likely act on this drive when he or she is headed toward clearly articulated behavioral goals perceived as challenging and improving one's health. However, not all motivated behavior is to reach a positive goal. Fear and anxiety also impel or drive behavior and may do so in a direction away from desired learning or goal attainment.

Function as Adaptive Performance

The person is an active and choosing agent who interacts with and acts on his or her environment. The environment responds to the individual and selectively reinforces behavior. Those behaviors that are reinforced will most likely recur. All behaviors can be broken down into observable, measurable actions or discrete steps. However, the occupational therapist is most often concerned with building or enhancing groups of task behaviors known as **skills**. Together, the skills that a person has create a skill repertoire that enables functional performance. These skills will be viewed as **adaptive** if they enable the individual to satisfy personal needs, live according to his or her values, achieve independence, achieve pleasure, and live in harmony with others in society.

Dysfunction as Skill or Performance Deficit

An important influence of behavioral therapy has been to challenge the supposition that deviant behavior is an illness. As identified in this model, dysfunction results from gaps in learning (skill deficits), failure to demonstrate learned skills (performance deficits), or learning in which undesirable behavior (maladaptive behavior) has been intentionally or inadvertently reinforced. That does not mean that persons with whom this model is used could not also have a psychiatric diagnosis that has influenced his or her behavior and ability for learning.

Skill Deficits

A **skill deficit** exists when a person lacks the ability needed to perform a task or skilled behavior (Murdoch & Barker, 1991, p. 80) or is unable to meet personal standards or external standards in performance (Holm, Rogers, & Stone, 1999, p. 481).

Consider the following: Blake is a young man who was trained as a welder. Although he has considerable experience in his field, he has never formally applied for a job. He decides to seek a new position and spies this ad in the classifieds: "Wanted: Welder. New electronics firm. Experience a must. $28/hr; 35hr/wk guaranteed. Send resumé." Blake neither knows what would be included in a job resume, nor has he ever written one. He has a skill deficit.

Skill deficits may occur when a client has never learned the skill or when the ability to use the skill has become impaired. These deficits may become apparent when clients encounter changing life circumstances, as from disease, trauma, or the aging process. The person who needs to learn to use a prosthetic device for dressing, grooming, and other daily living tasks following a limb amputation or the older widow who needs to learn how to change the oil in a car formerly maintained by her spouse has skill deficits.

A skill deficit represents a skill not currently in an individual's repertoire and, as such, cannot be encouraged by means of selective reinforcement alone. Rather, the therapist will combine various learning strategies such as modeling, shaping, chaining, and other forms of instruction and information-giving in order to teach the client the desired skill. Further, the therapist will create opportunities for the new skill to be practiced in multiple settings.

With uncorrectable skill deficits (the client cannot be taught the skill), compensatory strategies will be used to enable the person to function optimally in his or her environment.

Performance Deficits

With a **performance deficit**, the person is able to perform the desired skill but fails to do so in a situation that calls for it or fails to demonstrate the skill with the necessary consistency (intensity, duration, or frequency) (Murdoch & Barker, 1991, p. 82). There are many causes for performance deficits. Sometimes performance deficits result when a client is depressed or for other reasons lacks the energy or persistence to exhibit the targeted skill. For example, the widow knows how to change the oil in her automobile but has lacked the energy or desire to do it since her spouse died. There are other reasons clients may choose to not exhibit requisite skills (e.g., the child or adolescent who is asked to organize his sports cards by brand but fails to do so because he doesn't like being "told what to do").

Performance deficits may also occur when a client doesn't recognize that the skilled performance is needed (e.g., the client who fails to brush her teeth as often or carefully as recommended because she doesn't realize that teeth should be cleaned at least twice daily). With a change in the client's familiar environment, the client may not recognize that a specific skill (e.g., changing bed linens) is expected, as when a client moves from a residential care setting (which has house-keeping service) to a half-way house in which residents are responsible for changing their own linen. Another reason that skills or specific skilled behaviors might not be demonstrated is that they are not being currently reinforced in the client's environment.

Sometimes clients simply aren't comfortable performing skills that they haven't used in a long time or don't have much practice with (e.g., the adult who hasn't been on roller skates since he was a child may be hesitant to join his child in this activity). In this latter instance, the skill may have atrophied to the point where it is now a skill deficit.

Performance deficits relate to skills that are part of a client's skill repertoire and can be remediated through selective reinforcement, including words of support and encouragement from the therapist, the client's family, or peers. It is vital that the occupational therapist ascertains that a desired skill is actually in a client's repertoire before assuming that this person has a performance deficit and not a skill deficit. It may happen, for example, that a client—adult or child—will state that he or she could perform a skill if he or she "felt like it" or "really needed to do it," when, in fact, the person is unable to perform the skill. The best way to ensure that a skill is in a client's repertoire is to observe the individual performing the skill in the specific environment in which it is required.

Dysfunction as Behavior Excess

Both skill and performance deficits address problems in which the client or patient needs to learn or more consistently perform desired behavior. In contrast, behavior problems can also result from **behavioral excess**, wherein a behavior is occurring at too great a frequency, intensity, and/or duration (Murdoch & Barker, 1991, p. 78). As indicated previously, the way to eliminate or extinguish maladaptive behavior is to carefully avoid reinforcing it; however, not all behavioral excesses represent behavior that needs to be eliminated; rather, behavior may just need to be reduced. This begins with identifying what in the physical or social environment is acting as a reward for this behavior. The therapist can then teach and reinforce alternative (incompatible) behavior, teach self-control strategies, and/or reinforce behavior exhibited at the appropriate or a reduced rate of intensity.

Ineffective Discrimination

Maladaptive behavior, including behavioral excesses, can occur when an individual who is trying to act in an acceptable manner does not recognize that his or her behavior is unacceptable. This may happen, for instance, when a client fails to discriminate the behavior expected in a given situation. The person with poor social skills, for example, might not realize that the spontaneous conversation encouraged in client group meeting is inappropriate during a formal lecture. In this instance, the skill of carrying on social conversations is being used in too wide a range of settings.

Occupational therapists can help clients take responsibility for eliminating or modifying maladaptive behavior by helping these persons identify the discriminating features of various social or work environments and recognize what behavior and what rate of behavior is most acceptable.

Other Ways to Reduce Behavioral Excesses

Behavioral excesses are frequently seen in social behavior (e.g., behavior that is too aggressive, over-talkativeness, excessive alcohol consumption, etc). The occupational therapist may be in a position to teach new skills or coping strategies that would provide alternatives to these behavioral excesses. To illustrate, all three of the behaviors cited (talkativeness, aggressive behavior, and alcohol consumption) could be maladaptive responses used by a person experiencing unmanageable stress. Teaching the client healthier coping skills intended to substitute for these maladaptive behaviors could help reduce the undesired behaviors. As with building discriminatory skills, the therapist may be able to help the client take responsibility for reducing behavioral excess by increasing the client's awareness that these excesses exist. Other strategies that a therapist could use have been discussed previously and include punishment and selective reinforcement.

Role of the Occupational Therapist

The primary role of the therapist in the behavioral frame of reference is to facilitate the acquisition of desired performance skills that will enable the client to function optimally in his or her expected environment. This means that we expect, at least in part, the **person** to change in the **person-environment-occupation** triad. Facilitating change may occur through direct intervention or by means of consultation and education. The therapist may direct his or her attention to teaching desired skilled behavior through use of the various strategies for learning, as described. The therapist will be equally concerned with creating or maintaining an environment capable of supporting this learned behavior. As part of this process of facilitating skill acquisition, the therapist typically does one or more of the following:

- Identifies (or helps others identify) gaps in skilled performance and designs learning experiences in which these skills can be learned and maintained
- Helps manage or eliminate inappropriate behavior
- Serves as a role model for healthy behavior and skilled performance
- Selectively reinforces desired behavior
- Educates family and other caregivers in the use of behavioral strategies that will help maintain skilled occupational performance

Influencing Motivation and Acting as a Reinforcing Agent

The therapist uses various strategies to influence a client or patient's motivation. Clinicians can influence by:

- Giving explanations to the patient/client about his or her condition
- Providing explanations and assurance regarding the purpose of therapeutic activities
- Engaging the client in the goal-setting process
- Helping to establish moderately challenging goals and modifying goals to keep them appropriately challenging
- Offering support and affirmation that the individual can succeed

Although motivation is understood to be an internal phenomenon, it is recognized that an individual's belief that he or she can meet personal goals is an important requisite in goal setting and supports persistence in goal-directed behavior (Locke & Latham, 1990).

In residential and inpatient mental health settings, intervention teams, including the occupational therapist, frequently award privileges as a reinforcement when a client meets his or her goals (Boronow, 1986; Wilberding, 1993). The patient/client who fails to comply with intervention guidelines or to meet goals within the therapeutic milieu may be refused passes home, passes for community visits, or time free of staff supervision.

Rapport and a positive relationship between patient/client and the therapist is highly significant in this model, for it enhances the ability for therapist attention and approval to serve as an effective reinforcement. It may be that a desire to gain therapist approval is an early reinforcer during therapy;

once the client begins to experience success, the internal satisfaction of seeing one's self succeed can then become a more critical reinforcer. Barbara Borg shares the personal story that depicts the significance of the clinician in this model (see Significance of Therapist-Client Relationship).

SIGNIFICANCE OF THERAPIST-CLIENT RELATIONSHIP

My father had a below-the-knee amputation. It occurred following a critical block of blood flow to his lower limb, as a result of peripheral vascular disease. My dad had little time to prepare for the amputation. He went in to see his primary care physician on a Monday morning, which also happened to be his birthday; by Monday afternoon he was seeing a vascular specialist, and Thursday morning the leg was removed. Following the surgery, he became an inpatient on a rehabilitation unit. As he recovered from the surgery, he seemed more reserved than usual, perhaps somewhat depressed, though motivated to regain independence as quickly as possible. One of the obstacles standing in his way was residual nausea, which was presumed to be an after-effect of the anesthesia he had been given during surgery. Day after day he had difficulty holding down food, and as he said, "Food tastes of nothing." One concerned nurse approached my dad and asked him if he could think of anything that "sounds appetizing," adding, "It doesn't have to be on the hospital menu." After thinking for a few moments my father said, "A chocolate milk shake sounds good." From that day forward, each day this particular nurse was scheduled to work, she would stop at a fast-food restaurant, purchase a chocolate milk shake, and bring it to my dad. It took roughly 6 months of inpatient, then outpatient therapy before my father was able to walk independently and was permitted to drive a car. On the day he could go alone, he went back to the rehab setting to show this nurse that he had successfully regained his independence and to thank her.

Designing Client-Centered Learning Experiences

The behaviorally oriented occupational therapist can remain true to the professional commitment to be client-centered by sitting down with a new client or family and determining first what problems the client is experiencing and what is most important to the client in terms of therapeutic goals. The therapist then applies his or her knowledge and expertise to identify the specific skills necessary for these goals to be reached. The therapist must differentiate between those skills that have never been learned (**skill deficits**) and those that are not being used optimally (**performance deficits**). He or she can then design learning experiences that respect the client's preferences and that appreciate the strengths and limitations that are unique to the individual. We will be looking further at this process of teaching when we discuss specific intervention strategies later in the chapter.

Corrective Learning

In the psychiatric learning setting, the term **corrective learning** may be used to describe occupational therapy intervention in which clients learn to recognize inappropriate behavior and replace it with more adaptive behavior. This often occurs in the context of social skills and parenting experiences. For example, adults who were abused as children often reenact these abusive behaviors with their own children. The therapist may teach the client to recognize internal signals that he or she is losing control and then educate the person in alternative means of handling feelings, or the therapist may choose to build parent effectiveness by teaching the individual specific child-rearing skills. Frequently, the occupational therapist can enhance his or her role as instructor by modeling desired social and task behavior.

Therapist as Role Model

As a social role model, the therapist exhibits skills and behaviors from which the patient/client can learn. The learning process occurs as the client or patient identifies with and imitates the therapist. This is more likely to occur when the client respects and admires the therapist, has a positive relationship with the therapist, and/or can identify with the therapist in some way (as with gender, age, or other characteristic). The individual can learn verbal behavior as well as other specific skills, particularly social skills. This learning may occur quite naturally as the person observes the therapist in a variety of interactions within the intervention setting. The identification process in interactions is also apparent as we see one patient/client teach another a task skill, imitating what the therapist does or says.

Therapist as Coach

The occupational therapist may use specific learning activities that incorporate role-playing (also called **behavioral rehearsal**). Individual and group role-play experiences are used to teach new behaviors or to provide support to individuals in allowing them to explore multiple responses to problem situations. During role-plays, the therapist may demonstrate desirable verbal and nonverbal behaviors, which can later be mimicked by the patient/client when he or she role-plays a specific situation. As the role-play ensues, the therapist may stand next to the person who appears unable to generate a suitable response and cue or coach him or her in what to say or do. Within the context of coaching and providing cues, the therapist can also give immediate feedback and reinforcement to clients in regard to their behavior. Such coaching can be done with children as well as with adults.

Therapist as Consultant

Increasingly, occupational therapists are serving as consultants. The initial consultation may request the therapist to assess functional needs and to design a behavior program that will respond to the client's/family's performance goals. The occupational therapist may then train an aide, COTA, or other staff member to work cooperatively with the patient/client. The therapist may work directly with the family to advise them of client limitations, to help them establish reasonable expectations for therapy, and in order that they can implement the intervention plan.

Implementing behavioral strategies often requires diligence, especially where extra care is needed to selectively reinforce only desired behavior. This can wear on family members who may, for example, perceive inattention to negative behavior as being unkind or punishing. As a part of being a consultant, the therapist might use him- or herself as a model, showing care-providers how to best respond to behavior and/or how to build desired skills. For example, parents of children with chronic illness and disabling conditions often have difficulties setting limits and having behavioral expectations for the child. The occupational therapist is able to educate parents about developmentally appropriate behavior and model behaviors that incorporate limit setting and that expect appropriate responsibility-taking by the child (Kibele, Padilla, & Burton, 1998). The occupational therapist may also teach family members and care providers to set mutual goals through the use of contracts and to document progress. See Behavior or Learning Contract (Table 5-1) for an example of a learning contract format that can be used with clients.

When the therapist provides family members and caregivers information that helps them manage difficult behaviors or that ultimately leads to more successful interpersonal and goal behavior, it often helps the entire family unit to pull together and gain confidence that they can cope with the changes brought on by illness, trauma, or other challenges.

Activities as a Vehicle for Improving Occupational Performance

Building Skills

The heart of behavioral occupational therapy is the use of meaningful learning activities that comprise those occupations in which the client wishes to function.

Activities are used to teach performance skills, to serve as simulated learning experiences, to function as reinforcement, and to provide varied opportunities for practice of new skills. The therapist may initially break down activities into their component parts and must be aware of both the level of challenge presented to the patient/client and the skills required of

the individual when completing each step in the activity. As discussed previously, activities can be thought of as behavior chains in which one piece or component of the activity signals that it is time for the next link in the chain to ensue. A simplified example is provided here:

When we say someone has "independence in meal planning or preparation" we may expect that he or she has knowledge of and skills in budgeting, grocery shopping, meal preparation, serving, and clean-up. Each of these major components can then be further broken down into behavioral links. For example, "grocery shopping" could require that a person do the following:

- Make a shopping list that includes items from the major food groups and that would be sufficient in quantity to feed a given number of persons
- Access public transportation to get to the supermarket
- Demonstrate interpersonal skills that enable appropriate discourse in the community setting
- Use financial skills necessary for purchasing the food (e.g., making change)

It is important that the client be reinforced sufficiently while moving along this performance chain so that the desired functional outcome is achieved.

Activities are selected according to their interest and value to the client and to the degree in which they are consonant with sociocultural expectations. When operant conditioning is used, the expectation for performance must begin at the level of behavior that the patient/client is currently capable of demonstrating or performing. When modeling and imitative behavior are incorporated, activities can be selected that begin with novel, not previously demonstrated, behavior.

Splinter Skills and Functional Skill Training

A **splinter skill** is "a specific motor or mental skill that is performed only under specific circumstances and not integrated into a person's total behavior" (Banus, 1979; Becker & Banus, 1979). A splinter skill is non-stage specific and may be performed without the development of the enabling skills that are typically acquired in a chronological developmental sequence. Splinter skills are used in a specific context; they may be lost if not practiced continually and usually are not generalized (Nuse-Clark & Allen, 1985). For example, a child can memorize the alphabet song without understanding the concept and function of letters. He or she will forget the alphabet if the song isn't practiced frequently.

While occupational therapists would not typically want to build splinter skills, there are situations in which these may be desirable. Persons with developmental delay, cognitive impairment resulting from head injury, and other significant cognitive impairments may be able to be trained to function in a particular residential or vocational setting, engaged in work or other tasks that use splinter skills (Giles, 1992, 1998; Giles & Clark-Wilson, 1999; Neidstadt, 1994a, 1994b). In these instances, desired occupational tasks are

---

Table 5-1

BEHAVIOR OR LEARNING CONTRACT

Goal Target Date: _____ Goal Outcome Date: _____

Performance expected/mastered task/activity achieved and method to achieve goal:

1.

2.

3.

Expected consequence of meeting goal:

Client signature _____ Date: _____

Clinician signature _____ Date: _____

---

taught by first breaking down the task into component sub-skills. Each subskill is then practiced repeatedly through a process called **overlearning**. In order to enable each subskill to be learned, the therapist may supply cues or prompts. These cues are then gradually diminished (or **faded**) until the subskill can be done independently or with minimal prompting. Backward chaining is often used to establish the sequence in which subskills are taught, and selective reinforcement is used to maintain learning.

Behavioral Outcomes

Activities frequently used when applying this frame of reference include craft activities, task groups, prevocational or work experiences, relaxation experiences, assertiveness groups, social skills training, desensitization experiences, and tasks related to the use of token economies. The therapist uses activities to achieve an end (i.e., to reach a behavioral goal). When the focus is on the outcome, one asks the following:

- Can the person initiate a conversation?
- Can the client cook a meal?
- Is the person able to go to the bank and set up a new account?
- Did the group finish the task and accomplish its goal?
- Can the family manage behavior that is in conflict with environment expectations or out of context?

The focus is **not** on the process or what the person experiences during the activity, "What does it feel like to be in this group?" These feelings and process concerns are the primary emphasis in the psychodynamic model.

Activity Outcomes as Reinforcers

For many people, though not everyone, mastery of activities and one's environment becomes an internal reinforcer.

Although not directing the discussion to how the client or patient feels about a task experience, the occupational therapist recognizes that successful task experience and the sense of accomplishment that comes from task completion can be a source of reinforcement. He or she can further recognize the person's accomplishments with praise and appreciation for either the quality of the end product ("You did a great job reorganizing the storeroom. Thank you so much!") or the manner in which the task was carried out (e.g., "I know that you have worked hard to get yourself dressed and ready to go"). The therapist may also ask the client to affirm his or her accomplishments by identifying the skills that were acquired during the activity process. The therapist might ask, for example, "What did you see yourself do differently today in our pre-voc group, as compared to last week?"

Simulated Learning Experiences

Simulated experiences, also called **analogues**, are situations designed by the therapist to replicate the patient's or client's expected (post-intervention) or natural environment. In this analog context, the client can practice new skills that will, ideally, be easily transferred to the home.

For example, an area in which simulated experiences are frequently used in occupational therapy assessment and intervention is financial management. Financial management includes the ability to make money transactions, pay one's bills, plan a budget, and identify and use community and personal sources of income. To determine the ability to make banking transactions or to teach one to complete such transactions, the therapist asks the client to fill out bank deposit and withdrawal forms. Similarly, the client can be asked to use simulated checks to pay simulated bills or to create a monthly budget.

Learning is believed to be **situation specific** (Anthony, 1979; Palmer, 1988; Spiegler & Agigian, 1977; Watts & Bennett, 1983). For example, certain skills or repertoires of behavior are needed by a mother to care for her 3-year-old at home in the playroom. Different skills will be called for if the same child is being supervised on a bus ride. Because of this situation specificity, it is not assumed that what the client learns in a clinic or simulated setting will automatically transfer to the home setting. Even when skills are taught in the home setting, there will be differences in the tasks once the therapist is no longer involved. The encouragement or reinforcement at home may be vastly different once therapy ceases. Additionally, client emotions about the activity may vary within and outside of the therapeutic context. For this reason and in accord with principles related to generalization of learning, the therapist often encourages the client to practice in multiple or varied contexts and, when possible, may follow-up clinical intervention with home visits.

Theoretical Assumptions—Guide to Evaluation and Intervention

The theoretical assumptions (see Behavioral Theoretical Assumptions) are a summary of the basic beliefs about the person, activities or occupations, and the environment or context. These beliefs are adapted from the behavioral theories previously described in this chapter. The assumptions about the person-environment-occupation variables and their possible relationships guide evaluation and intervention in occupational therapy.

Evaluation

The behavioral frame of reference gives guides for identifying different behaviors and environments that influence the person's baseline of occupational performance. The assessment instruments integrate observation, interview, and task performance to identify observable and measurable behavior.

Goals of Evaluation

The behavioral assessment elicits measurable data that can be used to:

- Identify problems and target behaviors to be extinguished and skills to be learned
- Help identify viable intervention strategies
- Act as a baseline of performance against which progress can be measured

BEHAVIORAL THEORETICAL ASSUMPTIONS

Person and Behavior

1. A person's behavior is predictable, measurable, and objective.
2. A person's verbalization and self-descriptions are behaviors.
3. An individual's repertoire of skills determines the ability to engage in occupations that are personally meaningful and socially acceptable.
4. The person has a repertoire of behaviors, adaptive and maladaptive, that has been learned through selective reinforcement within the environment.
5. An individual can learn to modify and control his or her behavior through positive and differential reinforcement and the systematic application of learning techniques.

Environment/Context

6. The environment gives positive or negative reinforcement of a person's behavior.
7. Only demonstrated behavior can be reinforced.
8. New behavior can be established through the use of continuous or frequent and predictable reinforcement; however, the most stable behavior, and the most difficult to extinguish, is that maintained by intermittent reinforcement.
9. If maladaptive behavior is only occasionally reinforced, it is strengthened.

10. The therapist is concerned both with extinguishing maladaptive behaviors and with establishing adaptive behavior that will enable learning and desired occupational performance.

Activity/Occupation

11. In occupational therapy, through activity and occupation, the patient or client can learn new skills or refine present skills for occupational function.
12. In occupational therapy the patient or client can learn to manipulate the environment to problem solve and improve his or her occupational function.
13. Either through direct care, education, or consultation, the occupational therapist strives to increase the patient's/client's ability to transfer (or generalize) the behaviors learned during intervention to a broad range of environments and life situations.
14. Generalization is enhanced when skills are practiced in multiple settings and contexts.
15. Clear, concrete goals increase the client's understanding of the purpose of intervention and the achievement of occupational performance.
16. Clear, specific goals expedite the intervention process and facilitate the evaluation of the occupational performance outcome.

Because of the situation specificity of behavior and because there are practical limitations on what can be assessed, the assessment must precisely identify characteristics of the environment in which the learned behavior is to be used and the exact behaviors required for function in the expected setting. With this information, the therapist and client together identify areas of concern, goals, and resources.

Performance Baseline

In each area of concern, the therapist and patient/client will typically identify the following:

- Existing behaviors and skills that contribute to adaptive performance; this may include noting the intensity, frequency, and/or duration of this adaptive behavior
- Behaviors that interfere with adaptive performance, including their frequency, duration, and/or intensity
- Behaviors and skills necessary for adequate function in the person's natural or expected environment
- Cues for adaptive and non-adaptive behavior
- Current reinforcers for behavior and skilled performance
- Potential reinforcers for desired behavior and skilled performance
- The person's ability to discriminate among stimuli and to generalize learning effectively

From the preceding information, the occupational therapist often establishes a database, or performance baseline, sometimes depicted in a chart or graph, in which he or she notes the frequency and strength of specific behaviors during a limited time.

A characteristic of the behavioral evaluation is the specificity sought in designating the strength of behavior. For example, rather than making a general evaluative statement indicating that the patient "fails to ask for assistance in the clinic, as needed" or "tends not to clean up his work area," the therapist may indicate as part of the database that (the patient/client) "asked for assistance one time during a 50 minute session" and (the patient/client) "cleaned his work area one time during a five-session week."

Conditions of Assessment

As identified by Kazdin (1981), behavioral assessment occurs on a continuum according to the following conditions:

Naturalistic-Contrived Assessment

When **naturalistic assessment** occurs, the assessment environment has not been structured by the occupational therapist. Rather, the therapist observes the individual carrying out his or her normal routine. Such observation and assessment might occur, for example, in the individual's home, school, or place of employment. While such assessment is ideal insofar as it recognizes the situation specificity of behavior, the person being observed may not display the behaviors or skills in question. Unpredictable disruption or alterations in routines may also suggest that the skills and behaviors demonstrated during the assessment period were not truly representative of the person's best performance. Naturalistic assessment may not be possible due to limits imposed by short intervention or lack of funding for home/school/employment visits.

Simulated settings: In contrast, the therapist may assess the individual in a therapeutically structured environment, including a simulated setting. In some hospitals and residential settings, for example, the living unit or "ward" is structured to simulate an extended family home environment. Within such a setting, the occupational therapist can gain assessment data by observing the informal interaction that occurs among staff and residents, as well as from observing individuals engaged in daily routines. Many centers specializing in rehabilitation following traumatic head injury create an elaborate, simulated town known as Easy Street to allow clients to practice multiple functional skills. The client's daily progress in this simulated setting can be documented as evidence of progress toward goals.

The validity of assessment in a simulated setting is generally related to the extent to which the behavior performed within the assessment actually replicates that of the natural setting. The situation specificity of behavior cautions against assuming that performance in a simulated structure will be identical to performance in the natural environment (Kazdin, 1981, pp. 116-117).

Unobtrusive vs. Obtrusive Assessment

A second condition of assessment relates to whether or not the individual is aware of being assessed (e.g., as with clinical observation) or has knowledge of the skills and behaviors that are being assessed. Within an assessment battery, the therapist might ask the client to perform a specific behavior and tell the client what is being measured (**obtrusive assessment**). For instance, as part of the Kohlman Evaluation of Living Skills (KELS), the therapist requests, "Please show me how you would use this phone book to obtain the number of a movie theater."

In contrast, the therapist might observe a client during the client's participation in a therapy group and make specific observations regarding his or her performance. The individuals participating in the group may not realize that their behaviors are being documented in this manner (**unobtrusive assessment**).

Literature in the area of assessment reminds us that the knowledge that he or she is being observed can influence an individual's performance during a task (Kazdin, 1981).

Temporal Conditions

A third condition of behavioral assessment that can influence the utility of the data obtained relates to the time span over which the assessment occurs. Some behavioral assessments in occupational therapy are designed to be completed in one session (e.g., the KELS, as cited in the previous example.) Other assessments are designed to be completed over several therapy sessions, as with the Bay Area Functional Performance Evaluation (Williams & Bloomer, 1987). Assessments carried out over extended time periods or made in multiple situations can be more time-consuming and therefore less cost-effective; however, they have the advantage of being able to provide a more representative sampling of an individual's task behaviors. They are consistent with a commitment to ongoing assessment. This can be especially significant when a person's performance is highly erratic, as may occur with persons who have head injuries or struggle with mood disorders (Borg & Bruce, 1991, p. 55).

Method of assessment: Some common behavioral assessment formats include the structured interview, behavior rating scales, batteries of structured task experiences, observation of behavior in simulated settings, and natural setting observation.

Assessment can be **objective** (from the therapist's perspective) or **subjective** (from the client's perspective). Typically it is a combination of observation and rating of task performance along with an interview of the client, family, or other care-providers.

Behavioral observation guides are often used in the assessment of task behavior and to structure the interview. Structuring is believed to help objectify the data gathered, increase the likelihood that necessary information is not overlooked, and help minimize the impact of therapist-observer bias on the assessment process. The behavioral interview targets current problems and the context in which they occur, and is concerned with history only to the extent that history influences current behavior. In settings in which intervention is for acute problems only and in which intervention is to be very brief, the clear identification of existing occupational skills and of those lacking may be the extent of intervention.

Behavioral therapists emphasize that knowing what one wants to do or should do does not necessarily translate into the ability to take the desired action. Similarly, seeing where one has made a mistake in the past does not necessarily prevent one from repeating similar mistakes in the future.

The word **insight** is used when the behavioral therapist tries to increase the individual's recognition that a particular behavior has brought about a specific, predictable result.

Behavioral Database

Kaye, Mackie, and Hitzing (1970) gave one example of behavioral evaluation and goal setting in their article, "Contingency Management in a Workshop Setting: Innovation in Occupational Therapy." In describing their work with eight male patients with chronic impairment, they noted that all of the patients exhibited minimal social skills, "bizarre motor and verbal behavior," "tardiness and inattention" (Kaye et al., 1970). The patients participated for an hour each weekday in a workshop occupational therapy setting. During the baseline phase, the patients were observed for several weeks, and a list of undesirable behaviors (at least six per patient) was made up and restated in terms of a positive behavioral objective.

For example, the following behavioral goals were among those listed by the authors: (Client will be) "on time; clean up assigned work area; tell the truth; stay at the job with no pausing or pacing longer than... minutes per session; initiate relevant, appropriate conversation at least... times" (Kaye et al., 1970). The therapist tallied the six behavioral goals for each patient on a survey sheet. The authors included a sample behavioral survey sheet to illustrate the vehicle for weekly tallying (Table 5-2). The progress of each patient was then made visible by means of a graph (Figure 5-1 on p. 142).

This process concluded the establishing of behavior baselines. Baseline data surveys and graphs were then displayed prominently, and the therapist spoke to each patient about the goals of treatment and the responsibility of each for filling out his or her own behavior objectives survey, for being able to verbalize personal behavioral goals from memory, and to cite criteria for appropriate behavior. Reinforcement revolved around the accumulation of token points, as well as social reinforcements such as smiles and praise.

Behavioral Self-Inventory

The next example describes the use of an adapted behavior evaluation format that incorporates a behavioral checklist and an interview. Preceding the evaluation interview, the client was asked to complete a self-inventory. The one from which this excerpt is taken had 50 self-statements. The client, a 21-year-old woman, came to the interview somewhat carelessly dressed, appeared overweight, and had facial acne. She was asked to rate her performance as described by each of the 50 statements. The client assessed her performance by checking one of the following: always (A), frequently (F), sometimes (S), or never (N). The client was also asked to indicate if she was satisfied with her performance or if she wished to change her behavior (Table 5-3 on p. 142). The statements related to the client's behavior in interpersonal, self-care, task, community, and communication activities. The client and the occupational therapist then discussed the responses on the form to target behaviors for change, set treatment goals, and discuss the resources that were available for learning experiences in occupational therapy. It would not be unusual for individuals to rate themselves low on many areas of such a checklist and to desire to make multiple changes.

The self-inventory experience can be a huge blow to a person's self-esteem as well as an overwhelming experience.

Table 5-2

TYPICAL BEHAVIORAL OBJECTIVES SURVEY SHEET
OBTAINED DURING BASELINE

NAME   Joe Smith   Week of 5/19/69-5/23/69

DAYS

Behavior	M	T	W	Th	F	Weekly Total
1. On time: Present before 10:03			X	X	X	3
2. Stayed at job with no pausing or pacing longer than 5 minutes per session		X			X	2
3. Cleaned up assigned area(s)		X		X		2
4. Well-groomed; shaven, hair combed, clothes properly secured	X		X	X		3
5. Initiated relevant, appropriate conversation two times			X			1
6. Smiled (at least three times)	X				X	2
TOTALS	2	2	3	3	3	13

Therefore, the occupational therapist should use questionnaires judiciously and help clients and patients organize the information in a manner that helps them identify desired changes as well as their own strengths (adaptive behaviors), establish priorities for the desired changes, and identify sources that will culminate in a successful learning experience that will enhance the individual's sense of accomplishment.

Discussion of Client Questionnaire

The following excerpt is taken from the client-therapist dialogue that took place after the completion of the inventory. The reader can contrast this dialogue with the one in Chapter Four, even when there are similarities in the individual's concerns regarding physical appearance.

OTR: "On your list you have indicated that you'd like to change your appearance and your clothes and improve your physical coordination and skin condition."

Client: "I'm heavy and clumsy... I'd like new clothes... I need new make-up."

OTR: "I can't buy you new clothes or make-up, but in occupational therapy I can help you find ways to become more physically active, and I can help you plan a weight reduction program. You also can experiment with skin care and make-up and clothing selection in occupational therapy." (Pause) "Where would you like to begin?"

Client: "I can't decide."

OTR: "Let's talk about the first statement that you made about yourself, and I will help you begin. You first mentioned that you're 'heavy.' Are you interested in working toward a weight loss while you're in day care?"

Client: "I've tried. It's hard."

OTR: "Yes, it's difficult... and I think we have some supports here that can help you. We could look at both your eat-

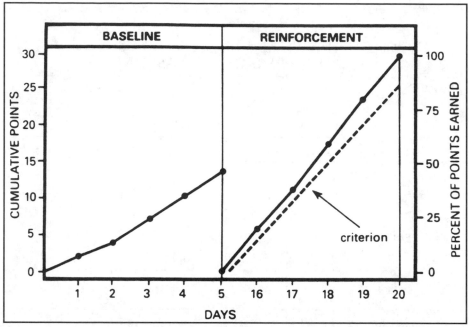

Figure 5-1. Cumulative graph points earned by Patient D during last week of base line and third week of reinforcement (reprinted from Kaye, J. H., Mackie, V., & Hitzing, E. W. [1970]. Innovation in occupational therapy: Contingency management in a workshop setting. *Am J Occup Ther, 24*(6), 415. © 1970 by the American Occupational Therapy Association, Inc. Reprinted with permission).

Table 5-3
EXCERPT FROM COMPLETED QUESTIONNAIRE

Behavioral Statement	Rating*	Selection
I am satisfied with my physical body (body weight and shape, muscle strength)	N	Want to change
I can find clothes that fit well and that are attractive and comfortable	S	Want to change
I am satisfied with my general appearance (hair style, skin condition, etc.)	S	Want to change
I am satisfied with my physical coordination (e.g., the way I walk, my ability to use my hands)	S	Want to change

*N = Never, S = Seldom

Reprinted with permission from Bruce, M., & Borg, B. (1993). *Psychosocial occupational therapy: Frames of reference for intervention* (2nd ed.). Thorofare, NJ: SLACK Incorporated.

ing habits and your level of physical activity. Have you spoken to your doctor about your weight concerns? He can order special weight reduction meals for you while you are here."

Client: "No. I don't like many foods. I thrive on junk food."

OTR: "If you decide that you want to work toward losing weight, you will need to speak to your doctor when you see him. Perhaps, too, you'll have to work on changing your eating habits."

Client: "I love the snacks in the cafeteria here, and when I have free time in my schedule, I like to go there to relax."

OTR: "To help you avoid the snacks here and at home we could write a contract. A contract is a written statement of your goals, such as, 'I want to lose 5 pounds.' Then you write down how you intend to reach your goal, and what your reward will be for doing it. You might contract to limit your in-between snacks to one or two a day, and reward yourself at the end of the week."

Client: "I'm not in the mood to write today; I'm tired."

OTR: "I think that we have done enough for today, and it is almost time to stop. Tomorrow in occupational therapy we will talk more about your specific goals and work on your contract for occupational therapy."

During this interview the therapist summarized one area of the questionnaire, and worked with the client to identify specific problems and establish priorities for desired changes rather than pursue the client's feelings about herself. Although the client was not ready to complete her contract, the therapist established that there would be an emphasis on changing behavior.

Assessment Instruments

The occupational therapy literature identifies the following behavioral assessments designed for use with clients having mental health issues: The Kohlman Evaluation of Living Skills (KELS), The Comprehensive Occupational Therapy Evaluation (COTE) and the KidCOTE, the Bay Area Functional Performance Evaluation (BaFPE), the Milwaukee Evaluation of Daily Living Skills (MEDLS), and the Scorable Self-Care Evaluation (SSCE). These assessments are summarized here. Details and specific protocol are available from the identified sources.

Kohlman Evaluation of Living Skills

The KELS (Thompson, 1992) was developed in an acute psychiatric setting for use with adult psychiatric clients. An occupational therapist (OTR) or certified occupational therapy assistant (COTA) under the supervision of an OTR may administer the KELS. Interview and tasks are used to determine the client's ability to function in everyday living situations. Administered in 30 to 45 minutes, this battery identifies 17 living skills that are categorized under the five broad headings of:

1. Self-care

2. Safety and health
3. Money management
4. Transportation and telephone
5. Work and leisure

The KELS requires performance of these living skills or knowledge of procedures in those instances where performance is not expected within the assessment. Reading and writing are evaluated in so far as they are used in some of the tasks. The test manual is available from the American Occupational Therapy Association, Products Division.

Comprehensive Occupational Therapy Evaluation and KidCOTE

The COTE (Kunz & Brayman, 1999) was developed in an acute psychiatric setting to reflect a focus on occupational performance, to improve communication with staff, and to improve the system of data formation and retrieval. According to Kunz and Brayman, readers familiar with the COTE will note "few changes since its introduction in 1975" (p. 260). These changes are limited to some format changes, changes in the definitions of some behaviors to better reflect current terminology, and the addition of one test item. The COTE identifies 26 behaviors that can be observed in occupational therapy and include those related to punctuality, organization, initiative, responsibility, dependability, attention to detail, interest, neatness, and concentration. They are organized under three major categories:

1. General behavior
2. Interpersonal behavior
3. Task behavior

The behaviors are rated on a 0 to 4 scale and are reported on a grid displaying numerical scores for each behavior.

The KidCOTE was developed in 1995 by an occupational therapist at the University of Texas Medical Branch at Galveston. It is also a performance assessment, formatted as a behavioral grid and designed for use with children having psychiatric problems (Kunz & Brayman, 1999, p. 267). The KidCOTE assesses 27 behaviors, which are organized into four broad areas:

- General behaviors (e.g., responsibility, reality orientation, attention/punctuality)
- Psychosocial behaviors (e.g., behavior related to self-concept, social conduct, coping, and insight)
- Cognitive behaviors (e.g., decision-making, following directions)
- Sensorimotor performance (e.g., sensory awareness, fine and gross motor skills, posture, gait, tone)

Task behaviors are observed during performance in occupational therapy and are scored on a 4-point scale (Kunz & Brayman, 1999). Both the COTE and KidCOTE have been examined for reliability and validity, which have been found to support their use.

Bay Area Functional Performance Evaluation

The BaFPE (Blooomer & Williams, 1979; Williams & Bloomer, 1987; Klyczek, 1999) was developed by Williams and Bloomer in 1977 at Langley Porter Psychiatric Institute at the University of California Medical Center to meet the need for a standardized occupational therapy assessment of functional performance. The current BaFPE has two subtests: the Task Oriented Assessment (TOA) and the Social Interaction Scale (SIS). The TOA begins with a pre-assessment interview designed to gain information about the client's previous and present function and to help establish rapport. The TOA consists of five time-limited tasks that are both structured and nonstructured: sorting shells, completing a money and marketing task, drawing a house floor plan, duplicating a block design, and drawing a person. The therapist then rates the following 12 functional behaviors:

- Memory for written and oral instructions
- Organization of time and materials
- Attention span
- Evidence of thought disorder
- Ability to abstract
- Task completion
- Errors
- Efficiency
- Motivation and compliance
- Frustration tolerance
- Self-confidence
- General affective and behavioral impression (Klyczek, 1999)

The SIS is a behavior rating scale, not a behavior checklist, that depends on the observation of the client in five specified situations and includes an optional self-report. Developed by Williams & Bloomer (1987), it is used to assess seven categories of social interaction:

- Verbal communication
- Psychomotor behavior
- Socially appropriate behavior
- Response to authority figures
- Independence vs. dependence
- Ability to work with others
- Participation in group or program activities

Klyczek (1999) summarizes numerous reliability and validity studies on the original and revised versions of the BaFPE. The test manual and materials are available from Consulting Psychologists Press, Inc. (*www.CPP-db.com*)

Milwaukee Evaluation of Daily Living Skills

The MEDLS (Leonardelli, 1988) is a functional assessment developed to measure the abilities of persons with serious (chronic) mental illness to do basic and more complex tasks of daily living. The individual for whom the MEDLS was intended was an adult, age 18 and above, with a history of mental illness of at least 2 years duration. The original MEDLS consisted of 20 subtests or skill areas, from which the test-giver could select, based upon the client's history and areas that appear to be at risk. There is a minimum of self-report on the MEDLS; most skills were assessed by having the client perform or simulate performance of the skill. Content validity and inter-rater reliability were established. Subtests in the original MEDLS were as follows:

1. Basic communication
2. Bathing
3. Brushing teeth
4. Denture care
5. Eyeglass care
6. Dressing
7. Eating
8. Hair care
9. Clothing maintenance
10. Make-up use
11. Medication management
12. Nail care
13. Personal health care
14. Safety at home
15. Safety in the community
16. Shaving
17. Time awareness
18. Use of money
19. Use of telephone
20. Use of transportation

An advantage of the MEDLS is that subtests are scored independently of other subtests (there is no cumulative score); thus, the assessor need only have the patient/client complete those subtests in which there is a concern about the client's skills.

Since the publication of the original MEDLS, author Haertlein has begun revision of the MEDLS, adding six new subtests, which include items related to cleaning (washing the dishes, taking out the garbage, changing bedsheets, dusting, vacuuming, and bathroom cleaning) and using a Rasch analysis of test items to determine item difficulty. Preliminary studies of the revised MEDLS challenge the notion that items that appear to be simple (e.g., dressing and brushing teeth) are easier for persons with serious mental illness than are more complex items, such as changing bed linen (Haertlein, 1994, 1999). The author states that the MEDLS lacks a sufficient number of difficult items to evaluate the abilities of more capable persons having serious mental illness (Haertlein, 1999, p. 254).

Scorable Self-Care Evaluation

A standardized self-care evaluation instrument designed by E. Nelson Clark and Mary Peters (1984), the evaluation is used to identify baseline performance in basic living skills (personal care, housekeeping, work and leisure, and financial management). The authors provide subtasks for each of the basic living skill areas, a format for administering subtasks, a format for scoring performance during subtasks, reliability studies and standard scores to assist in the interpretation of patient scores, and forms for communicating evaluation and progress data.

INTERVENTION

Behavioral theory influences the process for defining the problems, setting goals, and structured documentation in occupational therapy intervention. It increases our understanding of behavior management across the life span and in varied contexts. The learning principles of this frame of reference can be integrated into individual and group interventions for children and adults.

Establishing Goals

An important contribution of the behavioral frame of reference comes from the guidelines it has provided for writing therapeutic goals. Owing to the desire to establish efficacy of intervention and the requirements of third-party payers, most clinicians have been influenced by the behavioral goal-setting system. In general, goals must be observable and measurable.

Originally, the behavioral occupational therapist identified problems, determined the goals for treatment, and designed the intervention plan; this continues to be the process only when the client is believed to be incapable of contributing to goal setting. Even then, the client may include the family or other care-providers whose input will be sought. Most often, the client (child or adult) actively participates in the decision-making process and works cooperatively with the therapist to target his or her problems and determine the specific changes that need to occur in order for that performance to be optimized.

Defining Target Problems

The targeted problems must be defined in observable terms and as measurable outcomes and be individualized for each client. Multiple resources are available to aid the therapist in the goal-setting process (Foto et al., 1990; Lewin & Reed, 1998; Mager, 1962). This process is summarized as follows:

After the completion of the initial assessment, the therapist and the patient/client identify the changes that need to occur to improve the person's occupational performance within his or her expected environment. These changes may be stated in terms of the individual's feelings, desires, interests, or concerns and are usually general statements.

Next, the therapist takes the client's general statements and works to identify the specific behaviors that would indicate that this person had learned a new skill or otherwise addressed the changes desired. These behavioral statements, which are derived from an analysis of the tasks that relate to the patient's/client's broad concerns, must be understood by the individual and agreed upon as subskills of behaviors or steps in the learning process.

General Statements Become Observable Goals

After targeting behaviors, observable goals are established. The therapist and client establish behavioral expectations within a framework that may identify the context, time, and place in which skills will be learned or behavior changed and the significant persons involved in or affected by the behavior.

Having identified the observable behavioral goal, the patient/client and therapist then discuss the frequency of behaviors expected and the criteria that indicate success or failure to accomplish the goal. In this way, the observable behaviors become measurable goals.

The Goal-Setting Process

The goal-setting process is exemplified as follows: Let us take a frequent situation that occurs in psychiatric settings with persons having chronic problems and frequent outbursts of disruptive behavior. A young man's family decides that they can no longer cope with his unpredictable, childlike behaviors and inform the individual that he may not return home. The client's problem and concerns include, "Where am I going to live? How am I going to care for myself?" As the client and therapist discuss the concern, the following issues and skills that need to be learned are identified. These are described in Table 5-4.

In the process of establishing therapeutic goals, the individual and therapist will often identify behaviors that are not adaptive and that interfere with goal attainment.

Typically, the therapist will take note of these maladaptive behaviors and attempt to remove reinforcement for them. However, unless the therapist and the staff have complete control of the client's environment, eliminating such reinforcement is difficult and at times impossible.

Positive Statements

Goals are most often written in terms of what will be attained, not what will be eliminated. For example, the "childlike" behavior in our example might include excess time spent by the young man brooding in isolation in his room. Steps taken toward exploring community resources and gaining employment represent adaptive behaviors that can lead to needed skills and are opposite to brooding and isolating behaviors. These adaptive behaviors can serve as goals.

Setting Priorities

Usually, multiple issues, problems, and behavioral goals are present, as can be easily seen in the previous example. Also see Table 5-4 for an example of the behavioral goal-setting process. Therefore, the therapist helps the client figure out where to begin and to have realistic expectations. Being able to see larger goals as consisting of smaller, achievable steps helps the client feel empowered and helps him or her to feel less overwhelmed.

Table 5-4
GOAL-SETTING PROCESS

Concern

- Where am I going to live?

Issues

- What is important to me about where I live?
- How will I pay for the setting (apartment, boarding home, house)?
- What supports are available (financial, interpersonal)?

Necessary Skills

- Identify alternatives by scanning the classified advertisements and contacting community agencies.
- Clarify values and identify personal needs.
- Speak to personal and community resources regarding financial support.

Behavioral Goal Statements

- Client will identify two possible settings in which he could live.
- Client will speak to his parents regarding possible financial support.
- Client will participate in a values clarification group and identify in what type of setting he wants to live, with whom he wishes to live, and what kind of support group or social network he desires.
- Client will gain employment in order to be capable of meeting financial responsibilities.

As intervention progresses, these measurable statements are reviewed frequently to determine if the client is progressing toward his goals. Measurable goals and the review process allow the client, therapist, other staff and care-providers, and reimbursers to clearly identify the client's progress and to evaluate the success and limitations of the intervention plan.

Behavior Contract

Sometimes performance goals and intervention strategies are written in the form of a contract. A **contract** is a verbal or written agreement between the patient/client and the therapist (or other persons) that defines the roles of each during therapy, the behavioral goals, reinforcements and their schedules, the strategies that will be used to enhance learning, and other related negotiations. If written, both the therapist and the client sign the contracts. Contracts are time-limited and are reviewed, renegotiated, or terminated at agreed intervals.

Rules for Writing Sound Behavior Contracts

The following highlights characteristics of a sound contract (adapted from Brammer, L. (1979). *The helping relationship: Process and skills.* Englewood Cliffs, NJ: Prentice-Hall and Bower, S. A., & Bower, G. (1991). *Asserting yourself: A practical guide for positive change.* Reading, MA: Addison-Wesley) (see also Increase Your Understanding: Contracts):

- Contracts specify **both** what the client (helpee) and therapist (helper) will do.
- Contracts are **specific**: The helpee knows **what** behaviors are expected; exactly **where**, **when**, and **how long** they are to be exhibited; and the **consequences** of meeting or not meeting goals.
- Contracts are **impersonal**: This contract doesn't reflect on helper or helpee "liking" each other.
- Behaviors must be **feasible**: The client must be able to perform the specified behavior or skill.
- Attainment of the goal is **observable** and **assessable**. Ask for and reward specific accomplishments rather than general obedience or good intentions.
- Contacts often use **reward liberally**, especially at first.
- Contracts typically include a **time commitment**, or a time specified for renegotiating the contract.
- Contracts should be expressed in **positive terms**. Try to state what the client/helpee will do, not what he or she won't do.
- All parties should understand the contracts are **fair**.

INCREASE YOUR UNDERSTANDING: CONTRACTS

Contracts

Contracts are not only between client and occupational therapist. They may also be negotiated between client and employer, client and family member, or any other persons who wish to establish an agreement. The therapist may help two parties negotiate a fair contract, using the same rules for contracting that were previously listed.

Case Scenario

Marney is a 9-year-old girl who 18 months ago had a traumatic injury to her right arm and can use it only minimally for self-care. She has been taught to dress, groom, and do basic hygiene independently but over the past several weeks has been taking so long to get ready for school in the morning that her mother has begun dressing and grooming her.

The therapist recommends that Marney and her mother create a contract that will encourage Marney to resume independence in her morning routine.

Compare the following two hypothetical contracts. One is much better than the other. Which contract best follows the "rules" of good contracting provided? Which rules do you recognize?

Contract A: If Marney gets ready as she should in the morning, mom agrees to take Marney to a G-rated movie of her choice at the end of the week.

Signed: (Marney) Signed: (Mom)
Date: Date:

Contract B: For each morning this week of October 7 that Marney dresses herself completely and grooms herself fully (to include washing face, brushing teeth, and combing hair) without mother's help by 7:45 am, Marney will be allowed to watch 15 minutes of morning television. If Marney is fully dressed and groomed by 7:45 every morning for the next 7 days, Mother will take Marney to any G-rated movie of Marney's choice on Sat., Oct. 14. This contract will be re-evaluated on Sat., October 14.

Signed: (Marney) Signed: (Mom)
Date: Date

- The reward should be worth the effort or difficulty of the behavior being asked for. Therapists should do what they have promised as soon as possible.

Problem-Oriented Record

Along with mandates calling for specific, observable, and measurable treatment goals, and the growing interest in data-collection came the need for specific formats of documentation. One of these formats was the **problem-oriented record**

as described by Weed (1969). This format was not initially designed for occupational therapy or psychiatry. It was first used in general medicine settings but has influenced documentation in many medical, nonmedical, and occupational therapy intervention sites (Foto et al., 1990).

Components of the Problem-Oriented Record

The problem-oriented record has four major components. The **database** includes demographics; medical and social history; medical, laboratory, and psychological test results and related clinical reports; and a statement of the patient's chief complaint. The **subjective data** includes the views expressed by the patient and his or her family. The **objective data** includes staff observations and laboratory reports. Finally, the **problem list** includes past and present psychiatric and medical problems identified from the information in the other three components of the problem-oriented record.

Progress Note Format

For each problem listed by number and title, a diagnostic and treatment plan are listed. Progress notes are then keyed to a particular numbered problem and are written according to the "SOAP" format. SOAP is an acronym for the following: "S," the patient's subjective response to treatment and patient observations; "O," objective data from laboratory studies, diagnostic reports and objective assessments, and treatment; "A," the assessment or analysis of the subjective and objective data; and "P," the diagnostic, therapeutic, and patient education plan (Weed, 1969).

The influence of the problem-oriented record system and its adaptations is evident in the records and documentation in many mental health settings. The problem-oriented record is reflected in goal-oriented intervention in which there is a problem list, specific goals (long- and short-term), and intervention strategies specific to each problem on the list (Foto et al., 1990; Lang & Mattson, 1993).

The authors are also familiar with a system that uses a "NAP" note. NAP is an acronym that stands for "N," a narrative that combines the subjective and objective data; "A," the assessment that identifies the problems and states how they were determined; and "P," the plan, with the goals and intervention strategies that are used to resolve and identify problems.

Caveats

Behaviorally based occupational therapy is concerned with building skills that contribute to adaptive occupational performance while eliminating those that interfere.

The straightforward nature of this statement should not suggest that behavioral intervention is simple or necessarily the same across various settings. Although behavioral therapists hold in common the concern for observable, measurable behavior, the strategies and techniques used to modify and build specific behaviors vary. We wish to dispel the idea that just acknowledging a person's success in occupational therapy (as through smiles or privileges), ignoring maladaptive behaviors, and writing measurable goals suffice as behavioral intervention. The complexity of the human being is such that identifying and isolating everything that influences learning and functional performance is virtually impossible, at least in the practical sense. The behavioral therapist must be very diligent in the application of behavioral strategies if he or she hopes to successfully carry out a behavioral intervention plan, even in the most circumscribed learning setting. The therapist must also realistically evaluate the environment and contexts of intervention to identify the feasibility of implementing behavioral strategies.

Implementing a Plan

Having set learning goals, it is time to implement the plan. As suggested, behavioral intervention is the application of one or more of the learning strategies described previously. These include selective reinforcement, skill instructions, strategies designed to enhance discrimination and/or generalization, modeling, cues and coaching, role-play, and practice. The therapist designs an **optimum learning experience**, which is characterized as follows:

- The learning experience is compatible with the client's age, interests, values, societal expectations, and the expected duration of therapy.
- There will be an opportunity for the desired behavior or skill to be demonstrated (or modeled, shaped, chained).
- There is, when needed, an opportunity for trial and error problem solving and sufficient opportunity for repetition of adaptive responses (practice).
- The therapist and designated others can ensure that positive reinforcement be given, per schedule, for adaptive behavior; and reinforcement is withheld in response to maladaptive behavior.
- There is opportunity within the experience to move from continuous or frequent external reinforcement to more everyday (intermittent, internal) reinforcement.
- The individual can recognize the similarities between the behavior in the therapeutic environment and its enactment in the natural environment (the therapist may amplify salient features of both the therapeutic and natural environment to make these similarities clearer).
- The learner can perceive the differences between demonstrating the learned behavior in appropriate versus inappropriate settings (the therapist may help the client identify these differences).
- The therapist has specific criteria against which progress can be periodically measured.

Behavioral Communication

Regardless of the activity or techniques used, throughout the intervention process the occupational therapist informs the individual(s) of what is expected and the goal of each learning experience. The therapist uses a vocabulary and manner of explaining that are understandable to the client to accomplish this goal. For example, the therapist might indicate to a client, "I would like you to work on this leather key case so that you can practice following written instructions. I will be available for assistance if you need help; I want you to try this on your own first, so that you can become more accustomed to working independently." The therapist might tell a group of children, "Today our goal is to learn better ways to let our friends know when we are angry."

Behavior-Consequence Relationship

The therapist uses dialogue with the individual or group to assist them to recognize the relationship of their behavior to the consequences that result. The therapist does not attempt to deny or overlook the client's thoughts or feelings, but he or she responds to them in terms of the behavior that is demonstrated. Rather than telling an individual that he or she looks "sad," "angry," or "depressed," for example, the therapist may say, "The way you're throwing/grabbing your clothes looks angry," or, "You've spent most of the hour sitting by yourself, and it appears that you feel discouraged."

Constructive Feedback

Information that is given to the individual about his or her behavior is referred to as **feedback**. When relating to the client, the therapist tries to verbally recognize positive behavior and to specify expected behaviors. During a community outing, the therapist may begin by saying, "Please stay with the group when we leave the van and walk to the entrance of the YMCA. Enter the lobby, be seated, and wait for the Y program director to join us," rather than just saying, "Don't stray from the group."

To cite another example, when a client in a therapeutic cooking group is using a knife carelessly, the therapist will not only say, "Be careful." He or she will say, "Be careful; your hand is too far down on the knife blade. Here, let me show you." Then, the therapist proceeds to demonstrate the correct procedure. Even when giving criticism, the therapist avoids using blanket remarks that suggest something is bad, wrong, or ugly. Rather, he or she demonstrates how to use a tool or do a process correctly, or identifies what characteristics of a task or activity have been completed successfully and which may need improvement.

The therapist also uses dialogue to help persons generalize their learning to the natural environment. The occupational therapist encourages the clients to assume responsibility for personal behavior and strive to build a sense of self-control.

Application of the Behavioral Model Across the Life Span

Example 1: Adults with Mental Illness

Mt. Airy House is described as a group home for 16 mentally ill adults. It is a "quarterway house" for individuals aged 18 to 65, formerly hospitalized clients now taking a step toward community re-integration. Once a resident is accepted into the Mt. Airy program, a "careful assessment of his or her behavior is made." Behaviors are identified as either "behavioral deficits (absence of adaptive behavior); excesses (acting out, odd, or bizarre behaviors); or behaviors present or absent in functional skills areas" (Wilberding, 1993, p. 121) (see Excessive Behavior List). The philosophy at Mt. Airy House is based on the belief that "successful adjustment to community life requires understanding the specific and unique problems of each resident." In order to help residents learn "new and more adaptive skills and behaviors," program objectives include providing an atmosphere for the "learning and maintenance of the highest attainable levels of functioning" and "building social skills, (and) daily living skills." Staff, led by the director, who is a master's degree occupational therapist, are trained in providing both emotional support and task assistance. Techniques they use include behavioral reinforcement (verbal praise and encouragement), credits/money earned, privileges earned, clear expectations for behavior in the form of "house rules," written behavioral contracts, and skill instruction that includes the use of demonstration, redirection, written directions, and checklists (Wilberding, 1993).

Example 2: Child with Physical Injury and Psychosocial Outcome

Marney is a 9-year-old girl who lives alone with her mother. Her father died several years ago from complications of multiple sclerosis. Eighteen months ago, when Marney was 7-years-old, her right arm was severely injured in an automobile accident. The nerve damage left Marney's arm only minimally functioning. She received hospital-based OT and PT services designed to prevent flexor contracture, to enable her to use her arm in functional activities, and to educate her mother to help Marney be as independent as possible. Rehabilitation was discontinued approximately 1 year ago, although Marney continues to be checked frequently by her physician.

Shortly after her accident, Marney transferred to a small, private school, which contracted with both a speech and occupational therapist. Concerned about her school performance, her teacher and the school's principle recommended that they consult with the occupational therapist, and Marney's mother agreed. Her teacher

EXCESSIVE BEHAVIOR LIST

Following are some examples of "excessive behaviors" (Wilberding, 1993):

Impulsivity
- Money (impulsive or excessive spending)
- Massive consumption of anything
- Splitting (running away)
- Shoplifting
- Substance abuse
- Self-destruction
- Threatening others
- Destruction of property

Poor Boundaries
- Asking for things beyond what is reasonable
- Acting in an intrusive manner toward others
- Wandering off

Socially Inappropriate Behavior*
- Vulgar and rude comments to others
- Talking and/or laughing to yourself while out and about
- Dressing in bizarre ways
- Poor hygiene
- Inappropriate sexual behavior

Angry Outbursts
Dangerous Smoking
Inability or Unwillingness to Respond to Limits or Requests

*This means behaving in ways that would embarrass someone else, make someone else nervous, or attract unwanted attention to yourself.

reported that Marney has been averaging 1 or 2 days a week absence. She seldom speaks up in class, and when called upon to speak, speaks so softly that no one can hear her. On the playground during lunch and recess, she usually retreats to the top of the playground equipment and hides out among its nooks and crannies. The parent-helpers typically approach her, encouraging her to play. They say she refuses and appears fearful. Often she ends up sitting on the lap of a parent-helper or being pushed by one of them on a swing. With them, she appears content, even talkative. The other children have started teasing her and calling her a "baby." During organized games, she only participates if forced to. The games and activities often require use of arms, and teachers admit they aren't sure how best to include Marney. When Marney doesn't want to play she will sometimes say her arm "hurts" and teachers are reluctant to push her to participate.

Mom reports that Marney has said she doesn't like school and wants to be "home-schooled." Mom states that even though Marney is able to dress and groom herself independently, lately Marney has taken so long to get ready in the morning that mom has started dressing her, combing her hair, and brushing her teeth. Mom admits that on some days, rather than bring Marney to school late, she lets her stay home, adding, "She isn't going to be little for much longer, and I like being able to spend time with her."

First determining that Marney's physical condition has not deteriorated, the occupational therapist begins her intervention by identifying maladaptive behaviors. These include speaking softly, retreating in the playground, sitting in parent-helpers' laps, making excuses not to play, refusing to dress herself in a timely manner, and saying that her arm "hurts." The therapist next identifies what in Marney's home and school environments seem to maintain these behaviors and identifies time and attention from parent-helpers, being allowed to sit and watch during organized play, her mother's help and attention with grooming and dressing, being able to miss school, and time home with Mom.

A talk with mom and Marney enables the therapist to identify potential rewards for Marney's positive behavior. These include TV time, special time with mom, and praise and attention from parent-helpers. The therapist recommends a united school and parental plan in which Marney will be reinforced only for age-appropriate behavior, which includes dressing and grooming herself independently, speaking audibly in class, and interacting and playing with peers on the playground. The therapist provides Marney's teacher and the parent-helpers a list of games and activities that Marney should be able to do without difficulty and also adaptations that would enable Marney to participate in play with her peers. Parent-helpers are advised to not allow Marney to sit on their laps, but rather to create small play groups that include the parent-helper, another child, and Marney; and parent-helpers are advised to praise even the smallest steps taken by Marney toward increased participation.

Mom and Marney each sign a written contract for the first week that specifies that Marney's being able to watch television in the evening will depend on her getting herself ready for school and to school on time each day, and that at the end of a successful week, she and mom will spend a Saturday afternoon together at the city zoo.

Example 3: Adult Behavior Modification Program

A woman, formerly a prominent lawyer, has had a basilar stroke and is now living at home with her husband and daughter. Recently, the woman has become uncooperative in regard to both eating and engaging in her daily therapy. Occupational therapy referral requests that the occupational therapist work with a neuropsychologist to establish a behavior modification program that will enhance the client's participation. Specifically, the occupational therapist is asked to identify what might act as reinforcers for this woman's participation in home therapy and what might facilitate her eating (Borg & Bruce, 1997, pp. 103-104).

Behavior Programs in Multiple Contexts and Environments

In each of our three examples, occupational therapy has followed a behavioral model. In the first instance, the occupational therapist is a member of a residential, community transition team; in the second, the therapist consults with a small private school; and in the third instance, occupational therapy occurs in the context of home-based care. The age of the clients in these three examples extends across much of the life span.

Behavioral practices are based upon principles of learning and are not age-specific. Neither child nor adult need be verbal nor have high cognitive function for principles of selective reinforcement, generalization, and skill training or enhancement to be used. However, behavioral intervention, like any occupational therapy, must match the developmental needs and experiences of the person with whom it is being used. See Adapting Behavioral Intervention for a guide to meeting developmental needs.

Whether for a young child or for an adult, the therapist makes behavioral expectations clear and explicit. The clinician identifies reinforcements that are meaningful to the client and uses reinforcement selectively. Using client concerns and goals, the therapist creates learning experiences in which the child or adult can learn and practice age-appropriate skills and often incorporates peers as models for desired behavior and skills.

Behavior Management with Children and Adolescents

Behavior management is the systematic use of behavioral strategies to externally control undesirable behavior and to facilitate desirable behavior with those individuals who lack internal control. Examples of behaviors that might call for behavior management include disobedience, inattention, overactivity, destructive behavior, and aggressive behavior (e.g., bullying) (Charlebois et al., 1999, p. 137). Behavior management includes the following:

- Creating a clear structure
- Setting explicit rules, boundaries, and expectations
- Individual contracting
- The use of positive reinforcement
- The use of time-outs (Charlebois et al., 1999; McIntyre & Battle, 1998)

ADAPTING BEHAVIORAL INTERVENTION

When adapting behavioral intervention to the developmental needs of a client or group, consider the following:

1. The age-appropriateness of the behavior being required. As a general rule, only developmentally appropriate behavior or behavior appropriate in the expected environment will be reinforced.

2. The language being used to identify behavioral expectations to the client, if language is being used. Even young children can help set simple behavioral contracts, but the language in which these are stated must be understood by the child.

3. The length of time between the desired response and the reinforcement. The client must be able to associate one with the other. The younger the child, the more immediate the reward; "tomorrow" or "at the end of the week" is not meaningful to very young children.

4. The required duration of attention to a task (i.e., how long a behavior must be sustained before a reinforcement is given). Both frustration tolerance and the ability to postpone gratification increase with maturity.

5. The comparative use of external or tangible reinforcement (e.g., tokens, treats) as compared to internal rewards (personal satisfaction). Self-satisfaction becomes a more stable reinforcer with the older child and adolescent; young children may respond better to activity reinforcers and social reinforcers.

6. Whether differences and similarities in settings are very explicit or quite subtle. The ability to discern differences and similarities increases as we mature. Young children cannot be expected to discern subtle differences in cues or in performance.

7. The time set for a time-out. Time-out will be shorter for young children. Five or 10 minutes is experienced as a long time to a young child.

To illustrate, an occupational therapist working with a group of at-risk pre-adolescents might begin their weekly goal-setting meeting by reiterating the "rules" of the group: Each member will listen respectfully and not interrupt when others are talking; members are to remain seated until the group is finished; disruptive behaviors will not be tolerated and will result in expulsion from the group.

In principle, behavior management contrasts with but complements social skills training and self-control training, which are both designed to enhance internal control (Charlebois et al., 1999). Behavior management is used with both children and adults and includes a firm (but not provocative) tone of voice, direct eye contact, and other nonverbal indicators that a staff member has confidence in his or her ability to handle a situation, and faculty and staff present a united presence. A key premise in the use of behavior management techniques is that preventing problems is easier and more desirable than trying to reestablish control after it has been lost.

Behavior Management with Disruptive Behavior Disorders, Schizophrenia, and Serious Emotional Disturbance

Behavior management strategies are often used when working with those youth given a diagnosis of conduct disorder, learning disorder, attention deficit/hyperactivity disorder, and schizophrenia, and those youth identified as having **serious emotional disturbance (SED)**. Serious emotional disturbance is a nonmedical identifier used in the public education system to indicate that a child's educational performance is adversely affected by one or more of the following:

- An inability to learn that cannot be explained by intellectual, sensory, or health factors
- Inability to build or maintain interpersonal relationships with peers or teacher
- Inappropriate behavior or feelings under normal circumstances, pervasive unhappiness or depression, and tendency to develop physical symptoms associated with personal or school problems

The term also includes schizophrenia (Individuals with Disabilities Education Act, Public Law 101-47620, U.S.C. 1401(a)(1), p. 4802). Some students will carry the SED label in the school and have a concurrent psychiatric diagnosis. Serious emotional disturbance can be identified in elementary, middle, or high school and may result in these youth being sent to residential placements or being home schooled. Because these young people typically have difficulty adjusting to high school, both academically and behaviorally, many will fail to get their diplomas and will lack the life skills that will be needed to make a successful transition to young adulthood and to being self-supporting (Tobin & Sugai, 1999).

Three Behavioral Occupational Therapy Groups

We have selected three examples of behavioral group learning that we believe are representative of the current application of behavioral theory in occupational therapy. Although not all behaviorally oriented occupational therapy occurs in a group context, it frequently does. Each of the group experiences discussed here represents or is a composite of behavioral groups that we have observed or that have been part of the fieldwork experience of students we have supervised.

In behavioral group treatment, the therapist must structure the group and learning environment to ensure that specific target behaviors for each group member are facilitated and reinforced. The therapist has the same gatekeeping functions described in the previous chapters. Additionally, he or she must see to it that there is a means to monitor specific behaviors and to supply (or withhold) reinforcement. At times, this technique requires having other staff or aides present, all of whom coordinate their efforts.

Group I—Prevocational Group

The prevocational occupational therapy group in which each participant works on a shared or individual task typifies one type of behavioral group. The clients have in common a need to learn general task skills that will enable each to ultimately succeed in either supported or non-supported employment.

For example, in a shelter for homeless men in an urban area on Monday, Wednesday, and Friday afternoons from 1 to 3 p.m., there is a work group in which those clients who are not presently employed are expected to participate. The number of participants varies from 6 to 20 and includes "regulars" and men who will use the shelter only for 1 or 2 days. Behaviors that the therapist tries to promote include the following:

- The ability to initiate productive work
- The ability to pursue a task to completion
- The ability to work well alone
- The ability to cooperate with others
- Social skills related to sharing space and materials
- The ability to make timely decisions based on available data
- The ability to anticipate consequences
- The acquisition of habits related to punctuality, safety, and cleanliness
- The ability to identify and use available resources

The occupational therapist may contract with local agencies for simple jobs that clients can complete in a short time, including assembling cardboard boxes, packing machine or electronic parts in a container, collating printed materials, stuffing envelopes, folding linen, and sorting tasks. The men are reinforced for their productivity, as each is paid a small wage that is directly proportionate to the amount of work each completes.

In order to enhance the transfer or generalization of learning, the workroom is structured to be comfortable but employment-like. Expectations for performance are made verbally explicit, and there is a list of behaviors that clients must follow. These include respectful language, not being intoxicated while in the work group, preparing and cleaning up one's own workspace, and appropriate use of tools. Clients are provided a meal before joining the group, and if too tired to attend to the work project, must excuse themselves from the work setting. Socialization is encouraged during a designated coffee break during each work session.

The occupational therapist and volunteers are primarily responsible for monitoring work behavior and work quality, providing verbal praise, and paying participants.

Group II—Resocialization Group

The intervention process in the resocialization group begins with each member meeting individually with the therapist to target initial behavioral goals. In some instances, a new member may be assigned to the group for an initial observation period to identify significant behaviors to establish a baseline of targeted behaviors for change by the therapist. Ultimately, each group member and the therapist discuss and agree upon learning goals. In this instance, only those clients with similar social learning needs are placed in the resocialization group.

For example, at a local mental health facility, outpatients are periodically selected into "FAC" (Friday Afternoon Club). On Wednesday of each week, all group members and the occupational therapist meet. The group typically, but not necessarily, consists of five to eight younger unmarried adults, most of whom have been identified as having chronic mental illness. Members come and go from the club as their outpatient tenure dictates. Therefore, the group must constantly respond to changes in its membership.

All the participants share difficulty in either initiating or sustaining social conversation, lack familiarity with community resources, have little confidence (especially in situations involving the opposite sex), exhibit poor grooming and dressing habits, and/or exhibit poor habits in regard to keeping appointments or arriving on time for social engagements.

At the Wednesday meeting, each member reports to the entire group on his or her progress toward meeting weekly goals. Many weekly goals involve specific social skills that each client is to exhibit while at home. For example, one participant may have agreed to check out a book from the local library, to call a designated friend on the phone, or to obtain a brochure describing extension classes at the community college.

As an additional function of the Wednesday meeting, the group plans a Friday social outing at which the therapist is to be a participant-observer. Arrangements are made to meet at a specified locale (restaurant, skating rink, bowling alley) on Friday afternoon.

Each group member is to identify one short-term goal for the Friday engagement (e.g., to be on time, to order dinner independently, or to initiate a conversation with a group member or non-group member). Further, one or two short-term goals to be accomplished at home during the next week are verbalized by each client and recorded by the therapist.

At the social outing, therapy talk is kept at a minimum. This outing is intended to simulate as much as possible a natural social event. As a participant, the therapist models appropriate social behavior and helps stimulate casual conversation. Group members and the therapist provide natural social reinforcement, responding to the social overtures made by various members. Because participants have a large responsibility for reinforcing each other, the success of this group depends, in part, on the ability of individual clients to respond to each other positively and appropriately.

The therapist, who is often emulated, plays a key role through modeling, helping the client group to attend to the positive behavior of its members. The therapist identifies significant behaviors during the social outing that need to be addressed by the group at the next Wednesday meeting and is responsible for communicating with the other mental health center staff on the status of individual clients regarding goal attainment.

Group III—Assertiveness Training Group

A third type of behavioral group is an assertiveness training group. Assertiveness training is part of a broader behavioral application known as social skills training. Training in social skills is designed to teach interpersonal skills and to promote the generalization and maintenance of these skills (Liberman et al., 1993, p. 156). **Social skills training** systematically uses behavioral learning principles to build skills, as compared to other non-specific activity-based groups that might include socialization. Liberman et al. (1993) describe the use of skills training to reduce the high recidivism of chronically impaired adults, while others cite its use with children and adolescents (Murdoch & Barker, 1991; Charlebois et al., 1999).

In an assertiveness training group, the social skills being targeted are those based on the ability to articulate one's needs while respecting the rights of others. Persons who might be referred to such a group include those who cannot ask for what they need, those who cannot say "no," those who feel that they are pushed around or taken advantage of by others, those who are overly apologetic in their interactions with others, and those who feel guilty when they are angry.

An assertiveness training group might be structured as follows:

- All members join the group at the same time. The group is planned to last a given number of sessions (e.g., two times per week, 1 to 1.5 hours per session, for 4 weeks).
- At the first meeting, the therapist describes the function and purpose of the group, the expectations of each group member, and the therapist's role. The therapist begins by educating the group on what is meant by "assertiveness" as compared to "non-assertive" or passive behavior and as compared to aggressive behavior. Participants may be asked to complete one or more questionnaires in which they indicate the nature of those situations in which they have difficulty being assertive. Eventually, each member is asked to describe briefly in writing five social situations in which he or she feels unable to make his or her needs known. Participants are then asked to order these needs hierarchically from least to most difficult.
- The therapist collects all the data provided by each participant, becoming aware of the common features

in which members experience difficulty. Although the situations and the order of difficulty will vary for each individual, the therapist can establish a working hierarchy of situations that can be simulated and role-played in each meeting. The kind of situations frequently simulated, in a hierarchical order, include:
- —Responding to a stranger who pushes ahead of you in a grocery line
- —Asking for a refund at a store
- —Saying "no" when asked to be on a committee
- —Saying "no" to a sexual advance
- —Asking roommates to clean up after themselves
- —Asking persons in neighboring apartments to keep noise down
- —Saying "no" when asked to work overtime
- —Asking for a raise

While these situations are quite general, the therapist has the option of individualizing role-plays.

- In each subsequent group meeting, the therapist constructs one or more situations for practice in role-playing. The therapist may start each session by giving additional didactic information or modeling the appropriate use of skills to the group. In some instances, the group may begin with a brief relaxation exercise. The therapist then describes the first situation that will be role-played. For example, "You've been waiting for 5 minutes at the checkout line at your grocery store. Suddenly, you find a newcomer has squeezed his way ahead of you. Everyone in line with you appears to notice, but no one has chosen to say anything. How would you respond to this situation?"
- Participants take turns playing a variety of roles in the simulations so that they may be both the giver and the recipient of appropriate assertive responses. The therapist may ask for volunteers but attempts to ensure that all group members have opportunities to practice new behaviors. When appropriate, the therapist might interrupt the process to model an effective assertive response; he or she may also coach behavior and give or encourage others to give reinforcement. Group members learn not only by their active participation but also by the observation of others. In this kind of group, modeling is an important teaching tool.
- After simulations are complete, verbal feedback is exchanged among participants about the effectiveness of others' responses. Although feelings may be expressed, they are not the focus of the interaction. The therapist, through enthusiastic praise, reinforces the effective playing out of assertive behaviors. The therapist helps participants give feedback to each other and identify other situations that would be quite similar to the ones role-played in order to facilitate the generalization of learning. The principle of desensiti-

zation plays an important part, as members have a chance to try new behaviors in a setting that is typically less anxiety-producing than those in the natural environment. Further, each participant is given the opportunity to build on past learning and gain confidence, as each week he or she encounters increasingly difficult situations in role-playing.

- As the group meeting nears its completion, each participant targets one specific assertive behavior that he or she will endeavor to accomplish before the next meeting. Time is set aside at the end of every subsequent meeting for members to relate in brief whether they attained their weekly goal. The therapist records changes in individual goals and progress made toward their attainment.

Summary—Behavioral Intervention

The behavioral model for intervention in occupational therapy is one in which behavioral learning principles are systematically applied in order to enhance personal learning and ultimately occupational performance. These behavior principles may initially be used to modify or enhance general behavior in order that skilled learning can occur. The behavioral approach is one that views behavior/skills as observable, measurable, and functional within the environment in which they are used. The model pays particular attention to the attributes of that environment in which behavior is learned and sustained, the role of selective reinforcement, and to the precise articulation of behavioral/skill deficits and concomitant intervention goals. Although behaviorally based occupational therapy acknowledges biological, cultural, cognitive, and emotional influences, it is not primarily concerned with them.

Faulty Learning versus Illness

One can look at the emergence of the behavioral framework in the 1960s within occupational therapy in the context of mental health and see it in part as a response to the limitations of the psychodynamic occupational therapy that preceded it. Within psychiatry in particular, the psychodynamic model attributed maladjustment to mental illness, often using metaphorical language that was not necessarily understood by everyone in the same way. Often, the goal of occupational therapy within this model was to better understand the person's inner world, to promote psychological adjustment, and to provide a supportive environment while medications were being titrated. Many mental health patients would be readmitted to care facilities, however, and the mental health community questioned whether the psychodynamic approach was the best for managing symptoms and sustaining adjustment to community life. Add to that, the increased concern in regard to the cost of health care, and the mental health community was ready to look at alternatives for intervention (Anthony, 1979).

Occupational therapists followed with other health practitioners, leaving the psychodynamic approach and reframing their intervention in terms of behavior change. As behavioral principles became more familiar, they were applied in a variety of contexts. As tends to occur when any new intervention approach is embraced, however, there followed some disenchantment with the behavioral model. In hindsight, one can view the behavioral approach as it has been applied in occupational therapy more realistically, looking at both its strengths and limitations.

CONTRIBUTIONS AND LIMITATIONS OF THE BEHAVIORAL FRAME OF REFERENCE

Contributions

The behavioral approach in mental health, as well as more globally in occupational therapy, can be credited for increasing the scrutiny given to goals and the efficacy of intervention strategies. Many therapists who thought, perhaps intuitively, that their intervention was helpful were forced to look carefully and reevaluate their intervention outcomes systematically. Further, it has provided clients/patients a clear way to identify their own goals and measure their progress, as, for example, through the use of learning or behavior contracts.

Behavior Management

The systematic use of behavior management strategies has provided tools for working with clients who lack internal control. The use of behavior management principles allows therapists to create a safe and predictable environment in which learning can occur. In work with children having disruptive behavior and with adult clients who are confused, impulsive, and/or aggressive, straightforward expectations and consequences for behavior enable clients to take responsibility for their behavior. In the area of mental health in particular, discarding the use of psychiatric jargon and labels that could overwhelm or confuse the lay person, the behavioral approach gave back to the client the ability to make understandable choices about his or her own care.

Skill Building

Behavioral techniques appear to work best with individuals having skill deficits in daily functioning and can be used successfully for skill building (Anthony, 1979; Boronow, 1986; Mosey, 1970). Improvements in grooming, appropriate verbalization, work skills, and social skills have all been addressed repeatedly in the literature. Skill enhancement has been especially significant in the outreach to individuals who have required long-term, habitual, or residential care. Behavioral therapy has been credited for humanizing the conditions of many persons whose lives have been otherwise devoid of success or joy.

Reinforcement

The thrust of traditional behaviorism can be credited for spotlighting the importance of attention and approval as reinforcements and for the significance of modeling in the learning process. Behaviorism has acted as a springboard for those investigators who have since sought to better understand the probable intervening process of cognitive structuring and the heretofore undeveloped understanding of social learning.

Limitations

The behavioral approach does not appear as applicable when there is not a specific skill or performance deficit. For example, if a young man is performing well in school and generally doing what is expected by family and friends yet expresses the sentiment, "What is life all about?," the behavioral approach has to strain to address the issue and may, many feel, address it only tangentially. The behavioral approach is not concerned primarily with meaning, per se, but rather performance outcomes. The literature that is cited in this chapter documenting the use of a behavioral model in occupational therapy has described its use exclusively with skill or performance deficits.

Constraints on Generalization

The behavioral approach for managing behavior appears to work best in a closed or self-contained environment, and gains made in the closed system do not necessarily generalize to home or to a more open environment. In a self-contained environment, such as a residential care setting or half-way house, individuals are more directly impacted by staff injunctions and reinforcements. Further, there is more likelihood that reinforcement will be judiciously given, modeling carefully provided, and progress nurtured. Although behavioral therapists acknowledge that internal motivation, self-reward, or naturally occurring rewards must at some point take over if an individual is to make a successful transition to a more open community, this intervening step may not occur (Mosey, 1970; Murdoch & Barker, 1991). In the everyday world, one's peers may again reward his or her maladaptive behavior or fail to notice his or her accomplishments, and maladaptive behaviors re-emerge. Our previous citations provide evidence of success within highly structured settings but raise questions when the environment cannot be controlled, such as those in home and community environments (Borg & Bruce, 1997).

Complex Intervention Planning

Designing and implementing an effective behavioral program for one or many patients is not necessarily as simple as it might appear. Whereas targeting inappropriate behaviors may not be difficult, isolating these behaviors and rewarding only the appropriate responses can be difficult, especially when many patients or clients are working together at one time. Identifying suitable rewards can also be difficult. If all persons desired candy and cigarettes along with hugs and smiles, it would be less difficult. For many depressed and regressed individuals, however, the secondary, and at times unclear, gains that they receive from maintaining their regressed behavior seem to be more rewarding than anything staff have to offer. The therapist finds him- or herself offering time alone as a reinforcement to a patient whose goal is to spend less time alone or food to an adolescent with eating problems whose goal is to spend less time involved with food. Further, it is difficult to achieve the generalization desired, while not promoting undesirable response generalization. For example, a specific therapist might elicit increased verbalization from a patient/client, but this social gain may not be generalized to other staff or to significant others who await the individual's return to home.

Finally, the behavioral position that complex behaviors can be broken down into smaller, discrete steps may be true, but in practice the effort to do so can become unwieldy. To define the exact circumstances under which a problem such as depression or diffuse anxiety occurs, one tends to respond to the most superficial issues—the tip of the iceberg. To do otherwise requires the kind of lengthy, extensive therapy that behaviorism has sought to replace.

Focus on Cognition, Motivation, and Meaning Limited

There are variables that traditional behaviorism has not addressed to some practitioners' satisfaction. It has spoken little, for example, to the role of internal motivation to excel where simple competence might have otherwise sufficed, the motivation to practice until perfect, the pleasure of activity for activity's sake. In failing to do so, traditional behavioral concepts seem self-limiting. The role of curiosity (e.g., the pleasure of a child in discovery and the joy of learning to speak a first word) is not the concern of behaviorists, yet it seems so integral to our understanding of purpose when as occupational therapists we use the term "purposeful activity."

The traditional behaviorist also does not address the issue of cognitive structuring as an intervening variable in learning and in problem-solving. With much of the early impetus coming from those who studied the function of language (Chomsky, 1967, 1972), scientists and practitioners have increasingly felt that such cognitive processing is necessarily conceived and is a separate and meaningful activity in itself.

One might see many of the opposition to behavioral thinking as philosophical. Behaviorism is a reductionist approach to understanding the human being. If we describe all the pieces—all the behaviors exhibited—have we really described the person? Or, are behaviors the external display of a far more complex internal process that cannot be as easily discerned? Does behaviorism trivialize the human condition, or is it an honest, practical approach to complex problems? With these questions in mind, we turn to the cognitive behaviorists and others who are concerned with the role of cognitive structuring in learning and in therapeutic intervention.

REFERENCES

Abildness, A. (1982). *Biofeedback strategies* (p. 8). Rockville, MD: American Occupational Therapy Association.

Anthony, W. A. (1979). *The principles of psychiatric rehabilitation.* Amherst, MA: Human Resource Development Press.

Bandura, A. (1963). *Social learning and personality development.* New York, NY: Holt, Rinehart and Winston.

Bandura, A. (1971a). *Psychological modeling: Conflicting theories.* New York, NY: Adine-Atherton.

Bandura, A. (1971b). *Social learning theory.* New York, NY: General Learning Press.

Banus, B. (Ed.). (1979). *The developmental therapist* (2nd ed., p. 260). Thorofare, NJ: SLACK Incorporated.

Becker, M., & Banus, B. (1979). Sensory-perceptual dysfunction and its management. In B. Banus (Ed.), *The developmental therapist* (pp. 239-273). Thorofare, NJ: SLACK Incorporated.

Bloomer, J., & Williams, S. (1979). *Bay Area Functional Performance Evaluation (BaFPE): Task Oriented Assessment and Social Interaction scale manual.* San Francisco, CA: USCF.

Borg, B., & Bruce, M. A. (1991). Assessing psychological performance factors. In C. Christiansen & C. Baum (Eds.), *Occupational therapy: Overcoming human performance deficits* (pp. 540-586). Thorofare, NJ: SLACK Incorporated.

Borg, B., & Bruce, M. A. (1997). *Occupational therapy stories: Psychosocial interaction in practice.* Thorofare, NJ: SLACK Incorporated.

Boronow, J. (1986). Rehabilitation of a chronic schizophrenic patient in a long term private inpatient setting. *Occupational Therapy in Mental Health, 6*(2), 1-20.

Burgess, P., Mitchelmore, S., & Giles, G. (1987). Behavioral treatment of attention deficits in mentally impaired subjects. *Am J Occup Ther, 41*(8), 505-509.

Charlebois, P., Normandeau, S., Vitaro, F., & Berneche, F. (1999). Skills training for inattentive, overactive, aggressive boys: Differential effects of content and delivery method. *Behavioral Disorders, 24*(2), 137-150.

Chomsky, N. (1967). Review of Skinner's "Verbal Behavior." In L. Jakobovits & M. Miron (Eds.), *Readings in the philosophy of language.* Englewood Cliffs, NJ: Prentice-Hall.

Chomsky, N. (1972). *Language and mind* (enlarged ed.). New York, NY: Harcourt Brace Jovanovich.

Clark, E., & Peters, M. (1984). *Scorable self-care evaluation.* Thorofare, NJ: SLACK Incorporated.

Corey, G. (1982). *Theory and practice of counseling and psychotherapy* (pp. 119, 135). Monterey, CA: Brooks/Cole Publishing Co.

Cormier, W., & Cormier, S. (1979). *Interviewing strategies for helpers* (p. 430). Belmont, CA: Wadsworth, Inc.

Diasio, K. (1968). Psychiatric occupational therapy: Search for a conceptual framework in the light of psychoanalytic ego psychology and learning theory. *Am J Occup Ther, 22*(5), 400-414.

Drouet, V. M. (1986). Individual behavioural programme planning with long stay patients, Part 1: Programmes planned and followed in an occupational therapy department. Part 2: Social skills training. *British Journal of Occupational Therapy, 49,* 227-232.

Durham, T. M. (1982). Community living skills training. *British Journal of Occupational Therapy, 45,* 233-235.

Engel, J., & Rapoff, M. (1990). Biofeedback-assisted relaxation training for adult and pediatric headache disorders. *Occupational Therapy Journal of Research, 10*(5), 283-299.

Fine, S. (1988). Working the system: A perspective for managing change. *Am J Occup Ther, 42*(7), 417-419.

Foto, M., Allen, C., Bass, C., Moon-Sperling, T., & Wilson, D. (1990). Reports that work. In C. B. Royeen (Ed.), *AOTA self-study series: Assessing function.* Rockville, MD: American Occupational Therapy Association.

Geiser, R. (1976). *Behavior modification and the managed society* (p. 42). Boston, MA: Beacon Press.

Giles, G. M. (1987). A behavioral approach to the treatment of the severely brain injured adult. *Occup Ther Forum, 2*(5), 3.

Giles, G. M. (1992). A neurofunctional approach to rehabilitation following severe head injury. In N. Katz (Ed.), *Cognitive rehabilitation models for intervention in occupational therapy* (pp. 195-218). Boston, MA: Andover Medical Publishers.

Giles, G. M. (1998). A neurofunctional approach to rehabilitation following severe brain injury. In N. Katz (Ed.), *Cognition and occupation in rehabilitation—Cognitive models for intervention in occupational therapy.* Bethesda, MD: American Occupational Therapy Association.

Giles, G. M., & Clark-Wilson, J. (1999). *Rehabilitation of the severely brain-injured adult—A practical approach* (2nd ed.). Cheltenham, United Kingdom: Stanley Thornes (Publisher) Ltd.

Gorman, P. (1991). Mental retardation and mental illness—Behavioral approaches. *Occup Ther Forum, 6*(5), 4-5.

Haertlein, C. L. (1994). Rasch analysis of the Milwaukee Evaluation of Daily Living Skills. In *Dissertation abstracts international section A: Humanities and social sciences, 54*(11-A), 40-70.

Haertlein, C. L. (1999). The Milwaukee Evaluation of Daily Living Skills. In B. Hemphill-Pearson (Ed.), *Assessments in occupational therapy mental health* (pp. 245-257). Thorofare, NJ: SLACK Incorporated.

Hilgard, E., & Bower, G. (1974). *Theories of learning* (3rd ed.). Englewood Cliffs, NJ: Prentice-Hall.

Hilgard, E., & Bower, G. (1975). *Theories of learning* (4th ed., pp. 136, 601-605). Englewood Cliffs, NJ: Prentice-Hall.

Holm, M. B., Rogers, J. C., & Stone, R. G. (1999). Treatment of performance contexts. In M. E. Neidstadt & E. B. Crepeau (Eds.), *Willard & Spackman's occupational therapy* (9th ed., pp. 471-498). Philadelphia, PA: Lippincott, Williams & Wilkins.

Hoppes, S. (1997). Motivating clients through goal setting. *Occupational Therapy Practice,* June, 22-27.

Jodrell, R., & Sanson-Fisher, R. (1975). Basic concepts of behavior therapy: An experiment involving disturbed adolescent girls. *Am J Occup Ther, 29*(18), 620-624.

Kaye, J., Mackie, V., & Hitzing, E. (1970). Contingency management in a workshop setting: Innovation in occupational therapy. *Am J Occup Ther, 24*(6), 413-417.

Kazdin, A. E. (1981). Behavioral observation. In M. Herson & A. Bellack (Eds.), *Behavioral assessment* (2nd ed., pp. 101-124). New York, NY: Pergamon Press.

Kibele, A., Padilla, R., & Burton, G. (1998). The psychological issues of illness and disability. In E. Cara & A. MacRae (Eds.), *Psychosocial occupational therapy in clinical practice* (pp. 199-226). Albany, NY: Delmar Publishers.

Kielhofner, G., & Burke, J. (1985). Components and determinants of human occupation. In G. Kielhofner (Ed.), *A model of human occupation.* Baltimore, MD: Williams & Wilkins.

King, L. J. (1974). A sensory integrative approach to schizophrenia. *Am J Occup Ther, 28*(9), 329-336.

Klyczek, J. P. (1999). The Bay Area Functional Performance Evaluation. In B. Hemphill-Pearson (Ed.), *Assessments in occupational therapy mental health: An integrated approach.* Thorofare, NJ: SLACK Incorporated.

Kunz, K., & Brayman, S. J. (1999). The Comprehensive Occupational Therapy Evaluation. In B. Hemphill-Pearson (Ed.), *Assessments in occupational therapy mental health: An integrative approach* (pp. 259-274). Thorofare, NJ: SLACK Incorporated.

Lang, E., & Mattson, M. (1993). The multi-disciplinary treatment plan: A format for enhancing activity therapy department involvement. In R. Cottrell (Ed.), *Psychosocial occupational therapy: Proactive approaches* (pp. 69-76). Rockville, MD: American Occupational Therapy Association.

Leonardelli, C. A. (1988). *The Milwaukee Evaluation of Daily Living Skills: Evaluation in long-term psychiatric care.* Thorofare, NJ: SLACK Incorporated.

Lewin, J., & Reed, C. (1998). *Problem-solving in occupational therapy.* Philadelphia, PA: Lippincott.

Liberman, R. P., Massel, M. A., Mosk, M., & Wong, S. (1993). Social skills training for chronic mental patients. In R. Cottrell (Ed.), *Psychosocial occupational therapy: Proactive approaches* (pp. 155-163). Rockville, MD: American Occupational Therapy Association.

Locke, E., & Latham, G. (1990). *A theory of goal setting and task performance.* Englewood Cliffs, NJ: Prentice-Hall.

Mager, R. (1962). *Preparing instructional objectives.* Palo Alto, CA: Fearon Publishers Inc.

Martin, G. L. (1978). *Behavior modification* (pp. 22, 58-59, 173). Englewood Cliffs, NJ: Prentice-Hall.

Martin, M. (1972). Behavior modification in the mental hospital: Assumptions and criticisms. *Hospital and Community Psychiatry, 28,* 292.

McIntyre, T., & Battle, J. (1998). The traits of "good teachers" as identified by African-American and white students with emotional and/or behavioral disorders. *Behavioral Disorders, 23*(2), 134-142.

Mischel, W. (1968). *Personality and assessment.* New York, NY: Wiley.

Mischel, W. (1973). Toward a cognitive social learning reconceptualization of personality. *Psychol Rev, 80,* 252-283.

Mosey, A. C. (1970). *Three frames of reference in mental health.* Thorofare, NJ: SLACK Incorporated.

Mosey, A. C. (1986). *Components of psychosocial occupational therapy.* New York, NY: Raven Press.

Murdoch, D., & Barker, P. (1991). *Basic behaviour therapy.* Oxford, England: Blackwell Scientific Publication.

Neidstadt, M. E. (1994a). The neurobiology of learning: Implications for treatment of adults with brain injury. *Am J Occup Ther, 48,* 421-430.

Neidstadt, M. E. (1994b). A meal preparation protocol for adults with brain injury. *Am J Occup Ther, 48,* 431-438.

Norman, C. (1976). Behavior modification: A perspective. *Am J Occup Ther, 30*(8), 491-497.

Nuse-Clark, P., & Allen, A. (Eds.). (1985). *Occupational therapy for children* (p. 271). St. Louis, MO: Mosby-Year Book.

Ogburn, K., Fast, D., & Tiffany, D. (1972). The effects of reinforcing working behavior. *Am J Occup Ther, 26*(1), 32-35.

Overbaugh, T., Bradley, B., & Bucher, M. (1970). Use of operant conditioning to improve behavior of a severely deteriorated psychotic. *Am J Occup Ther, 24*(6), 423-427.

Palmer, F. (1988). Present context of service delivery. In S. Robertson (Ed.), *Mental health focus: Skills for assessment and treatment* (pp. 1.28-1.36). Rockville, MD: American Occupational Therapy Association.

Pintrich, P., & Schunk, D. (1996). *Motivation in education: Theory, research, and applications.* Englewood Cliffs, NJ: Prentice Hall.

Rogers, J. (1982). The spirit of independence: The evolution of philosophy. *Am J Occup Ther, 36*(11), 709-716.

Rotter, J. B. (1954). *Social learning and clinical psychology.* Englewood Cliffs, NJ: Prentice-Hall.

Sieg, K. (1981). Applying the behavioral model to the occupational therapy model. *Am J Occup Ther, 35*(4), 243-248.

Skinner, B. F. (1938). *The behavior of organisms: An experimental analysis.* Englewood Cliffs, NJ: Prentice-Hall.

Skinner, B. F. (1953). *Science and human behavior.* New York, NY: MacMillan.

Skinner, B. F. (1968). *The technology of teaching.* Englewood Cliffs, NJ: Prentice-Hall.

Skinner, B. F. (1971). *Beyond freedom and dignity.* New York, NY: Knopf.

Spiegler, M., & Agigian, H. (1977). *The community training center: An educational behavioral social systems model for rehabilitating psychiatric patients.* New York, NY: Brunner/Mazel.

Stein, F. (1982). A current review of the behavioral frame of reference and its application to occupational therapy. *Occupational Therapy in Mental Health, 2*(4), 35-62.

Stein, F., & Nikolic, S. (1989). Teaching stress management techniques to a schizophrenic patient. *Am J Occup Ther, 43*(3), 162-169.

Stein, F., & Tallant, B. (1988). Applying the group process to psychiatric occupational therapy. *Occupational Therapy in Mental Health, 8*(3), 9-28.

Thompson, L. K. (1992). *The Kohlman Evaluation of Living Skills* (3rd ed.). Rockville, MD: American Occupational Therapy Association.

Tobin, T., & Sugai, G. (1999). Discipline problems, placements, and outcome for students with serious emotional disturbance. *Behavioral Disorders, 24*(2), 109-121.

Tolman, E. C. (1951). *Collected papers in psychology.* Berkeley, CA: University of California Press.

Trombley, C., & Scott, A. (1984). *Occupational therapy for physical dysfunction.* Baltimore, MD: Williams & Wilkins.

Wanderer, Z. (1974). Therapy as learning: Behavior therapy. *Am J Occup Ther, 28*(4), 207-208.

Watts, F. (1976). Modification of the employment handicaps of psychiatric patients by behavioral methods. *Am J Occup Ther, 30*(8), 487-490.

Watts, F., & Bennett, D. (1983). Introduction: The concepts of rehabilitation. In F. Watts & D. Bennett (Eds.), *Theory and practice of psychiatric rehabilitation* (pp. 3-14). New York, NY: John Wiley and Sons.

Weed, L. (1969). *Medical records, medical education, and patient care.* Cleveland, OH: Case Western Reserve University Press.

Wilberding, D. (1993). The quarterway house: More than an alternative care. In R. Cottrell (Ed.), *Psychosocial occupational therapy: Proactive approaches* (pp.127-138). Rockville, MD: American Occupational Therapy Association.

Williams, S., & Bloomer, J. (1987). *Bay Area Functional Performance Evaluation* (2nd ed.). Palo Alto, CA: Consulting Psychologists Press.

Yerxa, E. J. (1991). Nationally speaking: Seeking a relevant, ethical, and realistic way of knowledge for occupational therapy. *Am J Occup Ther, 45*, 199.

Yerxa, E. J. (1992). Some implications of occupational therapy's history for its epistemology, values, and relation to medicine. *Am J Occup Ther, 46*, 79-83.

CHAPTER SIX

Cognitive-Behavioral Frame of Reference—Thought and Knowledge Influence Performance

KEY POINTS

✧ History and Current Theory
- Occupational Therapy and Cognitive-Behavioral Literature
- Bandura's Social Learning Theory
- Ellis and Rational Emotive Theory
- Beck's Cognitive Therapy
- Donald Meichenbaum's Cognitive-Behavior Modification
- Coping Model of Intervention

✧ Theory in Context of Occupational Therapy Practice
- Person's Knowledge and Beliefs Influence Behavior
- Competence, Incompetence, and Unrealistic Reasoning
- Occupational Therapist—Educator-Facilitator, Scientific Role Model, Collaborator
- Activities Identify Knowledge, Enhance Competence, and Form Education Modules

✧ Theoretical Assumptions Guide Evaluation and Intervention
- Evaluation
  - —Identify Automatic Thoughts, Life Theme, and Knowledge
  - —Assess Cognitive Structures
  - —Evaluate the Person-Environment Match
- Intervention
  - —Re-establishing the Cognitive System as Self-Regulating
  - —Teaching Problem Solving
  - —Changing Knowledge, Behavior, and Thoughts
  - —Education Experiences and Socratic Approach Throughout the Life Span
  - —Education Groups in Occupational Therapy

✧ Contributions and Limitations of the Cognitive-Behavioral Frame of Reference

FOCUS QUESTIONS

1. How do behavioral therapy and cognitive-behavioral therapy differ?

2. How do cognitive-behavioral approaches differ from other cognitive approaches (e.g., cognitive disabilities and dynamic interactional frameworks)?

3. What is the role of cognition in cognitive-behavioral assessment and intervention?

4. What is the difference between the theories of Beck and Meichenbaum?

5. Describe Bandura's social learning paradigm.

6. In what situations that you have observed has the occupational therapist applied modeling of gradual mastery in teaching clients new skills?

7. Describe the roles of activities in cognitive-behavioral theory.

8. What are the differing views regarding graded activity?

9. How can occupational therapists use cognitive-behavioral theory?

10. Describe the elements of a psychoeducational course model.

11. What is the difference between a coping model of learning and a mastery model of learning?

12. How can the therapist structure the therapeutic relationship and use activities to enhance the client's/learner's feeling of competence?

13. What characteristics do the various cognitive-behavioral problem-solving strategies share? How do they benefit the learner?

14. How is relapse prevention approached in the cognitive-behavioral model?

15. In what contexts might the occupational therapist use principles related to relapse prevention and health maintenance?

HISTORICAL UPDATE

Some readers may ask if there is a difference between behavioral therapy and cognitive-behavioral therapy. **Behavioral approaches** give primary attention to the behaviors that need to be changed through the use of reinforcement strategies. Secondly, the behavioral therapist considers the thoughts that may influence behavior. **Cognitive-behavioral approaches**, on the other hand, primarily seek to change the thoughts believed to result in or cause specific behaviors and to develop a knowledge base for problem solving.

During the 1970s, there was a growing interest in cognitive processes and self-control within behavioral and social psychology. **Self-control** refers to the person's ability to influence his or her own growth and development rather than being controlled by outside reinforcers. This interest in cognitive processes and self-control conflicted with basic tenets of

behavioral theory and therapy and led to many disputes and, ultimately, a polarization between cognitive behavior therapists and non-cognitive behaviorists. A special interest group for cognitive-behavioral research was formed within the Association for the Advancement of Behavioral Therapy and the Association for Behavioral Analysis. This special interest group supported cognitive research and the study of the inner person in behavioral psychology. Out of the differing opinions, the conflicting discussions, the research, and the literature came cognitive-behavioral psychology, as it is known today. Cognitive-behavioral, cognitive, and learning approaches have expanded and they increasingly have been used to direct crisis, acute, chronic, and preventive evaluation and intervention programs. The theories in this chapter may be used alone or combined with other theories to meet client needs for growth, compensatory, and adaptive learning.

In the second edition of this text, we suggested that cognitive-behavioral approaches were combined with occupational therapy principles to create a basis for psychoeducational approaches used in occupational therapy. The **psychoeducational approach** in occupational therapy aims to strengthen or establish a knowledge base and to change the patient's or client's thoughts about one's self from "incapable" to "capable" and "competent." Educational courses are designed to prepare clients to respond to life's daily challenges. These courses may also increase client awareness, build functional skills, and teach problem-solving strategies.

Shortly after publication of the second edition, some occupational therapists selected certain cognitive and behavioral concepts and related them to Allen's cognitive disability theory. They suggested that cognitive-behavioral theory is useful with persons who function at levels 5 and 6 (indicative of higher cognitive abilities) (Cole, 1998). This adoption of cognitive behavior principles into cognitive disability theory still occurs today (Duncombe, 1998).

In preparing this third edition, we found that cognitive behavior theory has been combined with other theoretical frameworks from psychology and occupational therapy, including psychodynamic and developmental theories, and with the model of human occupation (Henderson, 1998). Thus, we recognize the potential for such combinations when cognitive-behavioral principles are to be applied with children, adults, and older adults with varied problems and in health promotion and prevention programs. Some examples of these eclectic applications are referenced and described later in this chapter. Examples are also available in Appendix J.

When reviewing the literature for this third edition, we noted also that some professionals reference cognitive-behavioral therapy as "cognitive therapy." In occupational therapy, however, the term "cognitive therapy" is applied to any one of several cognitive approaches (Katz, 1998). In this text, we describe three different cognitive models: cognitive disability, dynamic interactional, and cognitive-behavioral. Each one has distinguishing characteristics, and each is discussed in its own chapter in our text. The reader will find that with each model, terminology may be used similarly or quite differently, and intervention principles may overlap or contrast sharply.

Of the many cognitive-behavioral theories, Albert Bandura's social learning theory has had a particularly significant impact on contemporary psychology and work in the areas of prevention and health education. The educational programs and strategies that incorporate social learning theory may or may not be identified as psychoeducational. They include learning for self-management, health maintenance, and prevention of disability and functional problems. Social learning theory also guides the evaluation of client's perceptions of one's self and the environment and contributes to our understanding of the role of self-efficacy in occupational therapy interventions. One's sense of efficacy is believed to influence client goals, problem solving, and participation in daily life. Beliefs around self-efficacy also influence therapy outcomes and contribute to the evaluation of therapy effectiveness.

Although Bandura's work has been cited in our discussion of behavioral therapy, in this chapter we emphasize its application in cognitive-behavior therapy and examine its utility in the practice of occupational therapy. Because social learning theory is comprehensive and has multiple applications in occupational therapy practice, we recommend that Bandura's work be given attention even if the reader chooses not to apply a cognitive-behavior frame of reference to plan intervention (Bandura, 1977; Rosenthal & Bandura, 1978).

In this third edition of our text, we provide additional examples that illustrate the role of cognition in daily life and support the use of cognitive-behavioral principles in occupational therapy practice. As noted in previous editions, there remains a need for occupational therapists to demonstrate the utility of cognitive-behavior theory and cognitive approaches when they are used in practice (Henderson, 1998). We hope that the extensive resources cited in the reference section at the end of this chapter can guide occupational therapists in the design of outcome and theoretical studies or can be used to support the efficacy of using cognitive-behavioral approaches in the context of occupational therapy. What we present in this chapter points to a basic premise, which is that social learning and cognitive-behavioral theories are compatible with basic occupational therapy principles and can be applied to enhance practice.

DEFINITION

Cognitive-behavioral theory is used not only in psychosocial contexts and settings, but in any intervention setting in which the goals are to broaden clients' knowledge, strengthen the application of knowledge in skill-building, or improve the ability to problem solve. It is a frame of reference that assumes that a person's cognitive function and beliefs mediate or influence his or her affect and behavior. As part of the assessment process, the individual's perceptions, thoughts, attitudes, values, and beliefs are solicited. How these interact will impact the person's emotions and day-to-day behavior. With this understanding, the clinician structures the therapeutic learning experience. Cognitive-behavioral theory recommends that intervention include both verbal and behavioral strategies. The goal of intervention is to change the person's thoughts, which in turn will change the person's behavior, ultimately improving the client's daily function and sense of self-efficacy. When applying this framework, the occupational therapist grades activities in order to provide progressive challenges and success experiences. The clinician uses activities expected to illustrate to the client the relationship between thoughts and behavior and to develop those cognitive abilities needed to enhance performance. Individual and group learning experiences are designed to expand clients' knowledge base as well as repertoire of problem-solving strategies. Clients are given multiple opportunities to practice new strategies and skills. An important outcome of cognitive-behavioral intervention is that of increased self-knowledge and a heightened sense of self-efficacy, as clients view themselves as capable of handling new situations that may arise.

THEORETICAL DEVELOPMENT

Occupational Therapy Literature

Cognitive-behavioral approaches are compatible with the theoretical foundation of OT practice. Since the beginning of the profession, the principles of social learning, behavioral, and cognitive theories and approaches have been valued. Meyer suggested that clients adapt by changing their behavior, the environment, or their thoughts. These changes were expected to help clients problem solve (Duncombe, 1998; Lidz, 1985; Meyer, 1922). Cognitive-behavioral theory and occupational therapy theory share several characteristics:

- Both value the person's perspective or "phenomenological experience"
- Both recommend that there be a collaborative relationship between client and practitioner during the evaluation and intervention process
- Both value cognitive awareness and the person's ability to problem solve
- Both integrate activity or tasks into the intervention process
- Both provide many opportunities for practice in varied contexts in order to increase generalization of function (Duncombe, 1998)

The influence of social learning theory is evident in recent occupational therapy models, which focus on the interactions and transactions among the person, activity/occupations, and environment/context (Christiansen & Baum, 1997; Dunn, Brown, McClain, & Westman, 1994; Kielhofner, 1995; Law et al., 1996). Cognitive-behavioral principles applied during groups are also compatible with the task-oriented group theory that has a long tradition in occupational therapy (Duncombe, 1998; Fidler, 1969). The combined use of tasks and activities with skill practice, feedback, and discussion is core to many group interventions in occupational therapy. Throughout our professional history, occupational therapists have designed interventions that influence client behaviors and/or the environment in a way that would enhance the person's meaningful participation in daily life. Whether the therapist has chosen to emphasize behavioral or cognitive approaches or combine the two was influenced, in part, by the dominant theories in the mental health community, the client's needs, and the clinician's ability to integrate occupational therapy and mental health perspectives.

Previously, the educational emphasis in intervention was on the use of psychoeducational programs in occupational therapy. Currently, the literature contains many examples of different types of educational programs intended to meet cognitive, psychosocial, and physical needs; however, these learning experiences may or may not be identified as "psychoeducational." Frequently, the emphasis in current occupational therapy educational interventions is on the whole person rather than one particular component of function (e.g., psychological, social, physical, or cognitive). These programs reference social learning and cognitive theories, and they emphasize the relationship between mind and body, the need to increase both the client's knowledge and skills for performance in daily life, and the person's general well-being. These educational programs (Bodenham, 1988; Greenberg et al., 1988; Gutterman, 1991; Kramer, 1984; Lenters, 1999; Missiuna, Malloy-Miller, & Mandich, 1998; Neistadt & Marques, 1984; Perry, Tarrier, Morriss, McCarthy, & Limb, 1999; Schaefer, 1999; Sharpe et al., 1996; Sladyk, 1990; Vernon, 1999a, 1999b; Weinstein & DeNeff, 1989) have been used in community and health care environments and are designed for children, adults, and family members. In this chapter there are examples of cognitive-behavioral interventions (Cox & Findley, 1998; Crist, 1986; Deale, Chaider, Marks, & Wessely, 1997; Giles & Allen, 1986; Lenters, 1999; Lillie & Armstrong, 1982; Missiuna et al., 1998; Rynne & McKenna, 1999; Salo-Chydenius, 1996) and educational approaches that are or could be used in occupational therapy practice. These clinical applications suggest that cognitive-behavioral approaches are compatible with occupational therapy models (Banks, Crossman, Boel, & Stewart, 1997; Chesney & Brorsen, 2000; Crist, 1999; Flaherty, 1999; Folts, 1988; Hayes, 1989; Kaufman, Daniels, Laverdure, Moyer, & Campana, 1988; Lenters, 1999; Roth, 1986; Sladyk, 1990; Stockwell, Duncan, &

Levens, 1988; Yeager, 2000; Zimmerman, 1999). They also suggest that cognitive behaviorism is adaptable to both mental health treatment and prevention (Blackburn & Twaddle, 1996; Brownell & Fairburn, 1995; DeMars, 1992; Diamond, 1998; Follette, Ruzek, & Abueg, 1998; Jao & Lu, 1999; Johnson, 1987; Marlatt, 1995; Olmsted & Kaplan, 1995; Taylor, 1988; Vitousek, 1995).

Cognitive-Behavioral Literature

Cognitive-behavior therapy, also called **cognitive therapy**, has drawn from basic psychology, applied psychology, and education. It represents the integration of multiple theories, beginning as early as 1935 with the work of Adler who suggested that the person's view of one's self and of the world influenced the person's behavior. Since this time, other theorists have built on this work and suggested that the person constructs an image of the world and of change that influences behavior and one's emotions (Kelly, 1955). Other theorists have proposed that the method in which the person processes information (Williams, Watts, McLeod, & Mathews, 1988) and assimilates and accommodates new information (Piaget, 1972) is the variable that influences a person's thoughts and, thereby, one's emotions and behavior. These basic theories as well as those that come from clinical literature suggest that cognition is related to behavioral and emotional change (Arnold, 1960; Lazarus, 1976) and that cognitive therapy can help the person control thoughts, behavior, and emotions (Beck, 1976; Ellis, 1962; Mahoney, 1974).

In the 1970s, contributions of rational emotive therapists, cognitive therapists, social psychologists, and some behavioral theorists merged to form cognitive-behavioral theory. The work of Ellis, Beck, and Bandura and the studies and writings of Davidson, Kanfer, Phillips, Lang, Lazarus, Mischel, Peterson, Mahoney, Meichenbaum, Goldfried, Kazdin, Wilson, and other cognitive-behavioral theorists are represented in cognitive-behavioral literature. The merger emphasized the role of cognitive processes in understanding behavior, developing self-control, planning assessment and intervention strategies, and furthering the efficacy of behavioral intervention (Stone, 1980). The psychologists who contributed to the cognitive framework of therapy have emphasized the importance of cognition in the mediation of behavior. They also interpreted classical conditioning and reinforcement in cognitive terms.

In the literature the terms "cognitive therapy" and "cognitive-behavior therapy" have been used interchangeably. We have used sources representative of both terms in our discussion of cognitive-behavioral theory and its application in varied intervention contexts.

Forms of Cognitive-Behavior Therapy

Mahoney and Arnkoff (1974) have identified three major forms of cognitive behavior therapy:

- Rational psychotherapies

- Coping-skills therapies
- Problem-solving therapies

The **rational psychotherapies** include Ellis' rational emotive therapy (RET), Meichenbaum's self-instructional training (SIT), and Beck's cognitive therapy (CT). **Coping-skills** therapies use existing methods to facilitate coping with stressful events. Methods include covert modeling (Kazdin, 1974), modified systematic desensitization (Goldfried, 1971; Lang, 1969), anxiety management (Suinn & Richardson, 1971), and stress inoculation (Meichenbaum, 1973).

Problem-solving therapies are exemplified by Fairweather's treatment program for institutionalized adults (Fairweather, 1984) and other programs (Davidson, 1969; D'Zurilla & Goldfried, 1971; Mahoney, 1977; Spivack, Platt, & Shure, 1976). The therapist teaches skills that are used to find specific solutions for a presenting problem as well as strategies that can be used to solve similar problems in the future. The emphasis in this approach is on the client and therapist collaborating to identify strategies for problem solving. In contrast, in the problem solving of the behavioral approach the therapist more often uses reinforcement methods to modify the patient's or client's behavior to solve problems. The focus on problem-solving therapy continues to increase in the clinically applied cognitive behavior literature (D'Zurilla & Nezu, 1999).

Occupational therapists use diverse cognitive and cognitive-behavioral strategies in occupational therapy intervention and prevention. In this chapter, we will summarize four major theories that are often cited in occupational therapy literature and contribute to intervention and health education strategies in occupational therapy practice. These are Albert Bandura's social learning theory, Albert Ellis' rational emotive therapy, Aaron Beck's cognitive therapy, and Donald Meichenbaum's cognitive behavior modification. We also provide examples from the psychology, counseling, and education literatures that represent innovative applications of these theories in mental health and behavioral health contexts. These examples are chosen because they incorporate activities, learning tasks, and strategies that are compatible with occupational therapy principles and can be used to enhance the client's performance throughout the life span.

BANDURA'S SOCIAL LEARNING THEORY

Albert Bandura conceives social learning as an interactive-interdependent paradigm. **Learning** is viewed as an outcome of the interaction between behavior, person, and environment. Behavior is not just the outcome of the interaction between the person in his or her environment or determined solely by the environment. Rather, behavior is seen as an **interacting determinant** of the outcome or response. In other words, how people react and their unique perceptions of the

environment act on the environment as much as the environment acts on them.

For example, the occupational therapist in rehabilitation frequently encounters spinal cord injured patients with lesions at the same spinal cord level who have similar physical abilities and limitations of function but who vary in their response to rehabilitation and what they accomplish in treatment and in life. This difference is due in part to the patients' unique views of their disability and what each hopes to accomplish, as well as their actions in the environment. A patient's behavior can elicit empathy, sympathy, dependence, anger, acceptance or challenge, and assistance from those with whom he or she interacts. The reaction of others will affect the individual's self-image and the opportunities that become available to him or her, as well as the individual's ability in the future to progress and cope.

In the mental health setting, this interactive-interdependent paradigm can be seen in an adolescent intervention setting in which several adolescents with similar problems may participate in the same therapeutic milieu, but each will vary in his or her response to intervention as well as in personal progress. The adolescent's view of problems, personal strengths, peers and adults, his or her beliefs about treatment, and personal values and expectations influences his or her behavior and ability to profit from intervention. This behavior influences what parents, staff, and peers expect and think of the client; the goals they hold for him or her; the support they offer; and the reactions that they have based on judgments of previous behavior. Ultimately, the adolescent influences and can control many of the current and future reactions of others through his or her behavior and can create an environment that will influence his or her quality of life.

From these examples we see that both environment and the person may regulate behavior and influence the outcome of interactions. It is the correlation rather than the pairing of events that determines behavior (Bandura, 1977). Through an increased understanding of social learning theory, the reader broadens his or her knowledge in multiple areas, which assists in developing effective occupational therapy interventions. Among these are the following:

- The role of internal and external reinforcement
- The role of cognition in mediating environment and person interactions
- The role of cognition in modeling and observation learning
- The role of self-control and self-regulation in learning social responses
- Principles of corrective learning
- Alternative sources of motivation for behavior and intervention
- The relationship between beliefs about self-efficacy and a client's activity and participation in daily life

The Importance of Cognition in Modeling

Traditional behaviorists acknowledge that learning may occur when an individual models his or her actions after observing another individual. Social learning theorists like Bandura emphasize that cognition plays a significant intervening role in modeling. They remind us, however, that people do not imitate or model every behavior that they observe. Rather, individuals actively think about and select those behaviors that they will try to reproduce. The behaviors they choose to imitate will depend largely on what Bandura calls **anticipated consequences** (Perry & Bussey, 1984). Understandably, individuals are more likely to model behavior that they believe will lead to something they want. They learn this in part by noticing the consequences that result when others engage in a particular behavior. For instance, if an adult sees another person being praised for the care given to a craft project or efforts to use compromised limbs, the adult (the observer) may choose to imitate this behavior. Likewise, children who observe a peer receiving a certificate of achievement for completing a volunteer project may want to volunteer also.

Modeling and Imitation

Modeling and imitation can play a part not only in skill building, but also in rule and attitude formation. The person who observes another patient/client or staff member consistently displaying certain attitudes (sharing, concern for others) may discern the common thread that runs through diverse situations and repeat a similar attitude in his or her own interactions.

As we have discussed previously in the text, an individual is more likely to imitate someone he or she perceives as similar (e.g., a male will more likely imitate a male; a member of one group will more likely imitate another group member) or someone highly regarded. However, individuals are unlikely to model behaviors that they feel incapable of (e.g., clients who believe they are incapable of mastering dressing techniques are unlikely to model after someone dressing no matter how high the regard they may have for the model). Bandura's work in this area is pertinent to occupational therapists. His studies suggest that if the observer (here, the patient or client) can see the model performing individual steps in the task while the patient/client imitates and practices each of these steps, the learner increases his or her own perception of self-efficacy. This process is referred to as **modeling of gradual mastery** (Bandura, 1977; Rosenthal & Bandura, 1978).

Cognition in Reinforcement

Both internal and external sources of reinforcement may stimulate and maintain behaviors and thoughts. Not only must the tangible outcome or measurable reinforcement be considered, but also the individual's expectations regarding the reinforcement. These expectations are modulated by the person's cognitive abilities, as discussed. In the social learning view, reinforcement can be an external, a vicarious, or a self-produced consequence (Bandura, 1977). **External reinforcers** are money, food, material goods, social approval, privileges, or penalties. **Vicarious reinforcers** are symbolic (those images that a person has as a result of observing and learning from others) and include the individual's values and images of success or failure (Bandura, 1977). For example, the student who is studying for a profession is reinforced for his or her efforts and the sacrifices that studies demand by the images held of mentors, the prestige of the profession, and the values and salary associated with the position he or she hopes to attain after graduation.

Successful performance during tasks leads to a sense of efficacy and competence. **Competence** means that the person has internalized behaviors, which are maintained even when external reinforcers are withdrawn. When a patient or client succeeds and feels competent, he or she gains a sense of self-control. **Self-control** further indicates that the person is capable of setting standards, judging personal behavior against these standards, comparing performance with previous performance, and maintaining an internal reward (Bandura, 1977).

Self-produced consequences, the third type of reinforcement, come from the individual's sense of accomplishment, sense of self-control, and sense of competence that result from success (Bandura, 1977). Stated simply, feeling competent and in control is a good feeling and is rewarding.

Hierarchy of Reinforcement

Social learning theory also conceptualizes a hierarchy of reinforcement based on the view that reinforcers acquire meaning and change as a result of developmental experiences. Think about the way in which children respond to different kinds of rewards as they grow. **Initial reinforcers** are more often external, such as smiles of approval, attention from significant others, and treats like candy (Bowlby, 1977a, 1977b). As cognition develops, symbolic reinforcers play an increasingly important part in influencing behavior. **Symbolic reinforcers** are memories, verbalizations, and internalized pictures (Bandura, 1977). For example, the child remembers the fun the family had when they went to the local amusement park, so Mom's promise that, "We will go this weekend if you are on your best behavior all week," is a powerful incentive for exemplary behavior. Conversely, the child learns self-control in part from parental discussion or reprimands that identify negative consequences of undesirable behavior. These may be identified as related to the laws of God, nature, or society as well as family. Both children and adults can control their behavior in part because they can create a mental picture of the negative consequences of lying, speeding, trespassing, or stealing.

Next in the hierarchy is social contracting. A **social contract** is the system that identifies rewards, privileges, and the punishments and censure that accompany specific behavior (Bandura, 1977). When an individual assumes roles and responsibilities of a job through written contractual agreement, the employer provides benefits and salary. When parents neglect or abuse a child, they violate the social contract for parenting and are punished by society.

Personal satisfaction, the last developmental step in the reinforcement hierarchy, is an intrinsic, self-produced reward and is the best reinforcement of behavior. Because personal satisfaction is probably the reward least dependent on changing, often fickle external circumstances, behavior based on this stage of the hierarchy is difficult to extinguish (Bandura, 1977). **Self-satisfaction** comes from self-evaluation and self-produced consequences. The person who perfects intellectual, creative, or physical skills or abides by the speed limit in order to please the self rather than or in addition to others gains personal satisfaction.

Whatever the reinforcement, cognitive theorists emphasize that the ability to think about or anticipate reinforcement frees the individual from needing an immediate reinforcement for behavior. Traditional behaviorists state that positive reinforcement should immediately follow a desired response. Cognitive behaviorists disagree with this requirement in general but do acknowledge that certain cognitive structures must exist for the individual to recognize and wait for a non-immediate reward.

Further Influence of Cognition in Social Learning Theory

Cognition influences motivation, goal setting and attainment, achievement of insight and acquisition, retention, and expression of behavior. Once a person has the ability to represent events symbolically (i.e., once he or she can create a mental picture of people, objects, and events), then he or she is able to identify similar personal experiences or experiences of others, remember previous outcomes, and evaluate these events to anticipate possible consequences of behavior. This symbolic process allows a person to learn from **vicarious experiences** (e.g., those heard or read) and to problem-solve in thought without needing trial and error learning experiences. In other words, the person can imagine "what would happen if..." and does not have to experience everything personally to learn from it.

Goals

The ability to anticipate the likely consequences of behavior influences the person's motivation and regulates the goals that the person tries to achieve. **Goals** are statements of the general standards of conduct that regulate behavior. People use goals to evaluate their performance and their accomplishments. In the application of social learning theory, behavior is evaluated by comparing the client's behavior with

his or her goals and by comparing present behavior with the previous behavior. Thus, goal accomplishment suggests increased competency. The client's or patient's behavior is not contrasted with that of other people or the norms for behavior.

As with traditional behavior therapy, goals should be specific enough to make identification of accomplishment possible; the conditions for behavior and the type and amount of behavior required should be stated. Consistent with the principle of creating moderate disequilibrium, goals should be moderately difficult. If they are too easy, the client loses interest; if they are too difficult, the person is unable to perceive the self as attaining them. Social learning theory emphasizes that the individual's perception of self as capable of goal attainment actually increases his or her ability to accomplish goals (Perry & Bussey, 1984).

Example—Child Self-Efficacy and Goal Setting

Recent occupational therapy literature discusses the effect of clients' sense of **self-efficacy** (their beliefs regarding their capability in specific situations) on goal setting. One study that illustrates this relationship is the study of the Perceived Efficacy and Goals Setting System (PEGS) by Missiuna and Pollock (2000). These researchers evaluated the relationship between children's beliefs regarding self-efficacy and their goals for therapy. Although occupational therapists might assume that they are working to achieve the child's goals, it appears that in many situations the goals that are the focus for intervention are actually set by parents or the clinician. Missiuna and Pollock used a picture card sort process to study goal setting with school-aged children and found that these children were capable of identifying goals; however, they sometimes overestimated their ability. Citing a study by Landry, Robinson, Copeland, and Garner (1993), the researchers proposed that this overestimation could be a motivator that helps the child create a challenge. It would then be the job of the clinician to assist in identifying subgoals that would enable successful accomplishment. When comparing child and parental goals, they identified similar desired changes. However, the priority given to the goal or the order in which goals would be pursued varied. Children selected both fine-motor and gross-motor goals and preferred to focus on self-care and leisure tasks. Parents chose predominantly fine-motor goals and preferred printing and drawing tasks as the focus for goals. This study supported the view that occupational therapists can use a child's self-efficacy beliefs to set and mediate goals and that including children in the goal-setting process could enhance goal attainment.

Subgoals

Goals are accomplished through the satisfaction of subgoals. **Subgoals** are the immediate goals that can mobilize effort and indicate what the client is to do in the here and now.

When successfully accomplished, they increase the image of self as capable and reinforce the expenditure of effort needed to attain remote goals. **Remote goals** identify behaviors desired or required in the distant future to produce self-satisfaction and control. They are not incentives for the present because they are usually too far removed from the present, which has competing demands for the person's attention. Clinicians use the process of **mediation** to connect subgoals and develop learning experiences that relate to the client's long-term or remote goals. The process provides the "just right challenge" for the person to achieve personal subgoals and goals.

Example—Mediation in Occupational Therapy

The occupational therapist's role in mediation is to provide an environment with adequate challenge for the client and to facilitate the client's learning experience to achieve both goals and objectives. The example of mediation that we discuss here comes from the study of Missiuna et al. (1998), who propose mediation guidelines be used with children and adults to teach problem solving. This example depicts a **top-down approach** to therapy (i.e., a plan of intervention that emphasizes performance in context [e.g., functional communication in a school or employment environment, skills for using a computer, or writing] not isolated practice of individual performance components, such as memory, attention, or strength). The mediation process is a cognitive approach based upon the work of Vygotsky (1962, 1987), Luria (1973, 1980), Meichenbaum (1977), and Meichenbaum & Biemiller (1998). The reader is referred to the original sources of these theories. Missiuna and colleagues integrate these theories of cognition and learning to form guides for mediation during occupational therapy intervention.

To facilitate mediation, the therapist follows five steps for planning a session:

1. Analyzes the task(s) related to the client's goal and your observation of the client's related performance.
2. Makes hypotheses about the client's possible performance and forms questions that will help him or her identify his or her performance problems.
3. Identifies possible performance strategies to achieve goals and structures the learning experience so that the client can discover them.
4. After the client selects a strategy, asks the client to practice it and evaluates the strategy's effectiveness.
5. Helps the client evaluate his or her performance by use of questions and feedback that relate to the performance context.

During the occupational therapy session, the clinician skillfully uses questions to increase the client's awareness of knowledge needed for the task and of those personal strengths and skills that are effective for the current inter-

vention situation as well as future occupational performance contexts. A guiding principle of these strategies is "Ask, don't tell" (Missiuna et al., 1998, p. 206). For example, ask the client to **predict, describe, evaluate, and identify variables** that influence his or her behavior (see Using Mediation—Sample Questions).

USING MEDIATION—SAMPLE QUESTIONS

For example, the therapist asks the client:

- What will be difficult to do during the task? (**Predict**)
- What will make it easier to perform the task? (**Description**)
- What did you do well? (**Evaluate** his or her performance)
- What do you need to do to improve your performance? (**Identify**)

Consider the following example: You have been working with a young woman who has recently had a CVA and has residual hemiparesis. She is discharged from the rehabilitation setting to return home. You ask what is important to her as she thinks about returning to her home, and she indicates that she wants to be able to prepare meals for herself and her husband, to be able to bathe independently, and to be able to do personal hygiene. We can use the example of meal preparation. The therapist might be inclined to tell her, "I expect that it will be difficult for you to stand at the sink or to go to and from the refrigerator and stove. Let's find a stable seat or tool that you could use," or "Let's rearrange your work space." Using principles of mediation, you would begin instead by asking this woman, "What do you think will be most difficult as you envision yourself returning to the kitchen?," and "What do you think will make meal preparation easier?" The woman might be permitted to try to retrieve items from the refrigerator or wash vegetables at the sink, and she could be asked, "How do you feel you're doing? What will make this easier?" This process gives the client more control in the therapeutic process and can help to increase his or her insight. The young woman is considered the expert who has ideas that influence performance.

Insight

A critical function of cognition is that it allows the person to accurately interpret reality and develop insight. As in traditional behavioral practice, social learning theory states that when a person has **insight**, he or she is aware of the relationship between contingencies, events, and what is reinforced

(Bandura, 1977). This knowledge is believed to enhance learning and increase insight; both are goals of many social learning strategies. When a patient or client knows the reason for and benefits of intervention, he or she is more inclined to try new experiences and is often more motivated to learn, provided the benefits are compatible with personal needs and interests. Insight also increases the ability for self-control.

Learning is also affected by the person's use of cognitive structures to interpret reality. An individual can misread reality, over-generalize, have false or rigid beliefs, or use faulty cognitive processing and thus misinterpret reality. Because a person's beliefs and his or her anticipation of the outcome of behavior are believed to govern behavior, such misinterpretations must be corrected if adaptive learning is to take place. For example, if a person falsely assumes that if he or she produces a well-organized resume, the first job applied for will be offered, then that assumption must be corrected.

Summary—Relevance of Bandura's Work to Occupational Therapy

As suggested by the examples and citations in this chapter, occupational therapists have supported the application of social learning theory in occupational therapy practice for years. Social learning theory is also evident in early as well as more recent theories that guide occupational therapy practice (Christiansen & Baum, 1991, 1997; Conte & Conte, 1977; Koestler, 1970; Law et al., 1996; Mosey, 1974). Bandura's work supports one of occupational therapy's underlying premises—that doing facilitates change. In his discussion of modeling and observation learning, Bandura proposes that the efficacy of intervention is increased by actual performance or cognitive-behavioral learning rather than by relying solely on cognitive verbal methods.

Model for Success

Bandura's work provides a circular, interactive model of intervention. To facilitate a relationship between the person and the activity to promote success, the clinicians can do the following:

- Change an individual's thoughts from "incapable" to "capable" (to facilitate engagement in activity).
- Use activities in which persons can experience themselves as capable. Grade these, use physical guidance, or use a model engaged in gradual mastery to ensure success while at the same time increasing patients'/clients' perceptions of themselves as capable.
- Use verbal techniques to help clients identify their success, generalize learning, and increase their sense of self-control and competence.

When a person experiences success, he or she increases his or her feelings of satisfaction, competence, and control. These thoughts and feelings help a person face and cope with other day-to-day and future demands (see Performance for Learning).

PERFORMANCE FOR LEARNING

The emphasis on actual performance during learning is similar to Jerome Bruner's concept of enactive learning. Bruner, often cited in education literature, emphasizes the importance of having physical experience as well as the opportunity to reflect on or talk about what one has just accomplished. This combination of enactive learning along with verbalization is thought to facilitate learning more than either action or talking alone.

Group Membership

Bandura's work on modeling raises a question about the typical grouping of participants in occupational therapy. For example, we often find that patients or clients performing at a similar level are grouped together. However, the clinician may consider the potential merit of pairing more functional, interactive clients with those who are perhaps less involved or less functional. If persons with limited function can identify with those who are more functional, they may profit. The clients may imitate the adaptive behaviors that they observe. More functional clients can take on the role of teacher or mentor and themselves gain from the experience. Therapeutic experiences of this nature have proved successful in remedying social learning problems with children (Perry & Bussy, 1984). This option of mixing level of ability is in direct contrast with Allen's cognitive disability model (Allen, 1985, 1994; Allen & Blue, 1998), which recommends that clients with similar ability be placed together to do activities graded in accordance with cognitive ability.

Sense of Control

Bandura's conclusions are consistent with the behavioral practice of incorporating both external and internal reinforcement. Bandura and social learning theorists go further, however, in proposing that clinicians actively help clients identify properties of anticipated reinforcements and that they assist patients in achieving a sense of control so that they can moderate their need for immediate gratification. Bandura's work also supports active intervention by the clinicians to assist patients and clients in identifying personal strengths, limitations, and the cognitions used to solve problems so that these individuals feel in control of and responsible for their own actions.

ELLIS AND RATIONAL EMOTIVE THERAPY

Of the identified cognitive therapies, rational emotive therapy (RET), introduced by Albert Ellis in 1955, may be the one best known. Ellis disagreed with the Freudian view that a person's instincts determine behavior. Nor did he endorse the existential view that the authenticity of and the acceptance by a therapist could change a patient's beliefs and habits. He believed that it was the client's perception of and beliefs about an event that influenced the person's feelings and ultimately his or her behavior.

When reviewing the literature for this third edition, we found that it is also called rational emotive behavior therapy and that there is continued and increased support for using rational emotive theory as a basis for interventions with adult and child populations. The intervention may be part of private practice, inpatient, community mental health, or school programs, or the theory may be the basis for prevention and health promotion programs for children and adults. The current emphasis in health promotion and education programs is toward the goal of enabling learners to take care of their "emotional health" as part of "growing up" (Vernon, 1999b). Therefore, in the section that follows, we summarize Ellis' theory and provide examples of Ellis' theory applied to children and adults. These examples illustrate strategies that occupational therapists can teach clients or care providers in order to increase the clients' participation in daily occupations of school, work, and promote health maintenance throughout the life span.

ABC Theory

Ellis was dissatisfied with the results of his psychoanalytical practice and decided to take a cognitive approach. This approach assumed that thoughts, feelings, and behaviors interact and have a reciprocal cause and effect relationship. The approach has been summarized in what is called the **ABC theory:** (A) A fact, *activating* event, behavior, or attitude causes or influences the *belief* (B), which determines the *consequence* (C). It is the belief, not the activating event, that determines the consequences. Therefore, the therapist uses interventions that dispute the client's self-defeating beliefs. For example, in order to dispute or challenge a person's belief that he or she is globally incompetent, the occupational therapist would recommend activities in which the client could succeed. He would also recommend activities that clearly illustrated those particular areas in which the client had difficulty and those in which he or she was strong.

Irrational Thinking

RET strives to help the individual develop a rational basis for living through disputing those irrational views that pro-duce what Ellis referred to as "neurosis" or problems in living or self-defeat. Ellis summarizes these irrational views in three statements called "**musturbatory thinking:**"

1. I must perform well and be approved by significant others. If I don't, then it is awful, I cannot stand it, and I am a rotten person.
2. You must treat me fairly. When you don't, it is horrible, and I cannot bear it.
3. Conditions must be the way I want them to be. It is terrible when they are not, and I cannot stand living in such an awful world (Corey, 1979).

In an occupational therapy context these may be expressed as, "I must do everything perfectly." The client who is transitioning back into the workplace states, "All I do is work all the time, and I never get recognition from my boss like everyone else does. What's wrong with my work? I just want to quit. Why try? I'll never please my boss. I am blamed for everything that goes wrong. I'd be better off staying home."

To counteract these irrational views and promote rational living, the rational emotive therapist does the following:

- Gets patients/clients to acknowledge the irrational ideas that motivate their disturbed behavior and challenges them to validate these ideas.
- Uses logical analysis to demonstrate the illogical nature of the person's thinking and to minimize these beliefs.
- Shows how the beliefs are self-defeating and how they will lead to future emotional and behavioral disturbances.
- Uses absurdity and humor to confront the irrationality of the patients' or clients' thinking.
- Explains how these ideas can be replaced with more rational ideas that are empirically grounded.
- Teaches the person how to apply the scientific approach to thinking so that he or she can observe and minimize present or future irrational ideas and illogical deductions that foster self-destructive ways of feeling and behaving (Corey, 1979, pp. 173, 176; 2000, pp. 403-406).

In occupational therapy, the therapist will often assign activity homework to help the client gather data that confirm or dispute particular perceptions and beliefs about one's performance. The client and clinician then talk about the activity experience and identify strategies that can be used to manage uncomfortable feelings or self-defeating thoughts in the future. A client having problems with an employer might, for instance, identify and could practice through role-play behaviors for responding to the problem situations in the work environment. The purpose would be to increase the client's sense of efficacy and control, with the emphasis on increasing the client's awareness of his or her faulty beliefs.

RET Techniques

Rational emotive techniques can be used with individuals and groups, and clients can help each other catch themselves expressing self-defeating beliefs. **Cognitive methods** include disputing irrational beliefs, cognitive homework, bibliotherapy, and using new self-statements (Corey, 2000; Ellis, 1973, 1979, 1996).

When disputing irrational beliefs, therapists help the client or clients see that it is their view of an event or belief about themselves that is causing their symptoms or sense of defeat. The therapist then asks clients to give evidence that supports their beliefs or interpretations of reality. Later, clients will be asked to do the disputing themselves and to work systematically to diminish their distorted views.

Ellis' homework assignments were given to patients to demonstrate the rational or irrational nature of their thoughts and behaviors. These included behavioral assignments, reading, or specific therapeutic tasks. For example, during a public demonstration of RET for marriage and family problems, Ellis gave an assignment to a woman who he had interviewed for 15 minutes during which they discussed her marital stress. He asked her to do the following: During the next week sit quietly, ask yourself these questions, then answer them:

1. "Why must I have a perfect marriage?"
2. State why it is that, "If I don't have a perfect marriage, I'm an awful person."
3. "What would I change to make the marriage more perfect?"

With this assignment Ellis tried to help the woman see that she had unrealistic expectations, that no marriage is perfect, and that while she may have feelings about herself and her contributions to the relationship, they don't make her an "awful" person. He also asserted that she must begin to identify what she can change in the relationship or what she would like her spouse to change. A similar strategy could be used when an OT client trying to learn to transfer from wheelchair to tub insists that he or she will "never be able to do this" or will "never be able to live by myself again." (An important caution, however, is that cognitive techniques such as these are not to be used in a manner that would appear to trivialize the client's concern or be punitive.)

Task and reading assignments (**bibliotherapy**) are used to diminish distorted thoughts and change behavior. Clients can be given articles or pamphlets that describe "ABC" principles or the physical effects of anxiety and strategies to manage anxiety or other symptoms that the client may have that interferes with daily life. Rational emotive therapists would be inclined to have clients read *Humanistic Psychology: The Rational Emotive Approach, A New Guide to Rational Living,* or *How to Stubbornly Refuse to Make Yourself Miserable About Anything—Yes, Anything!,* or other similar literature (Ellis, 1973, 1975, 1988).

The therapist may assign other homework as well (e.g., audio and videotape assignments, workbook pages, etc.). There may also be "real life" tasks that are usually completed between sessions or during the intervention sessions. They are used to help the individual manage anxiety and dispute irrational beliefs.

For example, a person who is afraid of heights might be asked to take an elevator to the top of a building, or a person who is afraid of crowds may be asked to go to a place in which a crowd of people are present. This strategy is controversial and is seldom used by occupational therapists who more often use graded tasks and bibliotherapy.

The occupational therapist leading a support group or consulting with a day program in which participants have such disabling conditions as multiple sclerosis or paraplegia might assign reading that demonstrates that persons with disabilities can succeed. In a community outreach program one participant was an African-American, single mother of three children who was abusing alcohol. She was assigned readings that depicted struggles by other African-American women who overcame adversity, as well as educational literature that would increase her knowledge of effective parenting and stress management strategies.

Emotive techniques used in RET include unconditional acceptance, rational emotive role playing, modeling, self-statements (which may be voiced aloud or said to one's self), rational emotive imagery, and shame taking. The therapist teaches patients/clients to accept themselves. The ideas that "We all make mistakes," that "We can learn from mistakes," that "Nobody is perfect," that "It's OK to be yourself," and that "One needs to learn to live with one's self" are emphasized to develop unconditional acceptance (Ellis, 1993a, 1993b, 1994; Ellis & Dryden, 1997; Ellis & Whiteley, 1979).

Within RET the therapist is a model for the patient or client. Therefore, he or she actively participates in therapy sessions to verbalize rational thoughts, model effective task behavior, model courage during new experiences and when taking risks, and model unconditional acceptance of one's self and the patient/client. Likewise, other patients or clients in the therapeutic group can serve as models for appropriate risk-taking behavior. For example, in a support group for persons with head injuries, a member may indicate that he is afraid of looking like a "freak" if he attends his upcoming high-school reunion. Other members voice that they have had similar fears when they first ventured out, but they challenge his need to be the "same guy" he was 20 years ago.

Imagery and role-playing allow the participant to try out the expression of new thoughts, feelings, and behaviors in thought or fantasy or in contrived (but safe) settings before risking their expression in the everyday world.

RET and Behavioral Techniques

Operant conditioning, self-management, systematic desensitization, instrumental conditioning, biofeedback, relaxation techniques, and modeling are behavioral techniques used by rational emotive therapists (Dryden, 1984; Ellis, 1996; Ellis & Dryden, 1997). Incorporation of these techniques into therapy reflects a broadened view of RET. Ellis has called this a second type of RET and sees it as the same as other cognitive-behavioral therapies. Not all cognitive-behavioral therapists agree with Ellis; however, his approach is used with clients of all ages, in many contexts, and may be combined with other learning experiences. The next three examples describe rational emotive behavior therapy for children and adolescents.

Example 1: RET with Child and Adolescent Populations

The theory and application of RET has evolved over a 40-year period. During this time it has been used primarily with adult clients; however, the more recent use of RET with children continues to grow. Vernon (1999b) indicates that rational emotive strategies are used in the United States, England, Australia, and Western Europe with child and adolescent populations. They are used to change disruptive, aggressive, fearful, anxious, withdrawn, and impulsive behaviors. They are used to improve the child's self-concept and interpersonal relationships and increase problem solving and achievement. They can be applied with individual clients or groups at school as part of health education, and for classroom management.

Example 2: Rational Emotive Behavior Therapy with Children and Adolescents

As summarized by Vernon (1999a, 1999b), practitioners using RET with children and adolescents believe that within the process of normal development children will need to be able to manage their behavior and emotions if they are to meet the challenges of growing up and problem solving in daily life. They believe that children's/adolescents' thoughts are a key influence on emotion and behavior. As with adults, it is the young person's thoughts about an event that interrupt goal attainment and may produce behavior that is incompatible or in conflict with social expectations at home or in school. The focus of assessment and intervention is the relationship of the child's thoughts to behavior and identifying whether thoughts are rational or irrational.

For example, if a child makes a mess in the kitchen and a parent becomes angry, the child need not assume, "I am a bad person," or "Mom and Dad don't like me." Rather, it means, "I made a mistake. Next time I will clean up even if my friend is here waiting for me to play." When an adolescent breaks off a relationship with a boy- or girlfriend, the person "being dumped" may feel that he or she is ugly, unlovable, and will never have another boy- or girlfriend. In situations such as these, clients are taught to evaluate their thinking and develop rational ideas that change their perceptions of themselves, the event, and their behavior within daily activities. The goal is for clients to "get better" not just "feel better." Behavior change, as evidenced by improved participation at school and at home, is the desired outcome.

Problem-Solving Strategies

Proponents view this approach as an efficient process that is easily understood by children of various ages. They propose that it is easily applied and provides opportunities for the child to learn basic strategies that he or she can use in daily life. Occupational therapists applying these principles are advised that they need not get extensive details about a problem situation. These details are not believed needed for effective problem solving. The approach has four major steps:

1. Get a clear statement of the problem
2. Identify the behaviors related to the problem
3. Identify the person's beliefs about the problem
4. Identify the emotional consequences of the problem

The therapist then collaborates with the child or adolescent, taking a rather directive stance that may vary with the age of the child. The therapist also injects the use of humor, warmth, and praise throughout the process. When the child or adolescent resists the idea of intervention, the therapist acknowledges this and lets the person know that this is a common reaction, and then gives an example of how others have felt similarly. The clinician shares with the client that others have questioned the value of intervention but chose to participate and ultimately had a positive outcome. The therapist may add, however, that the positive outcome did not necessarily mean that others got their boyfriend or girlfriend back. They did learn, however, about themselves and the qualities they have that make them likeable, and they did develop skills for developing new relationships.

Example 3: RET for Children

When RET principles are taught to children and adolescents this does not typically occur in a formal lecture, as frequently occurs in adult therapy groups. Instead, the clinician uses the child's issues (e.g., stresses, disappointments, or problems) and teaches the process informally. The youngster learns to identify the action (A), beliefs (B), and the consequences (C) of the action as he or she problem solves around a specific situation from his or her daily life. After learning the "ABC" format, RET strategies used with children are similar to those used with adults. The therapist challenges the child's beliefs and helps to reframe the experience for problem solving. The child and the therapist agree upon an experiment to test one's beliefs or practice problem solving at school or at home. The child may practice new behaviors during role play in a therapy session before the "real world" context. Children also can benefit from reading and homework assignments. Bibliotherapy is adjusted to the level of ability of the child or adolescent. Vernon (1999a) suggests assignments such as reading *How to Get Along with Friends* or learning experiences that can come from emotional education curriculum for children or adolescents (Vernon, 1989a, 1989b, 1989c, 1998a, 1998b, 1998c). We recommend that the clinician who works with children and adolescents becomes familiar with the popular literature of these clients and choose readings for children and families that support learning related to therapy goals and the client's desired outcomes.

Example 4: Rational Emotive Principles in the Classroom

In the classroom, children and adolescents may participate in RET in order to improve their problem solving, but the primary goal is to learn about one's emotional health and to develop attitudes and behaviors that can minimize psychosocial problems throughout life. Children learn about the relationship between their feelings and thoughts. They learn to distinguish facts from beliefs and can use this information to respond to stressful events in life. In doing so, they learn about their strengths and weaknesses and what they can reasonably be expected to accomplish. It is important also that they learn that their value lay not only in their accomplishments but in who they are as people. They learn to express their feelings and to adjust their behavior to meet the expectations of the current situation, for example, when to be assertive, or how to be a good team player, and so on.

Example 5: RET and the Adventure Challenge

Given their popularity, the reader is probably familiar with survival school experiences such as Outward Bound. These programs are available for adolescents and adults. Their focus varies from interventions geared to identified physical and psychosocial problems, to building management teams in corporations, and may include physically challenging activities such as backpacking, hiking, rock climbing, rafting, ropes courses, rappelling, and community service endeavors. The identified purpose of these programs may be recreation, education, fitness, or personal and interpersonal growth. The outcomes are not based in empirical findings, but those reported include changes related to therapy goals:

- Participants increase confidence and positive self-image
- Participants learn personal and peer group problem-solving
- Participants use effective communication

- Participants demonstrate increased skills for completion of group tasks

In the past, the primary model for these programs was experiential learning. Recently, Leeds (1999) and other professionals suggested that the benefits of the adventure challenge would be increased if experiential models were combined with a therapy model that incorporated group and personal therapeutic strategies such as those used in RET. It was recommended that professionals train adventure program personnel to use RET strategies in helping participants set personal goals and challenge dysfunctional (self-defeating) beliefs within the adventure experience. In general, they are trained to turn the participants' anxiety into eustress, or the positive energy from stress, which can motivate the person to meet challenges. Because of the clinician's expertise in task analysis and knowledge of the variables that influence a person's performance, this trainer role is one that an occupational therapist could fill.

Therapeutic strategies such as those in RET would be used to meet client-generated goals (i.e., adventure participants would identify personal goals related to increased knowledge and skills about survival and personal competence). They could decrease their sense of helplessness and dependency, enhance their feelings of self-worth, and increase their sense of control. Therapeutic programs that have successfully combined the adventure experiential-learning model with RET have been used with juvenile offenders, adolescent substance abusers, and others (Clagett, 1989, 1992; Davis-Berman, Berman, & Capone, 1994; Nadler, 1995).

BECK'S COGNITIVE THERAPY

As noted previously, there are differences in the application of cognitive theory in clinical situations. Ellis' RET differs from cognitive-behavioral therapy as conceived by Aaron Beck. We will briefly describe Beck's approach, then contrast Beck with Ellis, drawing the reader's attention to principles that are especially applicable to occupational therapy.

Beck has been a key contributor to cognitive-behavioral therapy (Beck, 1976, 1997; Beck & Haaga, 1992; Beck & Weishaar, 1994). He refers to his model as cognitive therapy (CT) and defines it as "an active, directive, time-limited, structured approach used to treat a variety of psychiatric disorders" (Beck, Rush, Shaw, & Emery, 1979, p. 3.) (e.g., depression, anxiety, phobias, pain and somatic problems). As with other cognitive-behavioral models, Beck's approach has an underlying theoretical rationale that an individual's affect and behavior are largely determined by the way in which he or she thinks about the world (Beck et al., 1979). Beck has four assumptions about the role of a person's cognition. He assumes that:

1. An individual's cognition influences how he or she perceives and experiences everyday events
2. One's cognitions are based on internal and external stimuli as well as past and present experiences
3. Cognitions (thoughts) influence personal feelings and behavior
4. Therapy can heighten the individual's awareness of these cognitions and how they influence his or her feelings and behaviors (Beck et al., 1979)

Scientific Approach

The techniques in Beck's cognitive therapy depend on a collaborative, here-and-now relationship in which the clinician uses behavioral strategies for multiple purposes. The clinician first helps the patient or client identify his or her beliefs or thoughts, then imagine other ways events can be interpreted. They also discuss the benefits and liabilities of changing or maintaining the client's present beliefs and behaviors. The cognitive and behavioral strategies combined with discussion help individuals develop a **scientific attitude**. This means that clients are taught to systematically test and/or find evidence in support of their assumptions, much as a scientist would do. In this way, clients can differentiate fact from beliefs and rational thoughts from irrational.

Cognitive Techniques

Like Ellis, Beck uses such **cognitive techniques** as graded task assignments, modeling, coaching, behavioral rehearsal, homework, stress inoculation, cognitive modeling, and scripting. These techniques are often used to help develop assertive beliefs and identify the client's personal rights. Other techniques include thought-stopping, role reversal, emotive imagery, and symbolic modeling. Educational methods may be combined with cognitive techniques to increase client awareness and control of his or her thoughts to achieve change and client goals (Rathjen, Rathjen, & Hiniker, 1978).

Contrast Between Ellis' RET and Beck's Cognitive Therapy

Both RET and cognitive therapy hold that change in behavior comes from cognitive change; if you can change how a person views an event or change one's self-perceptions, you can change behavior. Differences arise in the use of terminology, the therapeutic approach, the methodology used to re-examine beliefs, and the homework assignments given to clients (Table 6-1).

Rules for Living

Beck suggests that the therapist work with the person's **rules for living** (the patient's or client's entire philosophy of life) and not just the "musts" in life or the irrational thoughts, which are the focus of the rational emotive thera-

pist. The rational emotive therapist has a more forceful approach in which he or she is directive in identifying, confronting, and disputing irrational beliefs. Beck envisions the therapist engaged in a collaborative effort in which the client and therapist mutually explore the person's beliefs to identify those that lead to cognitive distortions and overgeneralizations. This awareness of one's thoughts is then used to mutually negotiate behavioral assignments.

Disputing Beliefs

Within intervention, the process for rethinking differs with the two therapies. The rational emotive therapist quickly identifies the "musts" in the patient's/client's life, evaluates these thoughts, and then goes about to dispute these "musts." The clinician's own philosophy of life is very influential in this process. Beck prefers using inductive questioning and a **Socratic dialogue method**. In this method of questioning, the therapist helps clients identify thoughts and find the evidence needed to support their beliefs. Clients and practitioners then work cooperatively to find the means to correct or change these thoughts. Later, the therapist proposes to clients that they evaluate these beliefs and, in some cases, consider changing their philosophy of life (Dryden, 1984).

Using Graded Tasks

Although both therapies use behavior assignments, Beck proposes that these assignments be negotiated by the client and the clinician. He would consider the person's present ability and function, then negotiate increasing demands for performance through graded tasks. Tasks are graded in difficulty, and work periods are increased. The rational emotive therapist does not use graded tasks, believing that they limit the person's capabilities. Instead, the therapist usually determines the homework assignment and asks for high performance or behavior contrary to that which a person currently demonstrates (Dryden, 1984). This difference in use of graded tasks poses an interesting question for the occupational therapist. Does the use of graded activities promote success? Does this approach convey to the person that he or she has limitations and cannot manage a greater challenge? In what instances might it be more (or less) helpful to impose limitations?

ABC Theory versus Scientific Theory

Clients engaged in RET are encouraged to undergo a logical analysis of their belief system based on the ABC theory. There is an activating event (A), which influences what a person believes (B), which in turn influences subsequent behavior or the consequence (C).

Beck's cognitive-behavioral therapy uses a scientific method to identify and test personal beliefs. The clinicians help clients make hypotheses about the reasons behind their behavior and then develop a plan to systematically test these hypotheses. Clients also negotiate and participate in corrective learning experiences much like the ones used by occupational therapists. These experiences are designed to promote

Table 6-1
CONTRASTING RATIONAL EMOTIVE THERAPY AND COGNITIVE THERAPY

	Rational Emotive Therapy	Cognitive Therapy
Treatment focus	Focus on "musts" and individual's irrational thoughts	Look at individual's philosophy of life
Nature of therapist interaction	Therapist is directive; challenging	Therapist collaborates with patient in mutual exploration
Role of the therapist	Therapist disputes irrational beliefs; models rational behavior	Therapist uses inductive methods; asks patient to support or dispute beliefs
How activities are determined	Therapist determines treatment activities	Therapist and patient collaborate to select treatment activities
Nature of therapeutic activities	Does not typically use graded tasks; patient confronts the task that he or she had been incapable of performing	Uses tasks graded in difficulty

Reprinted with permission from Bruce, M., & Borg, B. (1993). *Psychosocial occupational therapy: Frames of reference for intervention* (2nd ed.). Thorofare, NJ: SLACK Incorporated.

cognitive functioning and thereby enhance coping and problem-solving skills as well as develop or revise beliefs. Based on previous discussion in this text, it appears that the occupational therapist is more likely to incorporate social learning and cognitive-behavioral approaches similar to those of Beck rather than rational emotive techniques, which use emersion techniques rather than graded tasks. However, all have been influential in formulating cognitive and psychoeducational interventions. They may also contribute to health education and prevention programs.

DONALD MEICHENBAUM'S COGNITIVE BEHAVIOR MODIFICATION

A fourth highly influential contributor to cognitive-behavior theory is Donald Meichenbaum. His approach is referred to as **cognitive behavior modification**. The theoretical assumptions that influence the principles of cognitive behavior modification come from the work of Luria (1980) and Vygotsky (1962). Both Luria and Vygotsky describe the influence of language on behavior and suggest that the way we talk and interact with others changes the way we think and behave in our daily lives. The relationship between language and behavior changes throughout life from external to internal verbal guidance that controls behavior. For instance, parents guide the child's behavior when they articulate their expectations for behavior and when they give feedback, which helps the child meet these standards; standards that match what is generally expected by society.

Children internalize these rules and, in a real sense, tell themselves how to behave. With time and participation in daily life these rules become automatic and contribute to the child's increased ability to regulate and control his or her own behavior. A person's behavior is not a product of just reinforcement from the external environment, rather it comes from the transaction between the person and the social environment, the transaction being the interaction between the child's internal thoughts and speech and the expectations of his or her environment as they are articulated by parents, teachers, and significant others.

Because of the unpredictability of what will be expected in one's daily life, Meichenbaum believes that instead of just reinforcing a particular behavior we need to teach our children and our clients strategies that can be generalized and used in multiple situations. These strategies, such as his **Think Aloud protocol** for problem solving (see Think Aloud Protocol for Problem Solving), can be used to manage daily stresses. Cognitive behavior modification theory places less emphasis on skill mastery and more on mastering strategies that can be used in multiple contexts. The assumption is that by mastering strategies, one is better able to meet diverse challenges (Meichenbaum, 1979, 1985).

THINK ALOUD PROTOCOL FOR PROBLEM SOLVING

Using the Think Aloud method, the client is taught to ask him- or herself four questions that help in planning and monitoring behavior:
1. What is my problem?
2. What is my plan?
3. Am I using my plan?
4. How did I do (Meichenbaum, 1979, p. 42)?

Meichenbaum developed this theory to work with children who were "hyperactive" and had poor social behavior at home and at school. As his ideas have been researched and refined over the years, they have been used in regular classroom environments to assist with behavior management, to support learning, and to teach children to problem solve. They have also been used with adult clients having schizophrenia, persons with brain injury, and with persons needing to better cope with such emotions as anger, anxiety, and fear (Meichenbaum, 1979). Meichenbaum's theory influences the approaches used to manage acute reactions to various medical procedures, such as preparing for surgery or going to the dentist. The coping principles are also applicable for managing acute health conditions (e.g., burns) and such chronic health conditions as arthritis and obesity and for managing post-traumatic stress reactions that result from rape, disaster, and war (Meichenbaum, 1979). The literature further indicates that these principles have been incorporated into health promotion and stress prevention programs for professionals such as nurses, teachers, and the police to build their skills for problem solving, managing stress, using time, communicating effectively, and facilitating the creative process (Meichenbaum, 1985).

The goal is that the client stops and considers carefully the exact nature of the problem and how the problem will be solved. Think Aloud protocols have been used with children and adults (Meichenbaum, 1979, 1985). The Think Aloud method is practiced during a series of sessions, the number

depending on the person's needs for intervention and his or her ability to learn. Usually about a dozen trials, in the same or different contexts, lead to mastery of this strategy. When a child is the client, parents are also taught the strategy so that they can assist their children. When working with children, the therapist needs to be aware of the parent's thoughts as well as those of the child because all may influence the therapeutic outcome.

Self-Instruction

Another strategy developed by Meichenbaum (1979, 1985) is that referred to as self-instruction. It uses self-talk. Clients are taught to use **self-instruction** if they have not already internalized procedures and strategies for participation in daily life activities. Self-instruction incorporates mental and physical demonstration and practice of behavioral procedures. The client can think about situations and mentally problem solve, or the client can practice self-instruction procedures "in vivo." Persons of all ages and of varying abilities have used both mental and behavioral procedures. For those clients who need to master "in vivo" strategies, the following five-step model is used for changing behavior:
1. The clinician or teacher demonstrates (models) the desired behavior or task performance and simultaneously describes the procedure(s) out loud.
2. The client tries the same task while the clinician describes out loud the procedure(s) the child or adult is following.
3. The client then performs the task and verbalizes out loud self-cues that were learned from modeling in stages one and two.
4. The client performs the task and whispers the task or behavior protocol to one's self.
5. The client's performance is automatic, and the verbal cues are internalized and guide performance with minimal self-instruction (Meichenbaum, 1979, p. 32).

For those readers who have observed or participated in rehabilitation environments, this protocol may contrast with and is believed preferable to the one that you may have observed in which the therapist constantly gives verbal cues for performance. For example, occupational therapists assisting clients with safe gait might say, "Lift, step through... watch your right... etc." According to Meichenbaum, it is better to have clients self-cue. Initially, they can identify aloud the procedure to be mastered. When the protocol is mastered, they can describe it to themselves until the behavior to be mastered is automatic. If the client makes a performance error, then the therapist corrects the performance and, if needed, demonstrates the correct procedure.

On multiple occasions in outpatient rehabilitation, clients who had a stroke or head injury could be overheard sharing with clinicians, "I bet you think I'm nuts the way I talk to myself." The clients had noticed that since their injury they thought aloud. They were concerned that others (family, friends, and therapists) would see them as crazy. Clinicians assured clients that they were "not crazy" and that they were using a self-instruction strategy that assisted them in organizing their thoughts, problem solving, and following task procedures.

Purpose of Self-Instruction and Think Aloud Protocol

The self-talk method and Think Aloud strategies serve multiple purposes in treatment and in prevention contexts. Both can:

- Increase and hold the client's attention to the task
- Identify the task procedures and behavior needed to achieve a goal
- Help the client master task procedures and thus increase self-control
- Improve the client's efficient use of behaviors needed in social and task performance
- Contribute to mastery of information, skills, and rules used to problem solve
- Guide self-monitoring of behavior and task performance
- Increase the client's awareness of performance boundaries
- Increase the client's effective participation in his or her environment (Meichenbaum, 1979, pp. 17-32)

Task Analysis and Self-Instruction

Both Think Aloud and self-instruction require the client to analyze tasks in the context of his or her typical daily routine. Initially, the therapist helps the client break the task into parts, and together they identify the skills and procedures involved in doing the task. These are then translated into the verbal protocol that the client uses to improve performance during everyday situations. A frequently used strategy has four steps. The client asks the following:

1. What is my goal?
2. Do I have what I need?
3. What is my plan?
4. How did it work?

Using a previous example, an adult returning home from a rehabilitation setting may wish to prepare breakfast. The client asks him- or herself: "What is my goal?" Answers self: "To make myself scrambled eggs, toast, and juice for breakfast." Asks: "Do I have what I need?" Answers: "I have the eggs, margarine, milk, seasonings, bread, pan, toaster; I'll wait on the juice until the eggs are done." Asks: "What's my plan?" Answers: "I'll turn the burner on, whip my ingredients together, put bread in toaster, then scramble eggs in pan. Toast should pop up when I'm about done." Asks: "Am I using my plan?" Answers: "So far so good. Oops! I forgot to

get a bowl in which to mix up the eggs." (Person continues to evaluate the plan, making corrections as needed.) Asks: "How did it work?" Answers: "Not too bad. The toast is a little cool, but I'm on the right track. Next time I'll wait on the toast until the eggs are ready to serve." The client achieves the goal and reviews the strategies used to be successful. If they are unsuccessful, he or she applauds him- or herself for trying and requests assistance. Clients are advised that there is more than one way to do something or achieve a goal.

In a similar way, a child may use the protocol for tabletop activities: What is my goal? "To put together a small jigsaw puzzle in 30 minutes." Do I have what I need? "All of the pieces are out of the box. I'll follow the picture on the box top, and I can work here at the table where no one will bother me." What's my plan? "I'll start by pulling out all the pieces with straight edges and do the border first, then I'll work in." Am I using my plan? "I've got the whole border done; now I need to make a pile of dark pieces to work on the upper corner." (Child evaluates his or her work and its effectiveness and makes corrections or continues until completion.) How did it work? "I'm getting tired, but I got a lot done. I know I can finish it next time!" (Child achieves the goal and reviews the strategies used to be successful.)

Coping Model

The self-instructional methods used by Meichenbaum and others are based on a coping model rather than a mastery learning model. The **coping model** emphasizes learning from mistakes, while the mastery model strives for no errors. During training, the therapist helps the client learn those skills that are needed to perform the task (e.g., physical, social, or adaptive skills). The therapist also poses problem scenarios that require clients to think about alternatives if the skills learned don't work or if the skills are not adequate for the specific situation. The coping model is characterized by problem-solving strategies that:

- Include task evaluation (activity analysis)
- Provide opportunity to practice problem solving
- Provide opportunities to use self-talk in varied contexts
- Include practice in responding to failures
- Teach the person to identify possible problems and choose coping responses

There is a dual emphasis wherein the client learns what is required for the immediate situation as well as for future hypothetical situations. In order to identify these individual situations, coping strategies, and potential future contexts for performance, the therapist and client talk about what the client might expect to face in the future. This occurs through what Meichenbaum refers to as the **collaborative relationship**.

The Collaborative Relationship and Socratic Model for Coping

As conceived by Meichenbaum (1979), the collaborative process is combined with a Socratic model to develop coping strategies. The clinician and the client work together to identify the problems or areas that require new learning and change. They also work together to develop the intervention plan. To help clarify learning needs, some of the following questions may be posed to the client:

- How do you currently respond in the situation targeted for change? (How do you do the task? What are you doing now?)
- What is your perception of the situation? Is it stressful for you? Are others unhappy with your performance? Do you want to change?
- What are your reasons for managing the situation as you do currently? (What is working well?)
- What are your ideas for improving the situation? (How would you change what you do?)

This is reminiscent of the principles of client-centered intervention discussed earlier in the text. During the **Socratic dialogue**, the clinician and client identify possible changes or adaptations that would be expected to improve task or social performance, including any changes that could be made in the performance environment. They also discuss what would comprise the most effective and efficient use of the coping strategies. The goal is to help clients obtain the information they need in order to generalize their coping and problem-solving skills.

Related Coping Skills Techniques

Meichenbaum (1979) has summarized some of the methods used during coping interventions. He recommends that the therapist consider:

- Describing the benefits of the skill training to the client.
- Teaching the relationship between the presenting problem and the person's cognitions. Clinician uses a combination of didactic and self-exploratory approaches.
- Teaching a system of self-monitoring thoughts and behavior. For example, ask clients to keep a log, diary, or some written or computer format for recording behaviors and cognitions.
- Teaching a specific method of problem solving. Clients should define the problem, identify consequences of the problem and alternative solutions, and evaluate the feedback they receive from others and from their performance.
- Providing opportunities for modeling, rehearsal, self-evaluation of specific skills, as well as overall outcome of one's performance.

- Providing multiple opportunities for clients to practice specific behaviors related to the problem situation.
- Asking clients to complete behavioral assignments that are graded in difficulty in order to provide adequate challenge (pp. 143-182).

Whatever specific strategies are used, Meichenbaum and his colleagues emphasize the need for flexibility. A client-centered learning program integrates cognitive and behavioral strategies specific to the person, culture, and the specific environment. The therapist and the client need to keep in mind that even these factors may change over time and thus may necessitate ongoing adjustment. Meichenbaum recommends that the client engage in mental rehearsal before or along with actual practice in the physical environment. Finally, when in the real environment, he suggests clients practice in situations that are challenging but not so challenging that they will overwhelm the client; in other words, he recommends that we strive for a "just right challenge" (Meichenbaum, 1979, p. 149).

Stress Inoculation—A Coping Model

Some of Meichenbaum's writing has been in the area of stress inoculation. **Inoculation** here refers to a process similar to what we think about in medicine when one is "inoculated" against (prepared to fend off) a disease. He recognizes that individuals often need to face or confront a situation that they wish to avoid. He begins by teaching them that the symptoms of stress such as anxiety or over-eating are not the sign of impending illness, but rather signals that tell the person now is the time to use coping strategies. In this way, clients shift from viewing themselves as helpless and instead view themselves as resourceful agents who, through the acquisition of coping strategies, can problem solve and manage their symptoms. To achieve these outcomes, Meichenbaum (1979, 1985) structures this **coping model** into three major phases:

1. Conceptualization
2. Skill acquisition and practice
3. Application and follow-through

Although these are considered separate phases of stress inoculation training, they may occur simultaneously during training programs. These phases occur over a series of intervention sessions. The number of sessions for any one of the identified phases varies with the population participating and the focus of problems (e.g., pain, preparation for surgery, coping with cancer, stress in work environments, coping with trauma, etc.).

Conceptualization Phase

Conceptualization is the didactic phase of the educational experience. During this phase the clinician gives the client basic information, in lay terms, about the stressful situation (e.g., pain, anger, physical illness). The educator-clinician also helps clients conceptualize their individual responses to the source of stress. The clients' perceptions of stress are the focus of the intervention. In addition to the source of stress, the clinician helps clients identify their past and current responses to the stressful situation. Clients and clinicians collaborate to answer the following questions:

- Does the stress cause embarrassment or avoidance?
- Does it elicit feelings of helplessness and being overwhelmed?
- Are there related physical ailments or anxiety?

The therapist tries to get a sense of both physical and cognitive reactions because both types of responses will be addressed during treatment and prevention programs. The intervention is designed to increase the client's understanding and eventual control of physical arousal and to change those thoughts or self-statements that lead one to become overwhelmed by stress. The goal is for clients to learn that they can handle stress and will be rewarded for their efforts.

Skill Acquisition and Practice Phase

The second phase of the coping model is the **practice phase**. During this phase skills are acquired through rehearsal. Clients are prompted to challenge their thoughts as well as learn specific behaviors to manage stress. They practice using stress management strategies to firmly establish new methods of coping with pain, role conflicts, chronic illness, stressful environments, etc. Practice usually includes at least the following five steps:

1. First, clients gather information about the source of stress and methods that they could use to decrease physical arousal (e.g., muscle relaxation, diaphragmatic breathing).

2. Next they learn to do something with their discomforts; for example, they may be encouraged to change it into something positive (e.g., I can channel the energy from my anger to do something constructive instead of brooding).

3. Third, they select a positive response that would increase their sense of control of the situation (e.g., When my pain seems too much to handle, I know that if I lie down for 10 or 15 minutes or put my work aside and go to the breakroom, it will subside).

4. Fourth, they listen to their internal dialogue for adaptive and maladaptive self-statements (e.g., telling myself, "I can't stand this" only makes it worse). Clients are taught to monitor their dialogues to identify the content as well as the context of the thoughts. For example, "Since my head injury, I feel stupid when I go out with my friends because I never seem to know what they are talking about," or "My friends think that I'm weird because I am afraid of heights and can't snowboard," or "I hate going to school. I am a lousy student because I can't read as fast as everybody," or "I have no friends. I don't get asked to parties because I am a nerd and nobody likes me."

5. With help from the clinician, clients use their own self-statements to form a plan in which they will assess the reality of their situation (get the facts) and identify their perceptions of the threats that exist in the situation. The person then creates a plan for responding to his or her thoughts and self-defeating behavior.

Initially, the therapist may model proposed new behaviors in the "real world," and the client and clinician can rehearse these new behaviors or they can work together to problem solve. Rehearsal may engage the client in role-play in a "safe" (clinical) setting and gradually move into real life challenges. Clients can learn from films, each other, or examples taken from the clinical and popular literature. The goal of these varied experiences is to increase clients' sense of self-efficacy or their belief that they are prepared to meet a specific challenge successfully. Once the client has mastered the plan in a safe context, he or she is ready for the challenges of the "real world" stressful situation.

Application and Follow-Through

Meichenbaum (1985, 1986) believes that classes that teach stress management to groups but fail to take into account the specific circumstances of each person are likely to be unsuccessful. Therefore, in this third phase, as in the other two phases of the coping model, the therapist and client maintain a collaborative relationship. During this phase they create an intervention plan that is individualized for the person and his or her special circumstances. Clinicians help clients:

- Specify those stressful situations in which the clients will try out their newly acquired coping skills
- Identify what will be their homework assignments
- Identify and write the protocols for problem solving
- Determine how their success will be measured

During the later sessions of intervention and throughout follow-up, clients are involved in activities that consider the possibility of failure and re-occurrence of stress, or clients are assisted in revising what had been working well before and needs to be revised because life's circumstances are always changing. They are encouraged to see failure, reoccurrence, and modification as part of a normal change process and that these are opportunities for learning and modifying their coping plan and skills.

The clinician emphasizes that because problems change over time, it would not be unusual to return to therapy for "booster" sessions, using the analogy of the shots we receive to prevent physical illness. Clients may be given a checklist to complete periodically to help them review their coping status and identify possible need for such a "booster" session (Meichenbaum, 1985). They are told that there may be setbacks and to look at them as a normal part of life. This attitude—that setbacks are normal—is similar to the work done in substance abuse or the relapse prevention programs, which are discussed later in this chapter.

CURRENT PRACTICE IN OCCUPATIONAL THERAPY

Much of the recent occupational therapy literature describes programs that use cognitive-behavioral theories along with those specific to OT. While the programs are not typically identified as "cognitive-behavioral" the citations given in this literature in support of programming refer to recognized cognitive-behavioral theorists. In occupational therapy literature, the most frequently cited theory is Albert Bandura's social learning theory. However, we see compatibility between all of the theories in this chapter (themselves related to social learning) and current occupational therapy intervention as well as potential practice innovations. We provide recent examples from occupational therapy practice that illustrate how social learning, cognitive, and cognitive-behavioral principles integrate with those of occupational therapy.

The Person and Behavior

The therapist using cognitive behavior theory sees the person, child, and adult as someone who thinks, feels, and functions in multiple environments. According to the laws of normal development, throughout his or her life the individual participates in infinite life experiences as well as formalized learning experiences from which he or she acquires a knowledge base. This knowledge (both tacit and explicit) is stored and can be retrieved to create beliefs about one's self, others, and the world. This knowledge forms the basis for one's behavior and how one approaches daily tasks.

Sometimes, however, occupational therapy clients have delayed or inadequate knowledge development. They may have knowledge that is no longer effective for managing or for problem solving within their current situation. In the cognitive-behavioral frame of reference, it is the **person's cognition** (which includes his or her awareness of information, personal beliefs, and strategies for problem solving) that is the focus when identifying functional problems or managing the interactions and transactions among the person, their environment, and their occupations.

Sense of Safety

A person explores and learns from the environment when he or she senses that it is safe and permissible to do so. Ideally, this sense of safety is conveyed to the child by adult role models who provide a safe and consistent environment. These adults also communicate that they believe the child is capable of controlling the environment and can learn from exploration. In this safe, consistent, as well as appropriately stimulating environment, the person learns through exploration and gains the knowledge base that will shape his or her beliefs, future learning, and knowledge acquisition, including his or her unique approach to problem solving. Positive experiences lead to one's feeling capable, and, according to this model, believing one's self to be capable in the present actually increases one's capability in future endeavors. Negative experiences or limited exploration lead to many opposite outcomes. A person may learn to fear the environment or may have distorted or limited knowledge. He or she may develop a rigid and defensive attitude. If he or she believes the self to be incapable, it diminishes future capability. All this contributes to inadequate problem-solving skills, which in turn impair the ability to function in daily life.

Limited or Distorted Knowledge

Not all knowledge deficiencies come from limited exploration. Sometimes clients don't have access to accurate information, have misinformation, or have only part of the information they need, or physical changes may have impaired their ability to realistically appraise or use information. Whatever the cause, **cognitive dysfunction** may reflect misinformation, a misunderstanding of what is occurring around them, or an ineffective or inflexible problem-solving repertoire.

Competence Versus Incompetence

As the person grows and interacts in the environment, he or she not only gathers information about the environment but also about the self. This self-knowledge influences emotional development. **Emotional development** can be seen by the individual's position on multiple continuums that represent dependence and independence, self-interest and interest in others, the ability to be empathetic, identify with others, establish an autonomous identity, and the ability to express and control feelings. **Optimum function** depends on flexible thinking, adequate knowledge, emotional health, the belief that one can meet life's challenges, and the ability to problem solve in multiple situations. All of this is associated with feelings of competence.

Dysfunction is usually seen when the person's predominant behaviors are at the extremes of the emotional continuum or when cognitive function (knowledge, beliefs, and problem solving) does not enable one to meet personal and societal expectations. **Dysfunction** is associated with feelings of incompetence. The person thinks he or she is incapable of taking responsibility for one's own life, lacks a realistic understanding of his or her own abilities and limitations, has self-defeating beliefs or is unclear regarding one's own beliefs, or is unable to adapt and cope with changing circumstances.

Unrealistic Reasoning

The person with **distorted self-knowledge** often uses a reasoning process that is dogmatic or unrealistic. This method of reasoning may be illogical, not coinciding with reality, or may involve inferences that have no basis (Guidano & Liotti, 1983). For instance, the person may personalize information unnecessarily or perhaps view events from extremes (e.g., issues are judged as black or white, good or bad, possible or impossible). He or she may selectively abstract information and thus get a distorted view or may make global generalizations (e.g., all women [men] are bad, management doesn't care about employees, people in wheelchairs will never be able to enjoy life). The person's thoughts are uni-dimensional rather than holistic with multiple perspectives, and these thoughts cannot be easily reversed or varied (Beck, Rush, & Kovacs, 1976; Beck et al., 1979; Guidano & Liotti, 1983).

Cognitive distortions and deficiencies have also been identified within the context of specific diagnostic categories such as agoraphobia, depression, eating disorders, and obsessive-compulsive disorder (Bowlby, 1977a, 1977b). However, psychiatric labels are not necessary for the understanding and description of cognitive dysfunction. A person's beliefs impact his or her performance throughout the life span and influence a person's participation in home, employment, and community environments.

Role of the Occupational Therapist

The role of the therapist is not that of the expert and may include that of teacher, coach, and even "scientist." The occupational therapy literature suggests that the occupational therapist employ the Socratic method and continue to expand his or her role as educator. In this role, the therapist is a facilitator and sometimes participant-observer who designs and implements meaningful and corrective learning experiences for clients and their caregivers, teachers, and supervisors.

Educator-Facilitator

As an **educator-facilitator**, the therapist provides a vehicle for structured, experiential, or self-directed learning. The educational structure in occupational therapy intervention contexts is not like that in a traditional school setting. Rather, it is a structure in which clients help develop the course, identify their learning needs, and participate in determining the course content and homework assignments. This is analogous to **student-centered learning** in the classroom. The therapist designs or helps others design learning experiences that occur in a classroom atmosphere in healthcare, community, school, or other context.

During these learning experiences, the therapist-educator carefully explains the rationale behind the approaches and assignments and gives specific and frequent feedback regarding the client's thoughts, behavior, and accomplishments in relation to short- and long-term goals. Clinicians facilitate a learning process that helps learners gain new information and practice skills that increase their self-understanding and control of the environment. Learners are encouraged to identify and use new resources as well as familiar ones to problem-solve in daily life and manage current health conditions.

Modeling a Scientific Attitude

The reader should also consider the benefits that come from modeling the attitude of a personal scientist and using the Socratic method. The **scientific attitude** requires the client and occupational therapist to recognize the relationships between thought and behaviors and to create ways to prove or disprove inferences regarding these. Clients are expected to explore life and its multiple possibilities and probabilities and to question so-called "absolute certainties."

In modeling the **scientist**, the occupational therapist provides a secure base for exploration and encourages clients to explore life systematically, so they can hypothesize about and recognize cause and effect relationships in life. Learners then plan and carry through with experiments or learning activities to confirm or disprove their own hypotheses. As a personal scientist, the therapist helps the person step back from personal beliefs, postpone judgments of self and the world, and logically challenge beliefs.

Questioning Generalizations

The scientist attitude is illustrated in a response to comments frequently heard in occupational therapy: "I'm not good with my hands," or "I'll never get this." The occupational therapist replies, "What happened today that causes you to conclude that you're not good with your hands?" or "Are you referring just to occupational therapy activities, or have you had difficulties at work or home in the past?" With these responses the occupational therapist does not accept the person's statement as fact and asks the patient/client to either validate or question the generalization. Next, the therapist might ask the individual to perform specific tasks that do not relate to previous task failure. The therapist may serve as a model for skill mastery, breaking tasks down and demonstrating steps along the way to ensure success.

Introducing New Possibilities

The clinician strives to be flexible, to individualize learning experiences, and to adjust the intervention approach to the client. The goal is to find a style that fits the client's needs. Often, as a **participant-observer**, the occupational therapist provides support and gives feedback to the client in response to the thoughts and feelings that are communicated, as well as his or her behavior. The practitioner also shares his or her views of the problems confronted by the person. When observing the person, the therapist views the whole cognitive system and tries to increase the client's awareness of the interrelationships among thoughts, feelings, and behaviors, both past and present. When appropriate, the client is taught to come to new conclusions about one's self and others. This can be seen in the following example:

An 18-year-old young woman with a head injury had multiple physical and behavioral problems as a result of her injury. She shifted from childlike, attention-seeking, dependent behavior to acting-out, adolescent behavior. At times she also expressed concern regarding living independently, achieving an intimate relationship, and being employed. These interests were realistic provided she could gain control of her impulsive behavior. Acting out one day, she ran away from the rehabilitation center. It was not easy for this young woman to leave, given that she relied on her wheelchair for mobility and had many physical limitations.

The therapist decided to share with the patient her view of the experience. Instead of again reminding the client of the dangers of her behavior, as many other staff had done, the occupational therapist instead focused on the tremendous amount of energy required to run away. She challenged the young woman to learn to use this energy in a positive manner rather than in the negative, self-destructive manner that running away represented. This strategy helped avoid the client's usual authority struggle that had so often sidetracked constructive interactions and treatment.

In another example, a client who saw himself as superior was very intolerant of what he perceived as other clients' ignorance. One day the therapist chose to confront a statement the client had made to another person, "You mean you don't know that? Everybody knows that!" The therapist suggested to the client that he may know things that others don't, but rather than put others down for their lack of knowledge, he might see an opportunity to teach them and share his knowledge with others. She helped him recognize that he could gain respect for his knowledge from others rather than the contempt that he seemed to elicit for being bright.

Collaborative Relationship

In summary, in the **learner-teacher relationship**, the occupational therapist works collaboratively with the client to identify problems and to plan and implement learning activities. The therapist provides a nonjudgmental attitude and a secure base from which the client can reevaluate personal assumptions and test hypotheses. The therapist communicates respect to the client for his or her ability to learn and solve problems.

Function of Activities

The occupational therapist applying a cognitive-behavior frame of reference uses activities for multiple purposes. A client's performance during the task reflects the client's cognitive function, his or her knowledge, beliefs, specific skills, and use of problem-solving strategies. Therapists use meaningful activities to facilitate cognitive and skill development and practice of problem solving. Practice in multiple situations is very important because it forms the basis for the person to truly feel one's self as capable. Practice also assists in the generalization of learned skills. By seeing the outcome of their "doing" and with the clinician's or others' feedback regarding activity performance, clients can realistically assess their own performance abilities and boundaries. They expand their overall knowledge base and learn to prove or disprove personally held assumptions. Clients gain confidence in their ability to cope in current and future situations.

Assessing Knowledge and Skill Level

The client's current cognitive level is identified through his or her participation in activities in which beliefs and attitudes are verbalized. Activities also provide a vehicle for the person to demonstrate his or her **general fund of knowledge** (e.g., specific information content, the ability to read and write or use tools), as well as the skills and strategies used to apply this knowledge. In relation to knowledge, the therapist identifies strengths as well as limitations. Clients can learn wheelchair maintenance and practice using tools for making adjustments. Clients may learn employment preparation, practice completing job applications, and role-play interview responses. Adolescents in a community program for unwed mothers may learn childcare, life skills, and career information in preparation for managing the multiple roles of parent, student, and worker. This knowledge is then used in a supportive environment after the birth of the baby as the adolescent practices child care skills and activity planning to manage parent and school or worker roles.

Theoretical Assumptions—Guide to Evaluation and Intervention

The theoretical assumptions (See Cognitive-Behavior Theoretical Assumptions) are a summary of the basic beliefs about the person, activities or occupations, and the environment or context. These beliefs are adapted from the cognitive-behavioral theories previously described in this chapter. The assumptions about the person-environment-occupation variables and their possible relationships guide evaluation and intervention in occupational therapy.

Increasing Knowledge and Enhancing Competence

Cognitive development is facilitated through engagement in activities that provide opportunities to develop sensory, perceptual, motor, social, and academic knowledge and skills needed for competent role performance. The client's knowledge and skill competence increase the client's self-confidence and performance abilities in health care, home, and community contexts. Skill mastery and increased confidence in turn heighten the client's **sense of self-control**. Clients believe that they can manage day-to-day problems or find the necessary resources to assist them in problem solving.

Education Modules

Activities are often presented within the context of an **educational format**, which may be identified as a program curriculum, class schedule, or one-time information session. The occupational therapist develops course syllabi for the activities or educational modules presented. For example, syllabi have been developed in multiple areas including life skills, getting credit, consumer awareness, social networks and social support sys-

COGNITIVE-BEHAVIOR THEORETICAL ASSUMPTIONS

Person and Cognition

1. When you change thoughts and beliefs or enhance knowledge, you impact behavior and occupational performance.

2. People make decisions regarding their behavior based in part on what they expect will be the outcome.

3. A person's emotions and feelings are interdependent with what he or she knows and believes.

4. The person develops as a result of the interaction of the cognitive system, behaviors learned, and the social and physical environments.

5. Being willing to explore one's environment and try out new behaviors depends in part on one's belief that it is safe to make mistakes.

6. People have internalized "rules for living," life themes, and styles of problem solving that may or may not be aware to them but nevertheless characterize how they approach life's tasks.

7. Cognitive change is a gradual process; changing one's knowledge base and one's attitudes toward the self takes time.

8. The patient/client benefits from psychoeducational programs that integrate educational procedures and skill-building with psychological techniques.

9. When an individual learns new cognitive strategies to respond to the present, he or she is preparing to confront and solve future problems.

10. People are unlikely to participate in experiences in which they feel incapable.

11. Increasing one's beliefs about being capable increases one's capability and willingness to initiate tasks and risk change.

12. Beliefs about being capable and in control are more likely to increase when one experiences one's self successfully and is given responsibility for one's own learning.

13. One's thoughts are not always in conscious awareness; making thoughts aware makes them more amenable to change.

14. Learning is facilitated by practice in multiple and varied contexts.

Environment/Context

15. A learning format or context in which the person identifies the self as a learner is one that promotes exploration, openness to new experience, and a mindset toward enhancing knowledge and skills.

16. A learning context promotes the idea of life as a life-long learning process.

17. Cognitive function is influenced by the arrangement of the learning environment, which can facilitate cognitive development and stimulate problem solving.

18. The patient/client can benefit from a structured intervention setting that controls distractions and provides repeated opportunities for skill practice and problem solving.

Activity/Occupation

19. Therapeutic occupation is that which facilitates learning.

20. Practice in real-life contexts is a powerful accompaniment to learning in an analog or clinical setting.

21. Cognitive developmental theory can be applied when designing tasks to modify the complexity of the experience and to promote successful learning.

22. The therapeutic tasks used during educational experiences consider the learner's cognitive knowledge, level of cognitive function, and personal interests.

23. Goals that present a moderate challenge help hold the client's interest and facilitate participation in an intervention.

24. Intervention does not eliminate pathology but provides cognitive, affective, and behavioral learning experiences to teach skills, strategies, and methods of coping.

25. Intervention is more effective when specific techniques and skills are learned (e.g., when tasks and psychoeducational experiences are used) than when only verbal methods are used.

---

tems, job search, nutrition-on-a-budget, planning a diet, mastering work skills, increasing awareness, etc. to name a few (Brownell & Fairburn, 1995; Crist, 1999; Davis & Kutter, 1997; Donaldson, 1997; Greenberg et al., 1988; Kottman, 1999a, 1999b; Lillie & Armstrong, 1982; Lenters, 1999; Linroth, Zander, Forde, Hanley, & Lins, 1996; Precin, 1999; Salo-Chydenius, 1996; Toglia & Golisz, 1990). In general, courses have been grouped as basic living skills, community awareness, and personal growth and development.

Using Homework

Courses may include homework assignments. The counseling literature gives guidelines for increasing the effectiveness of homework and increasing the likelihood of its completion (Maultsby, 1971; Rathjen, Rathjen, & Hiniker, 1978). It is recommended that assignments:

- Be written using language compatible with the client's literacy level
- Identify the specific tasks to be completed by the client or, at times, by the client and therapist together

- Include the purpose of the assignment, instructions for the task, and other data that will enable the learner to determine when responsibilities have been fulfilled and the assignments completed
- Be individualized to meet each client's needs
- Allow for the learner's input at the time tasks are initially assigned (Beck et al., 1976; Maultsby, 1971)

The previous homework guides are also applicable for many of the home programs provided by occupational therapists in the various specialty areas of practice.

At the beginning of each intervention session, the therapist checks that assignments are complete and inquires regarding the client's thoughts and feelings about the assignment. Was the task too easy? Too difficult? Was it meaningful? If the person has not completed the tasks, the clinician tries to identify the reasons. To support the successful completion of assignments, the therapist may use follow-up reminders, phone contact, or contingency contracts.

Evaluation

As with other therapeutic approaches in occupational therapy, the therapist applying the cognitive-behavioral framework believes that assessment is an ongoing process and that assessment and change are interdependent (Guidano & Liotti, 1983; Meichenbaum, 1977). Therefore, the information that follows could be applied within the context of the initial or ongoing evaluation process.

Targeting Change

The cognitive-behavioral framework suggests that change be targeted in terms of four prongs:
1. In what environmental situation(s) would the patient/client like to feel more competent?
2. What thoughts (or attitudes) does he or she need to reassess?
3. What does the person need to know more about?
4. What skills/problem-solving strategies does he or she need to learn?

Automatic Thoughts

Our clients and patients may not always be aware of the information or skills they need, the thoughts to change, or even the situations in which they need to achieve competence. They may only be aware of their own feelings of discomfort or inadequacy, or others may indicate dissatisfaction with their performance. One reason for this lack of awareness is that many of the thoughts we have and behaviors we all engage in daily life are **automatic**; we do not routinely think about how we go about problem solving, evaluating our own performance, or recognizing our own internalized dialogues.

For example, when we drive a car and encounter problems suddenly presented by heavy traffic, poor road conditions, or a child running in the street, we respond without thinking about how we should react and problem solve. Our response is an automatic process. Nor are we necessarily aware of how stimulation influences our behavior. We are unaware of what determines how we formulate cause and effect relationships or the process of remembering.

This lack of awareness can again be illustrated in another automatic reaction—overeating. If you speak to people who overeat, they may tell you that they will eat if food is present without thinking about whether they feel hungry or whether their bodies require nourishment. Another example is the person who automatically withdraws from social interactions without considering the potential pleasure to be gained from, need for, or benefits of responding to family, friends, or new acquaintances. Finally, there is the person who expects to fail even before hearing instructions or initiating an activity.

Accessibility of Cognitive Process

An individual does not typically have immediate access to the rules of cognitive processing. Because the cognitive process is not in our immediate awareness in most instances, the therapist and the client make assumptions regarding the impact of cognition on behaviors and affect. They depend on keen observation of behavior and performance in order to gain an understanding of how thoughts are processed and to identify situations in which change would be desirable.

Assessing Cognitive Structures

The occupational therapist uses observation, testing, and interview to assess the effectiveness of the person's cognitive system for enabling functional performance. Formal assessment and observation are used to determine:
- The person's ability to remember, to perceive, and to attend within tasks.
- The person's ability to observe and accurately interpret behavior (the logic used in learning from events) including his or her ability to identify the historical data that relate to current problems and successes, the client's ability to identify stimuli (events, rewards) that support given behaviors, and the person's ability to identify personal, functional problems.
- The adequacy of the person's knowledge base; knowledge of information related to activities of daily living, vocational endeavors, and leisure pursuits (e.g., awareness of community resources and awareness of learning strategies).
- The strategies the person uses to problem solve and their effectiveness.
- The existence and effectiveness of specific skills needed for daily function.

Listening for a Life Theme

In addition to assessing specific cognitive structures and skills during assessment, the therapist tries to listen for the individual's life theme and **rules for living**. Internalized rules for living emerge from the person's behaviors and statements during the evaluation. Examples of "rules" include the following: I can take care of myself; I don't need my parents to run my life; people can't be trusted; I have to do as my spouse wants or he or she will get angry. Usually a theme will emerge (Guidano & Liotti, 1983). The **theme** is the message that underlies the rules for living and comes through consistently as the individual speaks and interacts in the interview and completes tasks. Typical self-defeating life themes include the following:

- I am a victim of circumstance.
- People and life have always been against me.
- I am unworthy.
- I have never been able to use my hands.
- My father thinks I'm stupid.
- I can't be independent.

Just as a person's thoughts convey a life theme, his or her problem solving may reflect a **lifestyle** such as a tendency toward patterns of behavior that are outgoing, withdrawn, intellectual, dependent, haphazard, or cautious. The therapist looks for indications of such a lifestyle, especially when this style tends to limit rather than enhance coping skills.

Evaluating the Person-Environment Match

The therapist also wants to assess the extent of the match between the learner and the environment. In this regard, the therapist may assess the following:

1. The person's view of self:
   - —What are his or her interests?
   - —Personal goals?
   - —What is the person's level of self-acceptance? Can he or she tolerate mistakes? Take risks? Can he or she exert self-control?
   - —In what areas does the patient/client feel capable, incapable?
   - —Do others' perceptions validate the person's self-image?
   - —Are his or her self-expectations reasonable?
   - —Is the person flexible, or does he or she respond rigidly?
2. The person's view of the environment:
   - —Is the patient/client aware of and interested in the environment?
   - —Does he or she see the environment as demanding, hostile, accepting, ignoring, or rejecting?
   - —What aspects of the environment receive attention?
   - —What kinds of situations and settings are preferred?
   - —What is expected of others?
   - —What is the level of tolerance of others?
   - —Does the set-up of the everyday environment enhance the person's function?
   - —Is the person aware of resources in the environment?
   - —Is his or her view of the environment and others realistic?
3. The person's learning style:
   - —Does he or she initiate tasks?
   - —Does the person sit back and observe?
   - —Who is admired?
   - —Does he or she have mentors?
   - —With whom does the person identify?
   - —Can he or she postpone gratification?
   - —Can he or she maintain diligence?
   - —What reinforcements maintain current behavior?
   - —What reinforcements might be used to build new behaviors?
   - —What strategies assist learning—verbal instruction, use of diagrams, hands-on-guidance, memory strategies?
   - —In what settings does he or she learn most easily—large group, small group, quiet, stimulating environment?
   - —Can he or she generalize learning?
4. What current and expected environmental/occupational demands is the individual preparing to meet?
   - —What knowledge and specific skills are required?
   - —What stimuli, cues, models, and reinforcements are available? What expectations will there be for patience, tolerance, self-control?
   - —To what degree will the person's rules for living enhance his or her success or diminish the likelihood of success?

In summary, the occupational therapist uses the assessment to learn more about the individual's cognitive structures (beliefs, internalized rules, and style of problem-solving), the extent of information and skills he or she possesses, and the "fit" the person makes with his or her everyday environment. With this information, the clinician and the client set priorities in each area and work to change thoughts, skills, knowledge, or specific situations. They also identify cognitive learning strategies that best match the person's learning needs.

Assessment Instruments

Task Check List (TCL)

The Task Check List designed by Lillie & Armstrong (1982) at the Life Skills Program is an adaptation of Hewett's hierarchy of educational tasks used to assess the learning needs of the adult psychiatric population (see Levels of Competence). The check list itemizes key behaviors for each of the seven learning levels identified by Hewett and Forness (1984):

1. Entry
2. Acceptance
3. Order
4. Relationship
5. Exploratory
6. Mastery
7. Achievement levels

LEVELS OF COMPETENCE

Frank Hewett (1984) is an educator who has numerous publications regarding educational approaches for the exceptional learner. Hewett identified six levels of competence that are necessary for effective learning to occur:

1. Attention—The level of competence associated with receiving and perceiving sensory stimulation, coming to, and sustaining attention and retention

2. Response—The level of competence associated with motor responding, verbal language skills, and active participation

3. Order—The level of competence associated with following directions and routines

4. Exploratory—The level of competence associated with gaining an accurate and thorough knowledge of the environment through sensorimotor experiences

5. Social—The level of competence associated with gaining the approval and avoiding the disapproval of others

6. Mastery—The level of competence associated with self-help skills, academic skills, and vocational and career development

---

The check list is used to develop an education plan for the patient (Lillie & Armstrong, 1982) (see Appendix K).

Beck Depression Inventory

In the 1960s, in an attempt to objectify psychiatric diagnosis, Aaron Beck developed the Beck Depression Inventory (Beck, 1976). Today's edition, the result of multiple revisions, is a self-report measure designed to assess the depth of an individual's depression. The patient or client is asked to choose from statements that describe levels of severity in depression. These choices identify the affective, cognitive, motivational, and physiological symptoms of depression that the person is currently experiencing. Since its introduction, health professionals from varied disciplines have used the inventory to identify pre- and post-intervention levels of depression. This inventory and Beck's Hopelessness Scale (Beck & Weissman, 1974) are cited in the occupational therapy literature. There are guidelines as to who can appropriately purchase and interpret findings from both Beck inventories, and occupational therapists are more likely to use these tools in collaboration with other health professionals.

Stress Management Questionnaire (SMQ)

In 1986, Franklin Stein developed the Stress Management forced-choice questionnaire (Stein, Bentley, & Natz, 1999; Stein & Cutler, 1998) to identify the symptoms, stressors, and coping activities that a person chooses to describe his or her stress and ways of managing stress. The 158 forced-choice questionnaire has test-retest reliability of .85 to .89. It has significant positive correlations with the Health Promoting Lifestyle Profile (Walker, Sechrist, & Pender, 1987) and the Survey of Recent Life Experiences (Kohn & MacDonald, 1992). The questionnaire is used to identify the person's stressors and reactions to stress. The data is used to plan an individualized stress management program.

The questionnaire helps the person consider physiological, cognitive, emotional, and behavioral symptoms of stress. Questions can identify the sources of stress—interpersonal and intrapersonal concerns, temporal conflicts, mechanical failures, performance demands, financial problems, illness, environmental stress, and complex or multiple roles. Queries pose options for managing stress—creative activities, construction or craft tasks, exercise, appreciation of the arts, self-care activities, social relationships, plant and animal care, performance activities, and sports. The questionnaire takes 20 to 30 minutes to complete.

Rotter's Internal-External Scale

The scale is a self-report forced-choice questionnaire that measures a person's perception of control; whether he or she is controlled by the variables in the environment or in control of his or her own behavior. The instrument can be completed in 15 to 20 minutes and has an answer key for scoring the responses. Therapists use Rotter's discussion (1966) and those of Robinson and Shaver (1973) to interpret scores that can guide changes in the environment or personal change.

Locus of Control for Children

This test measures the school-age child's perception of control. The scale has two forms (20 items each)—one for children in grades 1 through 6 and one for grades 7 through 12. The self-report questionnaire identifies if the child feels internal control or believes one's options are controlled by external variables (Nowicki & Strickland, 1973).

Other Assessment Instruments

Other assessment instruments cited in the occupational therapy literature include Young's Loneliness Inventory (Young, 1981), Zung's Self-Rating Depression Scale (Zung & Durham, 1965), Hamilton Rating Scale for Depression (Hamilton, 1960), State-Trait Anxiety Inventory (Spielberger, Gorsuch, Lushene, Vagg, & Jacobs, 1983), Beck Anxiety Inventory (Beck, Steer, Epleen, & Brown, 1990), and Dysfunctional Attitude Scale (Weissman & Beck, 1978).

Pre-tests and post-tests may also be used within the guides of this framework. Prior to participating in an educational group, patients or clients may take a pre-test to identify their current level of knowledge regarding a specific subject (e.g., knowledge of budgeting or knowledge of adult sexuality). The participant completes a post-test after the educational experience or series of groups to determine the change in level of knowledge or skill. These testing formats are also used in clinical research.

Intervention

Since the mid-1970s, multiple definitions of the **therapeutic intervention** for cognitive change have evolved. Guidano and Liotti (1983) provide six definitions. Of the six, two seem most applicable to occupational therapy: a *teaching relationship* in which the therapist facilitates the development of coping strategies and self-control (Goldfried, 1980), and a *scientific process* that helps the patient/client question personal beliefs and judgments and then systematically confirms or disproves his or her thoughts, a definition first used by Kelly (1955) and later by many other cognitive theorists (Guidano & Liotti, 1983; Lazarus, 1971; Mahoney, 1974, 1976; Mahoney & DeMonbreun, 1977; Meichenbaum, 1977; Mischel, 1968; Neistadt & Marques, 1984).

Re-establishing the Cognitive System as Self-Regulating

In general, the cognitive-behavioral change process in occupational therapy encourages shared authority and responsibility in intervention by patient/client and therapist. The goal of intervention is to facilitate cognitive growth and improve cognitive function to re-establish the cognitive system as a self-regulating system. To be a **self-regulating system**, the person needs a broad knowledge base; skills to function competently in the environment; knowledge of self, others, and the environment; and the ability to use knowledge for problem solving. The therapist frequently tries to improve the ability to problem-solve in a variety of daily situations, such as those proposed by Bara (1984) (see Categories of Problem Solving).

When individuals possess adequate knowledge and skills and perceive themselves as able to cope with a range of daily problems, they experience themselves as **competent**. The more competent they feel, the more able they are to act flexibly and respond to a broad range of available options. As a result, they become more competent.

Intervention Goals

As with other frames of reference, the cognitive-behavioral frame of reference sets behavioral goals to bring about behavior change and uses them to evaluate intervention outcomes. However, goals are intended to change a person's thoughts as well as his or her behavior.

Changing Behavior and Changing Thoughts

Although behavioral goals are used, it is not believed sufficient to have individuals change just their behavior; they must also change the way they think about themselves and their experiences (Mahoney, 1974; Reda & Mahoney, 1984). For example, the person may learn the skills for interpersonal interaction, such as how to initiate a conversation, communicate with peers at work, and be assertive with authority figures. In addition, however, he or she must have a sense of self-confidence in social situations and must be aware of when and how to use the communication skills learned.

Desired changes in the person's thoughts, attitudes, and values may also be written as goal statements. For example, "The client can verbally identify his or her interpersonal skills (abilities and limitations)," or "Can identify those situations in which the assertiveness skills learned in the course module are effective communication."

Shared Authority

The cognitive-behavioral framework strives for the release of power by the occupational therapist to clients in order to increase participants' responsibility for identifying intervention goals and strategies and for evaluating the efficacy of intervention outcomes. Therefore, authority tends to be more readily shared between patients and the clinician. In our previous discussion of techniques used to build problem solving, it was emphasized that the therapist collaborated with the client to create learning experiences responsive to the person's perceived learning needs. Lillie and Armstrong (1982) describe this model for psychoeducational programming in occupational therapy. Their Goal Attainment Through Education (GATE) group uses a process of group goal setting in which each participant selects his or her psychoeducational experiences based on personal needs and interests. The group is analogous to the high school homeroom group in which students meet, learn about the available courses, then set their goals for participation in the program. The clinician and client then collaboratively determine the types of learning experiences, courses, or groups that will support goal achievement.

Occupational Therapy and Cognitive-Behavioral Strategies

When the clinician integrates cognitive-behavioral approaches into occupational therapy intervention, he or she chooses a framework with an interactive focus rather than the traditional behavioral cause and effect relationships. That is, thoughts, feelings, and behaviors interact; the strategies the therapist selects emphasize this interaction. The clinician chooses approaches that change behavior, build knowledge, and develop problem solving.

Intervention for Peripheral or Deep Change

The occupational therapist keeps several issues in mind as he or she considers what strategies to use in order to bring about a change in the person's pattern of behaving or thinking. The therapist and patient/client must decide whether the goal is to bring about peripheral or deep change. **Peripheral change** results when the person is able to employ the problem-solving and compensatory approaches we have

CATEGORIES OF PROBLEM SOLVING

Bara (1984) identifies six categories of problem solving:

1. Formal
2. Mundane
3. Physical
4. Interactive
5. Personal
6. Self

Formal problem solving has limited application to clinical settings and uses mathematical and logical procedures.

Mundane problem solving uses "common sense" knowledge to interact in everyday life and solve day-to-day problems (e.g., the person has learned not to touch fire, not to run in the street in front of a car, and not to pick things up off the ground and put them in one's mouth).

Physical problem solving uses procedures that help us solve physical reality problems. For example, spatial and temporal orientation helps us see interrelationships among physical events. We know to put on our boots and raincoat when it is raining; we know we need a certain amount of space to walk through a doorway without hitting our head; we know to wear lightweight clothing when it is hot.

Interactive problem solving uses the social rules acquired from one's family and social network to understand and participate in social interaction such as the rules for interacting with one's parents, house rules that must be observed when one lives at home (e.g., time to be home, calling to notify parents that you will be late), or knowing how to greet a new acquaintance (e.g., shaking hands).

Personal problem solving, like interactive problem solving, uses social rules but adds a personal touch. Eventually, the person learns to interpret rules using a personal frame of reference rather than just doing what one is told or expected to do, and perhaps the person has learned to manipulate social rules. Therefore, personal experience and social rules are used to interact and problem-solve in social situations.

For example, the street person, the blue-collar worker, and the professional have each developed their own standards, style of interaction, and method of problem solving. All have learned from daily experiences or through observing their peers how to solve problems and the codes for interaction.

Self problem solving comes from experiences of problem solving. The person learns from his or her own personal experimentation. How often has a parent heard a child state, "Let me do it my way," or "I want to do this myself." Innovations may come from self problem solving. Self problem solving may reflect one's attitude toward one's self. In the previous example, the child is being assertive and seeking independence and permission to be a problem solver. This image of independence may be accurate or may differ from what the child actually thinks and feels.

---

described, which can manage symptoms that interfere with daily function. When working toward **deep change**, the therapist connects past with the present by listening for themes and relating the person's thoughts to such issues as trust, dependency, aggression, avoidance, and over-compliance (Blackburn & Twaddle, 1996; Guidano, 1987).

Level of Change and Socratic Approach

The content of questions varies with the level of change desired. The therapist who is using a **compensatory approach** to bring about peripheral change uses a problem-solving approach. To problem solve, the therapist uses questions that challenge the client to find or describe the evidence that supports the person's belief. For example, "What do people do that tells you they don't like you?" "What did your boss say that indicated his dissatisfaction with your work?"

When the clinician wishes to bring about a deep change or **change the client's schema** and personal identity, the questions emphasize the "meaning" of past and current events. "What does it mean to you if someone doesn't like you?"

Clients may respond that, "I'm a bad person," or "Something is wrong with me." Rather than ask for the evidence of work supervisor problems, the clinician asks, "What does it mean when a person with authority is unhappy with (or critical of) your performance?"

Modifying Personal Identity

A deep change necessitates a remodeling of personal identity. Remodeling requires continuous stimulation from experiences, which will enable the individual to gain knowledge and skills, form new self-statements, develop new rules for interaction, try various methods of problem solving, and then process these experiences to give data that enable a change in attitude toward self. This attitude and knowledge are integrated to modify personal identity. Working to modify core cognitive schemes and bringing about a deep change is more likely to occur in cognitive-behavioral intervention with children (ages 7 and older) whose self-identity is still actively being formed (Stark, Rouse, & Kurowski, 1994).

Modifying Thoughts and Behavior

In most instances, the occupational therapist does not work in the realm of deep structural changes. Instead, the client and therapist work to bring about a peripheral change. A **peripheral change** occurs as a result of a reorganization of attitude toward daily life. This reorganization need not include a change in personal identity but may lead to changes in attitude, behavior, and thoughts; increased adaptation to the environment; decreased emotional stress; and improved problem solving. While working toward this change of attitude, the therapist and learner should keep in mind three assumptions:

1. Cognitive change is a gradual process; to change one's knowledge base and one's attitude toward one's self takes time.
2. The therapist respects the patient's/client's personal thoughts, feelings, and views and encourages the person to openly express them. This does not mean that the therapist has to agree with them.
3. The therapist is aware of the patient's/client's history (thoughts, feelings, behaviors) because it will influence the learning experiences and their outcome.

Listening for Musts

Occupational therapy intervention does not focus extensively on "musts," nor does the clinician typically dispute the client's beliefs in the forceful manner described by Ellis. However, the occupational therapist listens for the "must" messages in the person's dialogue, such as might be communicated by the patient who "must" have a perfectly clean house despite the limitations imposed by a physical illness and then gives up trying when this goal cannot be met, or the child who must create the perfect picture. The therapist may ask the person to identify the things he or she "must" do during a typical week at home or on the job. The therapist then helps the client to see how these "musts" contribute to feelings of helplessness and defeat.

For example, the husband who shuns responsibilities and leaves home because he feels overwhelmed by his job, his family roles, and his need to be perfect in all of these roles can be helped to modify his standards. He can learn to express his feelings and learn to ask for help from his family. (This example also applies to the woman and her role in the family.) Through behavioral and activity experiences and feedback regarding performance, the therapist helps the person to gain control of his or her life through understanding the relationship between thoughts, problems, and behavior.

Homework

In occupational therapy, the occupational therapist more frequently assigns tasks rather than mental or verbal exercises like those of Ellis. These homework tasks typically can be accomplished quickly. For example, the client may be asked to make a draft of his or her resume before the next employ-ment-readiness class or to make a list of the geographical areas for finding an apartment and the benefits of each area before the next community transition group meeting. Children may be assigned work on a craft project or household chore that, when accomplished, concretizes their achievement and increases self-efficacy. The reader is referred to a more thorough discussion of the application of homework with children in this chapter in which we discuss the integration of cognitive-behavioral approaches for intervention with depressed young people.

Building Knowledge Through Reading

When using **bibliotherapy**, the occupational therapist is not likely to assign an entire book, as may the rational emotive therapist. Rather, the clinicians in psychoeducational programs more frequently use copied materials, short articles, or brochures that could describe a budget process, nutrition and meal planning, or first aid and emergency protocol. The occupational therapist, guest lecturers, community agencies, or service providers who work with the client can provide literature. Professionals from social service and community agencies invited to occupational therapy groups have provided literature about Medicare benefits, unemployment benefits, veterans benefits, the effects of alcohol, and weight control, to name a few. We also suggest that the occupational therapist consider the many educational resources "online" to plan educational groups and individualized learning experiences.

Individuals Learn Their Rights

When using cognitive-behavioral theory, the occupational therapist may use intervention strategies for developing assertive beliefs and identifying personal rights. The clinician may incorporate symbolic modeling and role reversal and may use instructional models. For example, these intervention strategies help the occupational therapist who is responsible for running assertiveness training or social skills training groups such as the two group formats described in this chapter and in Chapter Five.

The strategies are also used in individual intervention contexts to help clients learn to ask for what they need or be assertive within the context of any therapeutic activity. For example, the client who waits for the clinician to notice that he or she needs assistance is encouraged to express his or her needs. After a cooking group, the occupational therapist may discuss the experience with group members and ask them to verbalize their thoughts about working together, whether the burden of work was equally shared, and how different members went about getting the help they needed or their needs met.

Meichenbaum (1977, 1985, 1986) emphasizes that educational experiences used to increase assertiveness skills, like those addressing stress management or similar coping skills, need to be individualized to each client. Clients must identify those particular situations in which it is difficult for them to be appropriately assertive. Likewise, it is important that clients practice assertive behavior in real-life contexts.

Using Films and Visual Media

Films and videotapes can be used to demonstrate effective social interactions and task behavior. If social behavior is the focus, a narrator or the therapist can explain the "rules" for the competent social interactions exhibited in the film (Goldstein, 1973). In addition to the narrator's comments, a discussion typically follows the film or video to heighten participants' understanding of the film's content. Further, the client group may be given an opportunity to role-play similar social encounters. Videotapes of clients successfully performing rehabilitation skills such as transfers or employment skills are used in the same way and provide a form of modeling of desired performance.

Another way visual media can be used is to ask a client to predict how he or she will do in a given situation, then (with the person's knowledge and agreement) the client is videotaped. The client and the therapist can review the tape, and the client can see if he or she performed as was predicted. The therapist can facilitate this process by posing questions designed to bring the client's attention to especially salient features in the task performance. Seeing one's self on video can be a very powerful learning experience (sometimes very uncomfortable), and the therapist needs to use clinical judgment in choosing this learning tool.

Modeling and Role-Play

Three **dimensions of role-play** include rehearsal, modeling, and coaching. When using role-play, the therapist often actively participates in order to demonstrate effective methods for responding to problematic situations. The client then rehearses the verbal and behavioral techniques demonstrated, and the clinician and or other group members give verbal and nonverbal feedback. Role-play is used in multiple contexts in occupational therapy, often to prepare the client for prospective employment or social challenges. Through role-playing, for example, the patient/client can practice interviewing for a job, asking for a date, personal introductions for varied social situations, registering to vote, applying for a library card, and so on.

Prior to using role-play with children, the clinician considers the development level of the child, which must be judged to be at about age 7 or older for role-play to be used in the previously described manner. It is at this age that the child is able to clearly distinguish between real and pretend, can decenter, and imagine the view of others (Flavell, 1985). Children who have participated in role-play as a part of social skills training have responded positively to coaching, rehearsal, and corrective feedback (Frame, Johnstone, & Giblin, 1988; Frame, Matson, Sonis, Fialkov, & Kazdin, 1982; Petti, Bornstein, Delamater, & Conner, 1980). Role-play is a strategy used with children having behavior management problems and low self-esteem (Kolko, 1992; Stark et al., 1994). The development level of the person is also a consideration for the adult with developmental delay.

Modeling and Physical Guidance

Modeling is also used to build task skills, such as those involved in learning an unfamiliar job, self-care task, or sport. The clinician may act as a model or have a family member, staff person, or the client model the sequence of steps in a task, giving the client the opportunity to practice and achieve competence in each step before attempting the next. This exemplifies **modeling of gradual mastery**.

The therapist can also use **physical guidance**, placing hands on the patient's/client's hands as he or she attempts a motor act. Guidance is used to ensure success. As the person becomes more successful, the clinician gradually removes physical support. In addition, the therapist helps the individual verbally acknowledge his or her accomplishments and, when appropriate, identify the skills and reasoning used. It is hoped that through this process the person increases his or her awareness of information that can be generalized to future, similar situations.

Teaching Problem Solving

The occupational therapist can employ any of the problem-solving strategies or formats described earlier (such as those used in mediation, Think Aloud, task analysis, and self-instruction). A relatively simple four-step process that reflects these various formats is referred to by Meichenbaum as Goal-Plan-Do-Check (Meichenbaum, 1991). It is discussed in the occupational therapy literature by the Cognitive Orientation to Occupational Performance (CO-OP) Research Group (DCD Research Group, 1995). A child or adult uses this self-instruction process to do the following:

- Identify a problem and set a goal
- Create a plan of action
- Implement the plan
- Assess the outcome (Meichenbaum, 1977, 1991)

This process is used in the context of daily life experiences, not only for problem solving but also to teach the client to self-regulate behavior (Missiuna et al., 1998). The use of this cognitive-behavioral modification approach with children is documented in occupational therapy (Missiuna & Samuels, 1989; Wilcox, 1994) and education literatures (Hallahan, Kneedler, & Lloyd, 1983; Kendal, 1993). It can also be used with adults and may be combined with other frames of reference.

Creative Problem Solving

Another problem-solving format that has been discussed in the occupational therapy literature is referred to as creative problem solving (CPS) (Lewin & Reed, 1998). It is based upon the work of Alex Osborn (1963) and Sidney Parnes (1992). Osborn, an advertising executive regarded as the father of the term "brainstorming," created the model in the late 1930s, and Sidney Parnes, a psychologist, developed it further (Lewin & Reed, 1998, p. 20). The model continues to be researched and developed by individual scholars

(Firestein & Treffinger, 1983; Isaksen, Dorval, & Treffinger, 1994; Treffinger, 1996) and through the efforts of the Creative Problem Solving Institute.

The first step in creative problem solving is to determine what really is the problem; sometimes, when one is in a troublesome situation, it is not clear what exactly needs to be resolved. Please refer to Increase Your Understanding: Creative Problem Solving: What Is the Problem and Who Owns It? for details. Creative problem solving is to be used when there is not a pat solution or familiar protocol for solving the problem. Next, it must be established that the problem solver(s) "owns" the problem (i.e., he or she must truly want to work on resolving it and must be in a position to resolve the problem [some problems, no matter how troublesome, are realistically, out of one's hands]). If the problem meets these criteria, the next step is to generate as many ideas as possible to solve the dilemma. No idea is to be censored or evaluated until all ideas are generated; the goal is to defer judgment and generate as many possible solutions as one can because out of this comes insight or solutions that would have otherwise lay dormant. Then, each potential solution can be evaluated, as one considers, "What are the benefits of this idea?" "What are its drawbacks?" and "What more do I need to know about this idea to truly judge its merit?" In this process, prospective solutions may be combined or modified. Also important in this process of creative problem solving is the notion of **incubation**—giving one's self time to "sit on" an idea before choosing a solution.

There are other specific "thinking" strategies associated with the CPS process, which together create a rhythm of

INCREASE YOUR UNDERSTANDING: CREATIVE PROBLEM SOLVING: WHAT IS THE PROBLEM AND WHO OWNS IT?

Creative problem solving begins by identifying the problem and establishing ownership. A person or group of persons "owns" a problem when the problem meets the following criteria:

- The individual or group is aware that there is a difference between what is and what should be

- They are able to measure or specify that difference

- They have a need to solve the problem

- They have access to the internal and external resources needed to solve the problem and have the time and capability to use these resources (in other words, they are in a position to solve the problem) (Lewin & Reed, 1998, p. 156)

Sometimes it is quite clear what the problem is. Often, however, there are numerous ways a problem can be framed. Problems that are candidates for CPS are those in which the client is in a position to solve the problem and wants to work on the problem, and there is not already a set solution.

Consider the following scenario and list in the spaces provided additional "problems" that impact Pat. Consider for each whether or not these are good candidates for CPS. We have done three to get you started.

Scenario: Pat is an unmarried, 23-year-old young man who has struggled with recurrent bouts of schizophrenia since he was 14 years old. Pat lives in a group home with four other men. Pat's physician has indicated that it is unsafe for him to drive because he has unpredictable episodes of acute psychosis; therefore, Pat has never had a driver's license. Pat would like to get a job in the hub of the town in which he lives, but it is about 6 miles away. There are job openings in the immediate neighborhood in which Pat resides, but only in fast-food restaurants, and Pat views these as "dead-end" jobs. Pat lives about ¾ mile from the bus stop and could walk to catch the bus. Pat does not currently ride the bus but would like to be able to. He is reluctant because he has never ridden the bus by himself and is unfamiliar with the steps involved in accessing public transportation.

Possible problems:

Problem 1. Pat has unpredictable bouts of psychosis that keep him from obtaining his driver's license.

(A good problem for CPS? Not as stated. We have not read that Pat wants to resolve this problem, and it is doubtful that Pat has the internal and external resources to solve this problem. If more clearly defined, this problem might be able to be addressed.)

Problem 2. There are no jobs in businesses other than fast-food restaurants in Pat's immediate neighborhood.

(A good problem for CPS? No. Pat might like this to be different, but this is not under Pat's control.)

Problem 3. Pat views jobs in fast-food restaurants as "dead-end" jobs.

(A good problem for CPS? Possibly; we do not currently know that Pat views this as a problem, nor that he wishes to change his beliefs, but his beliefs are presumed to be within Pat's control.)

Problem 4. _____
_____

(A good problem for CPS?)

Problem 5. _____
_____

(A good problem for CPS?)

alternating between **divergent thinking** (generating all of the possibilities) and **convergent thinking** (selecting the best option). CPS is a process that has been taught to diverse groups, from healthy children and adults who wish to become better at coping with daily challenge (Keller-Mathers & Puccio, 1998; Lewin & Reed, 1998; Puccio, Keller-Mathers, & Treffinger, 1998), to inmates preparing to leave the prison setting (McCluskey et al., 1998; Place & McCluskey, 1995). Lewin and Reed (1998) describe the applicability of CPS to the clinical reasoning used by occupational therapists and also the merits of teaching CPS to clients (both child and adult) as part of occupational therapy intervention.

Identifying Cognitive Distortions

The occupational therapist may also help the person identify cognitive distortions and learn to test personal beliefs. Beck and his associates (1976) suggest that the individual write down thoughts, look for underlying themes, and then identify distorted thinking.

To identify cognitions, the occupational therapist can recommend that the person keep a log in which he or she records thoughts, feelings, and behaviors that occur during therapeutic activities or tasks throughout the day. For example, the patient taking a city bus for the first time might note a concern about missing his or her stop or a personal belief that other passengers were "looking at me strangely." The therapist then discusses these notes with patients/clients to help them understand their thoughts and their consequences. The notes and discussions also influence the subsequent choice of task and intervention strategies. Another way that thoughts can be monitored is by the therapist asking the client at random times during an intervention activity to state what he or she is thinking at that moment.

Testing Cognitions

Testing cognitions means that the person learns to distinguish thoughts or beliefs from facts. In the previous example, the therapist may ask the person to identify what happened or what people did that indicated people saw him or her as "strange." In this way, the therapist helps clients to confirm or negate their thoughts. Thoughts or beliefs are treated as hypotheses to be tested by inductive analysis, not as statements of fact. If indeed the client acted strangely, the therapist instructs or demonstrates acceptable behavior for riding the bus. Within the context of activity and the teaching relationship, the occupational therapist helps the client develop a scientific attitude and plan strategies for behavioral change.

Educational Experiences

Knowledge builds competence, and the occupational therapist can use a classroom format to increase knowledge. Sample education experiences suggested by Neistadt and Marques (1984) include money management (the participant learns to make a budget, open bank accounts, and manage a checkbook), movement and relaxation (the person may participate in exercise or aerobic sessions, learn body mechanics, and energy conservation and relaxation techniques), home management (the client learns meal planning and preparation or basic home repair), or time management (planning one's day, using a weekly calendar to coordinate family activities).

Other educational experiences (Sladyk, 1990) include memory training (the participant may learn rehearsal strategies and how to use external aids or cuing methods), effective communication (the client may learn to use the telephone, practice oral and written communication, and interact in dyadic and group situations), understanding sexuality (the person can learn about his or her own sexual needs as well as how to ask for a date, courting protocol, expression of sexuality, and means to ensure safe sex). Still other educational experiences might include anger management (Weinstein & DeNeff, 1989), learning to use community resources (Lillie & Armstrong, 1982), and vocational readiness (Kramer, 1984) in which the person can learn resume writing and job interview skills. These experiences may be planned and implemented by the occupational therapist or in cooperation with other health professionals. Other references are previously cited in Education Modules and in Appendices J and L.

Application with Children

Cognitive-behavioral strategies were originally conceived for adults but were subsequently adapted for use with children. We have referred to this throughout the chapter. These strategies include engaging children in a collaborative relationship to help them set their own goals and to help determine when goals have been achieved. The model is also used to teach children to employ problem-solving strategies (e.g., Think Aloud strategies, task analysis, and creative problem solving). The theory helps the clinician structure learning experiences for educating children in the use of relaxation and stress management techniques. The strategies include role-play, examination and reframing of one's beliefs, and assigning of homework, and are frequently used with children who have behavior management issues, social disorders, poor self-confidence, and depression. Important among the strategies with depressed children are those that engage children in challenging their self-defeating beliefs and assigning "homework," which requires the child to participate in enjoyable activities.

One must remember that cognitive-behavioral strategies are not just for children with emotional disorders. It is often very appropriate to teach stress management or other coping strategies to children who are coping with physical and learning challenges. Coping with chronic illnesses (e.g., asthma, arthritis, and cystic fibrosis), disabling conditions, and multiple medical procedures often creates tremendous additional stress for children. Learning simple but effective ways to reduce stress can help children manage frustration in a positive rather than self-defeating way and can thereby help them succeed and feel good about their accomplishments. In the applied literature we reviewed, instances of cognitive-behavioral application with children are described with children 7 years old or older (the most frequent examples we saw were age 9 and older). This coincides with the recommendation of Law et al. (1994), who authored the Canadian Occupational Performance Measure. They recommend that the semistructured interview be used to establish initial intervention goals with adults and children age 7 and older. Assuming then that we have child learners who are cognitively able to participate in these experiences, the following recommendations are a summary of what we found in the applied literature:

- Children at the developmental age of 7 and older are able to successfully use a cognitive behavior model.
- Children ages 7 through 11 can learn best from hands-on experiences; they easily become bored with too much talk.
- Parent support and cooperation is often critical to the success of cognitive-behavioral intervention with children. Parents can be taught the principles of cognitive behaviorism that are being used with their children, and their cooperation enlisted. They can be asked to praise accomplishment, support the completion of homework by the child, help the child verbalize thoughts, and help the child identify those situations in which it would be appropriate to use a coping strategy or problem-solving strategy. It is not unusual for parents of children having problems to need help knowing how to work and play with their children in a positive way, as well as be in need of resources for games, activities, and resources in the community for shared play and learning.
- Concepts, skills, and procedure are best presented in short, simple lessons with small goals that consider the child's shorter attention span.
- If presenting didactic information, use fun activities, cartoons, or other visual aids, and novelty to engage the child and maintain his or her attention.
- Children in the 7 to 11 age group particularly enjoy crafts and other projects in which they have a tangible outcome. These projects provide an excellent vehicle for learning about one's self, seeing what care and diligence to a task can produce. They can build tolerance for less-than-perfection, and they build beliefs around efficacy.
- Children in this age group can be taught to re-examine their beliefs and to engage in self-monitoring of their thoughts; however, they can become self-conscious if this monitoring is obvious to their peers.
- To participate in cognitive re-examination, children need to have the words with which to describe thoughts and feelings. Games and fun activities can be used with younger children to help them build an "emotional vocabulary."
- Children can be taught the same relaxation techniques as adults, provided the clinician uses the child's vocab-

ulary and considers the child's shorter attention span. The strategies taught to an adult in one or two sessions may take the child several or more sessions to learn (see Increase Your Understanding: Adult and Child Progressive Relaxation).

- Games are an excellent age-appropriate medium for children to learn about turn-taking, following rules, responding to frustration, winning and losing gracefully, and other skills related to social and moral development.
- If children are to reward themselves as part of a cognitive-behavioral program, rewards should be those that occur in their natural environment and something that they will be able to access. The cooperation of parents, teachers, or other adults is often needed to determine if rewards are appropriate.
- It is important that intervention extend into the natural environment. If the clinician cannot go into the child's home, similar context goals can often be accomplished through homework assignments (Schaefer, 1999; Stark et al., 1994; Vernon, 1999a, 1999b).

Group Intervention

Educational Groups

Because of the educational and didactic nature of the therapeutic experience, groups are frequently used in intervention. Depending on the nature of the activity, class groups are usually composed of 6 to 10 participants. Groups provide an opportunity for members to help each other and to discuss methods of problem solving. During class discussions the higher-level functioning member can help the lower-level functioning member. Participants can give each other support and support risk-taking, and they can give each other feedback about their thoughts, feelings, and behaviors. A group format also enables the use of role playing and modeling.

Sample Psychoeducational Group in Occupational Therapy

An example of a comprehensive psychoeducational group in occupational therapy is the Solving Community Obstacles and Restoring Employment (SCORE) program designed by Kramer (1984). The SCORE program identifies the participant as a student and the therapist as a teacher and uses an educational format to establish realistic career objectives; teach job seeking, social, and interpersonal skills; and improve self-presentation.

The program consists of 15 educational modules, which help the student-client assess the advantages and disadvantages of employment, evaluate work and leisure skills, and practice completion of employment forms. Clients learn to write resumes and job inquiry letters. They role-play and videotape employment interview questions and situations. Following work task performance, clients critique their job performance and that of peers.

INCREASE YOUR UNDERSTANDING: ADULT AND CHILD PROGRESSIVE RELAXATION

Progressive relaxation can be taught to both children and adults. It involves the deliberate, systematic tensing and relaxing of muscle groups of the body. Progressive relaxation can be taught through the use of purchased audiotapes or tapes made by the clinician or with the client's voice recorded as he or she reads the instructions aloud from a written script. The following are excerpts from two such scripts: one for the adult, the other for the child. They illustrate the difference in the way that instructions can be presented in accordance with the client's age and level of understanding. The clinician using relaxation strategies, whether with adults or children, is sensitive to the sexual stimulation these exercises can facilitate.

Adult Script (excerpt from Bower & Bower [1992])

Introduction:
Now is the time to try to relax. Find a nice comfortable position on a bed or on the floor mat and try to relax as much as you can right now. I'm going to ask you to tighten certain muscles and study the sensations that come from those muscles while they're tense, then notice what happens when you relax them... (p. 231)

Hands and Forearms:
To start with, clench your right fist and try to keep all the other muscles in your body relaxed. Your forearm will be down flat... Study the feelings of tension in your forearm. Notice the location of the muscles and how they feel when they are tensed... Relax now, all at once... (p. 231)

Forehead:
Now raise your eyebrows and pull your scalp down to meet your eyebrows so that you can feel the tension in your forehead and up across the top of your skull. Study the pattern of tension... (p. 232)

Child Script (Source unknown)

Introduction:
Today we're going to do some special kind of exercises called "relaxation exercises." These exercises help you learn how to relax when you're feeling uptight and help you get rid of those butterflies-in-the-stomach feelings.

Hands and Forearms:
Pretend you have a whole lemon in your hand. Now squeeze it hard. Try to squeeze all the juice out. Feel the tightness in your hand and arm as you squeeze it. Take another lemon and squeeze it. Try to squeeze it harder than you did the first one... Now drop your lemon and relax. See how much better your hand and arm feel when they are relaxed...

Face and Nose (forehead):
Here comes a pesky old fly... He has landed on your forehead. Make lots of wrinkles. Try to catch him between all those wrinkles. Hold it tight now. Okay, you can let him go....

The modules identify learning goals and provide the clinician-teacher (leader and co-leader) with guidelines for task presentation, implementation, and discussion. Teachers discuss relevant topics, give instruction in employment-seeking skills, and encourage discussion of tasks and feedback to peers. Modules may be presented in a flexible schedule, but Kramer recommends eight consecutive 3-hour sessions. Each student must complete 24 hours of class work and may do so outside of class time if necessary. Modules have some flexibility in presentation, which allows the course to be individualized to meet the student's needs. The reader is referred to the original source for detailed module descriptions. Included are sample forms and a comprehensive discussion of the group format used to assist the physically and mentally disabled person desiring reemployment.

Integration of Cognitive-Behavioral and MOHO Theory in a Group

In another example cited in the occupational therapy literature, cognitive-behavioral principles are combined with those from the Model of Human Occupation (MOHO) to provide group treatment in an acute inpatient psychiatric program for persons exhibiting substance abuse (Yeager, 2000). The author organizes educational groups around MOHO's habituation, volition, and performance subsystems. For example, there are groups responsive to problems in the performance subsystem, such as life skills, money management, nutrition for self and children, and safe sex. Subsystems groups also focus on coping skills, stress and anger management, and relaxation training for reducing addictive substance use. In some of the groups, clients learn from assertiveness training, practice identifying alternatives to violence, and learn time management. Groups related to issues around volition and personal causation include a creative group for expressing emotions, task groups to explore esteem, motivation, cause and effect, and the role of prayer and spirituality. Groups related to the habitation system include those designed to increase awareness of leisure and community resources.

Designing Educational Modules

When designing educational modules such as that described in the SCORE program and those intended for work with substance abusers, the occupational therapist uses task analysis to develop graded learning experiences (see Appendix J for an intensive outpatient program example). The experiences are selected to develop knowledge and skills and to provide opportunities to generalize new information and skills in different situations and settings. Within these multiple situations, the learner can recognize and correct errors, as well as identify and use personal strengths and abilities. Through these graded learning experiences, the learner masters new information and skills.

Education for Mastery

Mastery suggests that as a result of the learning experience, the client has acquired knowledge and skills, can identify a plan of action for a particular situation, is able to apply this knowledge effectively, and can use experience and knowledge to meet future demands. Mastery also indicates that the individual has met the goals that he or she set rather than those based on the norm or those of other participants in the group. Knowledge and skill mastery are the basis for the client's ability for self-management.

Increase Mastery for Self-Management

Self-management is frequently learned and practiced in a group context. Intervention groups for self-management focus on social skills, assertive communication, stress management, coping skills, and prevention skills. The assumption is that by giving client's information and teaching them specific skills to master, clients become empowered to take responsibility for managing their own lives. The goals identified for the different types of self-management groups described in Appendix L are just a sample of goals that may be set within these different groups. When leading these different types of groups the occupational therapist helps clients set individual goals and varies the learning strategies according to the clients' needs. The group descriptions in Appendix L are "generic" or general descriptions of cognitive-behavioral approaches that serve as a structure for many professionals who work in mental health or behavioral health. When the occupational therapist uses these educational groups, he or she usually conducts training in the context of the client's chosen occupational focus and performance environment. The therapist also considers the context of the intervention setting and adjusts intervention accordingly.

For example, the occupational therapist may adjust the general group formats in Appendix L when working with an adolescent group in a community or school setting to build social skills that support inclusion of students with disabilities. In a coping skills group, the clinician can problem solve with a small group of student-clients who are managing their disabilities in a school environment.

In an outpatient environment, the therapist who is leading a work readiness group may use social skills activities with clients who have an acquired brain injury and are transitioning to a modified work setting and have concerns about what to tell others about their injury. The occupational therapist may focus on daily and activity planning and time management in an outpatient couples group that serves the client and spouse after a traumatic injury. In couples groups, the clinician can also focus on lifestyle redesign to help couples manage the outcomes of trauma or chronic illness.

Stress Management

Most of the stress management approaches focus on mastery of specific skills. Earlier in this chapter, you read examples of relaxation approaches for coping with stress. Another approach suggested by Meichenbaum (1977, 1985, 1986) gives us a theory for stress management that goes beyond teaching the clients coping skills. He believes that skill training is necessary but not sufficient to manage stress over the long-term. According to Meichenbaum, we cannot eliminate stress from our lives, but we can change the way we view stress and its effects, which in turn will help us respond constructively to stressful situations. Thus, Meichenbaum describes an approach that gives equal emphasis to changing a person's perceptions and beliefs about stress and to developing and practicing skills for managing stress. Please see Appendix L for a brief description of the protocol for a stress inoculation group. Meichenbaum's approach can be especially useful when working with clients who are managing the stress of chronic illness and disease or long term disabilities.

Coping Skills Group

The previous types of cognitive behavior group approaches that we have described have a single primary focus for skill development and mastery. Lazarus (1971) describes another type of cognitive-behavioral group with multiple approaches. He believes that the therapist should have a repertoire of strategies for skill development and use them within a social learning group model to produce the desired change as identified by the client, not by the clinician or a program focus. He calls this approach "multimodal group therapy." In a sense, it is a generic group format that the occupational therapist can integrate within an activity context to build a variety of coping skills. This group approach could be used in support groups for clients and caregivers who are coping with chronic symptoms of illness and disease or long term disability. In educational and support groups that begin the process of coping with dramatic changes in the person's daily life during acute rehabilitation. See Appendix L for a coping skills group format.

Cognitive-Behavioral Model for Relapse Prevention

In occupational therapy, we have a major role not only in self-management but also in relapse prevention programs. When a person has a chronic condition or problem, whether it is related to physical or mental health, there is often a pattern of fluctuations in function, or a gradual decline in function over time. Some people view these changes as beyond their control because they are part of a biologic disease process. When these changes are seen as not within the person's control, the client may turn to a spiritual source or higher power to help or take control of the situation. Clients may assume that the medical community is responsible for the management of their health, illness, or impairment.

However, when the health condition is believed to be within the person's control, families, health care professionals, and the client may be critical of back-slides and may assume that the client needs to learn better self-management strategies to maintain optimum health and function and prevent future relapses (Marlatt, 1995). Even when an illness or physical condition cannot be totally controlled by the client, people often expect individuals having these conditions to take good care of themselves and avoid behaviors that would likely be detrimental to their own well-being.

With the increased emphasis on prevention of health problems or the management of chronic conditions, occupational therapists can contribute to interventions in multiple areas including substance abuse, eating disorders, and weight and fitness management for children, adults, and older adults. These disorders all include a potential for relapse. Although there are differences in programming, there exist underlying cognitive behavior principles that clinicians can use when planning and implementing programs aimed at minimizing the negative impact of these conditions and their relapses.

Meaning of Relapse

First, let us consider the term "relapse" and its meaning to the client and clinician before giving examples of relapse and prevention approaches. In medicine, successful management of a substance problem is often defined as total abstinence; **relapse**, which refers to resumption of use, signifies lack of success. In the cognitive behavior model, there is "absence" or abstinence, no unhealthy behavior. There is also **lapse**, meaning that the person on a one time basis breaks abstinence but does not return to baseline behavior, or there is relapse, meaning that the person returns to the pre-intervention condition of substance abuse, overeating, etc.

Chronic conditions such as diabetes, obesity, and cardiac disorders are all examples in which special diets and health regimens may be prescribed and in which relapse to

unhealthy behaviors is also a concern. In establishing a program to prevent return to habits that compromise health, the therapist takes into consideration the setting's and the client's definition of health, prevention, lapse, and relapse in regard to staying on course.

Prevention Model

The cognitive-behavioral relapse-prevention model emphasizes that abuse disorders in particular, while having a physiologic correlate, are in large part disorders of learning. Specifically, the abuser has established habits around substance use, eating, activity, etc. (McCrady, 1994). Because these habits have been learned over time, building new habits will also take time. Prevention of abuse and the goal of managing one's health and changing one's habits to increase health are both short- and long-term goals. The **relapse model** considers the person's thoughts, feelings, motivation, and ability to cope. It evaluates the social and cultural variables and the reinforcers that exist in the environment. It identifies biological factors that are related to the person's habits and health problems. All three of the variables (biopsychosocial) are evaluated and influence the intervention plan (Marlatt, 1995).

Lapse Not Failure

The advantage of allowing for a "lapse" in health maintenance and abuse management is that neither the person nor the helping staff need to see this as a failure. The client can choose to regain control rather than giving up or being dismissed from treatment. To help the client regain control and prevent similar lapses in the future, the client and the therapist work to identify the variables that led to the lapse of control. They identify future risks, and they formulate strategies for helping the person be more successful (Marlatt, 1995).

With substance abuse and unhealthy eating, for example, lapses are often related to social events and emotional changes. Celebrations such as weddings, office parties, or neighborhood picnics typically provide enjoyment associated with consumption of food and alcohol. These same events may be stressful for clients, can cause anxiety or sadness, and may trigger the lapse. In these situations, returning to one's old habits can serve as a form of "self-medication" (Marlatt, 1995). Additionally, there may be specific social expectations that promote lapse of self-control (e.g., the expectation that a person drink and consume rich food when entertaining business associates or business clients). To manage these occupational performance situations, occupational therapists can help the clients problem solve in prevention groups.

Goals of the Cognitive-Behavioral Prevention Model

The overarching goal of the health management program is to increase the client's self-efficacy for responding to the everyday challenges that can compromise one's health and participation in daily life. **Self-efficacy** means that the person has confidence that he or she has the knowledge and skills necessary for managing his or her health and changing personal habits (Marlatt, 1995; McCrady, 1994). In occupational therapy, clients can increase their sense of efficacy as they increase their awareness of the variables that challenge their ability to manage their behavior, symptoms, and health. In an occupational therapy prevention group they can share ideas with peers and develop a problem-solving plan that they use in or outside of the group. Clients practice skills and problem-solving strategies that they can then use when they are discharged or complete an educational group program. The problem-solving plan identifies individualized strategies for responding to daily life situations and for coping with the barriers that can limit occupational performance. When the client is aware of what to expect, has a plan for managing daily challenges, and has practiced what to do to meet his or her goals, the client's sense of self-efficacy is increased. This sense of self-efficacy helps prevent the sense of hopelessness or helplessness that tends to sabotage a person's healthy behavior and ability for self-management.

Relapse Intervention Guide

Intervention for changing one's habits and preventing a relapse to unhealthy behaviors is an ongoing process. As such, it provides the client the opportunity to periodically assess his or her own progress and to re-evaluate the strategies that the person is using. Within this on-going process, the person will need to re-commit to goals that have been set as well as identify and commit to new goals that accommodate to changes that occur over time. In this way, the prevention process helps the client develop and adapt a plan for achieving short- and long-term goals. Additionally, periodic review of and accommodation to changing circumstances can help sustain the person's interest and motivation for effective management of one's health condition (Marlatt, 1995).

Prevention Goals

As we have indicated, the goals for prevention and relapse programs must be individualized to meet specific client needs or those of the population. To make these programs more client-centered and bring about different kinds of change, the clinician can adapt any of the following general goals:

- To educate the client about the relapse process
- To increase the clients' awareness of their own patterns of behavior in their own lives
- To educate the client about the self-efficacy process and its place in successful health management
- To help the clients identify the risks in their own lives that interfere with healthy self-management
- To increase clients' awareness of their beliefs and rationalizations that either enhance or impede positive behavior change
- To identify the "what ifs" and develop a problem-solving plan to respond to lapses

- To teach clients alternative stress management or behavior management strategies (relaxation, exercise, deep breathing, spending time on an enjoyable activity)
- To increase clients' awareness of specific coping strategies and variables that interfere with their application (e.g., through use of a worksheet for self-monitoring, or a time line that depicts lapses or relapses and indicates under what conditions these occurred)
- To establish a system of social support for clients, especially one that supports abstinence
- To teach clients to evaluate personal goals, progress toward those goals (e.g., to help clients establish goals that are realistic and that can be observed), and reframe them if necessary
- To increase client awareness of the interactions among one's lifestyle, habits, and their consequences for controlling behavior and supporting health (Marlatt, 1995, p. 545; McCrady, 1994, p. 1162)

Developing the Relapse Prevention Plan

Blackburn and Twaddle (1996) summarize relapse prevention strategies for managing symptoms of depression, anxiety, and obsessive-compulsive and eating disorders. Some of the strategies are general guides and are summarized next because they can be used within occupational therapy in both individual and group contexts and in many specialty areas of practice. The strategies can also be used in health care and community support groups for populations with physical, psychosocial, and cognitive problems.

To develop a relapse plan for managing symptoms, clients may spend time during intervention sessions reviewing what they have learned and demonstrating their ability to use their knowledge and skills. Sample strategies used to develop the relapse plan during these sessions expect clients to:

- Review the sources or incidents that relate to the symptoms that interfere with their health, well-being, and participation in daily life
- Identify past and possible future sources of a problem and the factors that will maintain the problem
- Review and demonstrate the strategies that they learned for management of symptoms
- List the strategies they prefer and find most useful
- Demonstrate the ability to use the Socratic method for testing their self-efficacy beliefs and beliefs about others, the environment, and their activities
- Practice setting goals
- Develop a contingency plan for managing future challenges, such as substance abuse, over-eating, withdrawing, anger, and other symptoms that interfere with daily performance
- Agree to return for the next or follow-up sessions as recommended (Blackburn & Twaddle, 1996)

Occupational Therapy and Relapse Prevention

In summary, the cognitive-behavioral relapse prevention model provides guides that can be used in many occupational therapy contexts, both group and individual intervention. The model supports habit change, self-management, maintenance of healthy behavior, and measurable outcomes for persons with chronic conditions and addictive disorders. Even when the therapist is not employed in a setting directed at relapse prevention, occupational therapists often work with clients who exhibit self-destructive or unhealthy behaviors. Thus, prevention strategies can be used for managing these secondary conditions as well.

For example, clients seen in a home setting may lapse into eating that undermines weight control or using substances that compromise medical regimens. Both complicate the person's disability condition. Thus, the therapist may help clients manage new symptoms or problems that occur after illness, trauma, or physical disability. In these situations, therapists can help clients develop activity plans that support an individual's efforts to limit eating, alcohol use, tobacco use, or other substance use. They can develop fitness programs for health and weight management that integrate daily activities and activity planning. When negotiating these interventions, the clinician uses a cognitive-behavioral orientation for self-management and places emphasis on clients being pro-active. Both client and therapist adopt the attitude that clients learn from mistakes or lapse behavior rather than fail and are defeated by mistakes.

An example of a pro-active approach for healthy occupational performance is summarized next. The cognitive behavior principles applied in this exercise and fitness example can be used in other contexts. The following example is adapted from Brownell and Fairburn (1995, p. 476) and Grilo, Brownell, and Stunkard (1993, p. 366).

Cognitive-Behavioral Approach for Exercise and Fitness

Cognitive-behavioral approaches are used within fitness and exercise programs when it is believed that there are physical and/or psychosocial variables that interfere with consistent participation in the program. To respond to the client's physical and psychosocial needs, the therapist and client negotiate a fitness routine that supports health and meets standards for client self-efficacy. The program considers what the client feels is a reasonable goal for one's self. The goal choice helps the client increase fitness, and takes into account his or her age, physical health, and limitations. It is also manageable within the client's given life situation. Thus, the exercise routine is not built around external standards for maximum fitness. Instead, the routine includes enjoyable exercise and daily activities, things that the client is willing to commit to and is more likely to stick with. The clinician asks for a commitment from the client to adhere to the routine and helps the client establish a system to keep track of his or her progress. The client is also encouraged to establish a social network or "buddy" system that will support the exercise program (Brownell & Fairburn, 1995, p. 476).

When clinicians establish or carry out fitness programs for clients with a disability, they may recommend daily activity routines or connect clients to adaptive sports and fitness resources in the community. Overall, these fitness programs promote health through lifestyle redesign. They endorse a positive approach to "healthy doing" within daily living, work, and leisure occupations and try to encourage the development of new, healthier habits and physical routines that maintain optimum physical and emotional strength. These programs work to prevent secondary disabilities believed to result from sedentary life styles and poor health habits. In addition to the benefits for health and fitness, occupational therapists believe that fitness, recreation, and leisure activities help people learn about themselves, offer an opportunity for building friendships, and promote creativity (Buning, 1999; White, 1986).

Efficacy of Cognitive-Behavioral Approaches

The information in this chapter represents selected literature chosen by the authors to update the reader's knowledge of the relationship between cognitive and behavioral theories and their application in health care and occupational therapy. The marriage between cognitive and behavioral theories seems to be tenable for describing the interactive relationship among thoughts, affect, and behavior, and their outcome as functional performance. Although emphasizing the validity of subjective experience, the cognitive-behavioral therapist objectifies behavior change and uses such change to measure the effectiveness of psychosocial intervention. For some, this dual focus on thought as well as behavior is more comfortable than the perceived exclusivity of both psychoanalytic and behavioral therapies.

In occupational therapy, the integration of cognitive behavior approaches is recognized as effective (Bradlee, 1984; Campbell & McCreadie, 1988; Drouet, 1986; Duncombe, 1998; Eilenberg, 1986; Engel, 1992; Engel & Rapoff, 1990; Fine & Schwimmer, 1986; Friedlob, Janis, & Deets-Aron, 1986; Giles, 1985; Giles & Allen, 1986; Johnson, 1986; Lindsay, 1983; Moyers, 1988; Nickel, 1988; Stein & Nikolic, 1989; Stein & Smith, 1989; Stoffel, 1994). Given the focus on prevention and client education in today's practice environment, we assume that these approaches will continue to emerge as the profession builds on social learning principles that influence educational models for wellness and prevention in occupational therapy. We encourage the reader to explore cognitive behavior literature further and to evaluate its potential application in occupational therapy contexts. Next, we will share our impressions of cognitive-behavioral theory and its application, and make some conjectures about potential contributions and limitations of cognitive-behavioral theory as it is applied in occupational therapy practice. We also pose questions that have arisen from our study of the literature.

CONTRIBUTIONS AND LIMITATIONS OF THE COGNITIVE-BEHAVIORAL FRAME OF REFERENCE

Contributions

Compatibility With Occupational Therapy Philosophy

Cognitive-behavioral theory speaks primarily to enhancing occupational performance by changing the "person" in the person-occupation-environment triad. It does so by impacting cognition or "thinking." Collectively, it is theory that has been applied across disciplines, including psychology, education, and occupational therapy. What makes it especially appealing is that it is so compatible with occupational therapy philosophy, especially the emphasis given by cognitive behaviorism to collaborating with and empowering clients, engaging the client in experiential learning, and striving to change clients' beliefs about the self from incapable to capable. While we may not always view ourselves as engaged in impacting belief systems, one could argue that there is always a reciprocal relationship between clients being able to function capably and their perceiving themselves as capable. Occupational therapists are often in the position of teacher, whether they are engaged in direct or indirect service, and what cognitive behaviorism adds to their repertoire is specific techniques and strategies that facilitate the learning process and a basis for understanding why these strategies could be expected to be successful. The psychology literature summarizes research that supports the use of cognitive-behavioral strategies from middle childhood through the rest of the life span and with a variety of problems of living. Intervention strategies can typically be easily adapted to meet the child or adult learners' ability to understand and use information.

Increased Understanding of the Hierarchy of Reinforcement

The hierarchy of reinforcement, proposed by Bandura and influential in cognitive-behavioral therapy, has multiple applications in occupational therapy. These applications note the many levels of reinforcement that come into play in occupational therapy intervention and help us design successful learning experiences.

The application of cognitive-behavioral theory within educational programs promotes an education-learning focus rather than an illness-treatment focus and is compatible with the environment of many health and community settings. It, too, is proactive and promotes the attitude that life is a lifelong process of learning. In addition, an education or learning model is well suited to the area of prevention: a specialty that continues to be of interest to the occupational therapist.

The occupational therapist has adopted or adapted components of cognitive-behavioral strategies to enhance patients'/clients' basic knowledge and skills for personal self-care, social interaction, fitness, and work-leisure performance.

Problem-Solving Formats

The problem-solving formats that have evolved from cognitive-behavioral study are highly applicable to the work of occupational therapists in many environments, and especially those in which cognitive impairments, impulsive behaviors, and limited experience have made it difficult for clients to succeed in novel or familiar situations. One could, for example, use these principles to help coach head-injured clients trying to resume employment or teach aides or volunteers to be coaches. Because clients, both child and adult, help set and evaluate their own goals for the therapy experience, intervention can be individualized to meet the specific concerns of the client/learner. This, in turn, is expected to be more meaningful and motivating to the client. One could justifiably refer to this as a learner-centered or student-centered model.

Learning Process Is Facilitated

The educational strategies used in cognitive-behavioral intervention support "doing" or action through activities that provide graded challenges. This idea of grading tasks has been applied consistently by occupational therapists and is something that is enhanced by our expertise in task and activity analysis. Using graded tasks, modeling of gradual mastery, and homework, along with other techniques, promotes success and builds feelings of self-efficacy. If, as we contend, our goal in occupational therapy is to enable the client to be as independent and successful as he or she wishes to be, then these strategies appear to be very consistent with our mission.

The educational model promotes group intervention. Groups have been recognized as cost- and time-effective, as well as a useful vehicle for providing participants the opportunity to give to and support one another. The cognitive-behavioral frame of reference has the goal of promoting generalization, a goal clearly necessary if independence and reduced length of intervention is desired. Whether or not generalization is necessarily an outcome of education and intervention, however, is not so clear and needs to be pursued in research.

Limitations

Difficult to Document Change in Beliefs

The cognitive behaviorist says that improved performance is not enough—one must "think" differently. In the current climate of health care, community, and school intervention, the mandate for occupational therapy is to demonstrate improvements in client function; therefore, the therapist using this model is in somewhat of a dilemma. He or she may assume that beliefs have changed but whether and how to demonstrate (and document) this is another matter. In recent years, study in the fields of psychology, education, and medicine have broadened the definition of cognition and have increased our understanding of the growth, development, and function of cognition; however, much needs to be learned. We do not yet understand to what extent physiology, biology, heredity, environment, and experience contribute to cognitive growth, development, and performance. Although we know that cognition is a complex interactive process, we do not fully understand the interaction of the physical, environmental/contextual, and psychosocial factors as they impact occupational performance through the life span.

Limited Contribution to Understanding of Adult Cognitive Development

We do know that changes in cognition occur slowly and in a manner similar enough to be conceived as stage specific. Most research, however, has been in the area of child development. Researchers now must ask, "What factors influence cognitive development, knowledge acquisition, the evolution of beliefs, and performance during the adult years?" The burgeoning interest in education in the adult learner is an exciting development that may offer occupational therapists vital information about how to best meet the learning needs of their adult clients.

Given the status of theoretical development and research, the occupational therapist must acknowledge these limitations and the speculative aspect of practice. Questions that arise include how can the therapist easily and accurately assess and identify problems related to cognition and beliefs, and should this therapist try to assess this? To date, few cognitive-behavioral assessment tools have been developed in occupational therapy. Of those available in the field of psychology, most are more appropriately given by a psychologist. Future assessment tools must be able to help determine whether a particular cognitive skill has or has not been acquired. Cognitive performance may be identified with a particular developmental level but there are many degrees of function within that level; therefore, the therapist must determine whether the learner lacks knowledge or skill, whether he or she has adequate knowledge and skills but refuses to use them, or whether the person has knowledge and skills but uses them infrequently. When planning or supporting intervention with an individual or group, the therapist continues to ask, "What really influences the nature of and the growth rate of cognition? What strategies can enhance cognitive ability and performance?" Because science does not know exactly what happens between the presentation of a problem and the individual's response, it is difficult to accurately assess the impact of cognitive–behavioral strategies in the long run. We suppose, for example, that problem solving improves in future situations but we depend primarily on decreased recidivism as evidence of that.

Clients Need the Ability to Use Language

In addition to the previous issues, the occupational therapist must consider and ask, "Do participants need to function at a 'high' level to benefit from a cognitive approach?" It would appear that one could answer, "Not necessarily," although an expectation around the meaningful use of language exists. Is there perhaps a bottom or lower limit, a developmental age or level of cognitive ability that must be met for cognitive-behavioral strategies to be practical? The literature would suggest "yes," and this would be a developmental age of around 7. It is at this developmental age that we could expect the client to have the necessary abilities to sustain attention and verbalize thoughts and beliefs within learning experiences. When clients have information-processing problems, however, as one might see with head injury, vascular compromise, and mental illness, there is not this clear-cut developmental marker. Therapists might be left in the position of experimenting or trying cognitive-behavioral strategies to see what does and doesn't work. As with other frames of reference, the research available in the occupational therapy literature that describes the application of cognitive-behavioral learning strategies with persons who are cognitively compromised is limited. The nature of cognitive impairments is that they are unique to the person; therefore, they need individualized learning approaches and we could expect that performance-enhancing strategies based upon cognitive-behavior theory could be developed, used during interventions, then evaluated for their efficacy. Individualized strategy training is consistent with the findings and recommendation of occupational therapist Joan Toglia and discussed in Chapter Nine of this text.

Question if Compatible with Time Available for Intervention

Finally, we must pose a very practical question: Can the occupational therapist expect to have the time for intervention that is necessary to bring about enhanced knowledge, changes in beliefs, and the acquisition of new problem-solving strategies? An assumption of this model is that cognitive change takes time.

There is no simple answer. We know that in many direct care settings we have a role as teacher and, in fact, that educating our client (and families) so they can become responsible for carrying out recommendations is a vital role. In helping clients transition from the rehabilitation to home settings, for example, the therapist frequently provides the client/patient with a home program. Sometimes the time we are given to do this education is very short. In that respect, it would appear that any teaching tools that we have in our repertoire would be of potential benefit to us. As consultants, we can offer our expertise to care-providers, case managers, family members, residential supervisors, employers, and others to help them to create an optimum learning environment and/or design and carry out educational programming expected to lead to enhanced functional performance by persons in need. As occupational therapists, we know the nature of occupation and the vital place it has in health maintenance, prevention, and quality of life for persons of all abilities, especially those who have physical and emotional challenges. We can recommend adaptations that can facilitate these persons' engagement in meaningful occupation. If we can bring that expertise as well as knowledge of cognitive-behavioral strategies to such non-traditional settings and programs as those for prevention and health maintenance, outdoor adventure programs, to organizations like the Clubhouse, whose outreach is to the chronically mentally ill, and to after school programs for youth at risk, then we may find a context in which we have the time to fully develop occupational therapy based upon a cognitive-behavioral model.

REFERENCES

Allen, C. K. (1985). *Occupational therapy for psychiatric diseases: Measurement and management of cognitive disabilities.* Boston, MA: Little, Brown and Co.

Allen, C. K. (1994). Creating a need-satisfying, safe environment: Management and maintenance approaches. In C. B. Royeen (Ed.), *AOTA self-study series: Cognitive rehabilitation.* Bethesda, MD: American Occupational Therapy Association.

Allen, C. K., & Blue, T. (1998). Cognitive disabilities model: How to make clinical judgments. In N. Katz (Ed.), *Cognition and occupation in rehabilitation: Cognitive models for intervention in occupational therapy.* Bethesda, MD: American Occupational Therapy Association.

Arnold, M. (1960). *Emotion and personality, 2 volumes.* New York, NY: Columbia University.

Bandura, A. (1977). *Social learning theory* (pp. 97, 204). Englewood Cliffs, NJ: Prentice–Hall.

Banks, S., Crossman, D., Boel, S., & Stewart, M. (1997). Partnerships among health professionals and self-help group members. *Can J Occup Ther, 64,* 259-269.

Bara, B. (1984). Modifications of knowledge by memory processes. In M. Reda & M. Mahoney (Eds.), *Cognitive psychotherapies.* Cambridge, MA: Ballinger Publishing Co.

Beck, A. T. (1976). *Cognitive therapy and the emotional disorders.* New York, NY: International Universities Press.

Beck, A. T. (1997). Cognitive therapy: Reflections. In J. K. Zeig (Ed.), *The evolution of psychotherapy—The third conference* (pp. 55-67). New York, NY: Brunner/Mazel.

Beck, A. T., & Haaga, D. A. (1992). The future of cognitive therapy. *Psychotherapy: Theory, Research, Practice, Training, 29,* 34-38.

Beck, A. T., Rush, A., & Kovacs, M. (1976). *Individual treatment manual for cognitive/behavioral psychotherapy of depression.* Philadelphia, PA: University of Pennsylvania Press.

Beck, A. T., Rush, A., Shaw, B., & Emery, G. (1979). *Cognitive therapy of depression* (p. 3). New York, NY: Guilford Press.

Beck, A. T., Steer, R. A., Epleen, N., & Brown, G. (1990). Beck self-concept test. *Psychological assessment, American Psychological Association, June,* 191-197.

Beck, A. T., & Weishaar, M. (1994). Cognitive therapy. In R. Corsini & D. Wedding (Eds.), *Current psychotherapies* (4th ed.). Itasca, IL: Peacock.

Beck, A. T., & Weissman, A. (1974). The measurement of pessimism: The hopelessness scale. *J Consult Clin Psychol, 42,* 861-865.

Blackburn, I. M., & Twaddle, V. (1996). *Cognitive therapy in action.* London: Souvenir Press.

Bodenham, J. (1988). Rehabilitation of long-term mentally handicapped in community housing. In D. W. Scott & N. Katz (Eds.), *Occupational therapy in mental health—Principles in practice.* London: Taylor and Francis.

Bower, S. A., & Bower, G. H. (1992). *Asserting yourself: A practical guide for positive change.* Reading, MA: Addison-Wesley.

Bowlby, J. (1977a). The making and breaking of affectional bonds. I. Etiology and psychopathology in the light of attachment theory. *Br J Psychiatry, 130,* 201-210.

Bowlby, J. (1977b). The making and breaking of affectional bonds. II. Some principles of psychotherapy. *Br J Psychiatry, 130,* 421-431.

Bradlee, L. (1984). The use of groups in short-term psychiatric settings. *Occupational Therapy in Mental Health, 4,* 47-57.

Brownell, K. D., & Fairburn, C. G. (1995). *Eating disorders and obesity.* New York, NY: Guilford Press.

Buning, M. E. (1999). Fitness for person with disabilities—A call to action. *OT Practice, 4,* 27-31.

Campbell, A., & McCreadie, R. (1988). Occupational therapy is effective for chronic schizophrenic day patients. *British Journal of Occupational Therapy, 49,* 327-328.

Chesney, A. B., & Brorsen, N. E. (2000). Occupational therapy's role in managing chronic pain. *OT Practice, 5,* 10-13.

Christiansen, C., & Baum, C. (1991). *Occupational therapy: Overcoming human performance deficits.* Thorofare, NJ: SLACK Incorporated.

Christiansen, C., & Baum, C. (Eds.). (1997). *Occupational therapy—Enabling function and well-being* (2nd ed.). Thorofare, NJ: SLACK Incorporated.

Clagett, A. F. (1989). Effective therapeutic wilderness camp programs for rehabilitating emotionally disturbed, problem teenagers, and delinquents. *Journal of Offender Counseling, 11,* 79-86.

Clagett, A. F. (1992). Group-integrated reality therapy in a wilderness camp. *Journal of Offender Rehabilitation, 17,* 1-18.

Cole, M. B. (1998). *Group dynamics in occupational therapy: The theoretical basis and practice application of group treatment* (2nd ed.). Thorofare, NJ: SLACK Incorporated.

Conte, J., & Conte, W. (1977). The use of conceptual models in occupational therapy. *Am J Occup Ther, 31,* 262-265.

Corey, G. (1979). *Theory and practice of counseling and psychotherapy* (pp. 173, 176). Monterey, CA: Brooks/Cole Publishing Co.

Corey, G. (2000). *Theory and practice of group counseling* (5th ed.). Bellmont, CA: Wadsworth/Thomas Learning.

Cox, D. L., & Findley, L. T. (1998). The management of chronic fatigue syndrome in an inpatient setting: Presentation of an approach and perceived outcome. *British Journal of Occupational Therapy, 61,* 405-409.

Crist, P. H. (1986). Community living skills: A psychoeducational community based program. *Occupational Therapy in Mental Health, 6*(2), 51-64.

Crist, P. H. (1999). Community living skills: A psychoeducational community-based program. *Occupational Therapy in Mental Health, 6,* 51-64.

Davidson, G. (1969). Behavior modification techniques in institutional settings. In C. Franks (Ed.), *Behavior therapy: Appraisal and status* (pp. 220-278). New York, NY: McGraw-Hill.

Davis, J., & Kutter, J. (1997). Independent living skills and post-traumatic stress disorder in women who are homeless: Implications for future practice. *Am J Occup Ther, 52,* 39-44.

Davis-Berman, J. L., Berman, D. S., & Capone, L. (1994). Therapeutic wilderness programs: A national survey. *Journal of Experiential Education, 17,* 49-53.

DCD Research Group. (1995). *CO-OP: Cognitive orientation to daily occupational performance.* Unpublished manuscript, University of Western Ontario, London, Ontario, Canada.

Deale, A., Chaider, T., Marks, I., & Wessely, S. (1997). Cognitive behavior therapy for chronic fatigue syndrome, a randomized controlled trial. *Am J Psychiatry, 154,* 408-414.

DeMars, P. (1992). An occupational therapy life skills curriculum model for a native American tribe: A health promotion program based on ethnographic field research. *Am J Occup Ther, 46,* 727-736.

Diamond, H. (1998). Vocational decision making in a psychiatric outpatient program. *Occupational Therapy in Mental Health, 14,* 67-80.

Donaldson, G. (1997). Work programmes to enhance cognitive performance components. In J. Pratt & K. Jacobs (Eds.), *Work practice* (pp. 145-223). Boston, MA: Butterworth Heinemann.

Drouet, V. (1986). Individual behavioral programme planning with long-stay patients. Part 1: Programmes planned and followed in an occupational therapy department. Part 2: Social skills training. *British Journal of Occupational Therapy, 49,* 227-232.

Dryden, W. (1984). Rational emotive therapy and cognitive therapy: A critical comparison. In M. Reda & M. Mahoney (Eds.), *Cognitive psychotherapies.* Cambridge, MA: Ballinger Publishing Co.

Duncombe, L. (1998). The cognitive-behavioral model in mental health. In N. Katz (Ed.), *Cognition and occupation in rehabilitation* (pp. 165-192). Bethesda, MD: American Occupational Therapy Association.

Dunn, W., Brown, C., McClain, L., & Westman, K. (1994). The ecology of human performance: A contextual perspective on human occupation. In C. B. Royeen (Ed.), *AOTA self-study series—The practice of future: Putting occupation back into therapy.* Rockville, MD: American Occupational Therapy Association.

D'Zurilla, R., & Goldfried, M. (1971). Problem solving and behavior modification. *J Abnorm Psychol, 78,* 107-126.

D'Zurilla, T. J., & Nezu, A. M. (1999). *Problem-solving therapy—A social competence approach to clinical intervention.* New York, NY: Springer Publishing Co.

Eilenberg, A. (1986). An expanded community role for occupational therapy: Prevention depression. *Physical and Occupational Therapy in Geriatrics, 5,* 47-57.

Ellis, A. (1962). *Reason and emotion in psychotherapy.* Secaucus, NJ: Citadel.

Ellis, A. (1973). *Humanistic psychology: The rational emotive approach.* New York, NY: Harper and Row.

Ellis, A. (1975). *A new guide to rational living.* New York, NY: Harper and Row.

Ellis, A. (1979). The theory of rational emotive therapy. In A. Ellis & J. Whiteley (Eds.), *Theoretical and empirical foundations of rational emotive therapy* (pp. 33-60). Monterey, CA: Brooks/Cole.

Ellis, A. (1988). *How to stubbornly refuse to make yourself miserable about anything—Yes, anything!* Secaucus, NJ: Lyle Stuart.

Ellis, A. (1993a). Changing rational emotive therapy (RET) to rational emotive behavior therapy (RETB). *Behavior Therapist, 16,* 257-258.

Ellis, A. (1993b). Fundamentals of rational emotive therapy for the 1900s. In W. Dryden & L. K. Hill (Eds.), *Innovations in rational emotive therapy* (pp. 1-32). Newbury Park, CA: Sage.

Ellis, A. (1994). *Reason and emotion in psychotherapy (Revised and updated).* New York, NY: Birch Lane Press.

Ellis, A. (1996). Responses to criticisms of rational emotive behavior therapy by Ray DiGuiseppe, Frank Boyd, Windy Dryden, Steven Weinrach, & Richard Wessler. *Journal of Rational Emotive and Cognitive Behavior Therapy, 14,* 97-122.

Ellis, A., & Dryden, W. (1997). *The practice of rational emotive therapy* (2nd ed.). New York, NY: Springer.

Ellis, A., & Whiteley, J. (1979). *Theoretical and empirical foundations of rational emotive therapy.* Monterey, CA: Brooks/Cole.

Engel, J. (1992). Social validation of relaxation training in pediatric headache control. *Occupational Therapy in Mental Health, 11,* 77-90.

Engel, J., & Rapoff, M. (1990). Biofeedback-assisted relaxation training for adult and pediatric headache disorders. *Occupational Therapy Journal of Research, 10,* 283-299.

Fairweather, B. (1984). *Social psychology in treating mental illness: An experimental approach.* New York, NY: John Wiley.

Fidler, G. (1969). The task-oriented group as a context for treatment. *Am J Occup Ther, 11,* 43-48.

Fine, S., & Schwimmer, P. (1986). The effects of occupational therapy on independent living skills. *Mental Health Special Interest Section Newsletter, 9,* 2-3.

Firestein, R., & Treffinger, D. (1983). Ownership and converging: Essential ingredients of creative problem solving. *Journal of Creative Behavior, 17*(1), 32-28.

Flaherty, J. (1999). Community-based psychiatric services: A focus on function. *Mental Health, Special Interest Section Quarterly, 22,* 1-4.

Flavell, J. (1985). *Cognitive development* (2nd ed.). Englewood Cliffs, NJ: Prentice Hall.

Follette, V. M., Ruzek, J. I., & Abueg, F. R. (Eds.). (1998). *Cognitive-behavior therapies for trauma.* New York, NY: Guilford Press.

Folts, D. (1988). Social skills training. In D. W. Scott & N. Katz (Eds.), *Occupational therapy in mental health—Principles in practice*. London: Taylor and Francis.

Frame, C., Johnstone, B., & Giblin, M. S. (1988). Dysthymia. In M. Herson & C. G. Last (Eds.), *Child behavior therapy casebook* (pp. 63-81). New York, NY: Plenum Press.

Frame, C., Matson, J., Sonis, W. A., Fialkov, M. J., & Kazdin, A. E. (1982). Behavioral treatment of depression in a prepubertal child. *J Behav Ther Exp Psychiatry, 3,* 239-243.

Friedlob, S., Janis, G., & Deets-Aron, C. (1986). A hospital connected half-way house program for individuals with long-term neuropsychiatric disabilities. *Am J Occup Ther, 40,* 271-277.

Giles, G. (1985). Anorexia nervosa and bulimia: An activity-oriented approach. *Am J Occup Ther, 39,* 510-517.

Giles, G. M., & Allen, M. E. (1986). Occupational therapy in the rehabilitation of the patient with anorexia nervosa. *Occupational Therapy in Mental Health, 6,* 47-66.

Goldfried, M. (1971). Systematic desensitization as training in self-control. *J Consult Clin Psychol, 37,* 228-234.

Goldfried, M. (1980). Psychotherapy as coping skills training. In M. Mahoney (Ed.), *Psychotherapy process*. New York, NY: Plenum Press.

Goldstein, A. (1973). *Structured learning therapy: Toward a psychotherapy for the poor.* New York, NY: Academic Press.

Greenberg, L., Fine, S., Cohen, C., Larson, K., Michaelson-Baily, A., Rubinton, P., & Glick, I. (1988). An interdisciplinary psychoeducation program for schizophrenic patients and their families in an acute care setting. *Hospital and Community Psychiatry, 38,* 277-282.

Grilo, C. M., Brownell, K. D., & Stunkard, A. J. (1993). The metabolic and psychological importance of exercise in weight control. In A. J. Stunkard & T. A. Wadden (Eds.), *Obesity. Theory and therapy* (2nd ed., pp. 253-273). New York, NY: Raven Press.

Guidano, V. F. (1987). *Complexity of the self: A developmental approach to psychopathology and therapy.* New York, NY: Guilford Press.

Guidano, V., & Liotti, G. (1983). *Cognitive processes and emotional disorders* (pp. 131, 150). New York, NY: Guilford Press.

Gutterman, L. (1991). Day treatment program for persons with AIDS. *Am J Occup Ther, 44,* 3.

Hallahan, D. P., Kneedler, R., & Lloyd, J. (1983). Cognitive behavior modification for learning disabled children: Self-instruction and self-monitoring. In J. D. McKinney & L. Feagans (Eds.), *Current topics in learning disabilities* (pp. 207-244). Norwood, NJ: Ablex Publishing.

Hamilton, M. (1960). A rating scale for depression. *J Neurol Neurosurg Psychiatry, 23,* 56-61.

Hayes, R. (1989). Occupational therapy in the treatment of schizophrenia. *Occupational Therapy in Mental Health, 9,* 51-68.

Henderson, S. (1998). Frames of reference utilized in the rehabilitation of individuals with eating disorders. *Can J Occup Ther, 66,* 43-51.

Hewett, F., & Forness, S. (1984). *Education of exceptional learners* (p. 86). Boston, MA: Allyn and Bacon.

Isaksen, S., Dorval, K. B., & Treffinger, D. (1994). *Creative approaches to problem-solving.* Dubuque, IA: Kendall/Hunt.

Jao, H. I., & Lu, S. J. (1999). The acquisition of problem-solving skills through the instruction in Siegel and Spivack's problem solving therapy for the chronic schizophrenic. *Occupational Therapy in Mental Health, 14,* 47-63.

Johnson, M. (1986). Use of cognitive behavioral techniques with depressed adults in day treatment. *Depression: Assessment and update: Proceedings.* Bethesda, MD: American Occupational Therapy Association.

Johnson, M. (1987). Occupational therapist and the teaching of cognitive behavioral skills. *Occupational Therapy in Mental Health, 7,* 69-81.

Katz, N. (Ed.). (1998). *Cognition and occupation in rehabilitation.* Bethesda, MD: American Occupational Therapy Association.

Kaufman, C. H., Daniels, R. D., Laverdure, P. A., Moyer, R., & Campana, L. (1988). Pediatric occupational therapy within a cognitive-behavioral setting. In D. W. Scott & N. Katz (Eds.), *Occupational therapy in mental health—Principles in practice.* London: Taylor and Francis.

Kazdin, A. (1974). Effects of covert modeling and modeling reinforcement on assertive behavior. *J Abnorm Psychol, 83,* 240-252.

Keller-Mathers, S., & Puccio, K. (1998). *Big tools for young thinkers: Using creative problem-solving tools with primary students.* Sarasota, FL: Center for Creative Learning.

Kelly, G. (1955). *The psychotherapy of personal constructs.* New York, NY: Norton.

Kendal, P. C. (1993). Cognitive behavioural therapies with youth: Guiding theory, current status, and emerging developments. *J Consult Clin Psychol, 61,* 235-247

Kielhofner, G. (1995). *A model of human occupation* (2nd ed.). Baltimore, MD: Williams & Wilkins.

Koestler, F. (Ed.). (1970). *Reference handbook for continuing education in occupational therapy.* Dubuque, IA: Kendall/Hunt Publishing Co.

Kohn, P. M., & MacDonald, J. E. (1992). The survey of recent life experiences: A decontaminated hassles scale for adults. *J Behav Med, 2,* 221-236.

Kolko, D. (1992). Conduct disorder. In V. B. Van Hasselt & D. Kolko (Eds.), *Inpatient behavior therapy for children and adolescents.* New York, NY: Plenum Press.

Kottman, T. (1999a). Group application of Allerian play therapy. In D. S. Sweeney & L. E. Homeger (Eds.), *The handbook of group play therapy: How to do it, how it works, whom its best for* (pp. 65-85). San Francisco, CA: Jossey-Bass, Inc.

Kottman, T. (1999b). Play therapy. In R. E. Watts & J. Carlson (Eds.), *Interventions and strategies in counseling and psychotherapy* (pp. 161-179). Philadelphia, PA: Accelerated Development, Inc.

Kramer, L. (1984). SCORE: Solving community obstacles and restoring employment. *Occupational Therapy in Mental Health, 4*(1), 1-135.

Landry, S. H., Robinson, S. S., Copeland, D., & Garner, P. W. (1993). Goal-directed behavior and perception of self-competence in children with spina bifida. *J Pediatr Psychol, 18,* 389-396.

Lang, P. (1969). The mechanics of desensitization and the laboratory study of human fears. In C. Franks (Ed.), *Assessment and status of the behavior therapies*. New York, NY: McGraw-Hill Book Co.

Law, M., Baptiste, S., Carswell, A., McColl, M. A., Polatajko, H., & Pollock, N. (1994). *Canadian Occupational Performance Measure* (2nd ed.). Toronto, Ontario: CAOT Publications.

Law, M., Cooper, B., Strong, S., Stewart, D., Rigby, P., & Letts, L. (1996). The person-environment-occupation model: A transactive approach to occupational performance. *Can J Occup Ther, 3*, 9-23.

Lazarus, A. (1976). *Multimodal behavior therapy*. New York, NY: Springer.

Lazarus, A. (1971). *Behavior therapy and beyond*. New York, NY: McGraw Hill.

Leeds, S. (1999). Rational emotive adventure challenge therapy. In C. Schaefer (Ed.), *Innovative psychotherapy techniques in child and adolescent therapy* (2nd ed., pp. 189-228). New York, NY: John Wiley & Sons, Inc.

Lenters, D. H. (1999). Creating a thriving mental health program. *OT Practice, 4*, 49-51.

Lewin, J., & Reed, C. (1998). *Creative problem solving in occupational therapy*. Philadelphia, PA: Lippincott, Williams & Wilkins.

Lidz, T. (1985). Adolf Meyer and the development of American psychiatry. *Occupational Therapy in Mental Health, 5*, 33-53.

Lillie, M., & Armstrong, H. (1982). Contributions to the development of psychoeducation approaches to mental health service. *Am J Occup Ther, 36*(7), 438-443.

Lindsay, W. (1983). The role of the occupational therapist in the treatment of alcoholism. *Am J Occup Ther, 37*, 36-43.

Linroth, R., Zander, S., Forde, S., Hanley, M., & Lins, J. (1996). Ramsey county day treatment services: Day treatment to extended day treatment centers to focus groups. *Occupational Therapy in Health Care, 10*, 89-103.

Luria, A. R. (1973). *The working brain: An introduction to neuropsychology*. New York, NY: Basic Books.

Luria, A. R. (1980). *Higher cortical functions in man* (2nd ed.). New York, NY: Basic Books.

Mahoney, M. (1974). *Cognition and behavior modification*. Cambridge, MA: Ballinger Publishing Co.

Mahoney, M. (1976). *Scientist as subject: The psychological imperative*. Cambridge, MA: Ballinger Publishing Co.

Mahoney, M. (1977). Personal science: A cognitive learning therapy. In A. Ellis & R. Greiger (Eds.), *Handbook of rational psychotherapy*. New York, NY: Springer Verlag.

Mahoney, M., & Arnkoff, D. (1974). Cognitive and self-control therapies. In S. Garfield & A. Bergin (Eds.), *Handbook of psychotherapy and behavior change* (2nd ed.). New York, NY: Wiley.

Mahoney, M., & DeMonbreun, B. (1977). Psychology of the scientist: An analysis of problem-solving biases. *Cognitive Therapy Research, 1*, 229-238.

Marlatt, G. G. (1995). Relapse: A cognitive-behavioral model. In K. D. Brownell & C. G. Fairburn (Eds.), *Eating disorders and obesity—A comprehensive handbook* (pp. 541-546). New York, NY: Guilford Press.

Maultsby, M. (1971). Systematic written homework in psychotherapy. *Rational Living, 6*, 17-23.

McCrady, B. (1994). Alcoholics Anonymous and behavior therapy: Can habits be treated as diseases? Can disease be treated as habits? *J Consult Clin Psychol, 62*(6), 1159-1166.

McClusky, K., Place, D., McCluskey, A., & Treffinger, D. (1998). CPS gives aboriginal inmates a second chance. *Communique* (Vol. VI, p. 104). Buffalo, NY: Creative Problem Solving Group.

Meichenbaum, D. (1973). Cognitive factors in behavior modification: Modifying what clients say to themselves. In C. Franks & G. Wilson (Eds.), *Annual review of behavior therapy: Theory and practice* (Vol. 1, pp. 416-431). New York, NY: Brunner/Mazel.

Meichenbaum, D. (1977). *Cognitive behavior modification*. New York, NY: Plenum Press.

Meichenbaum, D. (1979). *Cognitive behavior modification: An integrative approach*. New York, NY: Plenum Press.

Meichenbaum, D. (1985). *Stress inoculation training*. New York, NY: Pergamon Press.

Meichenbaum, D. (1986). Cognitive behavior modification. In F. H. Kanfer & A. P. Goldstein (Eds.), *Helping people change: A textbook of methods* (3rd ed.). New York, NY: Pergamon Press.

Meichenbaum, D. (1991). *Cognitive behavior modification*. Workshop presented at Child and Parent Research Institute Symposium, November, London, Ontario, Canada.

Meichenbaum, D., & Biemiller, A. (1998). *Nurturing independent learners: Helping students take charge of their learning*. Cambridge, MA: Brookline Books.

Meyer, A. (1922). The philosophy of occupation therapy. *Archives of Occupational Therapy, 1*, 1-10.

Mischel, W. (1968). *Personality and assessment*. New York, NY: Wiley.

Missiuna, C., Malloy-Miller, T., & Mandich, A. (1998). Mediational techniques: Origins and application to occupational therapy in paediatrics. *Can J Occup Ther, 65*, 202-209.

Missiuna, C., & Pollock, N. (2000). Perceived efficacy and goal setting in young children. *Can J Occup Ther, 67*, 101-109.

Missiuna, C., & Samuels, M. (1989). Dynamic assessment of preschool children with special needs: Comparison of mediation and instruction. *Remedial and Special Education, 10*, 53-62.

Mosey, A. C. (1974). An alternative: The biopsychosocial model. *Am J Occup Ther, 28*, 137-140.

Moyers, P. (1988). An organizational framework for occupational therapy in the treatment of alcoholism. *Occupational Therapy in Mental Health, 8*, 27-46.

Nadler, R. S. (1995). Edgework: Stretching boundaries and generalizing experiences. *Journal of Experiential Education, 18*, 52-55.

Neistadt, M., & Marques, K. (1984). An independent living skills training program. *Am J Occup Ther, 38*(10), 671-676.

Nickel, L. (1988). Adapting structured learning therapy for use in a psychiatric adult day hospital. *Can J Occup Ther, 55*, 21-25.

Nowicki, S., & Strickland, B. R. (1973). A locus of control scale for children. *Journal of Consulting and Clinical Psychology, 40*, 148-154.

Olmsted, M. P., & Kaplan, A. S. (1995). Psychoeducation in the treatment of eating disorders. In K. D. Brownell & C. G. Fairburn (Eds.), *Eating disorders and obesity* (pp. 299-305). New York, NY: Guilford Press.

Osborn, A. (1963). *Applied imagination* (3rd ed. rev.). New York, NY: Charles Scribner's Sons.

Parnes, S. (1992). *Visionizing*. New York, NY: Creative Education Foundation Press.

Perry, A., Tarrier, N., Morriss, R., McCarthy, E., & Limb, K. (1999). Randomized controlled trial of efficacy of teaching patients with bipolar disorder to identify early symptoms of relapse and obtain treatment. *BMJ, 318*, 149-153.

Perry, D., & Bussey, K. (1984). *Social development* (p. 123). Englewood Cliffs, NJ: Prentice-Hall.

Petti, T. A., Bornstein, M., Delamater, A., & Conner, C. K. (1980). Evaluation and multimodality treatment of a depressed prepubertal girl. *J Am Acad Child Adolesc Psychiatry, 19*, 690-702.

Piaget, J. (1972). Intellectual evolution from adolescence to adulthood. *Human development—volume 1* (pp. 1-12). Switzerland: S. Karges.

Place, D., & McCluskey, A. (1995). Second chance: A program to support native inmates at risk. In K. W. McCluskey, P. A. Baker, S. C. O'Hagan, & D. J. Treffinger (Eds.), *Lost prizes: Talent development and problem solving with at-risk students* (pp. 137-146). Sarasota, FL: Center for Creative Learning.

Precin, P. (1999). *Living skills recovery workbook*. Boston, MA: Butterworth Heinemann.

Puccio, K., Keller-Mathers, S., & Treffinger, D. (1998). *Adventures in problem-solving (Grades K-3)*. Sarasota, FL: Center for Creative Learning.

Rathjen, D., Rathjen, E., & Hiniker, A. (1978). A cognitive analysis of social performance: Implications for assessment and treatment. In J. Foreyt & D. Rathjen (Eds.), *Cognitive behavior therapy*. New York, NY: Plenum Press.

Reda, M., & Mahoney, M. (1984). *Cognitive psychotherapies*. Cambridge, MA: Ballinger Publishing Co.

Robinson, J., & Shaver, P. (1973). *Measures of social psychological attitudes* (pp. 227-231). Ann Arbor, MI: Institute of Social Research.

Rosenthal, R., & Bandura, A. (1978). Psychological modeling: Theory and practice. In S. Garfield & A. Bergin (Eds.), *Handbook of psychotherapy and behavior change*. New York, NY: Wiley.

Roth, D. (1986). Treatment of the hospitalized eating disorder patient. *Occupational Therapy in Mental Health, 6*, 67-87.

Rotter, J. B. (1966). Generalized expectancies for internal versus external control of reinforcement. *Psychological Monographs, 80*, 1-28.

Rynne, A., & McKenna, K. (1999). Evaluation of an outpatient diabetes education programme. *British Journal of Occupational Therapy, 62*, 459-465.

Salo-Chydenius, S. (1996). Changing helplessness to coping: An exploratory study of social skills training with individuals with long-term mental illness. *Occupational Therapy in Mental Health, 8*, 21-30.

Schaefer, C. (Ed.). (1999). *Innovative psychotherapy techniques in child and adolescent therapy* (2nd ed.). New York, NY: John Wiley & Sons, Inc.

Sharpe, M., Hawton, K., Simkin, S., Surawy, C., Hackmann, A., Ivana, K., Peto, T., Warrell, D., & Seagroatt, V. (1996). Cognitive behaviour therapy for the chronic fatigue syndrome: A randomized controlled trial. *BMJ, 312*, 22-26.

Sladyk, K. (1990). Teaching safe sex practices to psychiatric patients. *Am J Occup Ther, 44*(3), 284-285.

Spielberger, C. D., Gorsuch, R. L., Lushene, R., Vagg, P. R., & Jacobs, G. A. (1983). *Manual for the state Trait Anxiety Inventory*. Palo Alto, CA: Consulting Psychological Press.

Spivack, G., Platt, J., & Shure, M. (1976). *The problem-solving approach to adjustment*. San Francisco, CA: Jossey-Bass.

Stark, K., Rouse, L., & Kurowski, C. (1994). Psychological treatment approaches for depression in children. In W. M. Reynolds & H. F. Johnson (Eds.), *Handbook of depression in children and adolescents* (pp. 275-307). New York, NY: Plenum Press.

Stein, F., Bentley, D. E., & Natz, M. (1999). Computerized assessment: The stress management questionnaire. In B. J. Hemphill-Pearson (Ed.), *Assessments in occupational therapy mental health*. Thorofare, NJ: SLACK Incorporated.

Stein, F., & Cutler, S. K. (1998). *Psychosocial occupational therapy*. San Diego, CA: Singular Publishing Group, Inc.

Stein, F., & Nikolic, S. (1989). Teaching stress management techniques to a schizophrenic patient. *Am J Occup Ther, 43*, 162-169.

Stein, F., & Smith, J. (1989). Short-term stress management programme with acutely depressed in-patients. *Can J Occup Ther, 56*, 185-191.

Stockwell, R., Duncan, S., & Levens, M. (1988). Occupational therapy with eating disorders. In D. W. Scott & N. Katz (Eds.), *Occupational therapy in mental health—Principles in practice*. London: Taylor and Francis.

Stoffel, V. (1994). Occupational therapists' roles in treating substance abuse. *Hospital and Community Psychiatry, 45*, 21-22.

Stone, G. (1980). *A cognitive-behavioral approach to counseling psychology*. New York, NY: Praeger Publishers.

Suinn, R., & Richardson, F. (1971). Anxiety management training: A nonspecific behavior therapy program for anxiety control. *Behav Res Ther, 2*, 510.

Taylor, E. (1988). Anger intervention. *Am J Occup Ther, 42*, 127-155.

Toglia, J. P., & Golisz, K. (1990). *Cognitive rehabilitation: Group games and activities*. Tuscon, AZ: Therapy Skill Builders.

Treffinger, D. (1996). *Creative problem solving and school improvement*. Sarasota, FL: Center for Creative Learning.

Vernon, A. (1989a). *Help yourself to a healthier you*. Minneapolis, MN: Burgess.

Vernon, A. (1989b). *Thinking, feeling, behaving—An emotional education curriculum for children grades 1-6.* Champaign, IL: Research Press.

Vernon, A. (1989c). *Thinking, feeling, behaving—An emotional education curriculum for children grades 7-12.* Champaign, IL: Research Press.

Vernon, A. (1998a). *The Passport program: A journey through emotional, social, cognitive and self-development, grade 1-5.* Champaign, IL: Research Press.

Vernon, A. (1998b). *The Passport program: A journey through emotional, social, cognitive and self-development, grade 6-8.* Champaign, IL: Research Press.

Vernon, A. (1998c). *The Passport program: A journey through emotional, social, cognitive and self-development, grade 9-12.* Champaign, IL: Research Press.

Vernon, A. (1999a). Application of rational emotive behavior therapy with children and adolescents. In A. Vernon (Ed.), *Counseling children and adolescents* (2nd ed., pp. 139-158). Denver, CO: Love Publishing Co.

Vernon, A. (Ed.). (1999b). *Counseling children and adolescents* (2nd ed.). Denver, CO: Love Publishing Co.

Vitousek, K. B. (1995). Cognitive-behavioral therapy for anorexia nervosa. In K. D. Brownell & C. G. Fairburn (Eds.), *Eating disorders and obesity* (pp. 324-329). New York, NY: Guilford Press.

Vygotsky, L. S. (1962). *Thought and language.* Cambridge, MA: MIT.

Vygotsky, L. S. (1987). *Mind in society: The development of higher psychological processes.* Cambridge, MA: Harvard University.

Walker, S. N., Sechrist, K. R., & Pender, N. J. (1987). The health-promoting lifestyle profile: Development and psychometric characteristics. *Nurs Res, 36,* 76-81.

Weinstein, B. D., & DeNeff, L. S. (1989). Hemophilia, AIDS, and occupational therapy. *Am J Occup Ther, 44*(3), 228-232.

Weissman, A. N., & Beck, A. T. (1978). *Development and validation of the dysfunctional attitude scale: A preliminary investigation.* Paper presented at the annual meeting of the American Educational Research Association, Toronto, Canada.

White, V. K. (Ed.). (1986). Health promotion. *Am J Occup Ther (special issue), 40.*

Wilcox, A. (1994). *Verbal self-guidance: An exploratory study with children with development coordination disorder.* Unpublished master's thesis, University of Western Ontario, London, Ontario, Canada.

Williams, J. M., Watts, F. N., MacLeod, C., & Mathews, A. (1988). *Cognitive psychology and emotional disorders.* Oxford, England: John Wiley & Sons.

Yeager, J. (2000). Functional implications of substance use disorders. *OT Practice, 5,* 36-39.

Young, J. E. (1981). Cognitive therapy and loneliness. In G. Emery, S. Hollon, & R. C. Bedrosian (Eds.), *New directions in cognitive therapy: A casebook* (pp. 139-159). New York, NY: Guilford Press.

Zimmerman, S. (1999). Occupational therapy service delivery to an apartment program. *Home and Community Health, Special Interest Section Quarterly, 6,* 1-3.

Zung, W. K., & Durham, N. C. (1965). A self-rating depression scale. *Arch Gen Psychiatry, 12,* 63-70.

RECOMMENDED RESOURCES

Assertiveness

Egley, J. (1987). *Self-advocacy and assertiveness for the learning disabled college student and how to use self-advocacy skills.* Lincoln, NE: Nebraska University, Barkley Memorial Center.

Rakos, R. F. (1991). *Assertive behavior: Theory, practice, and training.* London: Routledge.

Shaw, M. E. (1979). *Assertive-responsive management: A personal handbook.* Reading, MA: Addison-Wesley.

Shear-Goodman, M., Creager Fallon, B., & Gelles, R. J. (1987). *Pattern changing for abused women: An educational program.* Thousand Oaks, CA: Sage Publications.

Empowerment

Blanchard, K. H., Carlos, J. P., & Randolph, A. (1999). *The 3 keys to empowerment. Release the power within people for astonishing results.* San Francisco, CA: Berrett-Koehler Publishers.

Brownell, K. D., & Fairburn, C. G. (Eds.). (1995). *Eating disorders and obesity.* New York, NY: Guilford Press.

Follette, V. M., Juzek, J. I., & Abueg, F. R. (Eds.). (1998). *Cognitive-behavioral therapies for trauma.* New York, NY: Guilford Press.

Jones, S. (1999). *Developing a learning culture: Empowering people to deliver quality innovation and long term success.* London: McGraw-Hill Book Co.

Schaefer, C. (Ed.). (1999). *Innovative psychotherapy techniques in child and adolescent therapy.* New York, NY: John Wiley & Sons, Inc.

Vernon, A. (1999). *Counseling children and adolescents* (2nd ed.). Denver, CO: Love Publishing Co.

Self-Efficacy

Bandura, A. (1986). *Social foundation of thought and action—A social cognitive theory.* Englewood Cliffs, NJ: Prentice Hall, Inc.

Bandura, A. (1997). *Self-efficacy—The exercise of control.* New York, NY: W. H. Freeman and Company.

CHAPTER SEVEN

Model of Human Occupation— Systems Perspective of Occupational Performance

KEY POINTS

✧ History and Current Theory
- Occupational Behavior and Mary Reilly
- Model of Human Occupation
- System Theory, Behavioral, and Social Science Influences
- Motivation—Robert White and David McClelland

✧ Theory in Context of Occupational Therapy Practice
- Nature of Human Occupation
- Person: An Open System With a Heterarchy of Subsystems
- Volition, Habituation, and Mind-Brain-Body Performance Subsystems
- Person-Environment Interaction
- Occupational Performance—Development and Continuum
- Occupational Therapist Assists Change
- Occupation Restores Function and Balance

✧ Theoretical Assumptions Guide Evaluation and Intervention
- Evaluation as Data Gathering
  - —Data for Informed Decision Making
  - —Objective and Subjective Instruments
- Intervention
  - —Principles of Therapeutic Intervention—Assist Change
  - —Occupation Used for Intervention Across the Life Span
  - —Group Work Model and the Directive Group

✧ Contributions and Limitations of the Model of Human Occupation

Focus Questions

1. Identify several motivations for behavior.
2. What is subsumed in the MOHO term, **personal causation**?
3. Why are diagnostic labels of limited utility in this model?
4. Identify several reasons for the importance of habits and routines in one's daily life.
5. Why do lost habits and roles require "swift replacement"?
6. Viewing the person as a "system," how does this system relate to the environment?
7. How does the performance environment influence occupational behavior?
8. Why is participation in occupations of critical importance in this model?
9. Identify typical occupational changes that occur throughout the life span.
10. When using MOHO and whether using formalized assessments, observation, or informal interview, what is the occupational therapist trying to understand?
11. Discuss the rationale behind the principle "a change in skill" (as opposed to a change in underlying capacity) and why it should be the primary goal of therapy.
12. Why is it important for the occupational therapist to understand a client's life story?
13. In what way is the application of this model with children similar or different to its application with adults?

Historical Update

First articulated by Gary Kielhofner in his 1975 unpublished master's thesis, the model of human occupation (MOHO) is an occupational therapy practice model that has been vigorously elaborated throughout the last quarter century. Since our 1993 edition, occupational therapy theorist and educator Kielhofner (1995) has published a revised edition of *A Model of Human Occupation: Theory and Application* (2nd ed.). In this text, Kielhofner rearticulates the model's purpose, promising that the model will "provide an explanation of (human) occupation" (p. 2). As such, he writes, the model "focuses on the motivation for occupation, the patterning of occupational behavior into routines and lifestyles, the nature of skilled performance, and the influence of the environment on occupational behavior" (p. 2).

While holding to the essential principles of the model as identified in previous literature (Barris, Kielhofner, & Watts, 1983; Kielhofner, 1983, 1985a, 1988; Kielhofner & Burke, 1980; Kielhofner, Burke, & Igi, 1980), this most recent book is a product of its author's expressed desire to both streamline the model and make it easier to understand in a common sense way, while taking the reader to "successively deeper levels of understanding" (Kielhofner, 1995, p. 4). Some theoretical concepts have been condensed, others dropped, and still others modified to reflect advances in related fields. With considerable contributions from Dr. Anne Fisher and Trudy Mallinson from the United States as well as from practitioners and researchers in Canada, South America, and abroad, the 1995 edition offers an enriched cultural view of human occupation. Because this model pays considerable attention to psychological constructs and has been frequently referred to as the model of practice used to intervene with persons having identified mental health issues, we include it in our text.

As we indicated in the previous edition of our text (Bruce & Borg, 1993) this frame of reference has drawn from the work of hundreds of theorists, researchers, and practitioners in its evolution.

Definition

The model of human occupation (also referred to as the **model** and **MOHO**), which is an outgrowth of the occupational behavior frame of reference, is described as a holistic model for practice, education, and research. A highly eclectic model, it incorporates the views expressed by early occupational therapists and proponents of general system theory with ideas from existential and humanistic psychology, ego psychology, cognitive theory, sociology, biology, and social psychology. These ideas are combined to describe the nature of human occupation (also referred to as **occupational behavior** and **occupational performance**) as it develops throughout the life span. The model of human occupation takes a system's perspective of the person, emphasizing the constant transaction of person, task, and environment. Human occupation is believed to be innately driven and essential to human maintenance and self-organization.

Occupational therapy assists persons to engage in occupational behavior that will enable them to fulfill their capacity and live out meaningful life roles. To do this, the occupational therapist must strive to understand the client's unique life experiences and his or her abilities and constraints relative to occupational function. While MOHO provides general guidelines to help the therapist think about the client's circumstances, these guidelines are not prescriptive. It is expected that often in its application, the model will be judiciously combined with other conceptual practice models.

Theoretical Development

Occupational Behavior and Mary Reilly

During the late 1960s and throughout the 1970s, occupational therapy theorists, educators, and clinicians—many under the leadership of occupational therapist and educator Mary Reilly—emphasized the importance of occupation in one's life and in treatment and developed many of the occupational behavior views that continue to influence occupational therapy today. Through her work, Reilly encouraged the profession to adopt an occupational behavior paradigm. As defined by Kielhofner, a **paradigm** refers to the broad collection of assumptions or core concepts that give coherence to the profession (Kielhofner, 1995, p. 2). This paradigm emphasized the biopsychosocial nature of function and the need for human achievement. Reilly suggested that the paradigm become a framework, broader than that of the medical model and applicable to practice, education, and research. This paradigm for occupational therapy addresses the healthy nature of a person as well as the problems and incapacities that result from illness (Reilly, 1966, 1969, 1971, 1974).

Reilly urged occupational therapists to focus on occupation as the means of promoting adaptation and life satisfaction. She encouraged therapists to use the individual's healthy behavior to solve functional problems that result from disease and developmental delay. Therapists were exhorted to use healthy behavior and occupations to help patients explore and master their environment and learn to cope with their difficulties in daily living, work, and leisure (Reilly, 1966, 1969, 1971, 1974).

These views reaffirmed those of Meyer, Slagle, Barton, and Tracy, all founders of the profession. These earliest proponents of occupational therapy expressed their belief in the value of occupation; in the need for a balance of work, play, rest, and sleep; and in the importance of sound habits (Barton, 1917; Dunning, 1972; Dunton, 1917, 1919, 1928; Fuller, 1912; Meyer, 1922, 1977; Slagle, 1938a, 1938b; Spranger, 1928; Tracy, 1914, 1918).

During the 1970s, the occupational behavior body of knowledge expanded as Reilly worked with graduate students to develop an understanding of biopsychosocial function and human achievement. During this process, the works of ego psychologist R.W. White, psychoanalyst and developmental psychologist Erik Erikson, and psychologist, personality theorist, educator, and researcher David McClelland were used to form the basis of occupational behavior.

Model of Human Occupation

During the 1980s, occupational therapists worked diligently to build on occupational behavior theory. In addition to Kielhofner, who is most frequently recognized for his leadership in theoretical development and research, those who have collaborated with him in previous texts include Janice Burke, Cynthia Heard Igi, Roann Barris, and Ann Neville. Originally, Kielhofner and his colleagues retained the name "occupational behavior" frame of reference but later incorporated and refined concepts from this model to formulate

what they identified as the model of human occupation. Today, clinicians, educators, and researchers usually refer to it as MOHO or "the model."

In his 1995 text, Kielhofner states that, "the unique knowledge of occupational therapy is made up of both (1) a paradigm and (2) conceptual practice models" (p. 1). He goes on to state that MOHO is a "model of practice" containing knowledge to guide occupational therapy intervention (p. 2).

Therapists have applied the model of human occupation in many specialty areas, especially mental health. Earlier MOHO literature describes research in the area of assessment instrument development (Behnke & Fetkovich, 1984; Bledsoe & Shepherd, 1982; Brollier, Watts, Bauer, & Schmidt, 1989a, 1989b; Harrison & Kielhofner, 1986; Kaplan, 1984; Katz, Giladi, & Peretz, 1988; Katz, Josman, & Steinmetz, 1988; Kielhofner, Harlan, Bauer, & Maurer, 1986; Kielhofner & Henry, 1988; Oakley, Kielhofner, Barris, & Reichler, 1986; Watts, Brollier, Bauer, & Schmidt, 1989a, 1989b; Watts, Kielhofner, Bauer, Gregory, & Valentine, 1986). More recently, the work of Anne Fisher and her colleagues on the Assessment of Motor and Process Skills (AMPS) has been published (Bernspång & Fisher, 1995a, 1995b; Duran & Fisher, 1996; Fisher, 1995, 1997, 1999; Goldman & Fisher, 1997; Kirkley & Fisher, 1999; Pan & Fisher, 1994; Robinson & Fisher, 1996). Within this, much has been learned about the constituent skills needed for everyday function. Recent MOHO studies suggest continued development of measures (Henry, 1997), evaluation of reliability and validity (Henry, Baron, Mouradian, & Curtin, 1999), and construct identification (Mallinson, Mahaffey, & Kielhofner, 1998).

Early studies examined program effectiveness, comparative group outcomes, and the model's application in practice (Barris et al., 1986; Barris, Dickie, & Baron, 1988; Ebb, Coster, & Duncombe, 1989; Fitts & Howe, 1987; Katz, Giladi, et al., 1988; Katz, Josman, et al., 1988; Kielhofner & Brinson, 1989; Lederer, Kielhofner, & Watts, 1985; Smyntek, Barris, & Kielhofner, 1985; Spranger, 1928). In practice, the model has acted as a framework for programs in both community, residential, and home care settings and for child through older adult populations with varied disabilities. The broad application spectrum includes intervention with traumatic brain injury (Depoy, 1990; Series, 1992), pain management (Gusich, 1984; Padilla & Bianchi, 1990), chemical dependency (Scarth, 1990; Stensrud & Lushbough, 1988), pediatric mental health (Adelstein, Barnes, Murray-Jensen, & Skaggs, 1989; Sholle-Martin, 1987; Sholle-Martin & Alessi, 1990), pediatrics (non-mental health) (Kielhofner et al., 1983; Schaaf & Mulrooney, 1989; Takata, 1980), gerontology (Burton, 1989a, 1989b; Levine & Gitlin, 1993; Oakley, 1987; Olin, 1985; Tatham, 1992), HIV and AIDS (Pizzi, 1990; Schindler, 1988), adolescent psychiatry (Baron, 1987; Lancaster & Mitchell, 1991; Weissenberg & Giladi, 1989), adult psychiatry (Coviensky & Buckley, 1986; de las Heras, Dion, & Walsh, 1993; Gusich & Silverman, 1991; Kaplan, 1988; Khoo & Renwick, 1989; Kielhofner & Brinson, 1989; Muñoz, 1988; Neville-Jan, Bradley, Bunn, & Gehri, 1991; Salz, 1983; Weeder, 1986), anger management (Grogan, 1991a, 1991b), and developmental disability (Kielhofner & Takata, 1980). The model continues to have broad application in occupational therapy practice (Hagulund & Kjellberg, 1999; Laliberte-Rudman, Yu, Scott, & Pajoukandek, 1999; Neville-Jan, 1994; Rebeiro & Allen, 1998; Suto, 1998).

Research Designs

Group comparison, correlation, and single case studies are the more frequent research designs used to evaluate MOHO in practice arenas. Normal children, adolescents, and adults are compared with persons of similar age with psychiatric diagnoses, psychophysiological problems, various medical diagnoses, or chronic problems. These studies indicate that a person with occupational dysfunction exhibits problems related to his or her level of daily function, self-esteem, sense of control, role behavior, and everyday habits.

Program Outcome

When MOHO has been used to evaluate program effectiveness, assessment instruments specific to MOHO, as well as multiple standardized assessments associated with physical medicine, education, and psychology have been used to identify factors believed to contribute to occupational function ("order") and dysfunction ("disorder"). Parameters studied have included the subject's values, interests, goals, skills, roles, habits, locus of control, temporal orientation, physical and psychosocial abilities, and the perceived differences in quality of life before and after occupational therapy treatment. The outcomes of these studies describe the influence of the previously mentioned factors on the level of function and dysfunction, or the "order" and "disorder," of the person system.

Contribution to Occupational Therapy Theory

During the 1980s and early 1990s, much of the research focused on instrument development. As West (1990) noted, instrument development and the implementation of studies with stronger research designs has been a more recent emphasis in MOHO research. Previous MOHO research had been criticized for its small sample size, lack of reliability and validity measures, non-random samples, and unsophisticated statistical procedures (Curtin, 1990); however, because of their focus on occupation, all the studies are

believed to have contributed to the theory base of occupational therapy (Christiansen, 1981).

SYSTEM THEORY, BEHAVIORAL, AND SOCIAL SCIENCE INFLUENCES

In much of MOHO research, occupational therapy literature as well as system theory, personality theory, and behavioral and social science concepts are frequently referenced. For this reason, we briefly summarize the most influential of this literature. Those readers wishing a more in-depth understanding are referred to the original works, which are cited in the reference list at the conclusion of this chapter.

System Theory

From his earliest writing, Kielhofner described the person as an **open** or **dynamic system**, borrowing from system theory terminology. The term **system theory** may suggest a model, as shown in Figure 7-1.

This figure depicts the human being as like a machine or computer. Information comes into the system as **input**, is processed by the system as **throughput**, and is transformed to **output**, which produces information that comes back into the system as feedback. This model of man-as-machine, used by Heinz Werner (1948, 1957) and Allen Newell and Herbert Simon (1972), fails to convey the complexity, spontaneity, willfulness, and ability for adaptation inherent in the person system.

Kielhofner would refer to a more encompassing system theory—**general system** theory—as described by biologist Ludwig von Bertalanffy (1968). General system theory is used to describe the dynamics of open systems such as the complex human system, which consists of multiple component parts or **subsystems** (e.g., the musculoskeletal, digestive, and neurological subsystems), while being part of such larger systems as the family, neighborhood, or community.

Ludwig von Bertalanffy distinguished the open living system from the closed machine system. Critical in this idea of an open or dynamic system is the existence of constant give-and-take from the environment as well as give-and-take among subsystems (Kielhofner, 1995, p. 14). Other characteristics of the human (open) system that distinguish it from a machine are its ability to reorganize, adapt, and improvise in response to new task requirements. Behavior can change in response to internal (human) demands or changes in the environment. Because all systems—those within the person and those that make up his or her environments—are in continual contact and are interdependent, anything that affects the part will affect the whole (von Bertalanffy, 1968).

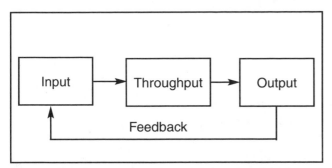

Figure 7-1. System theory model (reprinted with permission from Bruce, M., & Borg, B. [1993]. *Psychosocial occupational therapy: Frames of reference for intervention* [2nd ed.]. Thorofare, NJ: SLACK Incorporated).

Person-Environment-Occupation

As described by Kielhofner (1995) and in agreement with von Bertalanffy, the person, environmental context, and task or occupation in which the person is engaged create the **transactional paradigm** for human performance (Figure 7-2).

Behavior emerges from this dynamic interaction of individual, task, and environment; no one part is more important than the others in shaping behavior (Kielhofner, 1995, p. 21). As Kielhofner states, "Who, what, and where are inseparable in behavior." Further, the behavior that comes about is new and can never be fully predicted (Kielhofner, 1995, p. 21).

Theories of Motivation

As in other theoretical frameworks in occupational therapy, the model of human occupation has been influenced by knowledge advanced in the social sciences. In the model of human occupation, motivation theories borrowed from ego psychology and cognitive psychology have been highly influential. The model credits Berlyn (1960), Berlyn & Madsen (1973), Rotter (1960), DeCharms (1968), R.W. White (1959, 1971), David McClelland (1961, 1973), and most recently Csikszentmihalyi (1990, 1997). Csikszentmihalyi's work is discussed in Chapter Two, and it is White and McClelland who we will highlight here.

White

Before pursuing his interest in personality, Robert White taught history and government. Later, when working with Murray at Harvard and while teaching and doing research in psychology, White developed his views about personality and psychopathology. Based on his observations of psychotherapeutic interaction and from research, he identified two types of motivation: 1) **effectance motivation**—the person's desire to use one's own actions to cause an effect, and 2) **compe-**tence motivation—the person's attempt to become competent through one's experiences (Maddi, 1989).

The need to explore and have an effect has a biological basis and suggests that a person try, in a sense, to create or discover challenge. This process can be thought of as the need to create tension and disequilibrium as opposed to desiring balance, equilibrium, and tension reduction. Through exploration, a person gains experience and knowledge, which help him or her to perform competently in the environment and achieve a sense of competence. The need to continually explore and become more competent is felt to be innate or biological in origin and differs from the other biologic needs that might motivate behavior. These needs evolve and are expressed throughout life, initially through exploration, play, and make-believe, and later in adolescent and adult behavior as work and productivity.

McClelland

David C. McClelland has dedicated his career to teaching and researching personality development and more recently the application of his theory of personality in underdeveloped countries. His work focuses on the thoughts or cognitions that precede an individual's decision to engage in activity (Maddi, 1989; McClelland, 1973).

McClelland offers a rather unusual view of behavior. Although not a simple theory, its core can be simply stated as follows: People desire or crave small amounts of unpredictability in order to offset boredom, but they try to avoid large amounts of unpredictability (which would be perceived as threatening) (Maddi, 1989; McClelland, 1973).

McClelland describes three factors that influence function and personality development: motive, trait, and schemata. A **motive** is "a state of mind aroused by some stimulus situation that signals an imminent change that will be either pleasant or unpleasant" (Maddi, 1989; McClelland, 1973). McClelland assumes that the person will act either to increase pleasure or to avoid the anticipated unpleasant change. When the person anticipates pleasure, an approach motive exists; when he or she anticipates an unpleasant change, an avoidance motive exists (Maddi, 1989; McClelland, 1973). These motives correspond to a person's multiple needs. McClelland has emphasized the needs for achievement, affiliation, and power. Each of these needs may increase the likelihood of an approach or avoidance response (Maddi, 1989; McClelland, 1973). For example, in social situations the person who has a need for affiliation may be motivated to approach or participate in situations he or she anticipates will facilitate involvement with others. Those who wish to avoid affiliation may withdraw in social situations or avoid going to events expected to require social interaction. Approach and avoidance responses for achievement are referred to as **need for achievement** or **fear of failure**.

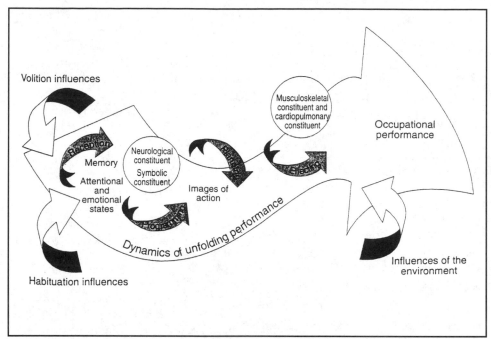

Labels within figure:
Volition influences
Musculoskeletal constituent and cardiopulmonary constituent
Occupational performance
Reception
Neurological constituent
Symbolic constituent
Memory
Attentional and emotional states
Images of action
Effection
Dynamics of unfolding performance
Habituation influences
Influences of the environment

Figure 7-2. The contribution of mind-brain-body performance subsystem, volition subsystem, habituation subsystem, environment, and task dynamics to the assembly of occupational performance (reprinted with permission from Kielhofner, G. [1995]. *A model of human occupation: Theory and application.* Philadelphia, PA: Lippincott, Williams & Wilkins).

McClelland does not address the development cycle per se. Through their history of experiences, however, individuals come to expect particular outcomes. If the expected outcome corresponds to the actual event and is positive, the person will have a pleasant feeling and will approach similar experiences in the future. If the expected outcome is very different from the actual experience or is unpleasant, the person may experience anxiety and avoid similar situations. The person's thoughts and experience can produce tension. Too much tension can cause a person to avoid the situation; not enough tension can cause a person to lose interest in the situation; adequate tension motivates the person to act (Maddi, 1989; McClelland, 1973). Over time, a pattern of thoughts and behaviors develops that may reflect approach and avoidance motives. This motivational pattern gives direction in one's life. **Approach motives** indicate the anticipation of success and lead to planned task behavior, which can produce effective, efficient outcomes and a sense of satisfaction. **Avoidance motives** usually emphasize the threats in the environment. They can yield ineffective, inefficient or obsessive thoughts and behaviors, passivity, or a sense of threat or dissatisfaction (Maddi, 1989).

McClelland, unlike other personality theorists, distinguishes between intentional and habitual functioning. **Intentional functioning** is goal-directed behavior and may cause a person to do something he or she has not tried before. **Habits** are consistent ways of behaving in particular circumstances and are learned through repetition; they are not the result of conscious planning. McClelland calls a collection of habits a **trait**. A trait is a "learned tendency in persons to react as they have reacted more or less successfully in the past in similar situations when similarly motivated" (Maddi, 1989; McClelland, 1973). A cluster of traits makes up a **role**. Traits and roles explain habitual functioning; motives explain intentional functioning (Maddi, 1989; McClelland, 1973). The third element of personality suggested by McClelland is the schema. The **schema** is a cognitive unit that symbolizes past experience. Schemata house one's values, ideas, and social roles, and thereby provide a guide for living and boundaries for the possibilities in one's life. According to McClelland, ideas and values concern primarily economic, aesthetic, social, political, religious, and theoretic realms (Maddi, 1989; McClelland, 1973). Social roles, previously identified by Linton (1945), are those related to age, gender, family position, occupation, and group membership (Maddi, 1989; McClelland, 1973).

In summary, McClelland's writing emphasizes the importance of expectancy in behavior as the person anticipates what lies ahead. As such, it is a highly cognitive, if eclectic, approach to understanding behavior. Although not described here, his work also provides guidelines for measuring the previously noted constructs in order to operationalize them. The reader is referred to the original sources for research approaches and the standard assessments used in these studies.

CURRENT PRACTICE IN OCCUPATIONAL THERAPY

As previously noted, occupational therapy publications reflect a broad application of the model of human occupation, suggesting that the model is being used as the theorists intended: as a generic frame of reference for practice. This chapter, however, focuses on the model's application in mental health.

The Person and Behavior

The person is first and foremost occupational or active by nature (Kielhofner, 1995, p. 27). Viewed as open systems, people are believed to engage in environments in which they constantly adapt to changing demands. People prosper physically and mentally because of their ability for this give-and-take. Despite the inevitable patterning of behavior into routines, people are viewed as unique and potentially unpredictable in their behavior. Behavior, in turn, is exquisitely personal and can be understood only as a reflection of the individual's personal (subjective) experiencing.

Nature of Human Occupation

Being engaged in **human occupation** means "doing culturally meaningful work, play, or daily living tasks in the stream of time and in the contexts of one's physical and social world" (Kielhofner, 1995, p. 3). Borrowing from occupational therapist and author David Nelson (1988), Kielhofner adds that the term "occupation" denotes the "action or doing through which humans occupy their worlds" (Kielhofner, 1995, p. 3). Occupational behavior arises from the choices one makes, which in turn reflect one's personal motives for occupation. It is important to remember that in this model it is believed that persons are, by nature, **occupational**—they need to be active.

Much of human behavior exhibits regularity. In other words, people are viewed as quite consistent in what they do and how they go about doing it. Changing one's patterns or habits often takes considerable effort and concentration.

Finally, human occupation expresses and depends upon one's underlying physical and cognitive capacity. An individual's capacity is not identical to his or her performance; a fact that will be important to bear in mind when helping persons achieve desired levels of performance.

HETERARCHY OF SUBSYSTEMS

The person as an open system has three subsystems. Addressing these simply for a moment, they are the:
- **Volition subsystem**, which chooses occupational behavior

- **Habituation subsystem**, which organizes occupational behavior into patterns or routines
- **Mind-brain-body performance subsystem**, which makes possible the skilled achievement of occupations

These three subsystems interrelate as a **heterarchy**, meaning that each contributes differently but in a complementary fashion to the function of the whole system. This idea of a heterarchal relationship represents a change from the previous MOHO view of these subsystems as existing in a hierarchical relationship (Kielhofner, 1995, p. 34).

Volition Subsystem: Understanding Motivation

In his 1995 text, Kielhofner states that the model's original conceptualization of volition was built largely on "trait theory" (Kielhofner, Borrell, et al., 1995, p. 39), which proposed that peoples' motivation would be highly influenced by their **interests** (what they find enjoyable), **values** (what they think is important to do), and their sense of **personal causation** (what they feel capable of). In 1995 he added the importance of "cultural common sense" in explaining human motivation. He elaborated this, writing that "...persons behave as they do because their behavior makes sense to them according to the way they experience the world as members of a particular culture" (Kielhofner, Borrell, et al., 1995, p. 40). Despite this addition to his theory, Kielhofner's 1995 discussion of motivation retains a strong basis in ego psychology and cognitive theory as described previously in this chapter.

The term **volition** implies both choosing to act and persistence. The intrinsic human drive to explore and the disposition to act urge volition. It depends in part on arousal, the person's view of his or her environment and the belief that it holds novelty, and on the expectation of success. Also referred to in the MOHO literature and slightly different in scope is the premise that the individual strives to have purpose and meaning in life. Basic survival needs are not denied, but the individual's striving to be creative and move toward greater complexity and self-enhancement is emphasized (Barrett & Kielhofner, 1998; Kielhofner, 1985a, p. 41, 1995, 1997).

The volition subsystem is conceived as bi-partite, having a volitional structure and a volitional process. **Volitional structure** is defined as "a stable pattern of dispositions and self-knowledge generated from and sustained by experience" Kielhofner, Borell, et al., 1995, p. 41). In other words, volitional structure consists of thoughts and beliefs. Volitional process "refers to the actual workings and procedures of anticipating, experiencing, choosing, and interpreting occupational behavior" (Kielhofner, Borrell, et al., 1995, p. 41). **Volitional process** implies acting upon one's motives.

Volitional Structure

Volitional structure consists of knowledge and beliefs related to the following:
- **Personal causation**

- **Values**
- **Interests**

These three areas have been discussed with considerable consistency in the MOHO literature.

Personal Causation

Kielhofner describes **personal causation** as a collection of dispositions and self-knowledge concerning one's capacities for and efficacy in occupations (Kielhofner, Borrell, et al., 1995, p. 43). It includes the person's awareness of his or her present and potential abilities and a sense of efficacy (his or her perception of control over one's own behavior, thoughts, and emotions, as well as a sense of control in achieving desired outcomes). We can see how personal causation impacts our choices if we consider that, all things being equal, we find ourselves more likely to undertake occupations in which we expect to succeed and avoid those that threaten us with failure (Kielhofner, Borrell, et al., 1995, p. 45).

Values

As defined in the 1995 text, **values** are "a coherent set of convictions that assign significance or standards to occupations, creating a strong disposition to act accordingly" (Kielhofner, Borrell, et al., 1995, p. 46). This reiterates previous discussions in which values have been defined as "images of what is good, right, and/or important to do" (Kielhofner & Burke, 1985, p. 17) and further as "commitments to performing in culturally sanctioned ways" (Kielhofner & Burke, 1985, p. 18). Values shape one's goals. They emanate from **personal convictions**, or beliefs about what matters in life, and from a **sense of obligation**, defined as a strong emotional bent to behave in what is perceived as the correct way to behave (Kielhofner, Borell, et al., 1995, p. 46).

Interests

Interests are defined as the "disposition to find pleasure and satisfaction in occupations and the self-knowledge of our enjoyment of occupations" (Kielhofner, Borrell, et al., 1995, p. 61). Having interests implies attraction to certain occupations and includes having preferred ways of performing occupations or activities.

Volitional Process

Volitional process is the enactment of one's beliefs as he or she goes about making occupational choices. What we choose to do depends in large part on what we anticipate will be the outcome, our feelings of efficacy, and what we value. We choose what to do this hour or this day, but in the larger scheme we think about our future lives and careers. In this regard, Kielhofner defines two levels of occupational choice:

1. **Activity choices**, which are of relatively short duration and determine how we are engaged in our more or less immediate futures
2. **Life occupation choices**, which are "nested in an unfolding life" or "life story" and mean deciding who we will become (Kielhofner, Borrell, et al., 1995, p. 51)

Habituation Subsystem

We are probably all quite familiar with the habitual nature of our own lives: the daily routines we follow day in and day out, often with minimum thought given. Kielhofner borrows from Young (1988) as he begins his discussion of the habituation subsystem, asking,

> Why then do people repeat themselves so much? Why do they do more or less the same thing every year at Christmas, or on their birthdays, or everyday as they go about their daily rounds... washing, dressing, getting breakfast, reading the paper... (Young, 1988, p. 75, as cited in Kielhofner, 1995, p. 63)

It is in understanding the habituation subsystem that we learn how occupational behavior is organized into patterns and routines and why successful habituation is so important to the individual. Like the volition subsystem, this subsystem consists of both structure and process.

Structure of the Habituation Subsystem

According to MOHO, the habituation subsystem is made up of **habits** and **internalized roles** (Kielhofner, 1995, p. 75).

Habits

Kielhofner cites Camic (1986) in describing a habit as a "...tendency to engage in a previously adopted or acquired form of action" (Kielhofner, 1995, p. 65). Habits are further understood as tendencies to repeat behavior or routines learned from previous repetitions and operating at a preconscious level (Kielhofner, 1995, p. 65). Behind habits are **habit maps** or frameworks for perceiving familiar events and context and guides for our habitual behavior (Kielhofner, 1995, p. 66). Some of the things we know about habits is that they are learned through repetition of behavior and that they serve several important functions.

Purpose and function of habits: Habits tend to guide human automatic behavior (e.g., that relate to grooming, dressing, making breakfast), and in so doing they allow people to do things without much energy expenditure. Because they don't typically require our conscious attention, habits allow two or more behaviors to go on simultaneously (Kielhofner, 1995, p. 67). For example, one can simultaneously eat and read the paper or file one's nails and talk on the telephone. When a person becomes depressed or physically disabled, however, he or she may need to consciously use energy in deciding what to wear or how to dress or may need to mobilize energy in order to pay attention to safety concerns while preparing meals. What was once habitual and easily accomplished often becomes difficult, even exhausting, when cognitive and physical disabilities disrupt habitual behavior.

Habits preserve the way people have learned to do things and tend to "weed out" ineffective or inefficient action (Kielhofner, 1995, p. 65). It is not that all habits are desirable habits, nor the best ways to accomplish mundane tasks, but habits tend to have a value in the environment in which they are performed. Habits shared by a society become a "custom" and in turn learning the group's habits allows one to become inculturated.

Habits bear a close relationship with temporal or time cycles. For example, how one organizes a typical day or week-day versus weekend of activity represents habits. The typical occupations and activities that a person does can provide desired structure and predictability for efficient participation in daily life.

Many people cling to and find comfort in their own habits. When people desire to change them, they often need to make a conscious effort to do so. Because habits tend to have a purpose specific to a given environment, familiar environments help maintain one's habits. When people change their environments (or "habitats"), a particular habit learned in a specific environment may become ineffective. This is one reason that a person may feel so out of step, even lost, if he or she moves from a familiar home, neighborhood, school, or job into a new setting (see Increase Your Understanding: Habits).

Despite its predictable nature, habitual behavior "requires improvisation" to accommodate novel elements in each new situation (Kielhofner, 1995, p. 65). If we were capable only of repetitive behavior, we would be helpless were we to drive a familiar route only to discover that road work required a detour, or if our housemate were to put the coffee pot slightly too far left or right from its familiar place on the kitchen counter.

Internalized Roles

MOHO literature has been particularly concerned with what are referred to as "internalized roles" (Kielhofner, 1995, p. 71). An **internalized role** is the "awareness of a particular social identity and related obligations" that together provide a framework for constructing the behavior viewed as appropriate to given situations (Kielhofner, 1995, p. 71). Behind roles are **role scripts** or ideas that people have about what behavior is expected of them in a particular situation within a particular role. Stated another way, you as the reader probably have a general idea of what is expected of you as a student in your educational setting or what is expected of you as a daughter or son in your own family (see Increase Your Understanding: Internalized Roles).

As a person forms habits and patterns of behavior related to role behavior, he or she internalizes expectations that come from his or her family, work, and social groups as well as from within one's self. The way I internalize a role will not be the way you do, so we each play out our roles uniquely. How we see ourselves in our role(s) becomes an important part of our self-understanding as well as how others respond to us. Like habits, roles also require improvisation. We cannot simply repeat identical role behavior in every similar situation.

INCREASE YOUR UNDERSTANDING: HABITS

1. Think about a time when you vacationed (went camping, traveled, etc.) or had a temporary illness or injury that forced you to alter your daily routines.

   a. List as many changes in your routines or habits as you can think of, starting with the time you first arose in the morning.

   b. Which of these changes in your routines were enjoyable? Which changes felt uncomfortable and/or disruptive?

   c. When you returned home or were able to resume your normal routine, what familiar routines were you glad to be returning to?

   d. Did you become aware of any habits or routines that you had not before recognized as important in your daily life? If so, what were these?

2. Talk with a friend or colleague who you know well to do this next exercise.

   a. Identify and write down three or more habits (routine ways of accomplishing daily tasks) that you are aware of in your own task or social behavior. Try to avoid applying labels of "good" or "bad" to these habits.

   b. Now ask a friend or colleague to identify one or more habit(s) of yours that they are aware of. Again, try to avoid applying labels to these habits. How do your colleagues' perceptions compare with your perceptions?

3. What daily habits/routines can you identify that you have maintained since childhood? (To get you started, think about eating, sleeping, and grooming/hygiene routines; for fun, think about how you approach games or how you engage in social activities.)

4. Have you ever made a conscious effort to break or interrupt a habit? How successful were you at making that change? What instigated, helped, or hindered your efforts?

Roles have what Kielhofner refers to as "varying **degrees of resolution**" (Kielhofner, 1995, p. 73). That is, roles with high resolution have clear and well-defined expectations about how they are to be carried out, while some with low resolution can be carried out more flexibly. For example, in some employment settings, the role of employer and employee may be spelled out very explicitly within written job descriptions, while the role of "friend" may be much less explicit.

INCREASE YOUR UNDERSTANDING: INTERNALIZED ROLES

1. Identify five roles that you currently hold, and write them down.
2. Consider each role, one by one. Create three sentences for each role that begin with the phrase "A good (brother, worker, etc.)..."
3. Look at the sentences you have written. Do you hold to each of these beliefs?
4. Think to yourself, where did I learn how these roles are to be carried out?

Purpose and function of roles: Roles enable the person to meet individual needs. They organize our occupational behavior by influencing our manner and style and even the content of our interactions with others (Kielhofner, 1995, p. 74). It is through one's role behaviors that he or she fits into social systems. Moreover, as the person internalizes expected role behavior and learns the "rules" associated with various roles, roles serve to direct behavior. Much of this becomes routine, and one can carry out many everyday roles quite automatically.

Habituation Process

Habituation includes the process of learning new habits and taking on new roles within the context of one's growth and maturation through the life span. New settings, new jobs, and evolving from child to parent, student to teacher require the acquisition of new habits and routines. Yet there are many routines (e.g., sleeping and eating patterns) that may remain surprisingly stable throughout life (Kielhofner, 1995, p. 77). As indicated, habits and role behaviors can be very resistant to change, and persons can feel quite disoriented when habits are disrupted or when they become unexpectedly unable to carry out familiar roles. This contributes to disruption created by acquired illnesses and disabilities.

Optimum Role Health

Earlier MOHO literature (Kielhofner, 1977, 1980a, 1983, 1985a) emphasized the importance of balance within one's role structure. This literature indicated that it was important to have neither too many nor too few roles; additionally, that there be a desirable balance between work and rest or leisure. Kielhofner's 1995 text emphasizes balance of a different type. It stresses the need for having a "well-organized but not overly rigid habituation structure" (Kielhofner, 1995, p. 76) that allows one to be stable and meet expectations and occupational demands, while being able to improvise and adapt to new situations.

Kielhofner's 1995 text proposes that for optimum function within the habituation subsystem, one needs also to periodically re-examine his or her roles and role-commitments. Again, the goal is to strike some kind of balance between needed "stability and consistency in (one's) everyday life" without being overly rigid and unable to change (Kielhofner, 1995, p. 79). Whether addressing one's behavior within a given role or the larger scope of roles taken during one's life time, role health requires flexibility and is unique to the individual person.

Mind-Brain-Body Performance Subsystem

Referred to in previous Kielhofner texts as the "performance subsystem," the third subsystem of the human open system is most recently identified as the **mind-brain-body performance subsystem**. This subsystem encompasses "what we have to perform with" (Fisher & Kielhofner, 1995, p. 83). Put another way, it is "an organization of mental and physical constituents which together make up the capacity for occupational performance" (Fisher & Kielhofner, 1995, p. 85). These constituents collaborate to process information and effect action in a manner that allows for behavior in concert with the rest of the organism and environment.

These physical and mental constituents are *not* the same as performance skills: one may, for example, have biologic capacity for skill but not exhibit the skill. The 1995 text identifies four categories or types of **constituents**:

1. Musculoskeletal—The bones, muscles, and joints that make up functional biomechanical units
2. Neurological—The central and peripheral nervous systems
3. Cardiopulmonary—The cardiovascular and pulmonary systems
4. Symbolic—Images that guide the person in his or her performance of occupational behavior

Key in the understanding of this mind-brain-body performance subsystem is that it is organized for efficient information sharing and effective acting upon the environment. There is a constant interchange of information amongst all constituents as well as with the environment in the processing of information for problem solving and action. We are reminded that this subsystem is part of an open system. Because constituents constantly "collaborate," one can't explain how one constituent is performing without explaining the relationship to the whole (Fisher & Kielhofner, 1995, p. 85). Figure 7-2 (p. 214) depicts the relationship of the subsystems with the environment and task to produce occupational performance.

PERSON-ENVIRONMENT INTERACTION

The model emphasizes that the person and his or her successful occupational performance is intimately linked to the environment, which creates the context for performance. No piece of this person-task-environment triad can be fully appreciated apart from the others. Nevertheless, there has been considerable discussion in MOHO literature particular to the environment and to how the environment can be expected to influence performance.

In earlier MOHO literature (Kielhofner, 1980a, 1980b, 1983, 1985a) the environment was discussed with particular attention paid to the stimulation that is **arousing** and that provides **press**, or expectation for given behavior.

Arousal is both physical and subjective; it is related to physiological output (e.g., rapid pulse rate) as well as to feelings of excitement relative to past or present experiences. In order for an environment to be arousing, the person must see it as interesting, novel, or challenging.

Once the individual is aroused and involved in the environment, he or she decides if what is available is compatible with personal values and interests and then makes occupational choices accordingly.

Feedback From the Environment as Press

The **press** of the environment is what it expects, "recruits," or demands (Kielhofner, 1995, p. 92). For example, the harsh environment of the homeless in winter requires that these persons change or adapt typical patterns of daily living in order to survive. The press in the local health club or gym is often for vigorous activity and exercise. The press for behavior in the sanctuary of a place of worship may be for quiet voices or for robust celebration, depending on the particular setting and culture.

In order to be fully adaptive within a given environment, the person must recognize press. When the individual either lacks an understanding of what behavior is expected within a given setting or lacks the skills needed to create this behavior, dissonance occurs.

Environmental Affords and Press

While not negating the importance of arousal, the more recent MOHO literature continues to emphasize the significance of **press** in the environment (what the environment expects) and contrasts this with what the environment **affords** (the potentials for behavior).

According to MOHO, when press is for behavior near the upper end of a person's capacity, it tends to evoke interest, attentiveness, and maximal performance (Kielhofner, 1995, p. 93). When press is for behavior well below capacity, boredom follows. When press is for behavior well beyond capacity, it tends to bring about anxiety. This is reminiscent of McClelland's writing, discussed earlier in this chapter. Both environmental press and what it affords will depend on what exists and/or is taking place within one's environment.

Physical and Social Environments

In describing what exists within or what creates environments, Kielhofner refers to two "dimensions" of the environment: the physical dimension and the social dimension.

The **physical dimension** includes the material environment, such as that made up of natural and fabricated spaces and objects (Kielhofner, 1995, p. 94). **Natural environments** might include, for instance, mountains, countryside, streams, or lakes. **Fabricated** or **built environments** are man-made.

Within physical environments are objects that in turn can make an environment arousing, comfortable, safe, practical, interesting, and aesthetically pleasing or uncomfortable, unsafe, and hard to maneuver through. We know that personal objects can take on great significance and meaning. Further, the way objects are arranged within an environment can either enhance or make performance more difficult. In the language of the model, objects are understood to both afford and press for behavior.

The **social dimension** is described as the world of interacting people and the things they do. This social environment consists of two elements: (a) gatherings or groups of persons that one joins (Kielhofner, 1995, p. 99) and (b) the **occupations** or **occupational forms** that persons perform.

OCCUPATIONAL BEHAVIOR SETTINGS

Physical and social environments are "intertwined" and create the "occupational behavior setting" or "context for performance" (Kielhofner, 1995, p. 104). The **occupational behavior setting** thereby comes to include "a composite of spaces, objects, occupational forms, and/or social groups that cohere and constitute a meaningful context for performance" (Kielhofner, 1995, p. 104).

We typically function in many often diverse environments and each one, with its particular people, spaces, objects, and occupations, affords and presses for behavior. Examples of familiar occupational behavior settings include home; school/work settings; neighborhoods; and gathering, recreation, and resource cites (e.g., museums, libraries, and churches). While participating in these environments, the person practices skills, develops patterns and habits, and becomes aware of personal abilities and limits. Through these interactions, the person participates in his or her life and finds meaning. In his 1985 text, Kielhofner emphasizes that when working with clients, therapists must consider carefully the availability of objects, tasks, and social structures. Part of the occupational therapist's job is to help create an environment that optimizes the client's natural urge to explore, master, and perform occupationally.

SKILLS USED IN OCCUPATIONAL PERFORMANCE

In order to engage in occupation, the person performs discrete behaviors, which together create **skills**. The model refers to three types of observable skills: motor skills, process skills, and communication and interaction skills. **Motor skills** are observable operations used to move one's self or objects. **Process skills** are the observable operations used to organize and adapt actions (e.g., to think about and plan what one will do next). **Communication and interaction skills** are the observable operations used to communicate intentions and needs and coordinate with others in what we consider as social behavior. These skills are related to physical and cognitive capacity but are conceptually different from capacity. Skill is manifested in actual performance. It may develop and improve with practice (Kielhofner, 1995, p. 113). Being able to identify and observe the skills used in actual performance helps describe what is actually happening when a person is unable to perform occupationally. While it is beyond the scope of this chapter to describe these skills in depth, the reader is referred to the work of Anne Fisher and her colleagues, who have contributed to the development of skill taxonomies in each of the three categories identified. They developed the Assessment of Motor and Process Skills (Fisher, 1999), a reliable and valid assessment tool that therapists can use to better identify a client's occupational strengths and limitations.

FUNCTION AND DYSFUNCTION

Health as Performance

In contrast to the traditional view of health as the absence of illness or disease, **health** in MOHO theory is the degree to which the physical, psychosocial, and environmental elements of the system work together to enable human occupation within the boundaries of health, disease, or disability. The presence of a psychiatric diagnosis or label does not tell anything about the extent of occupational function or dysfunction. In the face of disease and disability, the system tries to maintain meaningful occupations and maintain the well-being of the system. This process is similar to a concept in organismic theory that suggests that the organism will do the best it can to maintain balance and equilibrium. New demands on the system can be expected to bring about transformation and reorganization.

The person uses personal resources (such as knowledge, skills, and habits) to adapt and thereby meet the expectations of the community, maintain personal integrity, participate in the culture, and contribute to society. The person's ability to adapt is reflected in occupational performance (Kielhofner, 1985b, pp. 63-74; 1995, p. 19).

Occupational Performance Continuum

In earlier MOHO literature, a person's functional status was described as order or disorder. **Order** connotes a status of health and competent performance of daily living, work, and play tasks. **Disorder** is the inability to perform occupationally, decreased or absent role performance, and inability to meet role responsibilities (Barris, Kielhofner, & Watts, 1983). These dichotomies of performance have evolved into the occupational performance continuum.

The **occupational function-dysfunction continuum**, based on the work of Reilly, is expanded and refined to include six performance steps: achievement, competence, exploration, inefficacy, incompetence, and helplessness (Table 7-1). The person may slide along this continuum throughout the life span. This mobility suggests the flexibility and changing nature of the system's performance due to the dynamic process of the person-environment interaction.

Occupational Function

Occupational function suggests that the individual is able to choose, organize, or perform occupation of personal value and interest without undo difficulty. He or she is able to achieve a basic quality of life and meet reasonable environmental expectations (Kielhofner, 1995). This function depends in part on the ability to take the initiative to explore, achieve, and compete in the environment. In doing so, the person becomes aware of the expectations of others and his or her own abilities and learns and refines the skills needed for competence and role fulfillment. Occupational behavior flourishes. Throughout life, a person moves along a functional continuum as he or she develops and changes. It is as if there is a continuous cycle of exploring the environment, making choices, striving for competence to meet the demand of life's tasks, and achieving mastery. Then the cycle begins anew. The outcome of this cycle is a renewed sense of purpose, an enhanced system of values, a repertoire of interests, and skills and habits that support desired roles and responsibilities (Kielhofner, 1985b). In summary, **function** is viewed not as a state but as a process that reflects the ability for change and adaptation.

Occupational Dysfunction

On the negative side of the continuum is **occupational dysfunction**, which is reflected in impaired occupational performance. Dysfunction exists when an "individual has difficulty performing, organizing, or choosing occupations... also... when the pattern of occupational behavior exhibited by a person fails to provide a basic quality of life to the individual and/or meet reasonable expectations of the environment" (Kielhofner, 1995, p. 155). While dysfunction is not a precipitating disease or trauma, it can often include impair-

Table 7-1
FUNCTION-DYSFUNCTION CONTINUUM

Achievement	Competence	Exploration	Inefficacy	Incompetence	Helplessness
Actively involved in the environment; has established standards of performance; meets standards; assumes varied roles	Strive to improve to meet "press"; mastery of skills; formation of habits	Search for new experiences in safe and unfamiliar environments; investigation results in new skills	Decreased function; dissatisfaction with performance; decreases sense of control; changes interests, values, roles, and habits	No routine, does not consistently follow a routine; sense of loss of control; poor skill, habit, and role performance; decreased interests and values	Inadequate; poor or no function; few or no interests; few roles; few or disorganized habits; inadequate skills

Adapted from Kielhofner, G. (1985). Occupational function and dysfunction. In G. Kielhofner (Ed.), *Model of human occupation* (pp. 63-75). Baltimore, MD: Williams & Wilkins.

ment in the mind-brain-performance subsystem, as well as challenges in volition, disruptions in habits or roles, or difficulties with negotiating one's environment.

Emphasized in the more recent MOHO literature is that occupational therapists must appreciate the person's unfolding life story and manner in which it has been impacted by disease or disability. Like function, **dysfunction** is not a state but rather a process constantly changing over time. How each individual might be impacted by an acquired disability, chronic illness, or trauma—whether he or she will feel demoralized and out of control or remain invested and challenged—will depend in large part on each person's values and his or her perception of his or her own ability to reconstruct his or her life (Kielhofner, 1995).

Occupational Development Through the Life Span

MOHO approaches the development of occupation as a lifetime process of continual adaptation and renegotiation. Developmental change results from both changes within the person (e.g., skills and maturational changes) as well as from changes in the relevant environment, which both afford and press for particular occupational behaviors. These intrapersonal and social-environmental expectations require the system to learn, relearn, adapt, or otherwise respond to achieve or maintain an adequate level of function.

The model acknowledges the traditional developmental periods and the idea that there are normative or expected age parameters for developmental achievement. These are reflected in part by the obvious differences in typical occu-

pation through the life span (e.g., young children play; older children and adolescents attend school and perhaps hold down part-time jobs; adults typically work). Kielhofner emphasizes, however, the need to look at these developmental parameters flexibly. The process of occupational development is described as one of transformation in which periods of relative stability are followed by transition (instability), then a new order.

Periods of Occupational Development

As with other life span theories, the model identifies four periods of occupational development: childhood, adolescence, adulthood, and later adulthood. The occupational milestones described in the MOHO literature are consistent with those described by such theorists as Erikson (1959, 1968), Havighurst (1982), Levinson (1978, 1996), and Vaillant (1971, 1977) with emphasis given to changes within the volitional, habituation, and mind-brain-body performance subsystems. A summary of occupational development is outlined in Table 7-2.

Childhood

Childhood is viewed as a time of tremendous growth where new behaviors evolve and the system continually reorganizes to meet new challenges. As noted, play is a primary occupation through which children develop. Within this occupation, the child discovers and explores the environment, learns about his or her ability to make things happen, expands and hones skills, and learns about his or her own

Table 7-2
OCCUPATIONAL DEVELOPMENT

Period	Occupation	Outcome
Childhood	Play	Subsystems evolve and differentiate
Early		Autonomy
Middle		ADL skills
Late		Family role
		Role of student
Adolescence	Environmental interaction	Personal identity
		Refine skills
		Acquire and refine habits
		Increase roles
		Define and develop interests, abilities, and values
		Explore occupations
		Choose an occupation
		Begin pursuit of occupation
Adulthood	Career and work	Pursue a career
Early		Establish and maintain work skills
Middle		Manage multiple responsibilities
Late		Establish and maintain a lifestyle with work, home, and community occupations
		Personal achievement
		Economic gain
		Contribute to society
		Mentor role
		Change work focus to meet developmental needs

Reprinted with permission from Bruce, M., & Borg, B. (1993). *Psychosocial occupational therapy: Frames of reference for intervention* (2nd ed.). Thorofare, NJ: SLACK Incorporated.

abilities and limits. Also during childhood, the child develops occupational skills that enable increasing autonomy in self-care and other activities of daily living. The primary roles of the child are that of "player" and family member. Within his or her family, the child begins to develop habits as well as values and interests, much of which may be strongly linked to the values and routines within his or her family. As the child becomes older, he or she moves into other arenas that press for increasingly sophisticated social and occupational behavior. Opportunities expand for the acquisition of more roles and participation in an increasing number of occupations (e.g., those related to participation in sports, scouting, or church groups).

Adolescence

Adolescence, the bridge from childhood to adulthood, is understood to be another time of change, often including significant stress and turmoil. It is a period in which the adolescent has an increased urge for independence. Coincidentally, it is a time in which social, school, and family groups press the adolescent to take more responsibility for his or her occupational behavior. Adolescence affords many opportunities for the person to try out additional activities and occupations and to participate in new roles, often reflecting movement away from family activities. Within these new roles and occupations, the adolescent needs to establish habits that enable success and achievement. It is a time when family values will most likely be re-examined, and the adolescent moves to establish his or her beliefs.

How the person negotiates adolescence will have a powerful impact on his or her sense of efficacy. The adolescent who cannot find meaningful occupation, achieve at school, and/or is not involved in a worthwhile cause may enter adulthood with limited self-confidence.

Adulthood

As discussed in the MOHO literature, adulthood is closely tied to one's working life (Kielhofner, 1995, p. 146). It begins with the acquisition of more or less permanent full-time employment and ends with retirement. Through work, adults gain a sense of personal achievement, maintain economic stability, and are able to contribute to society. Within adulthood, there are significant transformations typified by two key periods:

1. An early period for establishing career skills, pursuing work/career goals, and establishing work skills
2. A latter period of evaluating one's achievements, reconsidering the personal meaning of work, and giving back to others

The adult most often has roles in addition to that of worker. These include roles related to family, as well as those inherent in community/leisure participation. The occupation of work, however, is considered to be the one "pervasive" feature of adult life, with the cultural expectation that adults contribute to society (Kielhofner, 1995, p. 148). Adults who will not or are unable to work may be stigmatized and find their opportunities for friendship and leisure curtailed as well.

Later Adulthood

Later adulthood is identified both by biological and societal changes. Entry into this period is marked by retirement from work and eligibility for social/medical benefits. It is a period associated with declining physical abilities, often with health conditions that affect capacity for performance, and decreasing opportunities to use one's abilities or pursue one's interests. The challenges of later adulthood include those related to the decline in physical ability, the need to replace lost roles (e.g., that of worker) with avocational occupation, and often loss of significant relationships. When there is also a decline in the ability for self-care and to live independently, the older adult may experience a diminished sense of self-esteem or self-efficacy. This in turn typically brings with it transformation in the person's values, with less importance given to productivity and more to equanimity.

Summary of Occupational Development

In summary, the course of occupational development, while highly variable, is characterized by the need for the person to constantly transform in response to both internal and societal changes. Rather than specify age-markers for each of the developmental periods discussed, the model identifies occupational markers associated with each period. Discussion in the MOHO literature emphasizes the importance of understanding developmental issues flexibly and appreciating that each individual will go through the developmental journey in his or her own way.

ROLE OF THE OCCUPATIONAL THERAPIST

The therapist's role within this model has been described in diverse ways through the last 25 years. In some respects it has been a striking evolution, as increased emphasis has been given to the therapist appreciating the life the individual has lived and might live in the future (Helfrich, Kielhofner, & Mattingly, 1994).

The occupational therapist is primarily responsible for evaluating clients' or patients' occupational performance and assisting them in making those changes they desire. In so doing, the therapist may take on specialized roles, including role model, teacher, mentor, counselor, supervisor, environmental manager, and consultant (Barris, Kielhofner, Neville, et al., 1985; Barris, Kielhofner, et al., 1983; Kielhofner, 1985a, 1995).

In Kielhofner's 1995 text, the role of the therapist is articulated quite simply and clearly. Therapy is described as helping persons to change, and it is the role of occupational therapist to *assist* or support change with the understanding that patients and clients accomplish most of that change through their own efforts (Kielhofner, 1995, p. 251).

It is proposed that occupational therapists can help persons make desired changes by striving to understand the changing landscape of their unique experience. The process of what therapists do then becomes one of personal engagement, experimentation, and problem solving, as they appreciate the impact that disease or trauma has had in a person's life and adapt general intervention guidelines to suit the client's life situation.

The therapist cannot expect to alter the human system directly (as a physician might with medication); consequently, the therapist carries out his or her role by producing a change in the client's relevant environment: altering the physical setting, providing assistive devices or technology, providing or monitoring social groups in which the client can participate, or helping to make available meaningful occupations (Kielhofner, 1995, p. 261).

ROLE OF OCCUPATION

In previous discussions, the terms "activity," "occupation," and "occupational behavior" have been used somewhat interchangeably in the MOHO literature as well as our own texts. For the sake of clarity, we will refer here only to occupation.

Formerly, participation in occupation was viewed as a means to restore normal function and a balance among work, play/leisure, and daily living tasks (Barris, Kielhofner, et al., 1983; Kielhofner, 1977, 1980a, 1980b, 1983, 1985a, 1988). The idea of "balance," per se, appears no longer as important as that occupation be meaningful and satisfying to the client and acceptable to his or her cultural group.

Another principle espoused was that of grading occupation from simple to complex and less demanding to more demanding, depending on the client's impairments and abilities (Barris, Kielhofner, et al., 1983). This idea of linearity has also been modified and replaced with the proposition that change does not mean simply more or less: it means a different organization (Kielhofner, 1995, p. 256). As Kielhofner writes, "...the idea of grading activities implies that change involves an incremental process in which a person simply acquires more ability, more confidence, and so on. Only when viewing parts of the human system in isolation is it possible to conceive of change as occurring in this linear fashion. When the person is considered as a whole system, we recognize that change is much more than a process of incremental improvement" (Kielhofner, 1995, p. 256).

Participation in occupation is the crux of therapy, as it begins the process of "self-driven change" (Kielhofner, 1995, p. 256). Participation in occupations helps the client to reorganize skills following a disruption of function. Because occupations provide "information-rich and meaningful contexts," they help to elicit maximal skilled performance. The occupations chosen should be those that the person enjoys and values. They should also be those that allow opportunities to either explore, improve skills, or achieve mastery depending on where the person functions relative to the function-dysfunction continuum (see Table 7-1). It may not always be possible for the person to achieve mastery within the context of time-limited therapy, but the principle remains that it is only through one's active participation in occupation that feelings of efficacy and mastery can be achieved.

Theoretical Assumptions—Guide to Evaluation and Intervention

The theoretical assumptions (See Model of Human Occupation Theoretical Assumptions) are a summary of the basic beliefs about the person, activities or occupations, and the environment or context. These beliefs are adapted from the theories that form the model of human occupation that are previously described in this chapter. The assumptions about the person-environment-occupation variables and their possible relationships guide evaluation and intervention in occupational therapy.

DATA GATHERING (ASSESSMENT)

Purpose of Data Gathering

There has been a consistent theme in the discussion of assessment throughout the evolution of the model. It is that assessment needs to be holistic; that it is the functioning of the entire human system and not any one portion that must be appreciated.

Kielhofner's 1995 text uses the term "data gathering" to evoke the sense that gathering information for informed decision making is an "interactive," "analytic," and "theoretically informed" process. The purpose of data gathering is to "reason about patients and their life circumstances" (Kielhofner & Mallinson, 1995b, p. 189). Further, occupational therapists must recognize that the data they collect will be used to "make moral judgments" about what *should* be done or what is *best* for the client. Endeavoring to make this judgment requires the occupational therapist to have enough information to understand the "dynamics of a person's dysfunction" and to "grasp the essential features of a person's life" (Kielhofner & Mallinson, 1995b, p. 189). Given that in data-gathering the therapist becomes an "investigator," therapists are advised to approach data in two ways: first, to use data to find out *about* a client (i.e., from the viewpoint of an outsider looking in on the client's circumstances); second, to collect and use data to help themselves understand how clients see themselves and their worlds (the subjective view) (Kielhofner & Mallinson, 1995b, p. 201).

This process of data gathering can be expected to go on throughout the course of therapy. Readers of Kielhofner's 1995 text are reminded that sound reasoning is not predicated on the use of a particular MOHO assessment instrument; rather, the therapist uses concepts from the model as a guide for answering those questions created by the model (see Sample Questions to Assist Reasoning on p. 226).

As described in the 1995 text, MOHO proponents recommend data gathering be done through both structured and unstructured means. **Structured means of data gathering** refers to the use of assessment instruments having a formalized protocol and basis for interpreting the data obtained. Less formal methods, which the authors refer to as "**situated methods of data gathering**," are those that allow the therapist to be more spontaneous and informal (Kielhofner, Mallinson, & de las Heras, 1995, pp. 205-206). This would include the therapist observing the client's performance in his or her everyday environments, engaging in dialogue with the clients' significant others, and so on.

MODEL OF HUMAN OCCUPATION THEORETICAL ASSUMPTIONS

The following theoretical assumptions are in some instances quite different than those identified in previous editions of this text. As such, they reflect the most recent comprehensive revision of MOHO theory (Kielhofner, 1995, 1997).

Person/Open System

1. The person can be compared to an open or dynamic system that is able to take what it needs from the environment, adapt, and transform itself.

2. The human system (person), the task in which it is engaged, and the environment all contribute to human behavior (occupational performance); a change in one necessarily affects the others.

3. Human behavior has a fluid, improvisational character spontaneously organized in context.

4. Human behavior tends to become patterned into habits and routines.

5. Daily routines and habits help people function efficiently and provide necessary stability to a person's life.

6. Patterns of behavior that have stabilized tend to resist change; changing habits and routines takes considerable effort and concentration by the person.

7. New habits and routines are often required in new situations.

8. Change in human behavior can be expected to be non-linear, irregular (even chaotic), and often unpredictable.

9. It is the nature of people to be "occupational" or active.

10. People strive to have meaning and purpose in their lives; when faced with disease or disability, the person system tries to maintain meaningful occupation and the well-being of the system.

11. People strive toward greater complexity, novelty, self-enhancement, and challenge.

12. Too much challenge discourages exploration.

13. The human system's organization is constantly being transformed through time in the process of life-development.

14. Transformations of the human system involve not only linear changes (more or less) but also changes in organization.

15. The person or human "system" can be viewed as composed of three subsystems (volition, habituation, and mind-brain-body performance), each of which contributes to the integrity and function of the system as a whole.

16. Functional occupational performance by the person is not a state but a constantly changing process.

17. Dysfunctional occupational performance by the person is not a state but a process in which unfolding behavior both reflects and contributes to dysfunction.

Environment/Context

18. The environment has two key influences on behavior: it provides opportunities and it imposes expectations.

19. There are two dimensions to the environment: the physical (natural and fabricated spaces and objects) and the social (world of people); when combined, they create the occupational behavior setting.

20. Therapeutic contexts (intervention programs) should provide choices for relevant occupations and provide social and physical environments that offer consistent and relevant expectations and opportunities for performance.

Occupation

21. Therapeutic occupation and the goal in its use is to provide opportunities for persons to promote self-organization.

22. Therapeutic occupation is the means by which individuals can perform, reflect on, organize, and adapt/change their occupational behavior.

23. Occupations provide information-rich and meaningful contexts and are the medium through which clients are therapeutically assisted in the process of self-maintenance and self-change.

24. Meaningful occupations are ones that provide opportunities to explore skills and/or achieve mastery and are something that the person enjoys or values.

25. In order to use occupation therapeutically, the therapist must understand its place in the patient's/client's life story.

SAMPLE QUESTIONS TO
ASSIST REASONING

- How has an illness, trauma, or disability impacted the person's view of his or her own abilities and sense of efficacy?

- What strategies does the person use to maintain a sense of control?

- What does this person look forward to and enjoy?

- How has illness or disability affected habits and roles?

- What values give the person's behavior coherence?

- Have values changed? What is the source of value change?

- What occupations have been impaired, or what adaptations have been made?

- What barriers exist in the environment?

- What particular activities have become difficult or impossible to complete?

- What occupation would this person like to return to? (Kielhofner & Mallinson, 1995b, pp. 190-191)

Of the common structured data collection methods, many have been developed for use in association with the model and fall into three major categories:

1. Observational measures
2. Self-report questionnaires and checklists
3. Structured interviews

Data-Gathering Instruments

There has been extensive instrument development within MOHO over the past quarter century, much of it carried out through the work of masters' students. In our previous edition (Bruce & Borg, 1993) we chose to list only those instruments that were discussed in juried publications. In Kielhofner's 1995 text, information is provided for obtaining all of the assessment instruments listed here, many of which are available through the Model of Human Occupation Clearinghouse, University of Illinois at Chicago. In addition, the formal assessment instruments we list here are described in greater detail in Kielhofner, 1995. Extensive citations are provided and the instruments' development discussed.

Observational Measures

Assessment of Motor and Process Skills

The AMPS (Asher, 1996; Fisher, 1999) was developed to measure the motor and process skills associated with the model. It is an assessment of occupational performance, not of underlying capacity or impairments (Fisher, 1999, p. 100). The AMPS is an assessment that has been vigorously researched both within and outside of the United States.

The AMPS employs observations of patients engaged in familiar occupations. It is preceded by an interview with the client and/or caregiver to ensure tasks will be relevant.

The client engages in IADLs as he or she would normally perform them, performing two or three familiar tasks from a choice of 56. Tasks typically take 10 to 20 minutes for each performance. Rating is of 16 motor skills (skills one needs to move the body and objects during performance) and 20 process skills (skills related to attention, organization, and adaptiveness used during the task).

Raw scores are subject to Rasch analysis to allow for adjustments on the score related to the relative ease or challenge of the task as well as for rater leniency. Therapists interested in using the AMPS validly and reliably must be trained and calibrated in its administration and interpretation.

Numerous studies (Bernspång & Fisher, 1995a, 1995b; Dickerson & Fisher, 1995; Doble, 1991; Fisher, 1994; Goldman & Fisher, 1997; Kirkley & Fisher, 1999; Pan & Fisher, 1994; Robinson & Fisher, 1996) have supported the validity and reliability of the AMPS, including its internal consistency, the stability of the AMPS over time, inter-rater reliability, and validity for differentiating motor and process abilities among various test populations.

Assessment of Communication and Interaction Skills

The ACIS (Asher, 1996; Salamy, Simon & Kielhofner, 1993) is intended to measure social interaction and communication skills and, to date, has been used predominantly with clients having psychiatric illness. It is based upon the observation of clients and carried out during a group activity (30 to 60 minutes). Behavior is rated according to 18 social and interaction skills. The ACIS reflects an instrument early in its development. Preliminary studies (Simon, 1989) indicated moderate inter-rater reliability (Kielhofner, 1995, p. 234).

Volitional Questionnaire

This measure (Asher, 1996; de las Heras, 1993a, 1993b) was created to obtain data related to volition from persons who could not report effectively and was originally developed for use with clients having chronic psychiatric disabilities or cognitive impairments. One observes and rates clients while they engage in work, leisure, or daily living tasks. The author recommends that clients be observed for a combined total of five sessions, with each session scored separately. The score indicates the amount of spontaneity (versus passivity or need for support and encouragement) and includes a brief narrative summary by the assessor detailing the client's interests, values, and the amount and kind of support needed for him or her to accomplish a task.

While a 1994 study does support its construct validity (Chern, 1994), the measure is still being studied. This instrument is available from the Model of Human Occupation Clearinghouse (Kielhofner, 1995, pp. 247-248).

Self-Report Measures (Checklists and Questionnaires)

Role Checklist

This written inventory (Asher, 1996; Oakley, Kielhofner, & Barris, 1985) identifies 10 roles and asks respondents to indicate for each role whether they have held the role in the past, whether they are now or expect to be in the role, and how much they value the role. It is intended for adolescents through adults of all ages.

Research done early after the instrument's development indicated both its content validity, and test-retest reliability (Oakley et al., 1986). Since then it has been used frequently in research to measure changes in role performance in clients with various disorders as well as with normal adults (Kielhofner, 1995, pp. 245-246). Copies of the Role Checklist can be obtained from the National Institutes of Health, Bethesda, MD.

Interest Checklist

The original checklist (Asher, 1996; Kielhofner & Neville, 1983; Matsutsuyu, 1969; Scaffa, 1981) has 68 leisure interests or activities to which the respondent indicates "strong," "casual," or "no interest." Modified versions allow respondents to indicate how their interests have changed and whether or not these are activities in which they now participate or would like to participate in the future. Studies have not supported the formal scoring of the instrument, but rather its use to help therapists understand clients' pattern of interests (Kielhofner, 1995, pp. 238-239). It is noted that the avocational interests listed reflect "middle-class, mainstream American interests in 1969," which may limit the instrument's relevance (Kielhofner, 1995, p. 217). The Modified Interest Checklist is available from the National Institutes of Health, Bethesda, MD.

Occupational Questionnaire

This is a pencil and paper activity configuration (Asher, 1996; Smith, Kielhofner, & Watts, 1986) that asks respondents to report, in half-hour blocks, what (waking) activities they are performing. Each activity is then rated by the respondent regarding whether he or she considers the activity to be work, leisure, daily living task, or rest. Respondents indicate how much they enjoy the activity, how important the activity is, and how well they do the activity. It can be filled out during the course of the day or at the end of the day. The therapist can also use it to guide a semistructured interview. Early research suggested adequate test-retest reliability and concurrent validity, but little psychometric work

has been added since then (Kielhofner, 1995, p. 244). The instrument has been used extensively in clinical research studies to compare patterns of time—use between dysfunctional and functional adults (Kielhofner, 1995, p. 244).

Self-Assessment of Occupational Functioning

The adult version of the SAOF (Asher, 1996; Baron & Curtin, 1990) (for persons 14 years and older) and its corresponding children's version (for children age 9 and older) (Curtin & Baron, 1990) were developed to assist collaborative treatment planning between patient/client and therapist.

It consists of a series of self-statements that correspond to MOHO constructs. The respondent rates each statement as an area that represents strength, as being adequate, or needing improvement. Two studies of content validity suggest that the instrument is theoretically sound.

Both the child and adult version are available from the MOHO Clearinghouse (Kielhofner, 1995, pp. 246-247).

Interviews

Each of the four interview instruments that follow have been developed for use with the model of human occupation. While each has a distinct format and focus, all are semistructured interviews with specific areas designated around which information must be gathered. Each also has a rating scale that the therapist-assessor must complete once the interview has concluded.

Occupational Case Analysis Interview and Rating Scale

The OCAIRS (Asher, 1996; Cubie & Kaplan, 1982; Kaplan & Kielhofner, 1989) was originally designed for discharge planning with clients in short-term inpatient psychiatric settings but has been used in other settings. It employs a semistructured interview, which is expected to take about 20 to 35 minutes to complete. Questions focus on personal causation, values and goals, interests, roles, habits, skills, and environment.

The therapist-assessor rates the client on a 5-point ordinal scale for each of 14 components, plus completes a brief one-page summary form. Early studies established content validity and acceptable inter-rater reliability.

Assessment of Occupational Functioning

The original AOF (Watts et al., 1986) was designed for use with clients involved in long-term care. A more generic version (Watts et al, 1989b) has been used with a broader range of populations.

This semistructured interview is designed to identify strengths and limitations in occupational function. The interview is expected to take 30 to 40 minutes to complete. There have been two revisions of the AOF, the most recent being tested with clients who abuse alcohol (Kielhofner, 1995, pp. 221, 237-238).

Occupational Performance History Interview

The OPHI (Kielhofner et al., 1998) was developed in response to funding by the American Occupational Therapy Association (AOTA) to create a generic history-taking instrument that could be used by occupational therapists across practice areas. It guides the therapist interview in five content areas: organization of daily routines; life roles; interests, values, and goals; perception of abilities and responsibility; and environmental influences.

By comparing information that the respondent gives about present with previous life concerns, it provides a historical perspective and allows for the development of a life story (Kielhofner, 1995, pp. 242-243). A revision of the OPHI in 1998 resulted in significant changes in how data is recorded. The OPHI is available from the AOTA.

Worker Role Interview

The WRI (Asher, 1996; Velozo, Kielhofner, & Fisher, 1990) was originally designed to obtain information regarding the psychosocial and environmental component with work-hardening clients. It combines information from the interview with observations made during a work capacity assessment. It is described as still in the early stages of development, but preliminary reliability and validity studies support its use (Biernacki, 1993; Kielhofner, 1995, pp. 249-250). This instrument is available from the Model of Human Occupation Clearinghouse.

INTERVENTION

Assisting Change

General guidelines for intervention have been provided in Kielhofner's 1995 text. A belief that has consistently guided intervention in this model is that therapy means helping people change; that it is through the clients' engagement in occupation that positive change occurs and that the aim of intervention is to enhance the function of the "open" system, which is capable of making the adjustments it needs to make. Also key in approaching intervention is that intervention *not* be based upon diagnostic labels. While the discussion of intervention in earlier literature (Kielhofner, 1985a) was often framed by the diagnostic information, this is less evident in Kielhofner's 1995 and 1997 texts.

The principles that follow represent the next step in the evolution of the model. In many respects, there is more flexibility in these most recent guides as compared to some of the mandates in earlier MOHO literature. In providing these guidelines, which he refers to as **principles for intervention**, Kielhofner adds a few caveats. First, that these principles are neither exhaustive nor prescriptive of what to do; rather, that these principles provide a means to "think about" therapy. Second, that these principles have some empirical support but are "not demonstrated facts." And third, that these general-

izations take on significance only in their unique application to the individual client (Kielhofner, 1995, pp. 250-252).

The aim of the model of human occupation is to help the therapist understand how volition, habituation, the mind-brain-body performance subsystems, and the environment contribute to adaptive and maladaptive occupational function and further to problem solve as part of planning and implementing therapy. The reader will find in these principles a re-statement of the assumptions and theoretical beliefs Kielhofner articulates throughout his 1995 text. These principles become a springboard for putting these beliefs into practice.

Principles of Therapeutic Intervention

- **Therapy is an event that comes into a life in progress and must be understood and undertaken in that context** (Kielhofner, 1995, p. 253): In articulating this principle, Kielhofner proposes that occupational therapists need to consider the special life situation of each client. He cautions against trying to apply the same solution to what may appear to be similar client problems. He also exhorts therapists to truly get to know their clients.

- **The focus for change should be the action or process underlying the human system** (Kielhofner, 1995, p. 254): Occupational dysfunction is a disorder of process; therefore, therapists want to enable an adaptive process that replaces a maladaptive one. Occupational therapists need to look at how the client—child, adolescent, or adult—is able to function or perform in his or her everyday environment, as opposed to focusing on particular structural (physical or cognitive) impairments in the human body.

- **Change does not mean simply more or less; it means a different organization** (Kielhofner, 1995, p. 256): Any change in any part of the human system will affect the whole; it is therefore impossible to think simply in terms of more or less. When people acquire disabilities, they will necessarily go about doing things differently. When endeavoring to assist persons with acquired illnesses and disabilities, therapists will need to help them alter the way in which they go about doing things, or otherwise change their relationship to their environment. One must always look at the whole.

- **Change can and should occur in many aspects of the human system simultaneously** (Kielhofner, 1995, p. 258): One can use the example of the child who becomes incapacitated by a muscular disorder that prohibits him from walking. Not only are the legs affected, so too will be the child's ability to play, his sense of esteem and control, and the interests he may be able to pursue in school. While it may appear easier to address one problem at a time or to address problems sequentially, occupational therapists are advised to capitalize on the natural interrelationships within the system.

- **Change is often disorderly** (Kielhofner, 1995, p. 259): This principle reiterates the idea that transitions can bring periods of chaos; progress can be uneven and often includes periods of stability followed by instability. According to Kielhofner, at times the role of therapy may be to provide a "place to re-group" after a setback and encouragement to go on (Kielhofner, 1995, p. 260).

- **Therapy should involve experimentation to find best solutions** (Kielhofner, 1995, p. 260): This principle reminds therapists that what works for one client may not work for another, and the best solution for an individual may not be apparent. The therapist is expected to be a problem-solver—one who will offer his or her client opportunities to experiment with alternatives to discover best solutions.

- **The only tool that therapists have at their disposal is to change the relevant environment to support or precipitate a change in the human system** (Kielhofner, 1995, p. 261): Occupational therapy does not directly alter the human system, unlike medications or surgery; therefore, therapists must direct their intervention toward modifying the physical setting, recommending adaptations that can be made in families or social systems, and/or helping make occupations available that give the client opportunities to learn or practice desired performance. Therapists must look at opportunities afforded by and behavior pressed for within therapeutic environments, whether these are at home, school, the workplace, or other setting.

- **Change in skill (as opposed to underlying capacity) should be the primary target of therapy** (Kielhofner, 1995, p. 262): While increasing strength, memory, or perceptual ability is an example of the kind of goals frequently set in therapy, it is more efficient and effective to aim for improvements in skilled performance. One could, in reality, achieve an improvement in underlying capacity without increasing a desired functional skill; plus, whatever changes are achieved in underlying capacity are believed to be best achieved in the context of functional performance.

- **Change in performance can involve learning to call upon different configurations of skills** (Kielhofner, 1995, p. 262): This principle suggests that as therapists we frequently assist a person to find new ways of achieving desired performance outcomes, often by substituting remaining skills for those lacking.

- **Occupational forms have a powerful influence on changes in skill** (Kielhofner, 1995, p. 262): Because they are meaningful, socially understood forms of action with coherent rules and purposes, occupations

provide "rich contextual information" for re-learning skills (p. 262). This is in contrast to requiring mere repetitions of behavior, exercise, or rote learning.

- **Habits and roles are naturally resistant to change because their basic function is to preserve patterns of behavior; sustained practice is necessary to cement change in habituation** (Kielhofner, 1995, p. 262): When the goal of therapy is to establish new roles or habits, the therapist needs to look for many opportunities for the client to practice new behavior. This may include finding opportunities beyond the therapy session, given the often short therapy duration.

- **Habituation organizes behavior for specific ecologies; new habits must often be learned in new ecologies** (Kielhofner, 1995, p. 263): As therapists, we need to see if a client's habits fit well with the environment in which he or she will be functioning. If not, we need to help make adjustments in the environment. It is best if clients can learn new habits in the environments in which they will be used. When clients are children, the focus of intervention may be establishing habits for the first time. Thus, it is vital that these new habits suit the values and life styles of the families and culture in which the child participates.

- **The loss of role and habits requires swift replacement** (Kielhofner, 1995, p. 264): This principle exhorts occupational therapists to move quickly when roles and habits have been disrupted. Habits and roles are viewed as a source of security, familiarity, and identity for individuals, and a disruption of habituation is believed to be potentially disorienting, disorganizing, and very uncomfortable. Sometimes former habits and roles will need to be replaced because they have lost their utility. At other times, clients may need help restoring familiar habits and roles.

- **Acquiring a new role script and related habits is a process of socialization and negotiation** (Kielhofner, 1995, p. 264): Therapeutically assisted change must provide opportunities for many and varied social interactions, which in turn provide opportunities for the client to get feedback and thereby learn what others expect of him or her in this new role. As with habits, it is best if new roles and social skills can be practiced in the real-life setting (e.g., home, school, or work place) in which the role is to be carried out. One way the therapist can assist in this process is to go to the natural environment with the client and serve as a role coach and/or help the client to determine what new behaviors are needed for a specific context.

- **Volitional anticipation, experience, interpretation, and choice are at the core of what is referred to as meaning in therapy** (Kielhofner, 1995, p. 265): If therapy is to be meaningful and truly assistive to the client, therapists need to enable occupations that are relevant to their clients. They need to "stay in touch" with the client in order that they have a sense of what he or she is experiencing in therapy. They should also encourage clients to reflect on the course of their therapy experiences in order that clients can make choices that reflect what is important to them.

- **Volitional change means finding a direction for one's personal narratives** (Kielhofner, 1995, p. 267): When faced with occupational dysfunction, persons typically need to figure out where their life will go next. Clients need to fit experiences into a new life story that, while representing a change in their life saga, continues to have meaning and coherence with the life they have lived previously. For many, this will mean learning to live with a disability, with the goal of achieving a quality of life.

- **Therapeutic programs should include occupations that are relevant to the client and allow the client to interact at his or her level of function (exploration, skill-building, or achieving mastery)** (Muñoz & Kielhofner, 1995, pp. 345-347): Participation in occupation is self-organizing and permits the client to move along this functional continuum, to adapt and change, and to learn about him- or herself as an occupational being. It is the availability of meaningful occupations that characterizes this as occupational therapy intervention.

- **Occupational therapy programs should provide social and physical environments that offer consistent and relevant expectations and opportunities for performance** (Muñoz & Kielhofner, 1995, pp. 345-347): The maintenance or creation of patterns of behavior as habits or roles is essential to the overall well-being of the person and is assisted by regularity and predictability within the environment.

Application Depends on Judgment

Early MOHO literature contained recommendations about the manner in which treatment would be carried out. Therapists, for example, were advised to focus on activities (occupation) as a means for the client to achieve an end product or to gain functional skills. The therapy session was not the time to be talking about feelings (Kielhofner, 1980a). This evolved to the suggestion that how a client viewed his or her accomplishments could be as important as the functional outcome (Kielhofner, 1985a), and one might wish to engage the client in a discussion regarding his or her perceptions. In his most recent text, Kielhofner (1995) does not tell the therapist how to carry out the therapy process. To the contrary, Kielhofner writes, "There is no standard way to operationalize theory into practice; the process always depends on the therapist's judgment as guided by theory" (Kielhofner, 1995, p. 341). He cautions, "This does not mean that therapists... pick and choose or impart their own

meanings to concepts that the book has taken pains to define and illustrate... (it) means that the therapist must be able to move between the concepts and the person receiving therapy, being the final arbiter of how theory is best applied to each individual" (Kielhofner, 1995, pp. 341-342). The following case example, summarized from Kielhofner's 1995 text where it is described in more detail, serves as an example of one application of the model and is illustrative only.

Adult Application

As described by occupational therapist and author Frances Oakley, Carl was a 32-year-old man with a history of chronic schizophrenia. Carl had stopped taking his medications about 6 weeks prior to his admission to an inpatient facility. At that time he had decompensated, was hearing voices, and was unable to care for himself. The occupational therapist was aware that upon resumption of his medications, Carl's thinking would clear and his symptoms would remit, but she had several concerns regarding Carl. Did he have any interests and experiences that would suggest a potential life role for Carl? How could he meaningfully fill his time and ultimately achieve an identity and satisfaction in life? The therapist was aware that having a daily schedule and life roles around which to organize his time could help Carl stay internally organized and perhaps lessen his relapses. Until now, Carl spent most of his day at home watching television and occasionally would go the local park and pick flowers. Initially, Carl was too confused to give meaningful information about himself, so the therapist talked to his family, who suggested that plants and flowers were of interest to Carl. As soon as he was able, Carl was invited to come to the occupational therapy setting and was asked to care for the plants there. Carl immediately perked up, and the therapist used his interest in caring for the plants as a motivator for him to improve his self-care; it was agreed that a condition of his coming to OT was that he properly dress and groom himself, which he did. As Carl's thinking cleared, the occupational therapist used both the Interest Checklist and the Role Checklist to better determine Carl's interests. Gardening and horticulture emerged as the most consistent and strongest of his interests. The therapist envisioned the role of "hobbyist" for Carl, and he agreed that this was a role he wanted to pursue. Since his hospitalization would be brief, they used the remainder of his OT sessions to help him develop this role. The therapist talked to Carl's parents, who agreed he could have responsibility for the plants and yard at home, and they would buy him supplies to pursue this hobby. Following discharge from the acute setting, Carl began as a patient at a day treatment center. The therapist apprised the staff of Carl's interest and gave them suggestions on how Carl might use his skills at this setting. Carl was soon recognized as the official "florist" at the day treatment center (summarized from "Carl:

Finding a Life Role" by Frances Oakley, MS, OTR/L, pp. 284-286, in Kielhofner, G., & Mallinson, T. (1995a). Application of the model in practice: Case illustrations. In G. Kielhofner (Ed.), *A model of human occupation: Theory and application* (2nd ed., pp. 271-342). Baltimore, MD: Williams & Wilkins).

Intervention Across the Life Span

In addition to its application in broad-spectrum age groups, descriptions of the model's application include those specific to children (Adelstein et al., 1989; Baron, 1989; Kielhofner, 1985a, 1995; Sholle-Martin, 1987; Sholle-Martin & Alessi, 1990; Woodrum, 1993), adolescents (Baron, 1989; Kielhofner, 1985a, 1995; Lancaster & Mitchell, 1991; Sholle-Martin, 1987; Weissenberg & Giladi, 1989), adults (Neville-Jan, 1994), and the older adult (Burton, 1989a, 1989b; Kielhofner 1985a, 1995; Levine & Gitlin, 1993; Oakley, 1987; Olin, 1985; Tatham, 1992).

Evident across these diverse application studies is the emphasis on a collaborative therapeutic process in which decisions are made *with* and *not* for the client and the client is actively engaged in the problem-solving process. The model is used to understand clients' motivation and values as well as behavior. The model is a guide for adjusting the intervention approach to the individual client and the environment and contexts of treatment.

Specific Recommendations for Use of the Model with Children

One can take the term "child" and legitimately substitute it for the term "person" throughout the previous discussion in this chapter. The understanding of the child and adult and principles for application of the model are identical. However, it is critical that intervention with young people reflects the clinician's knowledge and expertise in the area of child development, wherein he or she knows the tasks and skills appropriate to a child client's age.

Provide Opportunity for Play and Exploration

Children, like adults, are viewed as innately motivated to explore and master their environments. Indeed, anyone who has been around young children cannot help but see the obvious delight children experience in exploring their environment and their clear enjoyment in learning new skills. For the younger child, much of this occurs through the occupation of play. For this natural process to unfold, the child needs to be present in a physical and social environment that affords opportunities for play and exploration (i.e., one with materials/toys, play equipment, space, and age-mates).

When working with children, it is important for the occupational therapist to include family members and to make certain that they are familiar with developmental play activities compatible with the age and abilities of the child. Well-meaning parents may need help learning how to play with their child, and the clinician may model play behavior, including the parent(s) in therapy sessions. Therapists may provide parents with educational material or identify inexpensive avenues for play such as community settings in which the family can play together.

Provide a Safe Environment

Going back to MOHO's functional continuum of exploration-competence-achievement, one is reminded that exploration is the first step toward mastery; however, exploration requires that the child feels safe, both physically and emotionally. Children with physical limits or those who have cognitive impairments that somehow distinguish them from their peers may have difficulty handling themselves in normal play environments, may become uncomfortable, even fearful, and may become reluctant in play. Further, they learn very quickly that they are not as "good at" normal play as their peers, and their self-esteem and beliefs in their own efficacy suffer. Whatever the reason for the psychosocial referral, the occupational therapist will pay special attention to creating an environment in which the child is safe and can succeed at play, can express and follow his or her preferences, and begin to build those feelings of internal control and mastery necessary for child's occupational function. In so doing, the child is able to identify interests and develop values as well.

Develop Habits for the Environment

Not everything is play for the child, and the young child needs to learn age-appropriate roles and ADL behaviors. The occupational therapist must become familiar with what is expected of the child in his or home and can typically do this most easily by interviewing the parents. As the child moves into the role of preschooler or student, the therapist may interview teachers as well to identify the skilled behaviors and "habits" necessary for the child to function successfully in his or her school environment. This idea of having established "good habits" is important if children are to be successful. The older the child and the more roles he or she has, the more important it becomes that the child has an adaptive routine and habits that enable smooth, daily functioning. As the young child learns to perform these routines independently (e.g., dressing and bathing him- or herself) he or she gains confidence and pride in his or her own abilities.

Provide Opportunity for Occupation and Interests

Older children (7 or 8 years and above) not only have self-care and routines that they will be performing independently, many have other responsibilities as well. These children may have chores at home, for example, may have homework or engage with social groups in which they are expected to cooperate with others for task accomplishment. Additionally, the older child develops interests related to being productive (e.g., making crafts or becoming a collector or hobbyist). These occupations facilitate the further acquisition of routines and habits that will enable future successful performance as a worker. The therapist working with the latency-age child can use competitive games, craft activities, or activities related to community outreach to provide opportunities for the child to explore his or her interests and to establish a sense of competency and achievement. As with the younger child, the therapist needs to have available activities, supplies, and space that permit the child to pursue his or her interests. The clinician may involve parents and teachers, both to learn about routines expected of the child in his or her natural environment and to encourage follow through at home and school. It is often with the older child and with the adolescent that the child comes to the attention of the helping community because he or she does not exhibit established routines, habits, and behaviors expected and acceptable for children his or her age. Those instances draw attention to Kielhofner's exhortation to provide a therapeutic environment in which expectations are clear and routines are consistently followed.

Pediatric Application

The following summarizes an example of the model's application by therapist Kim Bryze, MS, OTR/L, with a youngster named Nathan. It is abbreviated here, with emphasis given to the salient features of the model's application. The reader is referred to the case's description in its entirety.

Nathan was 7 years and 4 months old and attended regular second grade in a middle-class suburb. One day Nathan came home from school with a troubled look on his face, saying, "Mom, something is wrong with me." At first his mom inquired about possible physical ailments, but Nathan clarified, "No, Mom, something is wrong with me! I'm not like other kids. I am afraid." Exploring his concerns with Nathan, the mother learned that group activities and physical games at school were intimidating for him and that he worried about participating in these; after participating, he felt like a failure. She learned that he felt isolated and "different." Nathan's mother talked to Nathan's teacher and other professionals and was referred to a pediatric occupational therapist that specialized in working with children who had problems similar to Nathan's. The therapist first talked to Nathan and his mother and suspected that Nathan had sensory processing difficulties. Observing Nathan's motor performance, taking a complete sensory-motor development history, and performing additional components of a sensory-integration evaluation, the therapist determined that Nathan was hypersensitive to touch and was dyspraxic, especially evident during fine motor tasks and during movement that required bilateral integration, sequencing, and antic-ipatory motor control (e.g., as used in throwing and catching a ball). The therapist also discerned from his performance and negative self-report that he expected to fail and often avoided or rushed through physical play in order to circumvent the painful experience of failure. He would not take even moderate risks that might have given him opportunities to learn better motor patterns, and in avoiding opportunities for physical engagement, he lost opportunities for socialization as well. His physical constraints led him to play mostly with younger children, and his interests were restricted to activities that involved minimal movement, such as video games and reading. Even in carrying out responsibilities at home, Nathan was constrained. For example, he wanted to help carry groceries, but he often dropped them, making a mess.

Following the model, the therapist paid attention to both Nathan's sensory-integration problems and his volition. She determined that she needed to create situations in which his personal causation could be increased and his fears and anxieties minimized. The overall aim of therapy was to halt and ultimately reverse the negative cycle of avoidance, negative emotions, and negative self-appraisal. Therapeutic goals were developed in collaboration with Nathan and his mother and related to the volition, habituation subsystems, as well as performance skills in the area of sensory-motor integration. These included the following:

- Each day Nathan will make positive activity choices in school, home, or therapy.
- Nathan will develop more varied interests at school and home.
- Nathan will be able to successfully help in family chores.
- Nathan will be able to complete self-care without aversive responses.
- Nathan will demonstrate age-appropriate play skills.

The approach in intervention was to provide opportunities for Nathan to explore and experiment with different equipment and toys in the occupational therapy environment, free from therapist pressure for Nathan to perform or be "good enough." This safe atmosphere enabled Nathan to try out and develop new skills. Nathan was given a great deal of control regarding what activities and games they would play, as well as in guiding the intensity and frequency of sensory input. As he began to feel in control and empowered in these therapeutic situations, he gained confidence in coping with sensory challenges in other environments. Nathan and his mother worked with the therapist and learned that certain times of the day and specific adaptations to his self-care routine at home enabled Nathan to be more comfortable and successful in ADL. They experimented with modifications to the environment, identifying optimum lighting, and organization in his physical work-space that would help Nathan either calm himself or get organized. All of this contributed to a positive cycle in which Nathan became more comfortable with physical play, learning ways to enhance his own performance. The family began to take him to a local park in which he could practice in a safe environment (without the competitiveness of peers), and his father built a backyard tree-house structure for such play. As therapy wound down, the therapist advised both Nathan and his family that Nathan could expect to have some lingering sensory-integrative difficulties. The therapist framed these as challenges unique to Nathan, reminding him that we all have challenges. With his greater competence, confidence, and understanding of how he could compensate for his limitations, it was Nathan who recommended that therapy cease, saying to the occupational therapist, "You know I can do everything here. I think I don't need to see you so much anymore" (Kielhofner, & Mallinson, 1995a, pp. 323-327).

Mental Health Group Programs

Extensive descriptive literature exists on the use of the model to guide mental health group programming. Many programs have been carried out within mental health facilities or with individuals experiencing mental health issues, including those related to anger management (Grogan, 1991a, 1991b), chronic pain (Gusich, 1984; Padilla & Bianchi, 1990), stress management (Affleck et al., 1984), dementia (Oakley, 1987; Olin, 1985), low self-esteem (Lancaster & Mitchell, 1991), mother-child attachment (Burke, Clark, Dodd, & Kawamoto, 1987), co-dependency (Neville-Jan et al., 1991), life-threatening illness (Pizzi, 1990; Schindler, 1988), chemical dependency (Scarth, 1990), adolescent conduct and behavior disorders (Baron, 1987; Lancaster & Mitchell, 1991; Weissenberg & Giladi, 1989), attention-deficit problems (Woodrum, 1993), eating disorders (Shimp, 1989), sexual abuse (Froehlich, 1992), and in child psychiatry (Adelstein et al., 1989; Baron, 1989; Sholle-Martin, 1987; Sholle-Martin & Alessi, 1990). While these therapeutic groups are not easily identified as different than other therapy groups described in this text, they pay particular attention to the essential MOHO constructs of volition, roles and habits, performance, and environment.

An Example of MOHO Adult Group Intervention

Occupational therapist Kathy Kaplan describes the use of the model in her intervention with clients who have psychiatric impairments and are low-functioning and often confused (Kaplan, 1988). She sees the group as providing an environment that can arouse interest in occupational function through the introduction of meaningful activities and careful articulation of goals based on the patient's needs, goals, and roles. She recommends that patients at similar functional levels be treated in three groups designed to address this specific level of function. These groups she identifies as achievement, competence, and exploratory groups. Each group has specific goals and involves group experiences consistent with the abilities of its members.

The Directive Group

One such group is the directive group. The **directive group** is a group experience for persons with varied problems and of various ages and diagnoses, but all participants are in the acute stage of illness. The group is structured and designed to support maximum participation from patients who function at a minimum level.

The group follows a consistent format:

- Orientation—The introduction of a brief activity to inform patients about where they are and what to expect in the group.
- Introduction of new members—Approached in a manner likely to stimulate interest and mobilize the participants, for instance, throwing a ball to each member and asking each to state his or her name.
- Warm-up exercises—Usually spontaneous movement exercises.
- Core or theme activity—Motor, cognitive, social-interactive, sensory, food-centered, or craft experience.
- Wrap-up—Activity is used to bring group closure, often with group or member goals and their attainment underscored.
- Post-group—Plans or directions for future groups are discussed.

The reader may recognize this group sequence as similar to that of Ross and Allen; however, Kaplan sees these groups as different in nature and theory from the directive group.

Of the 69 activities recommended for possible use in directive groups, the following is selected to illustrate a sample group exercise. Facts of Three (or Five) is a cognitive game that can be used to assess cognitive skills, increase interests, build knowledge, and emphasize the cooperative and competitive nature of roles when organized as team play.

Patients are given a copy of a grid sheet, which they complete as the game ensues (Figure 7-3). When the activity portion of the group begins, participants identify a three-letter word and three categories, then play begins. Participants take turns filling in the grid by identifying words that begin with the identified letter and satisfy a particular category. The game can be made more complex, may involve score keeping, or can require performance within time constraints. In this and other ways it can be adapted to meet patient needs.

Later, as clients improve and have increased processing ability, this type of game can be used as a warm-up activity, for a group of clients who are able to problem solve, role play,

Letters/ Categories	A	C	T
Occupation	Actor	Chiro-practor	Therapist
Places to Visit	Austria	Catskills	Texas
Feelings	Appalled	Calm	Terrific

Figure 7-3. Sample grid (reprinted with permission from Kaplan, K. [1988]. *Directive group therapy*. Thorofare, NJ: SLACK Incorporated).

and practice social skills. For example, clients could identify strategies to remain calm when one is upset or "appalled." Clients could practice social skills when they role-play initiating a conversation and share information about places they visited as they practice listening skills or recall of information.

Group Model for Occupational Performance

In addition to the examples of mental health groups, in the literature Kielhofner (1997) suggests that MOHO theory can be used in conjunction with another group model that emphasizes occupational performance in many social contexts as well as in traditional intervention environments. The group work model described by Howe and Schwartzberg (1988, 1995) is such a model. This model is applicable to family, school, work, and other social environments. It emphasizes the use of occupations in a group context. Occupations help the person adapt in a group and also contribute to the "energy field" that facilitates client participation in the group. Occupations, activities, and tasks give structure to the group and can provide roles for clients to assume. During groups, the occupational therapist-leader uses group dynamics to facilitate occupational behavior and helps clients learn the effects of group process on occupations, their roles, and their performance in groups. During group interventions, clients have the opportunity to choose activities, learn skills and adaptive behavior, practice problem solving, and influence their health. The reader is referred to Howe and Schwartzberg (1995) for model details and discussion of its application in practice.

CONTRIBUTIONS AND LIMITATIONS

Contributions

Strongly Researched Model

The model of human occupation presents a strongly researched and carefully articulated theoretical model for practice. Although described as a generic model, it is not surprising that it has been heavily applied in mental health settings and with mental health issues. The model concerns itself in large measure with what can be described as internal issues such as the person's values, motivations, and belief about efficacy. It also provides a framework for addressing problematic role and habitual behavior, both frequent concerns in persons having chronic mental illness. These issues also emerge after a person experiences trauma or is coping with chronic disease or a disability.

Many of the questions that we raised previously (Bruce & Borg, 1987, 1993) have been addressed in Kielhofner's most recent edition. These could generally be grouped as inconsistencies in language or how theoretical concepts tied together, and/or have been depicted schematically. Kielhofner and his colleagues have taken what he refers to as great "pains" to address theoretical constructs clearly.

Systems Model

The model is holistic and appreciates the highly complex interplay of systems within and outside of the individual, but it does not suggest that the therapist addresses every problem that a client or patient might have. It concerns itself with occupational function/dysfunction and the everyday routines of life that surround these functions. When first articulated, the model led the way for a return by occupational therapy as a profession to its professional roots and to the focus on occupation as the vehicle for healing. Other models have followed, but none are more carefully crafted than this model. Additionally, the large number of contributors, with diverse backgrounds and cultural heritages, brings richness to the understanding of the model and its application.

Development of Assessment Instruments

Many assessment instruments have been developed in support of the model. While the AMPS is the most rigorously researched, the availability of other instruments serves as an invitation to practicing therapists who would like to make use of these data-gathering instruments and contribute to the literature.

Breadth of Application

The model is one that emphasizes the subjective nature of occupational performance, while not negating the necessity of objective data gathering. It is consistent with, and in fact depends upon, a client-centered practice. It assiduously divorces itself from a medical and/or mechanical model and is as easily implemented in medical as nonmedical and nontraditional environments. It also takes a developmental approach to the understanding of occupational changes through the life span and is applicable with children and adults of all ages. It is noteworthy that, to date, a significant number of programs have been described in the literature for children and adolescents having mental health issues. With the many published articles that describe MOHO's application, it becomes clear that the model has a breadth of application.

In summary, the model provides a thorough theoretical framework for therapists to "think about" their clients' occupational dysfunction and to frame their intervention as they and their clients go about the task of problem solving to enable clients to resume meaningful engagement in occupation.

Limitations

The model guides the therapist in what to think but carefully avoids telling occupational therapists how to implement these guides in practice. If we compare this model to the behavioral or cognitive-behavioral frameworks, for example, we will find neither the techniques nor the intervention activities provided in these other two frameworks for practice.

Limited Intervention Guidance

Because of the internal nature of what is addressed by much of the model, therapists have to give careful thought to how they can best articulate intervention objectives for third-party payers. It is as if the model creates a background for intervention planning, in particular for assuring that intervention is meaningful to the client, while other theoretical practice models might need to come to the foreground in the writing of behavioral objectives. The model shares some of the problems associated with other frames of reference described in this text. When addressing values, motivations, habits, and roles, all may require considerable time for discernable change to occur. Kielhofner appears correct when he suggests that much of what is set into motion through the application of the model needs to be followed through by the client following the cessation of formalized therapy.

Unclear Application for Prevention Model

This model addresses both function and dysfunction but seems overall more focused on dysfunction. It is not clear how or if the model would serve as a basis for interventions that have a prevention focus.

Multiple Definitions of Terms

There is much attention given to defining terms specific to the model, but the desired term(s) remain unclear at times when discussing particular constructs. In some instances, terms seem to mean different things. This was evident in early MOHO literature and occurs in more recent literature as well. For example, the distinction between "role," "internalized role," and "role script;" between an "occupation" and "occupational form;" and between a "habit" and "habit map" (Kielhofner, 1995) are not always evident.

Throughout his 1995 book, Kielhofner advises the reader to approach the text in chunks; to read and perhaps re-read in order to gain a thorough understanding of the material therein. The model of human occupation theory is not now, nor has it been historically, easy reading. That should not take away from the often evocative and always thought-provoking content.

REFERENCES

Adelstein, L. A., Barnes, M. A., Murray-Jensen, F., & Skaggs, C. B. (1989). A broadening frontier: Occupational therapy in mental health programs for children and adolescents. *Mental Health Special Interest Section Newsletter, 12,* 2-4.

Affleck, A., Bianchi, E., Cleckley, M., Donaldson, K., McCormack, G., & Polon, J. (1984). Stress management as a component of occupational therapy in acute care settings. *Occupational Therapy in Health Care, 1*(3), 17-41.

Asher, I. E. (1996). *Occupational therapy evaluation tools: An annotated index* (2nd ed.). Bethesda, MD: American Occupational Therapy Association.

Baron, K. (1987). The model of human occupation: A newspaper treatment group for adolescents with a diagnosis of conduct disorder. *Occupational Therapy in Mental Health, 7*(2), 89-104.

Baron, K. (1989). Occupational therapy: A program for child psychiatry. *Mental Health Special Interest Section Newsletter, 7*(2), 89-104.

Baron, K., & Curtin, C. (1990). *A manual for use with the Self-Assessment of Occupational Functioning.* Unpublished manuscript, Department of Occupational Therapy, University of Illinois at Chicago.

Barrett, L., & Kielhofner, G. (1998). Meaning and misunderstanding in occupational forms: A study of therapeutic goal setting. *Am J Occup Ther, 52,* 345-353.

Barris, R., Dickie, V., & Baron, K. (1988). A comparison of psychiatric patients and normal subjects based on the model of human occupation. *Occupational Therapy Journal of Research, 8,* 3-37.

Barris, R., Kielhofner, G., Burch, R., Gelinas, I., Klement, M., & Schultz, B. (1986). Occupational function and dysfunction in three groups of adolescents. *Occupational Therapy Journal of Research, 6,* 301-317.

Barris, R., Kielhofner, G., Neville, A., Oakley, F. M., Salz, C., & Watts, J. (1985). Psychosocial dysfunction. In G. Kielhofner (Ed.), *A model of human occupation* (pp. 253, 258-259). Baltimore, MD: Williams & Wilkins.

Barris, R., Kielhofner, G., & Watts, J. (1983). *Psychosocial occupational therapy: Practice in a pluralistic arena.* Laurel, MD: Ramsco Publishing.

Barton, G. E. (1917). Inoculation of the bacillus of work. *Mod Hosp, 8,* 399-403.

Behnke, C., & Fetkovich, M. (1984). Examining the reliability and validity of the Play History. *Am J Occup Ther, 38,* 94-100.

Berlyn, D. (1960). *Conflict, arousal, and curiosity.* New York, NY: McGraw Hill Book Co.

Berlyn, D. E., & Madsen, K. B. (Eds.). (1973). *Pleasure, rewards, preference: Their nature, determinants, and role in behavior.* New York, NY: Academic Press.

Bernspång, B., & Fisher, A. G. (1995a). Differences between persons with right or left CVA on the Assessment of Motor and Process Skills. *Arch Phys Med Rehabil, 76,* 1144-1151.

Bernspång, B., & Fisher, A. G. (1995b). Validation of the Assessment of Motor and Process Skills for use in Sweden. *Scandinavian Journal of Occupational Therapy, 2,* 3-9.

Biernacki, S. D. (1993). Reliability of the worker role interview. *Am J Occup Ther, 47,* 797-803.

Bledsoe, N. P., & Shepherd, J. T. (1982). A study of reliability and validity of a Preschool Play Scale. *Am J Occup Ther, 36,* 783-788.

Brollier, C., Watts, J. H., Bauer, D., & Schmidt, W. (1989a). A concurrent validity study of two occupational therapy evaluation instruments: The AOF and OCAIRS. *Occupational Therapy in Mental Health, 8,* 49-59.

Brollier, C., Watts, J. H., Bauer, D., & Schmidt, W. (1989b). A content validity study of the Assessment of Occupational Functioning. *Occupational Therapy in Mental Health, 8,* 29-47.

Bruce, M. A., & Borg, B. (1987). *Frames of reference in psychosocial occupational therapy.* Thorofare, NJ: SLACK Incorporated.

Bruce, M. A., & Borg, B. (1993). *Psychosocial occupational therapy: Frames of reference for intervention* (2nd ed.). Thorofare, NJ: SLACK Incorporated.

Burke, J. P., Clark, F., Dodd, C., & Kawamoto, T. (1987). Maternal role preparation: A program using sensory integration, infant-mother attachment, and occupational behavior perspectives. *Occupational Therapy in Health Care, 4*(2), 9-21.

Burton, J. E. (1989a). The model of human occupation and occupational therapy practice with elderly patients, Part 1: Characteristics of aging. *British Journal of Occupational Therapy, 52,* 215-218.

Burton, J. E. (1989b). The model of human occupation and occupational therapy practice with elderly patients, Part 2: Application. *British Journal of Occupational Therapy, 52,* 219-221.

Camic, C. (1986). The matter of habit. *American Journal of Sociology, 91,* 1039-1087.

Chern, J. S. (1994). *The validity and reliability of the Volitional Questionnaire: A Rasch analysis.* Unpublished master's thesis, University of Illinois at Chicago.

Christiansen, C. H. (1981). Editorial: Toward resolution of crisis: Research requisites in occupational therapy. *Occupational Therapy Journal of Research, 1,* 115-124.

Coviensky, M., & Buckley, V. (1986). Day activities programming: Serving the severely impaired chronic client. *Occupational Therapy in Mental Health, 6*(2), 21-30.

Csiksentmihalyi, M. (1990). *Flow: The psychology of optimal experience.* New York, NY: Harper Collins Publishers, Inc.

Csiksentmihalyi, M. (1997). *Finding flow: The psychology of engagement with everyday life.* New York, NY: Harper Collins Publishing, Inc.

Cubie, S., & Kaplan, K. (1982). A case analysis method for the model of human occupation. *Am J Occup Ther, 36*(10), 645-656.

Curtin, C. (1990). Research on the model of human occupation. *Mental Health: Special Interest Section Newsletter, 13*(2), 3-5.

Curtin, C., & Baron, K. (1990). *A manual for use with the Children's Self-Assessment of Occupational Functioning.* Unpublished manuscript, Department of Occupational Therapy, University of Illinois at Chicago.

DeCharms, R. (1968). *Personal causation.* New York, NY: Academic Press.

de las Heras, C. G. (1993a). *Validity and reliability of the Volitional Questionnaire.* Unpublished master's thesis, Tufts University, Boston, MA.

de las Heras, C. G. (1993b). *The Volitional Questionnaire.* Unpublished manual, Santiago, Chile.

de las Heras, C. G., Dion, G. L., & Walsh, D. (1993). Application of rehabilitation models in a state psychiatric hospital. *Occupational Therapy in Mental Health, 12*(3), 1-32.

Depoy, E. (1990). The TBIIM: An intervention for the treatment of individuals with traumatic brain injury. *Occupational Therapy in Health Care, 7*(1), 55-67.

Dickerson, A. E., & Fisher, A. G. (1995). Culture-relevant functional performance assessment of the Hispanic elderly. *Occupational Therapy Journal of Research, 15,* 50-68.

Doble, S. (1991). Test-retest and inter-rater reliability of a process skills assessment. *Occupational Therapy Journal of Research, 11,* 8-23.

Dunning, H. (1972). Environmental occupational therapy. *Am J Occup Ther, 26*(6), 292-298.

Dunton, W. R. (1917). History of occupational therapy. *Mod Hosp, 8,* 380-382.

Dunton, W. R. (1919). *Reconstruction therapy.* Philadelphia, PA: W. B. Saunders.

Dunton, W. R. (1928). The "three Rs" of occupational therapy. *Occupational Therapy Rehabilitation, 7,* 345-348.

Duran, L. J., & Fisher, A. G. (1996). Male and female performance on the Assessment of Motor and Process Skills. *Arch Phys Med Rehabil, 77,* 1019-1024.

Ebb, W. E., Coster, W., & Duncombe, L. (1989). Comparison of normal and psychosocially dysfunctional male adolescents. *Occupational Therapy in Mental Health, 9,* 53-74.

Erikson, E. (1959). Identity and the life cycle. *Psychol Issues, 1,* 1-171.

Erikson, E. (1968). *Identity, youth, and crisis.* New York, NY: Norton & Co.

Fisher, A. G. (1994). Development of a functional assessment that adjusts ability measures for task simplicity and rater leniency. In M. Wilcox (Ed.), *Objective measurement: Theory into practice* (Vol. 2, pp. 145-175). Norwood, NJ: Ablex.

Fisher, A. G. (1995). *The Assessment of Motor and Process Skills.* Unpublished manuscript, Colorado State University, Fort Collins, CO.

Fisher, A. G. (1997). *Assessement of motor and process skills* (2nd ed.). Fort Collins, CO: Three Star Press.

Fisher, A. G. (1999). *Assessment of Motor and Process Skills manual* (3rd ed.). Fort Collins, CO: Three Star Press.

Fisher, A., & Kielhofner, G. (1995). Mind-brain-performance subsystem. In G. Kielhofner (Ed.), *A model of human occupation: Theory and application* (2nd ed., pp. 83-90). Baltimore, MD: Williams & Wilkins.

Fitts, H., & Howe, M. (1987). Use of leisure time by cardiac patients. *Am J Occup Ther, 41,* 583-589.

Froehlich, J. (1992). Occupational therapy interventions with survivors of sexual abuse. *Occupational Therapy in Health Care, 8*(2/3), 1-25.

Fuller, D. (1912). The need of instruction for nurses in occupations for the sick. In S. Tracy (Ed.), *Studies in invalid occupation.* Boston, MA: Whitcomb & Barrows.

Goldman, S. L., & Fisher, A. G. (1997). Cross-cultural validation of the Assessment of Motor and Process Skills (AMPS). *British Journal of Occupational Therapy, 60,* 77-85.

Grogan, G. (1991a). Anger management: A perspective for occupational therapy (part 1). *Occupational Therapy in Mental Health, 11*(2/3), 135-148.

Grogan, G. (1991b). Anger management: A perspective for occupational therapy (part 2). *Occupational Therapy in Mental Health, 11*(2/3), 149-171.

Gusich, R. (1984). Occupational therapy for chronic pain: A clinical application of the model of human occupation. *Occupational Therapy in Mental Health, 4*(3), 59-73.

Gusich, R. L., & Silverman, A. L. (1991). Basava day clinic: The model of human occupation as applied to psychiatric day hosptitalization. *Occupational Therapy in Mental Health, 11*(2/3), 113-134.

Hagulund, L, & Kjellberg, A. (1999). A critical analysis of the model of human occupation. *Can J Occup Ther, 66,* 102-108.

Harrison, H., & Kielhofner, G. (1986). Examining reliability and validity of the preschool play scale with handicapped children. *Am J Occup Ther, 40,* 167-173.

Havighurst, R. (1982). The world of work. In B. B. Wolman (Ed.), *Handbook of developmental psychology.* Englewood Cliffs, NJ: Prentice-Hall.

Helfrich, C., Kielhofner, G., & Mattingly, C. (1994). Volition as narrative: Understanding motivation in chronic illness. *Am J Occup Ther, 48,* 311-317.

Henry, A. D. (1997). Development of a measure of adolescent leisure interests. *Am J Occup Ther, 52,* 531-539.

Henry, A. D., Baron, K. B., Mouradian, L., & Curtin, C. (1999). Reliability and validity of the self-assessment of occupational functioning. *Am J Occup Ther, 53,* 482-488.

Howe, M., & Schwartzberg, S. (1988). Structure and process in designing a function group. *Occupational Therapy in Mental Health, 8,* 1.

Howe, M., & Schwartzberg, S. (1995). *A functional approach to group work in occupational therapy* (2nd ed.). Philadelphia, PA: J. B. Lippincott.

Kaplan, K. (1984). A short-term assessment: The need and a response. *Occupational Therapy in Mental Health, 4*(5), 29-45.

Kaplan, K. (1988). *Directive group therapy: Innovative mental health treatment.* Thorofare, NJ: SLACK Incorporated.

Kaplan, K., & Kielhofner, G. (1989). *The occupational case analysis interview and rating scale.* Thorofare, NJ: SLACK Incorporated.

Katz, N., Giladi, N., & Peretz, C. (1988). Cross-cultural application of occupational therapy assessments: Human occupation with psychiatric inpatients and controls in Israel. *Occupational Therapy in Mental Health, 8,* 7-30.

Katz, N., Josman, N., & Steinmetz, N. (1988). Relationship between cognitive disability theory and the model of human occupation in the assessment of psychiatric and nonpsychiatric adolescents. *Occupational Therapy in Mental Health, 8,* 31-44.

Khoo, S. W., & Renwick, R. M. (1989). A model of human occupation perspective on the mental health of immigrant women in Canada. *Occupational Therapy in Mental Health, 9*(3), 31-50.

Kielhofner, G. (1977). Temporal adaptation: A conceptual framework for occupational therapy. *Am J Occup Ther, 31,* 235-242.

Kielhofner, G. (1980a). A model of human occupation (part 2). Ontogenesis from the perspective of temporal adaptation. *Am J Occup Ther, 34,* 657-663.

Kielhofner, G. (1980b). A model of human occupation, part 3. Benign and vicious cycles. *Am J Occup Ther, 34,* 731-737.

Kielhofner, G. (Ed.). (1983). *Health through occupation—Theory and practice in occupational therapy.* Philadelphia, PA: F. A. Davis.

Kielhofner, G. (Ed.). (1985a). *A model of human occupation.* Baltimore, MD: Williams & Wilkins.

Kielhofner, G. (1985b). Occupational function and dysfunction. In G. Kielhofner (Ed.), *A model of human occupation: Theory and application* (2nd ed., pp. 63-75). Baltimore, MD: Williams & Wilkins.

Kielhofner, G. (1988). Model of human occupation. In S. C. Robertson (Ed.), *Focus.* Rockville, MD: American Occupational Therapy Association.

Kielhofner, G. (1995). *A model of human occupation* (2nd ed.). Baltimore, MD: Williams and Wilkins.

Kielhofner, G. (1997). *Conceptual foundation of occupational therapy* (2nd ed.). Philadelphia, PA: F. A. Davis.

Kielhofner, G., Barris, R., & Bauer, D. (1983). A comparison of play behavior in non-hospitalized and hospitalized children. *Am J Occup Ther, 37*(5), 305-312.

Kielhofner, G., Borell, L., Burke, J., Helfrich, C., & Nygard, L. (1995). Volition subsystem. In G. Kielhofner (Ed.), *A model of human occupation: Theory and application* (2nd ed., pp. 39-62). Baltimore, MD: Williams & Wilkins.

Kielhofner, G., & Brinson, M. (1989). Development and evaluation of an aftercare program for young and chronic psychiatrically disabled adults. *Occupational Therapy in Mental Health, 9*(2), 1-25.

Kielhofner, G., & Burke, J. (1980). A model of human occupation, part 1. Conceptual framework and content. *Am J Occup Ther, 34*(9), 572-581.

Kielhofner, G., & Burke, J. (1985). Components and determinants of human occupation. In G. Kielhofner (Ed.), *A model of human occupation* (pp. 14, 17-18, 24-34). Baltimore, MD: Williams & Wilkins.

Kielhofner, G., Burke, J., & Igi, C. (1980). A model of human occupation (part 4). Assessment and intervention. *Am J Occup Ther, 34*(12), 777-788.

Kielhofner, G., Harlan, B., Bauer, D., & Maurer, P. (1986). The reliability of a historical interview with physically disabled respondents. *Am J Occup Ther, 40*, 551-556.

Kielhofner, G., & Henry, A. D. (1988). Development and investigation of the occupational performance history interview. *Am J Occup Ther, 42*, 489.

Kielhofner, G., & Mallinson, T. (1995a). Applications of the model in practice. In G. Kielhofner (Ed.), *A model of human occupation: Theory and application* (2nd ed., pp. 271-342). Baltimore, MD: Williams & Wilkins.

Kielhofner, G., & Mallinson, T. (1995b). Gathering and reasoning with data during intervention. In G. Kielhofner (Ed.), *A model of human occupation: Theory and application* (2nd ed., pp. 189-203). Baltimore, MD: Williams & Wilkins.

Kielhofner, G., Mallinson, T., Crawford, C., Nowack, M., Rigby, M., Henry, A., & Walens, D. (1998). *Occupational performance history interview (II).* Chicago, IL: Model of Human Occupation Clearinghouse, Department of Occupational Therapy, University of Illinois.

Kielhofner, G., Mallinson, T., & de las Heras, C. G. (1995). Methods of data gathering. In G. Kielhofner (Ed.), *A model of human occupation: Theory and application* (2nd ed., pp. 205-231). Baltimore, MD: Williams & Wilkins.

Kielhofner, G., & Neville, A. (1983). *The Modified Interest Checklist.* Unpublished manuscript, University of Illinois at Chicago.

Kielhofner, G., & Takata, N. (1980). A study of mentally retarded persons: Applied research in occupational therapy. *Am J Occup Ther, 34*(4), 252-258.

Kirkley, K. N., & Fisher, A. G. (1999). Alternate forms of reliability of the Assessment of Motor and Process Skills. *Journal of Objective Measurement, 3*, 53-70.

Laliberte-Rudman, D., Yu, B., Scott, E., & Pajoukandek, P. (1999). Exploration of perspectives of persons with schizophrenia regarding quality of life. *Am J Occup Ther, 54*, 137-145.

Lancaster, J., & Mitchell, M. (1991). Occupational therapy treatment goals, objectives, and activities for improving low self-esteem in adolescents with behavioral disorders. *Occupational Therapy in Mental Health, 11*(2/3), 3-22.

Lederer, J., Kielhofner, G., & Watts, J. (1985). Values, personal causation, and skills of delinquents and nondelinquents. *Occupational Therapy in Mental Health, 5*(2), 59-77.

Levine, R. E., & Gitlin, L. N. (1993). A model to promote activity competence in elders. *Am J Occup Ther, 47*, 147-153.

Levinson, D. (1978). *The seasons of a man's life.* New York, NY: Ballatine.

Levinson, D. (1996). *The seasons of a woman's life.* New York, NY: Ballentine Books.

Linton, R. (1945). *The cultural background of personality.* New York, NY: Appleton-Century-Crofts.

Maddi, S. (1989). *Personality theories: A comparative analysis* (5th ed., pp. 355, 651-652). Chicago, IL: The Dorsey Press.

Mallinson, T., Mahaffey, L., & Kielhofner, G. (1998). The occupational performance history interview: Evidence for three underlying constructs of occupational adaptation. *Can J Occup Ther, 65*, 219-228.

Matsutsuyu, J. (1969). The Interest Check List. *Am J Occup Ther, 23*, 323-328.

McClelland, D. (1961). *The achieving society.* New York, NY: Free Press.

McClelland, D. C. (1973). *Personality.* New York, NY: Dryden Press.

Meyer, A. (1922). The philosophy of occupational therapy. *Archives of Occupational Therapy, 1*, 1-10.

Meyer, A. (1977). The philosophy of occupational therapy. *Am J Occup Ther, 31*, 639-642.

Muñoz, J. P. (1988). A program for acute inpatient psychiatry. *Mental Health Special Interest Section Newsletter, 11*, 3-4.

Muñoz, J. P., & Kielhofner, G. (1995). Program development. In G. Kielhofner (Ed.), *A model of human occupation* (2nd ed., pp. 343-372). Baltimore, MD: Williams & Wilkins.

Nelson, D. (1988). Occupation: Form and performance. *Am J Occup Ther, 38*, 777-788.

Neville-Jan, A. (1994). The relationship of volition to adaptive occupational behavior among individuals with varying degrees of depression. *Occupational Therapy in Mental Health, 12*, 1-18.

Neville-Jan, A., Bradley, M., Bunn, C., & Gehri, B. (1991). The model of human occupation and individuals with co-dependency problems. *Occupational Therapy in Mental Health, 11*(2/3), 73-97.

Newell, A., & Simon, H. (1972). *Human problem-solving.* Englewood Cliffs, NJ: Prentice-Hall.

Oakley, F. (1987). Clinical application of the model of human occupation in dementia of the Alzheimer's type. *Occupational Therapy in Mental Health, 7*(4), 37-50.

Oakley, F., Kielhofner, G., & Barris, R. (1985). An occupational therapy approach to assessing psychiatric patient's adaptive functioning. *Am J Occup Ther, 39*, 147-154.

Oakley, F., Kielhofner, G., Barris, R., & Reichler, R. K. (1986). The role checklist: Development and empirical assessment of reliability. *Occupational Therapy Journal of Research, 6*, 157-170.

Olin, D. (1985). Assessing and assisting persons with dementia: An occupational behavior perspective. *Physical and Occupational Therapy in Geriatrics, 3*(4), 25-32.

Padilla, R., & Bianchi, E. M. (1990). Occupational therapy for chronic pain: Applying the model of human occupation in clinical practice. *Occupational Therapy Practice, 1*(3), 47-52.

Pan, A. W., & Fisher, A. G. (1994). The Assessment of Motor and Process Skills with persons with psychiatric disorders. *Am J Occup Ther, 48*, 775-780.

Pizzi, M. (1990). The model of human occupation and adults with HIV infection and AIDS. *Am J Occup Ther, 44*, 257-264.

Rebeiro, K. L., & Allen, J. (1998). Voluntarism as occupation. *Can J Occup Ther, 65*, 279-285.

Reilly, M. (1966). A psychiatric occupational therapy program as a teaching model. *Am J Occup Ther, 20*, 61-67.

Reilly, M. (1969). The education process. *Am J Occup Ther, 23*, 299-307.

Reilly, M. (1971). Occupational therapy—A historical perspective: The modernization of occupational therapy. *Am J Occup Ther, 25*(5), 243.

Reilly, M. (Ed.). (1974). *Play as exploratory learning*. Beverly Hills, CA: Sage Publications.

Robinson, S., & Fisher, A. G. (1996). A study to examine the relationship of the Assessment of Motor and Process Skills (AMPS) to other tests of cognition and function. *British Journal of Occupational Therapy, 47*, 298-301.

Rotter, J. B. (1960). Generalized expectancies for internal versus external control of reinforcement. *Psychological Monographs: General Applications, 80*, 1-28.

Salamy, M., Simon, S., & Kielhofner, G. (1993). *The Assessment of Communication and Interaction Skills (research version)*. Chicago, IL: Department of Occupational Therapy, University of Illinois.

Salz, C. (1983). A theoretical approach to the treatment of work difficulties in borderline personalities. *Occupational Therapy in Mental Health, 3*(3), 33-46.

Scaffa, M. (1981). *Temporal adaptations and alcoholism*. Unpublished master's thesis, Virginia Commonwealth University, Richmond.

Scarth, P. P. (1990). Services for chemically dependent adolescents. *Mental Health Special Interest Section Newsletter, 13*, 7-8.

Schaaf, R. C., & Mulrooney, L. L. (1989). Occupational therapy in early intervention: A family-centered approach. *Am J Occup Ther, 34*, 745-754.

Schindler, V. J. (1988). Psychosocial occupational therapy intervention with AIDS patients. *Am J Occup Ther, 42*, 507-512.

Series, C. (1992). The long-term needs of people with head injury: A role for the community occupational therapist? *British Journal of Occupational Therapy, 55*(3), 94-98.

Shimp, S. L. (1989). A family-style meal group: Short-term treatment for eating disorder patients with a high level of functioning. *Mental Health Special Interest Section Newsletter, 12*, 1-3.

Sholle-Martin, S. (1987). Application of the model of human occupation: Assessment in child and adolescent psychiatry. *Occupational Therapy in Mental Health, 7*(2), 3-22.

Sholle-Martin, S., & Alessi, N. E. (1990). Formulating a role for occupational therapy in child psychiatry: A clinical application. *Am J Occup Ther, 44*, 871-881.

Simon, S. (1989). *The development of an Assessment for Interaction and Communication Skills*. Unpublished master's thesis, University of Illinois at Chicago.

Slagle, E. C. (1938a). Occupational therapy. *Trained Nurse and Hospital Review, 100*, 375-382.

Slagle, E. C. (1938b). The training of occupational therapists for work with mental patients. *American Association for the Advancement of Science, 9*, 408-415.

Smith, N. R., Kielhofner, G., & Watts, J. (1986). The relationship between volition, activity pattern, and life satisfaction in the elderly. *Am J Occup Ther, 40*, 278-283.

Smyntek, L., Barris, R., & Kielhofner, G. (1985). The model of human occupation applied to psychosocially functional and dysfunctional adolescents. *Occupational Therapy in Mental Health, 5*, 21-40.

Spranger, E. (1928). *Types of men* (W. Pigors, Trans.). Halle, Germany: Niemeyer.

Stensrud, M. K., & Lushbough, R. S. (1988). The implementation of an occupational therapy program in an alcohol and drug dependency treatment center. *Occupational Therapy in Mental Health, 8*(2), 1-16.

Suto, M. (1998). Leisure in occupational therapy. *Can J Occup Ther, 65*, 271-278.

Takata, N. (1980). Introduction to a series: Occupational behavior research for pediatric practice. *Am J Occup Ther, 34*(1), 11-12.

Tatham, M. (1992). Leisure facilitator: The role of the occupational therapist in senior housing. *Journal of Housing for the Elderly, 10*(2), 125-138.

Tracy, S. E. (1914). Invalid occupation in the curriculum of the training school. *Mod Hosp, 3*, 56-57.

Tracy, S. E. (1918). *Studies in invalid occupation*. Boston, MA: Witcomb and Barrows.

Vaillant, G. (1971). Theoretical hierarchy of adaptive ego mechanisms. *Arch Gen Psychiatry, 24*, 107-118.

Vaillant, G. (1977). *Adaptation to life*. Boston, MA: Little, Brown and Co.

Velozo, C., Kielhofner, G., & Fisher, A. (1990). *A user's guide to the Worker Role Interview (research version)*. Department of Occupational Therapy, University of Illinois at Chicago.

von Bertalanffy, L. (1968). *General system theory: Foundations, development application* (Rev. ed.). New York, NY: George Braziller.

Watts, J., Brollier, C., Bauer, D., & Schmidt, R. (1989a). A comparison of two evaluation instruments used with psychiatric patients in occupational therapy. *Occupational Therapy in Mental Health, 8*, 7-27.

Watts, J. H., Brollier, C., Bauer, D., & Schmidt, W. (1989b). The Assessment of Occupational Functioning: The second revision. *Occupational Therapy in Mental Health, 8*(4), 61-87.

Watts, J. H., Kielhofner, G., Bauer, D., Gregory, M., & Valentine, D. (1986). The assessment of occupational functioning: A screening tool for use in long-term care. *Am J Occup Ther, 40*, 231-240.

Weeder, T. (1986). Comparison of temporal patterns and meaningfulness of the daily activities of schizophrenic and normal adults. *Occupational Therapy in Mental Health, 6*, 27-45.

Weissenberg, R., & Giladi, W. (1989). Home economics day: A program for disturbed adolescents to promote acquisition of habits and skills. *Occupational Therapy in Mental Health, 9*(2), 89-103.

Werner, H. (1948). *Comparative psychology of mental development.* Chicago, IL: Follett.

Werner, H. (1957). The conception of development from a comparative and organismic point of view. In D. Harris (Ed.), *The concept of development.* Minneapolis, MN: University of Minnesota Press.

West, W. L. (1990). Nationally speaking—Perspectives on the past and future (part 2). *Am J Occup Ther, 44,* 9-10.

White, R. W. (1959). Motivation reconsidered: The concept of competence. *Psychol Rev, 66,* 297-333.

White, R. W. (1971). The urge toward competence. *Am J Occup Ther, 25,* 271-274.

Woodrum, S. C. (1993). A treatment approach for attention deficit hyperactivity disorder using the model of human occupation. *Developmental Disabilities Special Interest Section Newsletter, 16*(1), 1-2.

Young, M. (1988). *The metronomic society: Natural rhythms and human timetables.* Cambridge, MA: Harvard University Press.

CHAPTER EIGHT

Cognitive Disability Frame of Reference—Acknowledging Limitations

KEY POINTS

❖ History and Current Theory
- Questioning the Generalist Approach
- Organic Cause of Disability
- Cognitive Hierarchy: The Cognitive Levels
- Cognitive Modes of Performance Create the Allen Cognitive Level Scale (ACLS)

❖ Theory in Context of Occupational Therapy Practice
- Cognitive Function Is Central to Understanding the Person
- Motivation: Distinguishing Cannot From Will Not
- Therapist: Assessor, Expert, Environmental Manager, Consultant
- Activity: Measurement of Cognitive Processing, Success Experience, Diversion
- Environmental Compensation: Changing the Task or Activity

❖ Theoretical Assumptions Guide Evaluation and Intervention
- Evaluation
  —Role of Diagnoses and Medication
  —Cognitive Screen and Cognitive Assessment
  —Allen Diagnostic Modules (ADM)
- Intervention
  —Phases: Prevent Complications, Establish Cognitive Level, Specify Maintenance
  —Therapeutic Groups—Similar Cognitive Levels

❖ Contributions and Limitations of the Cognitive Disability Frame of Reference

Focus Questions

1. According to Allen, what is wrong with the generalist position in occupational therapy?
2. How does Allen's definition of cognition compare to that used by other frames of reference in this text?
3. Compare and contrast Allen's six cognitive levels with the behaviors subsumed in Piaget's sensorimotor period.
4. Why are persons with cognitive disabilities not expected to learn or improve as a result of occupational therapy intervention?
5. What is the **key** role of the occupational therapist?
6. What do **management** and **maintenance** of a cognitive disability mean?
7. What does a cognitive level predict?
8. What behavior(s) might one expect from a patient who is presented a task beyond his or her cognitive ability?
9. At what cognitive level is a person expected to learn new information and manage novel situations?
10. How does one establish **task equivalence**?
11. Why are occupational therapy services necessary, even when they may not contribute to a patient's improvement?
12. What service does the occupational therapist provide to the caregiver? To other professionals?
13. How is this model humanizing? How can individual differences be lost?

Historical Update

The cognitive disabilities frame of reference is the outcome of the professional work of occupational therapist Claudia Allen and her associates. It represents over a quarter century of study by Allen, whose early practice was largely with the psychiatric population. Recognizing at that time that many adults with mental illness reappeared at the doors of mental health settings and were, by definition, chronically mentally ill and unable to function normally in their environments, Allen began her exploration to discover the nature of the cognitive impairments that seemed to limit the functional abilities of these persons. Six levels of cognitive function were identified out of her study (eventually to be broken down further into sublevels). Through assessment of a patient's functional performance, the nature of his or her cognitive impairment could be described. By recognizing and accepting the limitations imposed by cognitive dysfunction, Allen's ultimate task, as she would write, became to "improve the quality of life of the cognitively disabled person" (Allen & Blue, 1998, p. 264).

In her early writing, Allen described the similarities she recognized between Piaget's sensorimotor stage of cognitive development and the mental processes used by the psychi-

atric patients whom she was treating. In the first edition of this text, Claudia Allen's theoretical approach to date (1985) was discussed as one example of a developmental frame of reference because her cognitive levels were, at that time, predicated on Piaget's sensorimotor period (Allen, 1982). In subsequent literature, Allen stated that Piagetian theory (Piaget, 1952, 1971, 1972, 1978, 1980), which was based upon normal development, was inadequate for explaining the mental processing of persons whose cognitive function was not normal. She then looked to the literature of cognitive psychology for a plausible theoretical base (Allen, 1987, 1988; Allen & Allen, 1987; Vygotsky, 1962). More recently, she has credited both Piaget and information processing theory as influences (Allen, 1991a, 1999; Allen & Blue, 1998).

Allen's work continues, and information about use of the model is disseminated through workshops/conferences available to occupational therapists. Although her model has historically been referred to as the cognitive disabilities model, Allen has consistently written that the cognitive levels describe a global measure of **ability** to function as well as severity of functional **disability** (Allen & Blue, 1998; Allen, Earhart, & Blue, 1992). In recent literature, Allen (1999) describes the underlying cognitive structures that guide normal behavior and refers to these as the Functional Information Processing System (p. 1). This suggests further movement toward a cognitive abilities rather than a disabilities model. As Allen writes, finding a theoretical base has "met many obstacles and few resources" (Allen & Blue, 1998, p. 264). Nevertheless, in her study, Allen has made a significant contribution to the profession's understanding of the nature of cognitive impairment, specifically as it compromises the abilities of persons to function normally in the everyday environment. Perhaps best known for the Allen Cognitive Levels, an ordinal description of cognitive processing abilities and disabilities, Allen's work has had a significant influence on practice both within the United States and internationally.

Definition

The cognitive disabilities frame of reference is one that describes the nature of cognitive processing impairments that compromise the ability for normal function and identifies adaptations that will optimize the ability of cognitively disabled persons to function in their everyday world. It has been used primarily with adults and assumes that individuals having cognitive disorders include not only those with chronic mental illness, but potentially any person whose condition includes a central nervous system disorder.

Cognitive disability leads to a reduction in normal task performance, which is debilitating for many individuals and requires that these persons have the assistance of family or other caregivers if they are to be safe in the community. As an alternative to expecting improvement, the therapist's primary goals are the following:

- To assess patient/client cognitive level
- To identify activities at which the patient can succeed
- To advise other professionals and caregivers about the limitations on functional performance that are imposed by cognitive disability
- To make environmental recommendations compatible with functional level.

Unlike other frameworks, activities are not expected to bring about behavior or cognitive change. Rather, they may be used as a vehicle for ongoing assessment of cognitive level and to engage the individual in activities that are realistic, relevant, and safe to perform.

THEORETICAL DEVELOPMENT

With her earliest publications (1982, 1985), Allen expressed dissatisfaction with the prevailing psychodynamic, behavioral, sociological, and sensory-integrative models used by occupational therapists practicing in mental health settings. Basing her conclusions on observations made with her own patients, she proposed an intervention model that would make better use of the activity focus basic to occupational therapy. The model would be primarily concerned with patients' cognitive abilities, especially as these influenced the ability to learn.

Questioning the Generalist Approach

In this early material and in later publications, the author was highly critical of a holistic, or what she termed a "generalist" approach taken by occupational therapists who practiced in mental health care (Allen, 1982, 1985).

> I have been frustrated by our generalist approach to identify the parameters of practice... our professional discussions contain the implicit assumption that a therapist needs to read every book in the library and offer services to every person in the community... (Allen, 1985, p. 17)

Compounding the problems of a generalist approach, Allen suggested that most psychiatric patients fit into one of the following two categories:
1. They are unlikely to show improvement
2. If they do improve, it is not likely to be due to their involvement in activity

In Allen's early work, the patient population was specifically identified as either "schizophrenic" or "psychotic." She would later write that the population she was addressing represented many persons who, subsequent to de-institutionalization, were chronically mentally ill (Allen, 1985, 1994; Allen & Allen, 1987; Allen et al., 1992).

Sensorimotor Stage and Cognitive Impairment

Piaget's first developmental stage, known as the sensorimotor stage and used to describe the development of cognition in infants age 0 to 2 years, was initially selected by Allen to describe adult patient problem-solving as used in task behavior. She concluded that these adults had a cognitive impairment and were unable rather than unwilling to perform adequately in many of the tasks they faced.

Cognitive Disability in a Medical Model

In 1982 and 1985 publications, the population of patients judged to have a potential performance deficit due to cognitive impairment was expanded to include most of the psychiatric population. Allen supported the view that the cognitive and behavior changes of mental illness result from biological changes in the brain. Seeking to define cognitive impairment in a way that would be objective and verifiable, Allen identified **cognitive disability** as a "restriction in voluntary motor action originating in the physical or chemical structures of the brain and producing observable limitations in routine task behavior" (Allen, 1985, p. 31). A cognitive disability, she wrote, inhibits task performance, prevents goal achievement, and promotes idle behavior. These problems result in a poor adaptive response and limit independent function in the community (Allen, 1982).

Organic Cause of Disability

In her 1985 book, Allen used professional data to conclude that roughly 80% of the patients treated by occupational therapists have "disorders with potential for a cognitive impairment," and by definition attributable to an organic cause (Allen, 1985, p. 13). **Organic** in this usage referred to impairments within the central nervous system. These disorders include developmental, mood, behavior, anxiety, substance abuse, and personality disorders and schizophrenia.

Criteria for Treatment

In developing her framework, Allen distinguished between those illnesses with an **acute component** (e.g., bipolar disorder and depressive psychosis), in which cognitive limitations were more likely to resolve with the use of medication, and **chronically disabling disorders** (e.g., chronic schizophrenia), in which patients would need help in compensating for residual disability. She proposed that those psychiatric patients with a cognitive disability were the population that occupational therapists working in mental health should treat because occupational therapy is expert in treating disorders that impair function. Other mental health professionals would treat those patients who did not have a cognitive disability.

Assessing Voluntary Motor Behavior

To objectify the extent of cognitive disability, Allen proposed using guided observation of the patient engaged in a specified motor task. The assessments developed by Allen and her associates during the 1980s included the **Allen Cognitive Level Test**, in which the patient is asked to imitate and thereby learn two leather-lacing stitches; the **Lower Cognitive Level Test**, which asks the patient to imitate the therapist's clapping hands; and the **Routine Task Inventory**, in which the patient's cognitive performance is assessed as he or she completes numerous activities of daily living. These tests have all undergone revision and are discussed in more detail later in the chapter. The patient's performance in one or more of these tests enabled the therapist to identify his or her level of cognitive function and in turn predicted the ability to do familiar activities and learn new ones. It also helped caretakers anticipate the most suitable post-treatment placement for the patient (Allen, 1987).

Cognitive Hierarchy: The Cognitive Levels

Cognitive function was initially classified on a scale of six levels, ranging from severe disability at the first level to normal ability at level six (Table 8-1). These levels were described as an ordinal description of functional states as delineated by the sensorimotor association used to guide voluntary motor actions (Allen, 1982, 1985, 1987). "**Ordinal**" means that the levels are in a hierarchical order, but the distance between the levels is not necessarily equivalent. These cognitive levels were also described as a "measure of competence as observed during task performance" (Allen, 1985, p. 79). In more recent literature, Allen has written that these six cognitive levels measure "inferred mental processes. The inference is based on (the person's) attention to environmental cues (**input**) and observed verbal and motor behavior (**output**). The mental process (**throughput**) is the (person's) capacity to translate the cue into activity performance" (Allen, 1994, p. 8).

Cognitive levels predict what a person will realistically be able to do, as well as the severity of a functional disability (Allen & Blue, 1998, p. 226). They can also be used to determine appropriate teaching methods or to indicate when learning cannot occur (Allen, 1994, p. 8). Use of cognitive levels "helps occupational therapists understand what the world looks like to a person who is cognitively disabled" (Allen, 1994, p. 9).

Using this expanded definition for the cognitive levels, Allen has further proposed that these six cognitive levels "predict (the patient's) awareness of problems in mental function, willingness to accept assistance from others, and capacity to set realistic goals" (Allen, 1994, p. 9). While these levels have undergone revision in order to make them more sensitive and descriptive of patient performance, we have in this chapter retained an overview of these six basic levels as they provide an informative summary of what is frequently observed in client performance (see Table 8-1).

Movement Away from Piaget and Developmental Precepts

As previously indicated, Allen, in her earliest work, wrote that Piaget's sensorimotor period was the basis for identifying her cognitive hierarchy. One could see important points of departure, however, since many of the behaviors described by Allen in case examples were adult behaviors not yet learned by the child, and many of the affective postures of the cognitively disabled as noted by Allen were not the healthy, exuberant faces or postures of a normal child. Perhaps more fundamentally problematic, although not discussed in her work, was that the behaviors that spanned Allen's "sensorimotor" hierarchy (specifically the higher cognitive levels) were not consistent with Piaget's "sensorimotor" period, but rather were indicative of much higher developmental levels in Piaget's model.

In 1985, Allen elaborated about her dissatisfaction with Piaget's general developmental postulates regarding the manner in which cognitive skills are built. Citing and in apparent agreement with Mounoud (1982), Allen stated that the development of cognitive abilities is a "maturational process that depends only very indirectly on the interactions of the child with the environment... and that... it is strongly determined by genetic regulation"(Allen, 1985, p. 32).

Allen added that she also wondered to what extent the rules of normal cognitive development could be applied to understanding cognitive disability and its remediation. The conclusion drawn was that the rules are not the same.

Is Skill-Building a Reasonable Goal?

Staying with her line of reasoning, Allen proposed that skill-building was not a reasonable goal for adult patients who have a cognitive disability. As she wrote,

> Changes in cognitive level are observed in acute conditions. (These changes are not) explained by the patient's experiences in the occupational therapy clinic... (and) have alternative explanations... the effectiveness of psychotropic drugs, the natural healing process, and the natural course of the disease... (Allen, 1985, p. 32)

The role of treatment by the occupational therapist was to assess cognitive level, observe for behavior changes that would suggest that medications are working to clear the condition, and identify and make available activities and environmental conditions in which the patient can succeed.

Table 8-1

OVERVIEW OF COGNITIVE LEVELS

Level 1: Automatic actions	The patient is conscious but responding to internal stimuli. He or she does not experience self as separate from the environment. Behavior appears to be instinctive and/or habitual, and the patient can be engaged only to a minimum extent in his or her own care. Grooming, dressing, bathing, and other nursing care must be provided, and the person is often restricted to bed. Level 1 functioning may be seen in patients having head trauma, stroke, and severe dementia.
Level 2: Postural actions	The patient is motivated to maintain a state of comfort and at times becomes involved in bizarre posturing. He or she appears to have a primitive sense of self as separate within the environment. The patient may be able to assist the caregiver in some self-care tasks but may also become suddenly distressed and resistive. The patient may follow others in walking to a destination but may also engage in aimless pacing and wandering. Twenty-four-hour nursing care is still required. Diagnoses often associated with Level 2 functioning include severe psychosis, head trauma, CVA, and dementia.
Level 3: Manual actions	The patient can respond to tactile cues with manual actions in order to produce an interesting result. Often, he or she engages in repetitive, seemingly pointless or inappropriate actions. Long-term repetitive training may enable a limited function of routine tasks. Patients may need much reminding in order to see a task to completion, and 24-hour supervision is suggested. Level 3 functioning is commonly seen in patients with dementia, acute mania, toxic psychosis, and acute schizophrenic episode.
Level 4: Goal-directed actions	At Level 4, actions are sequenced into goal-directed activity that can be identified and remembered (Allen, 1994, p. 8). The person functioning at Level 4 can carry out familiar routines but is unable to problem solve in novel situations. He or she pays attention to what is visible and tends to not notice what is out of sight. Training can be used successfully with this person if it is situation specific. Level 4 is commonly ascribed to patients with mild dementia, acute manic episodes, and chronic schizophrenia. It is important to note that patients at this level who have a well-established routine may appear to cope well day-to-day, but they cannot anticipate and adequately cope with unexpected events, thus requiring caregiver assistance. *(continued)*

Table 8-1 (Continued)

Level 5: Exploratory actions	The patient can use overt trial and error and experimentation to problem solve. New learning is occurring, and inductive reasoning enables new ways of performing activities (Allen, 1994, p. 8). Because he or she has to see the results of his or her actions on the environment, problems may occur when the need to anticipate or plan is required for performance. Vital tasks such as dressing, eating, etc. are accomplished without difficulty, but in such chores as those related to cooking, money management, shopping, or traveling, problems with planning may be evidenced. The ability to decenter and empathize with others becomes evident at Level 5 (Allen, 1994, p. 8). Level 5 may be "the usual level of function" for some (about 20% of a control population) and a "distressing disability for others (about 80%)" (Allen, 1987). Level 5 functioning has been attributed to persons with remitting affective disorders, personality disorders, and "good prognosis schizophrenic disorders" (Allen, 1987, p. 188).
Level 6: Planned actions	Level 6 describes the absence of disability. Symbolic cues guide motor action. The person can think of hypothetical situations or do mental trail and error. Future events can therefore be planned well in advance. Behavior is organized, verbal and written instructions can be followed, and the therapist need not demonstrate. At this level, the individual can consider the "greater good" of society (Allen, 1994, p. 8). If a cognitive impairment had existed, Level 6 would indicate full recompensation to normal ability.

Task Equivalence

In order for the therapist to provide those activities in which the patient could be expected to succeed, he or she must be able to analyze the cognitive demands of the activities in which the patient would be involved. Only then could activities be matched to the patient's cognitive level, a process referred to as creating **task equivalence**. According to Allen, task analysis allows the establishment of criteria that can be used to demonstrate that one activity is the cognitive equivalent of another. In other words, the cognitive processing demands are alike. If, for example, a patient is involved in putting together a tossed salad on one day and doing a copper tooling the next day, the therapist would have a means to judge if differences in that patient's performance on those 2 days was due to changes within the patient or due to the inherent differences in the tasks at hand. Just as important, if the person is able to succeed at making a salad, and the copper tooling craft makes the same cognitive demands, he or she could be expected to succeed at it also.

The same attributes that specify the cognitive levels for patients are used to describe the task's cognitive demands, although slightly regrouped in their presentation. As with cognitive performance level, the task analysis described in earlier literature addressed:

1. The sensory cues used in the activity
2. The nature of the motor actions, including the number of steps involved, the extent and type of tool used, and the nature and relative use of verbal and demonstrated instruction
3. The kind of reasoning employed (Table 8-2)

Allen also suggested that the therapist consider patient preferences and the role of past experiences in the patient's performance on selected tasks, but this was not specifically included in the task analysis. In subsequent literature, task and activity analysis included guidelines in regard to the assistance persons would be expected at the various cognitive levels, as well as specifying treatment goals and a safety precautions related to task accomplishment at the various cognitive levels (Allen et al., 1992).

Table 8-2
ATTRIBUTES OF MOTOR BEHAVIOR

Attention to sensory cues	The cues to which the patient attends (e.g., internal or visceral cues as opposed to touchable or visible ones) and the ability to ignore irrelevant stimuli.
Motor actions	The extent to which motor behavior appears consciously planned and executed, and the extent of imitation.
Conscious awareness	The motives that compel behavior, the sensations produced, and the kind of reasoning employed in problem solving (e.g., inductive as opposed to deductive, covert versus trial and error), as well as the ability to attend to a task over time.

Adapted from Allen, C. (1985). *Occupational therapy for psychiatric diseases: Measurement and management of cognitive disabilities.* Boston, MA: Little Brown and Company.

Allen has continued to emphasize the importance of task equivalence. By understanding the underlying premise of task equivalence, she suggests, the therapist can predict those activities at which the client can be expected to succeed and to predict his or her functional behavior. She has stressed, however, that this is different from changing functional behavior (Allen, 1994, p. 29).

New Theoretical Directions

In the late 1980s, Allen further disavowed Piaget, as she wrote:

> The search for measurable treatment objectives turned up Piaget's sensorimotor period which was modified for clinical purposes... Unhappily, an extensive critical analysis of Piaget's work suggested (he) was cooking his own theoretical soup in the form of equilibrium, adaptation, assimilation, and accommodation. (Allen, 1988, p. 320)

Allen had earlier underscored, however, that a "strict adherence" to the literature to which she referred was "not essential nor even beneficial" because the "detection of tautologies and the special needs of occupational therapy's patient population justify departures from the original sources" (Allen, 1987, p. 4).

Information Processing Model

The late 1980s found Allen exploring the literature of cognitive psychology, especially Soviet psychology (Kotarbinski, 1965; Leontyev, 1978, 1981). One influence

of this study appears to have been the increased emphasis Allen has since placed in her writing on the need for therapists to understand the special meaning of activity to their patients/clients.

However, it was Anderson's information processing model (1992) that Allen selected to serve as a more encompassing theoretical basis for explaining the performance abilities and disabilities she had been describing. She credits Anderson for bringing together both developmental and information-processing models (Allen & Blue, 1998, p. 10).

Adding the Cognitive Modes of Performance to Create the Allen Cognitive Level Scale

As her model evolved, an important addition was the expansion of the original six cognitive levels (from 0, coma through 6, normal) to include a **decimal subsystem**, which was added as a way to make the cognitive scale more sensitive and descriptive of small changes in functional performance (Allen et al., 1992, 1996). Starting with level 0.8 and stopping at Level 6.0, the remaining five levels were further divided into nine sublevels. In other words, Level 1 was subdivided into Level 1.0, 1.1, 1.2, 1.3,... 1.9; Level 2 became Level 2.0, 2.1, 2.2, 2.3,... 2.9, and so on. According to Allen, "the even number after the decimal point rates information that is translated into action," (something the person can do) and the "preceding odd number gives the patient credit for attention to a cue that is not translated into action (4.3 gives partial credit for 4.4.)" (Allen, 1994, p. 14). These sublevels are referred to as the **modes of performance**.

Each mode within these six large levels is "built around" the same cognitive framework and describes the person's abilities as related to attention (what he or she is attending to), processing speed, verbal/propositional abilities, visual spatial abilities, and memory (Allen, 1999; Allen & Blue, 1998).

The six main levels plus the decimal system are currently referred to collectively as the **Allen Cognitive Level Scale (ACLS)**. While the six levels currently have 52 possible modes of performance, Allen has written that the odd numbered modes are not typically used and the scale more often assesses performance according to 26 and not 52 modes (Allen & Blue, 1998, p. 226).

Allen recommends use of the decimal system during the initial evaluation when occupational therapists need to "detect and document" change in functional performance (Allen, 1994, p. 14). Further, she has suggested that by using the performance modes the therapist can create the "just right challenge" for clients (Allen, 1994, p. 16). Once cognitive function has stabilized, however, she indicates that reference to the original six levels may be an adequate guide for caregiver education and discharge planning (Allen, 1994, p. 14).

Research

Early research using a cognitive disabilities framework was conducted with a depressed population (Katz, 1985), patients with senile dementia (Heying, 1985; Wilson, Allen, McCormack, & Burton, 1989), adolescents (Katz, Josman, & Steinmetz, 1988), persons with schizophrenia (Allen, 1985), chemical dependency (Partida & Price, 1988), and a broader psychiatric population (Averbuck & Katz, 1988; Heimann, Allen, & Yerxa, 1989; Landsmann & Katz, 1988). Far more research has been conducted in an effort to establish reliability and validity of the assessments associated with the framework. These are referenced later in the chapter when we take a closer look at the assessment instruments. Research continues to refine the descriptions of cognitive levels and the analysis of activities. It also evaluates the application of the model with populations in and outside of mental health settings.

CURRENT PRACTICE IN OCCUPATIONAL THERAPY

The Person and Behavior

Because Allen consistently applies the term **normal human function** when she refers to the activity of nondisabled persons, this term is used in this text. The focus in this frame of reference has not been primarily on normal human function; therefore, our discussion of this dimension is somewhat brief.

Cognitive Function Is Central

As conceptualized by Allen, the person is one in whom all activity appears clustered about cognitive function. **Cognitive function** relates to the "mental control of behavior to do activities" (Allen, 1994, p. 12). Cognitive capacity as a brain-regulated process responds to chemical and structural brain changes and is not significantly affected by the person's interaction with the environment. Cognitive abilities are believed to develop in an invariant sequence that is "universal, cross-cultural, and handed down through evolution" (Allen & Blue, 1998, p. 237). The success and breadth of human performance depends on the level of cognitive function and the compatibility of cognitive skills with expectations for performance within the environment. **Normal human function**, a "qualitative capacity" that "can be measured by the cognitive levels," is defined as the "use of mental energy to guide verbal and motor behavior to do meaningful and durable activities. Function occurs in an ever-changing environment" (Allen, 1994, p. 12). Function in this model has also been described as the ability to do the mental processing necessary for engagement in occupation (Allen & Blue, 1998, pp. 226-227). These mental processes consist of mental structures that "direct the actions and activities of people" (Allen, 1999, pp. 4-6).

If this description of human function is contrasted with others, it becomes apparent that personality, feelings, thoughts or beliefs about the self, and social skills are not being emphasized; however, this does not mean that these other dimensions of human experience are ignored by this model. Allen states that her model targets the "whole person" (Allen, 1999, p. 9; Allen & Blue, 1998, p. 237). The capacity to think, she writes, has a "pervasive effect, impacting every aspect of the person's life" (Allen, 1999, p. 4; Allen & Blue, 1998, p. 236).

According to Allen, occupational therapy specifically works with functional problems that are a consequence of a medical problem (i. e., the limitations in function that Allen is addressing in her model are believed to be created by biological impairments in or restraints on cognition [Allen & Blue, 1998, p. 12]).

Normal cognitive function is designated as the ability to do cognitive processing at cognitive level 6.0 in Allen's cognitive hierarchy and is characterized as the ability to use symbols to think about, anticipate, and plan action.

Motivation: Distinguishing Cannot from Will Not

In agreement with what she refers to as an "organismic world view," Allen proposes that people regulate their own behavior and will do the best they can given their situation (Allen, 1985, p. 95). One's best or what a person is capable of is referred to as his or her **capacity** and includes his or her present abilities (physical as well as cognitive) and potential to develop new abilities (Allen, 1988). Although social feelings and skills are not cited as a part of capacity, Allen acknowledges that the ability to carry out acceptable social roles is influenced by cognitive and physical capacity.

What a person is capable of doing (what they "can do") must be made before a determination can be made that he or she is unwilling to engage in an activity ("will not do"). Too often people with cognitive impairments and those having chronic mental illness are judged by family members or other professionals as not trying when, in fact, they are doing the best they can. Capacity has to be present before a problem with motivation can be assumed (Allen, 1994, p. 16).

Normal human function produces results that affect material objects and people. These results are achieved within the context of the person's history and social group, and the person's ultimate satisfaction with what he or she has accomplished in activity may depend on the extent to which this activity fits with the social group's values. Seeing his or her own success can be expected to carry over as a positive motivator for continued task performance.

Dysfunction

Dysfunction assumes that a physiologic abnormality results in impairment, disability, or handicap, in turn reflecting compromise in the ability for functional performance. Early in her theory development, Allen defined **dysfunction** as an impairment in sensorimotor information processing (Allen, 1982, 1985) and referred to persons having permanent cognitive limitations as persons having a **cognitive disability**.

In Allen's educational video "Why Occupational Therapists Use Crafts" (1991b), Allen describes cognitively disabled persons as often childlike and "demanding," yet "wanting the privileges of adults." Other early literature suggests similar personality characteristics frequently associated with cognitive disability. For example, "Verbally facile patients are particularly troublesome if their motor performance does not match their verbal abilities" (Allen, 1985, p. 5).

> ...People who are depressed are suffering, and some of them complain a great deal... One can get very tired of listening to the same complaints over and over... There is a tendency to get mad at the patients or ignore them. (Allen, 1985, p. 140)

More recently, Allen and Blue (1998) have written that cognitively disabled persons are ones about whom, "We must assume that what they think and feel is both similar to and different from the way we think and feel" (p. 236). They have a "limited capacity to think" (p. 236). It is this difference in thinking that leads to the cognitive disability. The authors write, "People with cognitive disabilities are those whose ability to think and feel has been impaired by a medical problem. The impairment in thinking and feeling is

observed in behavior" (Allen & Blue, 1998, p. 225). More specifically, dysfunction is viewed as an impairment in information processing that occurs within the brain and that results in a compromised ability to carry out everyday activities (Allen, 1988, 1999, pp. 2-3; Allen & Blue, 1998, pp. 239-241).

Dysfunctional behavior is represented within the cognitive hierarchical scale from level one through lower level five. Even persons with normal cognitive abilities may use lower cognitive level skills to get through daily routines, but the person with a cognitive dysfunction cannot call upon more sophisticated cognitive skills when a situation might call for it (Allen, 1991b). Persons with cognitive disability are regarded as limited in their ability to adapt to new situations in everyday life and to learn.

Having a cognitive disability implies a cap on overall cognitive ability and what a patient can be expected to do. This limit remains constant (or, in the case of progressive diseases, could worsen). Early in her writing, Allen challenged the hope given to improvements based upon "brain plasticity." She emphasized that more studies in this area were needed, and, even where recompensation does occur, it may be very difficult to achieve and take so long that it is not practical in the scope of therapy (Allen, 1985, p. 95).

Individuals having focal brain lesions may have specific additional deficits based upon the site of those lesions, but the cognitive levels Allen is addressing refer to predominant ways of processing information and the general capacity to function (Allen, 1994, p. 9). While Allen acknowledges that fluctuations in level of function may occur, she says that these fluctuations can typically be explained as one having more or less energy, changes in clarity of thinking as related to medication, changes in stamina, or more or less effort being applied depending on the meaningfulness of the activity to the person (Allen, 1994, p. 16). If the therapist can offer an activity to the client that has the "just right challenge," in which activity demands match the individuals current capacity to function, the client is expected to feel comfortable and have a sense of mastery and well-being (Allen, 1994, p. 16).

Role of the Therapist

As in other theoretical frameworks in this text, the occupational therapist can assume multiple roles during intervention, and some may dominate more than others, depending on the needs of the clients. The cognitive disability framework describes the roles of the clinician in assessment, activity analysis, and managing the environment. It also describes the roles of consultant and advocate.

Therapist as Assessor

In all of the frames of reference discussed in this book, the role of the therapist is, of course, to assess, plan, and carry out intervention. In the cognitive disabilities framework, however, the role of therapist as assessor is so central that we identify it as the pivotal therapist role. Referring to assessment of a person's place according to the Allen Cognitive Level Scale, Allen and Blue write, "Scales are incredibly important because everything that the therapist does is based on the scale" (Allen & Blue, 1998, p. 226). Allen has never wavered from her earlier proposal that within compensatory treatment the "ideal role of the therapist is to evaluate the disability with accuracy and precision in order to specify areas where change in capacity or community support can be realistically achieved" (Allen, 1987, p. 565). The therapist is an **observer-assessor** throughout the patient's tenure, documenting changes in function and cognitive level when they occur.

Therapist as Expert

The therapist is the **expert** who knows the cognitive demands of activities and the patient's capabilities. Further, the therapist recognizes the long-range limitations imposed by the various levels of cognitive disability; therefore, the therapist knows which activities are feasible for the patient and the nature of the structure and guidance needed by a patient in order for him or her to be safe within the environment. Allen and others associated with her model have available resource information that describes in detail those activities at which patients can be expected to succeed, as based upon their cognitive level (Allen et al., 1992, 1996; Allen, Earhart, Blue, & Therasoft, 1996). Patients having cognitive impairments are not expected to know what activities are feasible and, rather, are believed to generally have a very unrealistic understanding of their own limitations (Allen & Blue, 1998, p. 237). Their input is elicited to identify activities that they enjoy and that are meaningful to them.

Therapist as Environmental Manager

Using his or her expertise, the therapist selects or modifies tasks in the environment so to enhance patient success. Allen refers to this as **environmental compensation** and writes, "Compensation is done by (the therapist) matching the complexity of the task to the patient's cognitive ability so that the patient has the opportunity to experience the successful manipulation of material objects"(Allen, 1985, pp. 25-27). Simplifying the task is in contrast to what she refers to as **biological compensation** (changing a person's biological make-up) and **psychological compensation** (teaching a skill) (Allen, 1985). In other words, Allen states clearly that hers is a compensatory rather than a restorative model. As an **environmental manager**, the therapist maintains a treatment environment in which the patient will be safe, and the aim is to foster pleasant experiences. Once the patient is discharged, the therapist recommends adaptations to the expected home/work environment that will enable optimal, safe function within the least restrictive environment possible (Allen & Blue, 1998).

Therapist as Consultant, Educator, and Advocate

"Very few people understand what a cognitive disability is and how it can affect daily life" (Allen & Blue, 1998, p. 229). Family members, even other professionals, have a "tendency to ignore, rationalize, and deny long-term cognitive disability" (Allen & Blue, 1998, p. 229). Following careful observation to support the presence of a disability, the therapist can educate other staff and caregivers in realistic expectations, helping them distinguish "cannot" from "will not." Therapists can also provide educational materials that describe the risks, safety concerns, and environmental adaptations that will foster safety and function (Allen & Blue, 1998; Allen, Earhart, Blue, & Therasoft, 1996).

If it is determined that a life-long cognitive disability exists, the therapist helps identify the extent of community and caretaker support that is required. By reporting to social service or legal agencies regarding the patient's cognitive level, the therapist contributes to the process of establishing legal competency, if needed.

In summary, according to Allen, "the therapist can offer an opportunity for positive experience in the task environment; the patient decides whether or not to accept that opportunity" (Allen, 1985, p. 96).

Function of Activities

The use of activities in the cognitive disability framework is used to measure change in occupational performance, provide opportunity for success, and give an opportunity for diversion. Activities also have a primary role in helping the person compensate for loss of cognitive performance.

Measurement

Activities consist of behaviors or outcomes that can be analyzed according to the level of cognitive demand they impose as well as the expected assistance that will be needed (as based on participants' cognitive level), and the nature of hazards imposed by the activity (Allen et al., 1992). Activities provide a vehicle for measuring an individual's ability for cognitive problem solving in order that mental processing (level of cognitive function) can be measured and cognitive change objectively demonstrated. A patient's ability to carry out familiar activities of daily living is *not* considered the best way to evaluate current cognitive capacity because familiar activities are typically "overlearned" and are done by habit (Allen & Blue, 1998, p. 228). For cognitive capacity to be assessed, the patient must be engaged in an activity that "demands the processing of new information" (Allen, 1994, p. 15). According to Allen, crafts work well as assessment tools because they can be readily graded to control the required standard of performance, they present varied problems for patients to solve, and patients often enjoy crafts (Allen, 1991b). While assessment instruments associated with this model use specified ADL tasks as well as a variety of crafts (available as kits from Allen resources), a therapist who has used this model to analyze the cognitive demands made by a particular task can use that activity to evaluate cognitive function.

Success Experience: Realistic Activities

Therapeutic activities are activities within the limits of the patient's cognitive capacity. Allen proposes that any functional activities that a person wants to do—"as long as they are legal"—are within the scope of therapeutic activity (Allen, 1985, p. 93). Those activities described consistently in Allen's work are those commonly referred to as activities of daily living (ADLs) and crafts. Allen has written that being asked to engage in an activity that has too complex task demands can bring about "catastrophic reactions... when patients recognize, to some degree, that they are unable to do a simple task and the personal disaster of a mental disorder becomes apparent" (Allen, 1985, p. 185). She has also written that steps in a task beyond the patient's ability will be refused or ignored (Allen, 1985, p. 190). Perhaps most consistent is the point that patients cannot do activities beyond their abilities. To expect more than a person is capable of may lead to "blaming" by the therapist and other professionals (Allen, 1994, p. 16).

In her earlier work, Allen strongly advocated for using crafts with the cognitively disabled, writing that she had been "struck by a consistent clinical pattern: at Levels 3, 4, and 5 the most popular tasks are crafts" (Allen, 1991a, 1991b). In more recent literature, she writes that crafts may not always be meaningful to persons with cognitive disabilities.

Activities that are the cognitive equivalent of a person's capability provide a vehicle through which the person can experience success. In this respect, use of the model enables therapy to be a humanizing experience. Caregivers and family members can create expectations of which the person is capable, and the client can feel a sense of mastery by completing a task.

Environmental Compensation: Changing the Task

Therapeutic activities become part of a task environment that can compensate for a patient's cognitive disability by using his or her remaining abilities in a way that enables the individual to achieve results that are personally satisfying and socially acceptable. Activities that have been altered to allow an individual to succeed are part of **environmental compensation**. Used in this way, a "therapeutic activity can be viewed like a piece of adaptive equipment" (Allen, 1985, p. 26).

Activities that are appropriately matched to the patient's cognitive level may reduce anxiety and discomfort associated with the disease. For example, if a patient experiences hallucinations or disturbing thoughts, the focus on a task may help interrupt and redirect disturbing stimuli. A person who engages with material objects through touching and manipulating might find it comforting and reality orienting to participate in an activity that involves use or handling of objects (e.g., as one might expect with an individual functioning at Level 3).

Diversion

Although admitting that references that credit occupational therapy for its ability to "keep the patients busy" can be slightly annoying, Allen purports that the statement is true and may help the patient to be more comfortable while medications are gradually taking effect (Allen, 1985, p. 227). Using depressed patients as an example, she writes, "Being spoken to as if they were children or being given projects with childish connotations can be upsetting to anyone and is especially upsetting to people who are depressed. Furthermore, people who are depressed are suffering. One can get very tired of listening to the same complaints over and over and over again. There is a tendency to get mad at the patients or ignore them. One way of coping with the complaining is to reassure them that the complaint is going to get better and then direct their attention to a task. The task helps to pass the time until diverting their attention away from the source of the pain reduces their mental anguish. The palliative powers of the task are temporary and discomfort will resume again, but the task does seem to help for a short period of time" (Allen, 1985, p. 140).

Assessment

Assessment is a here-and-now process of identifying a person's level of cognitive function, including assets and limitations. It is ongoing and is inseparable from treatment (Allen & Blue, 1998, p. 235).

Preliminary Assessment

According to Allen, assessment should begin with a review of the patient's medical chart to identify the reason for admission and to establish initial occupational therapy goals. The therapist needs to be knowledgeable about diagnoses (their symptoms, treatment, and probable course) so that he or she might contribute to establishing a diagnosis, if it is in question, and to recognize and document changes in the disease process.

Role of Diagnoses

Physicians provide diagnoses and typically prescribe medications. Occupational therapists can use that diagnostic information to anticipate likely affect on the ability to function. The therapist might, for example, ask him- or herself, "Is this condition typically temporary or permanent; is it likely to stabilize, improve, or worsen? What medication has been prescribed, and how might this medication be expected to impact function?"

When a patient's cognitive level does not improve as expected in response to medication, the therapist can alert the physician or case manager, and the decision may be made to re-evaluate medication type or dosage. In this way, therapists may provide input that bears on the **titration of medication** (Allen, 1985, p. 108).

Table 8-3
SEMI-STRUCTURED INTERVIEW GUIDE

- Past history
- Recent living situation
- Current social support system
- Responsibility for self-care tasks
- Work and educational history
- Interests (past and present)
- Patient's perception of abilities
- Patient's perception of limitations
- Patient's goals

Adapted from Allen, C. (1985). *Occupational therapy for psychiatric diseases: Measurement and management of cognitive disabilities.* Boston, MA: Little Brown and Company.

Theoretical Assumptions—Guide to Evaluation and Intervention

The theoretical assumptions (See Cognitive Disability Theoretical Assumptions) are a summary of the basic beliefs about the person, activities or occupations, and the environment or context. These beliefs are adapted from the theories of the cognitive disability frame of reference previously described in this chapter. The assumptions about the person-environment-occupation variables and their possible relationships guide evaluation and intervention in occupational therapy.

Chart Review

Chart review acts as an initial screening tool in determining who is appropriate for participation in occupational therapy. By reading the notes and documentation of other professionals and care-providers, the occupational therapist may get clues about patients' ability to function and their awareness of their own abilities and impairments. It is the occupational therapist who would be expected to report on the individual's capacity to function. Patients at Level 0.8 to 1.0 would not attend the clinic, nor would patients who might behave unpredictably, present an elopement or suicide risk, are refusing, are in restraints, or are mute (Allen, 1985). Chart review also helps the therapist make a decision about what would be the most appropriate assessment tool to use in his or her initial screening.

Interview

As in other frames of reference, Allen proposes using a semi-structured interview to become better acquainted with the person, to better understand how the disease process has

effected the patient's lifestyle, and to learn about what the person finds meaningful (Allen & Blue, 1998, p. 11). The therapist is advised to gain performance information in the areas outlined in Table 8-3. If needed, the interview can be postponed until the patient can provide an accurate self-appraisal. Allen suggests that the therapist takes notes during the interview and shows them to the patient if he or she requests (Allen, 1985, p. 118).

Assessment Instruments

Allen has developed several screening and on-going assessment tools over the years. In more recent literature she describes the Allen Battery, which is a compilation of resources for assessment as well as caregiver education (Allen & Blue, 1998, p. 227). The Allen Battery includes instruments for initial assessment and projects for monitoring change.

Initial Assessment

Initial screening tools are used to get a first impression of the patient's general ability. The particular screening tool selected would depend on the therapist's knowledge of the patient's presenting condition. Some tools are designated for persons functioning at lower or higher cognitive levels.

Allen Cognitive Level Screen and Large Allen Cognitive Level Screen

Originally developed by Allen and refined by Moore, the ACLS is the second revision of a standardized tool to be used by occupational therapists who have "studied the references and know how to interpret the scores" (Allen, 1996, p. 2). It is based on the complexity of the leather-lacing stitch that a patient is able to learn and the manner in which that learning occurs. Given his or her performance, the patient is

COGNITIVE DISABILITY THEORETICAL ASSUMPTIONS

The Person and Cognition

1. Cognition is observable as everyday behavior regulated by information processing in the brain.
2. Cognitive processing capacity develops in an invariant order of complexity.
3. Cognitive disability is caused by a biologic (central nervous system [CNS]) deficit.
4. Impairments in cognitive processing are present in a majority of persons having mental illness and many other persons who have physical conditions that affect the CNS.
5. Persons with cognitive disabilities have ways in which they think and process information differently than normal persons, which in turn impedes their routine task behavior.
6. Limitations in a person's task behavior can be described hierarchically by cognitive levels that reflect universal thought processes, acquired in a predictable, developmental sequence (Allen & Blue, 1998, p. 227).
7. The individual's cognitive level predicts the behavior that he or she can safely do.
8. Reduction in cognitive processing ability can result in impairment, handicap, or disability.
9. Patients will do the best they can given their situation. A determination of "can" and "cannot" must be made before "will" and "will not" can be inferred (Allen, 1994, p. 16).
10. Persons with cognitive disability are limited in their ability to learn and to adapt to changing circumstances.
11. The level of function of persons with cognitive disability would be expected to improve only if psychotropic intervention or the course of the disease process brings about a change in brain function.
12. Persons with a cognitive disability may have progressively declining functional performance if their disability is a progressive disease.
13. Function is the use of mental energy to guide verbal and motor behavior.

Environment/Context

14. The individual's ability to function safely in his or her environment is determined primarily by his or her ability to process new information and reason in novel situations.
15. The task environment may have a positive or negative effect on a patient's ability to function safely.
16. Patients with cognitive disability attend to those aspects of the task environment that are within their range of ability and ignore those that are not.
17. Therapists try to identify what will be the least restrictive environment; one that maximizes "the use of remaining abilities while protecting the disabled person from hazardous encounters with limitation" (Allen & Blue, 1998, p. 227).

Activity/Occupation

18. Steps in a task that require abilities beyond the patient's cognitive level will be either ignored or refused.
19. Assessment of cognitive level requires that the person demonstrate new learning; performance of familiar tasks can be misleading and suggest a higher cognitive level than the person actually has.
20. Participation in activity does not change cognitive level.
21. Therapists can select and modify a task so that it is within the patient's cognitive ability through the application of task analysis and the principle of task equivalence.
22. A just right challenge matches the (cognitive) demands of an activity with patients' cognitive abilities and enables successful task completion and feelings of mastery.
23. Treatment sessions should use activities that are realistic and practical and provide a sense of overall contentment.

Other

24. For patients with a cognitive dysfunction, and therefore for the majority of psychiatric patients treated by occupational therapists, management and maintenance are more tenable goals than skill-building or change in cognitive level.
25. The assessment of cognitive level can contribute to decision-making around prospective discharge placement, environmental adaptations, and establishing legal competency.

assigned a cognitive level on the ACLS. The assessment was designed for use with adults, although it has been studied with adolescents. Because the tool reflects developmental stages of cognition, children at younger ages would not be expected to have reached the higher cognitive levels on the ACLS. The therapist prepares the pre-punched leather by completing three stitches, which are then demonstrated to the patient. As part of the assessment, errors are made in the lacing, and the patient is asked to point out and correct those errors.

The ACLS is designed to assess the patient's ability to learn something new, so an important criteria that must be established before the instrument is used is that the patient is not already familiar with how to do these lacing stitches. If already familiar with the activity, the person's performance may be guided by habit. As such, it may lead the assessor to conclude that the individual is functioning better than he or she really is (Allen & Blue, 1998, p. 228).

The Large Allen Level Screen (LACLS) is identical to the ACLS except that the materials are larger. It is designed for individuals having visual or motor impairments.

Allen indicates that the ACLS and LACLS are intended for use with persons judged to be functioning at Levels 3.0 though 5.8. Thus, it would not be appropriate for patients who are confused or, conversely, those who are functioning at a very high level.

The current ACLS (and LACLS) represents modifications of earlier instruments using leather-lacing and designed to establish a cognitive level. Allen and her associates, plus others in the field, have carried out research to establish the reliability and validity of the ACLS/LACLS. They report that inter-rater reliability for both versions of the instrument is and "always has been high" (Allen & Blue, 1998, p. 230; Penny, Musser, & North, 1995).

Validity studies for the instrument have been conducted in regard to its ability to test what it purports to measure—in this case cognitive processing, overall ability to function, and severity of disability (Allen & Blue, 1998, p. 231). Studies suggest positive correlation with the Block Design and Object Assembly portions of the Wechsler Adult Intelligence Scale (Katz, 1985; Mayer, 1988), verbal ability as tested by the Shipley Institute of Living Scale (David & Riley, 1990), portions of the Riska Object Classification (ROC) (Williams, 1981; Wilson, 1985), the Brief Psychiatric Rating Scale (Moore, 1978), the Mini-Mental Status Exam (Heying, 1985; Wilson, 1985), the Developmental Test for Visuomotor Impairment (Shapiro, 1992), the Lowenstein Occupational Therapy Cognitive Assessment (Katz & Heimann, 1990), and the Wisconsin Card Sorting Test (Secrest, Wood, & Tapp, 2000). Other studies have been conducted to establish the ability of the assessment to differentiate persons having psychiatric disorders (Josman & Katz, 1991; Katz, Josman, & Steinmetz, 1988; Katz, 1985; Katz & Heimann, 1990).

Lower Cognitive Level Test

In this assessment developed by Allen, the patient is asked to follow the therapist's lead and clap three times in specified rhythms. This tool is designed for use with low functioning individuals. This assessment is described in Allen's *Occupational Therapy for Psychiatric Diseases: Measurement and Management of Cognitive Disabilities* (1985).

Routine Task Inventory and Routine Task Inventory-II

The original Routine Task Inventory (RTI) (Allen et al., 1992; Allen, Earhart, Blue, & Therasoft, 1996) was described as an observation guide, although it was recommended that either patients or caregivers provide the information covered to avoid the lengthy time that would be needed to observe patient performance. Fourteen task areas

were covered in the original RTI and were said to be taken from an inventory developed by Lawton and Brody for assessing the elderly (Lawton, 1970, 1971). Task performance was assessed in the areas of bathing, dressing, grooming, walking, food preparation, housekeeping, finance, medication compliance, and travel. In the revised RTI, tasks have been expanded to include those in the areas of therapeutic exercise, child care, communication (written and verbal skill), and work (including skills related to following a schedule, following instruction, and getting along with others) (Earhart & Allen 1988). The patient's performance is scored according to the ACLS.

The original RTI was examined for reliability and validity as part of master's theses, and high test-retest and inter-rater reliability were established (Heimann, 1985; Wilson, 1985).

Positive correlation between the RTI and the ACL have been demonstrated (Heimann et al., 1989; Wilson et al., 1989), as well as positive correlation with the Mini-Mental State and the RTI (Wilson et al., 1989).

Cognitive Performance Test

The Cognitive Performance Test (CPT) (Burns, 1991, 1992) is a standardized functional assessment designed for the evaluation of Allen Cognitive Levels in persons having Alzheimer's disease. It measures the performance of common activities of daily living for which "the information processing requirements can be systematically varied to assess levels of functional capacity" (Burns, 1991, p. 1, 1992, p. 46). The tasks on the CPT are identified as dress, shop, toast, phone, wash, and travel. Each task is presented with a standardized set-up and directions for administration. The level of disability is determined by evaluating the types of cues that capture the patient's attention and the manner in which behavior is organized for problem solving.

Administration of the CPT includes sequential elimination or provision of sensory cues and assistance when the patient is having difficulty completing a task. Depending on the type of cue and information the client can profit from, the therapist can identify the level of cognitive function. According to Burns (1991, 1992), the specific tasks that are selected, while having face validity, are less important than the manner in which patients are able to respond to tasks of varying complexity. While a particular patient would be expected to score at or close to same level on all six tasks (the task scores may differ), the total CPT score is used as the average representation of performance (Burns, 1992, p. 47).

Validity and Reliability Studies

Preliminary studies of the CPT were conducted at the Minneapolis VA Medical Center's Geriatric Research, Education, and Clinical Center with 75 patients having mild to moderate Alzheimer's disease and 15 normal control elderly persons. Both inter-rater reliability and test-retest reliability were reported to have been respectable (Burns, 1992). Data from a 4-year follow-up period showed that scores on the CPT declined with progression of the disease (Burns, 1992).

Work Performance Inventory

As described by Earhart (1985), this assessment was developed to improve communication with sheltered workshops, vocational counselors, and other non-occupational therapists. It describes the patient's work habits, work relationships, and emotions as they affect work performance. It assigns a cognitive level from 1 through 6 and makes recommendations regarding the patient's needs in task selection and therapist supervision.

Projects to Monitor Change

Allen Diagnostic Modules

The Allen Diagnostic Modules (ADM) (Allen, Earhart, & Blue, 1993) are a collection of sensory stimulation kits and craft projects used to verify the assessment of ability to function (Allen & Blue, 1998, p. 228; Allen et al., 1993). The *ADM Manual* (1993) describes the set-up and scoring of these activities; additionally, many of these craft projects can be purchased as kits and come with standardized instructions based upon Allen's cognitive levels. When a patient's ability to function is improving, the ADM is used to measure change; **probes** (cues given to see if improvement has occurred) are used. Probes attempt to direct attention to cues usually noticed at the next higher mode of function (Allen & Blue, 1998, p. 228). Crafts are described as an especially good way of assessing ability to function within Levels 4.0 to 5 because they are motivating (the person is making something concrete for self or others), because they are cost effective, and because if mistakes are made, they are usually without serious consequence (Allen & Blue, 1998 p. 228). Projects that have been selected are expected to appeal to adolescents and adults of both gender (Allen, 1994, p. 15).

Intervention

Overall, treatment in this model is said to aim at "making life with a disability as nearly normal as possible" (Allen & Blue, 1998, p. 228). To meet this objective, Allen conceives two complementary types of intervention: **management** and **maintenance**. Together, management and maintenance stand in distinct contrast to a goal of restoration or "fixing" the patient. **Management** occurs in the early phases of therapy when the therapist first meets the patient, establishes the level of cognition, and concomitantly determines the patient's performance capability. Part of management includes providing activities that patients can succeed at and helping them to remain relatively comfortable while their cognitive level stabilizes. **Maintenance** begins when it has been determined that improvement in cognitive level (and corresponding level of function) is not expected. Goals during maintenance therapy are those associated with setting up and/or conducting long-term care (Allen, 1994, p. 10).

Within this two-prong intervention plan, Allen delineated four distinct phases (acute, post-acute, rehabilitation, and long-term care) that create a **continuum of intervention** (Allen et al., 1992). Though more recent literature does not consistently refer to these phases by name, it continues to recognize the sequence described in the 1992 publication.

Acute Phase: Preventing Complications

During the **acute phase**, the patient is often not medically cleared for occupational therapy activity. The occupational therapist may be asked to estimate the person's cognitive level, particularly when precautions are being determined to insure the patient's safety. Because patients in this phase may be very confused and functioning at Level 1 and 2, it would not be appropriate to use the ACL, CPT, or RTI assessments. Patients having an acute psychotic episode, toxic substance reactions, recent stroke, or head injury are examples of persons in whom the acute phase is very obvious. The occupational therapist may, however, make an initial contact, and treatment may be aimed at preventing impairments (e.g., the therapist provides resting splints or maintains range of motion). Treatment at this phase emphasizes the prevention of complications (Allen et al., 1992, p. 20).

Post-Acute Phase: Establishing Cognitive Level and Keeping the Patient Comfortable

The **post-acute phase** begins when the patient has been medically cleared to engage in activities. During this phase, the therapist establishes short-term goals related to management of cognitive impairments. The medical condition may still be improving. Assessing cognitive function is a primary role of the therapist. This may include assessment with the ACL, RTI, or CPT, as well as use of Allen Diagnostic Modules to identify any changes in cognitive level, including those subsequent to medications. Typically, patients will be functioning between Level 3 through 5 during this phase. It is important to use the decimal system (modes of performance) when documenting changes at this phase. It is during the post-acute stage that cognitive level is expected to stabilize (i.e., no more improvement is occurring; therefore, therapists are able to begin discharge planning).

In this phase, therapists may be explaining to patients and their caregivers what is meant by their particular level of disability and type of caregiver assistance anticipated to ensure safety. According to Allen, the therapist needs to document the following:

- Symptoms of the disease as demonstrated in functional performance
- Symptoms of any other medical diagnosis that may assist with differential diagnosis
- The cognitive level at the time of referral as well as changes in cognitive level
- An estimate of the predicted cognitive level at discharge

• An estimate of the least restrictive environment that the patient can be expected to function safely in at the time of discharge (Allen et al., 1992, p. 22 [refer to both OT Progress Note and Table 8-4])

OT PROGRESS NOTE

Patient: M. Martin (fictitious name)
Pt. # 124-56-7890
Age: 48
Gender: F
Attending physician: Smith, Elizabeth
Admission date: 02/21/00
Service: Occupational Therapy Cognitive Group
Pt. Response: "I like to do crafty things at home; I always have lots of projects going"
Activity: Key chain
Functional observations: Patient engaged in task having familiar and novel steps for approximately 45 minutes. She was able to follow written instructions for unfamiliar steps. She worked quickly, was talkative, and became distracted from task several times. Initially, she failed to recognize flaws in her work but recognized when these were pointed out to her. She made some adjustments to correct errors, but these were not sufficient to correct her mistakes. When therapist pointed out remaining errors, patient at first was unable/unwilling to correct/refine her work. Again, given cues regarding errors in surface details, she responded by making corrections and completed project. She expressed pride in final outcome.

Assessment/plan: ACL at 5.0, with signs of next level emerging. This is same score as seen in previous sessions, with some signs of improvement; significant improvement since initial assessment at 4.2 on 02/23/00. Patient continues to demonstrate signs of manic behavior including impulsiveness, talkativeness, and pressure to move ahead in tasks. Continue to assess cognitive level and impact on functional level as patient responds to medical interventions. Next session 02/28/00.

Therapists are advised to recognize that during this phase when cognitive improvements are being observed, it is not due to the occupational therapy intervention. Nevertheless, the therapist has an important role in describing to other professionals the meaning of changes in cognitive level (i.e., what the changes mean in terms of ability for function and independence).

Rehabilitation Phase: Specifying Maintenance Outcomes

According to Allen, the **rehabilitation phase** signals the beginning of longer-term maintenance goals. In this phase, the individual is medically cleared to engage in all the activities that he or she is still able to do. The medical condition has stabilized, and there is little or no improvement in signs of the illness, improvement in function, nor change in cognitive level. Therapists contribute to the optimal performance and quality of life by providing caregivers and the patient with adaptive equipment, arranging for protective environments, and teaching caregivers how to provide the structure and guidance needed to help the patient stay safe in his or her home or work environment. The therapist in this phase may set up a **maintenance program** designed to be as nearly normal as possible.

The goal is to create the **least restrictive environment:** one which maximizes "the use of remaining abilities while protecting the disabled person from hazardous encounters with limitation" (Allen & Blue, 1998, p. 227). Allen advises the therapist to get a description of a typical day from the patient, a family member, or friend. The primary skilled service is that of teaching lay people how to maximize the functional abilities of the cognitively disabled person (Allen et al., 1992, p. 24). Allen and associates have created resources that include lists of activities cognitively disabled persons can be expected to do, common injuries, and accidents grouped by cognitive level (Allen, Earhart, Blue, & Therasoft, 1996; Allen et al., 1996). These resources can be given to caregivers, placed in the patient's chart, or provided to team members through in-service education. It is important in this phase to document what the patient can do spontaneously and what he or she can do when cued by the therapist. When the patient can do an activity safely with the prompting of a care provider, then skilled care is no longer needed (Allen et al., 1992, p. 24). Treatment effectiveness can be documented by an increase in the number or scope of activities that the patient is able to perform and with reduced injuries or accidents (Allen et al., 1992, p. 22).

Documentation during this phase should include:

• Changes in the patient's ability in respect to prior and present functional history
• Nature of the patient's social support system
• Symptoms of the presenting illness as expressed during present performance
• Degree of cognitive assistance required at the present time, with an estimate of any expected change
• Identification of activities that are important to the patient and caregiver
• Long-term treatment goals that identify the activities selected and the estimated assistance needed at discharge

Table 8-4
CASE EXAMPLE: AN INITIAL EVALUATION

Occupational Therapy Evaluation Date: 5/09/99

_X_ First Admission   _____ Re-admission

Diagnosis: depression/suicidal ideation

Reason for hospitalization/history: Pt. is a 29-year-old male brought to E.R. by police when he was found staggering in mall with apparent drug overdose; speech was slurred; this is pt's 3rd known suicide attempt; second hospitalization for depression; has history of rickets and scoliosis; lower back pain.

Assessments: _X_ Allen Cognitive Level Test   ____ Basic Living Skills Battery

____ Cognitive Performance Test   ____ Other: OT evaluation task group

_X_ OT interview

Occupational Functioning

Employment/education: Pt. describes 1 yr. liberal arts community college; currently works with uncle in construction and landscaping as back pain permits; has held other manual jobs; describes interest in computers and getting more technical training.

Living arrangements: Moved to Montana 2 years ago from Idaho; lives with uncle and uncle's girlfriend; has the "downstairs" (basement apt), which he is to keep clean; meals prepared by others in the house; pt. responsible for light meal preparation when others aren't home; states chronic back pain has kept him from holding full-time employment over past 2 years; has not yet qualified for disability benefits; awaiting response to his application; describes past interests as fishing, reading computer magazines, "browsing" the net, and bowling; pain has kept him from bowling, and sitting at computer aggravates back pain.

Support systems: Uncle and uncle's girlfriend; occasionally goes drinking with guys after work but states he "mostly hangs out" by himself; no other in-state family.

Results of ACL: Level 5.2

Explanation of Allen Cognitive Test Results

Level 5.2: Exploratory actions:

Client at this level:

Strengths: Uses trial and error to problem solve; learns by doing; can generalize information learned in one situation to another.

Limitations: Some difficulty with abstract reasoning; may not anticipate problems in future.

Work/school: Roles that require flexibility may pose a problem; able to follow series of demonstrated directions; can understand directions given in oral, written, or diagram form.

Living skills: Indep. with self-care; budgeting and other future-oriented life skills may be difficult due to problems anticipating future events or needs.

Medications: Independent with medications; can adjust to changes in schedule and dosage; may have difficulty understanding or anticipating specific side effects of medications.

Functional recommendations: Learns new information and skills through education, practice, or role-playing; benefits from individual or group problem solving; might need concrete directions/support from others during stress or change.

Assessment/Interpretation

Pt. observed in small OT group interacted minimally with other group members; asked for therapist's guidance regarding how he could help group as they prepared a light meal; appeared persistent in attempt to find way to open several hard-to-open jars, but needed therapist's suggestions when his initial efforts failed.   _(continued)_

Table 8-4 (Continued)

Recommendations

Future OT services to explore leisure interests; educate client in avenues for future employment; educate regarding lower back pain and protective techniques; identify community resources for increased social support.

Therapist: Sam Smith

Patient Name: John Jones (fictitious name)

123-45-6789

- Short-term treatment goals that identify methods used and the sequence in which activities will be presented, including the safety hazards expected (Allen et al., 1992, p. 25)

Allen writes that it is a myth that third-party payers will not reimburse rehabilitation. Within Medicare, rehabilitation of this type would be referred to as "setting up a rehabilitation program." Safety would be the critical component (Allen et al., 1992, p. 22).

Long-Term Care

Long-term care is defined as the "provision of a community-based activity program designed for people who are functioning at cognitive levels 3 and 4" (Allen et al., 1992, p. 25). The purpose of the program is to reduce the handicap imposed by having no occupation, maintaining the patients' maximum level of function and preventing further complications (Allen et al., 1992, p. 25). The therapist providing service within such a program tries to offer activities that are enjoyable to the participants, structured in a manner that respects what they can and cannot do, replicate as much as possible the social climate and culture that is comfortable to the group. Participation in such a program would be voluntary, requiring the cooperation and motivation of the disabled participants (Allen et al., 1992, p. 26).

Application of the Model with Children

The cognitive disabilities model was not created for use with children; however, Allen and Blue (1998) propose that cognitive screening using the model would be a way to determine that cognitive abilities had or had not reached a "ceiling" (p. 243). In other words, the ACL could be used as a developmental screen in which developmental changes could be demonstrated. The ACL can also be used to set treatment goals and methods that match a child's current level of function (Allen & Blue, 1998, p. 243).

Therapeutic Groups

Similar Cognitive Levels

Allen and her associates suggest grouping patients according to cognitive level. As a general rule, patients at Levels 1 and 2 will not be seen in the clinic environment, although the therapist may assess their cognitive function on the treatment ward. Allen suggests that patients in occupational therapy activity groups be at a Level 3 or higher and that they be predictable, nonviolent, and cooperative (Allen, 1985). Earhart (1985), however, describes a movement group for patients at Level 2. Level 3 and 4 groups typically extend for an hour and use activities that have familiar tools and materials and obvious visual and tactile cues. Such groups might be devoted to basic crafts, ADLs, basic woodworking, basic sewing, or grooming. Patients within these groups who are doing craft projects can be given instructions at a level that closely matches their particular cognitive abilities when crafts are from the Allen Diagnostic Modules. Earhart recommends that these groups meet at the same time each day, 5 days per week, and do not exceed 10 patients per group (less if more than half the group members function within Level 3) (Earhart, 1985, p. 238).

Safety

Because people with a cognitive disability are characteristically in need of supervision, the therapist must carefully monitor the treatment environment, including tools and supplies, to ensure patient safety. Allen (1985) and Allen, Earhart, and Blue (1992, 1996) provide specific recommendations regarding the use and storage of occupational therapy materials. These recommendations are consistent with safety precautions as addressed in other frameworks.

Higher Level Groups

Patients functioning at Levels 5 and 6 are offered special interest groups, as typified by a work group (using a limited number of vocational skills), a senior group for patients over age 55, and a medication group. Groups with persons functioning at higher levels can be up to 20 in number and can be supervised by one occupational therapist and one aide (Earhart, 1985, p. 263).

Patients at the two highest levels, 5 and 6, are given an opportunity to learn new craft and sewing skills at an advanced level; however, patients at these higher levels are not those to whom this framework is primarily aimed. According to Allen, other professionals, presumably psychologists and social workers, treat higher functioning patients.

Summary

Knowledge pertaining to the practice of occupational therapy is expanding dramatically. Specialization has been one consequence, and, in a sense, the cognitive disabilities frame of reference represents one kind of specialization. The thrust of intervention of this frame of reference is toward the assessment of cognitive level, particularly of cognition as it manifests in everyday functional performance, and the recommendation of adaptations that respect cognitive limitations.

Activity Focus

Having identified activity as a focus, the therapist must ask the following: "Based on the patient's cognitive ability, at what activity can he or she succeed?" Occupational therapy intervention is not expected to influence the disease process; however, the identification of cognitive level can:

- Document changes in patient function
- Help promote success experiences for the patient
- Monitor effects of medical intervention on the disease process
- Assist in the creation of home maintenance programs and/or the determination of appropriate post-discharge placement

Challenging Occupational Therapy Assumptions

The cognitive disabilities framework challenges many of the assumptions on which other frames of reference and occupational therapy have rested. Primary among these assumptions is that occupational therapy should serve patients who function at a full-spectrum of cognitive ability. Another assumption that is challenged is the belief that occupational therapy can or should expect to improve patient's ability to function. It disputes more specifically behavioral and holistic assumptions about the ability of a cognitively impaired person to learn, as well as psychological and cognitive behavioral theories that place importance on feedback, insight, and increased awareness.

Cognitive disabilities as a framework shares with several models an adherence to the traditional medical model. The belief is that diagnosis of specific psychiatric diseases is integral to the assessment and management of patients and that impairment has a physiologic basis.

Chronic Cognitive Disability

The cognitive disabilities frame of reference identifies itself as especially suited for use in response to the problems of chronically cognitively disabled persons in the context of an acute care setting. In fact, occupational therapists without experience are advised to avoid the "confusing and often demoralizing" area of chronic care practice (Allen, 1985).

CONTRIBUTIONS AND LIMITATIONS OF THE COGNITIVE DISABILITY FRAME OF REFERENCE

Contributions

Gathers Data for Understanding Functional Performance

The thrust of this frame of reference has been to gain objective data about patients' abilities to perform motor behavior in a controlled environment and, by implication, to function in their everyday environment. Cognitive disabilities proponents have embarked on the arduous task of implementing research that can be expected to provide an increasing amount of information about the role of cognitive limitations on functional performance during daily tasks and craft activities.

Because the role of occupational therapy is limited to cognitive assessment of the specific type discussed, the therapist is guided in compiling concise data that he or she can share with colleagues and that establishes a sound basis for documentation around functional performance. This approach is well-suited to the increased pressure in acute care to assess and place patients. This circumscribed role also helps keep the therapist from trying to be all things to all persons and thereby has a practical advantage. Similarly, data obtained through a relatively straightforward assessment process have become increasingly accepted as a means to identify appropriate placements and to decide competency issues. As a result, the therapist has something workable and specific to offer among a plethora of treatment services.

Guides for Client Success

By creating an environment in which the patient can be expected to succeed, the therapist provides a humanizing and positive treatment experience that may build patients' confidence and acceptance of their own limitations. Much of the more recent work in this model has been in developing guidelines to be given to care givers of cognitively disabled persons. By not only helping family members and other care providers to accept the limitations of the cognitively disabled person, but additionally providing very specific guides in regard to what adjustments need to be made in the home and work setting, the model is expected to be very helpful to caregivers who otherwise may be at a loss as to interating with and helping the patient be successful.

Roles for the Clinician when Client Change is Unlikely

The model has contributed to the occupational therapy profession as well in its articulation of specific contributions that occupational therapy can make even when improvement in patient/client abilities is not expected. As Allen underscores, the occupational therapist does not need to take credit for improvements in order to serve an important function in the rehabilitation process. Emphasizing instead the therapist's role as educator, consultant, and advocate, the model is very compatible with changing mandates within the profession.

Although originally developed as a model for treating persons with identified mental illness, the model is applicable with any person(s) in whom a physical condition has affected the ability for cognitive processing, such as those having Alzheimer's dementia, cerebral vascular disease, multiple sclerosis, and Parkinson's disease, and may help caregivers who work and live with persons having these disorders anticipate a means to manage their disabilities.

Limitations

Recommends Limited Intervention Role

Some of the limitations of the cognitive disabilities frame of reference are self-imposed. Its advocates decry the involvement of occupational therapy in trying to treat too broad a range of problems. Increasingly in the literature, this framework is discussed in relation to patients placed on the continuum of sublevels comprising Levels 3 and 4. Allen says, quite clearly, that because the majority of mental health patients seen by occupational therapists aren't going to improve in her view, occupational therapists should get out of the business of trying to improve them. For individual therapists to limit their practice as suggested is, of course, their choice, but when Allen's exhortation is to the profession to limit itself, the issue becomes much more complex. With many mental health patients currently seeking treatment who are not cognitively disabled by Allen's definition but nevertheless having functional impairments, and with other information demonstrating that even persons who are cognitively disabled can continue to learn, such a limitation of practice could be short-sighted. The issue is complicated, too, because proponents of this framework, using cognitive disability guidelines, have influenced public policy in some states regarding third-party reimbursement.

Allen's assertion that people with a cognitive disability cannot be expected to improve as a consequence of occupational or social intervention challenges the position taken by adherents of other models of practice, most directly the multi-context model, sensory-motor framework, and behavioral models as discussed in this text. Future research and the increased call

for evidence-based practice may help to strengthen the arguments made by all of these treatment frameworks.

Although medication can help patients think clearly and can alleviate symptoms, it is not a magic cure, as evidenced in the many patients who continue to require care. The medical literature frequently expresses the view that chronic patients need to improve both their social and work-related skills. Such skill building is judged as important in helping to shorten the length of hospitalization, to avoid future hospitalization, and to build patient confidence.

Suggests Generalization Without Documented Support

This framework trusts that the response to craft activities can be generalized to home and community environments, but the literature rarely describes this relationship. Given that the person's response to a leather or other craft provides evaluation data that contribute to major decisions that affect a person's life (e.g., conservatorship), the link between patient responses in hospital and community environments needs to be carefully evaluated.

Unexplained Dissonance

Even cognitively limited patients may function well and problem solve at a higher level on occasion or in different environments. Allen credits this to over-learning or habit. Although Piaget's 2-year-old has never been capable of adult-level understanding, an adult now demonstrating a predominantly lower level of cognitive function may have integrated many adult experiences, memories, and behaviors into his or her learning repertoire. No direction is given within this framework to help the therapist make positive use of instances of higher functioning or to respond to the cognitive dissonance that may result when these instances are ignored. It is this dissonance that is perhaps at the heart of one of the biggest limitations of this model.

Activities May Not be Client-Centered

Allen and Blue (1998) write, "The trouble with (providing) lists of realistic activities for the cognitively disabled is that they may not contain activities that the person would normally want to do, like driving, working, socializing, getting married, and having children. The cognitively disabled rarely understands why common activities may not be realistic for them. They understand, however, that they are being deprived of activities that they consider normal for them" (p. 237). Thus, there is a need for evaluations for driving and other occupations that a person wishes to perform.

Levels Threaten Individual Differences and Client-Centered Focus

Since publication of her earliest material and through the present, Allen refers to adults with cognitive disabilities as wanting the privileges of adults yet often being demanding like children and not having the ability to make good choices for themselves. Frequently, the language used to describe these adults has a tenor of irritation. It has only been recently in the literature that the definition of cognitive disability has been expanded to include impairments in "feeling." What is meant by the proposition that people with cognitive disabilities have an "impaired" ability "to feel" is not clear; however, the assumption of client-centered practice rests on the belief that people are the experts in their life. Given that Allen and her associates articulate with consistency the wish to put the person's best interests at the forefront, this model takes the position that the therapist knows more about the patient than he or she knows about him- or herself. The reader is left with some uneasiness about how client concerns will be addressed. Assuming, as we will, that cognitive impairments are very, very complex, one would be concerned about how the decision can best be made that people cannot participate in the "normal" activities of life. When people are grouped into "levels," there would appear to be a danger that individual differences will be lost.

Lack of Consistent Theory Base

As noted earlier, theoretical postulates continue to evolve within this framework, and the door remains open to address these issues in the future. However, Allen's practice of using theoretical concepts loosely, as with those of Piaget (1952) and Anderson (1992), makes it difficult to identify a theory base and to compare it to other established theories. Although it may be tempting to take advantage of the practical benefits and relative ease with which this framework can be used with patients, the lack of rigor and consistency in the theory base could seriously weaken its position in the future.

REFERENCES

Allen, C. K. (1982). Independence through activity: The practice of occupational therapy (psychiatry). *Am J Occup Ther, 36*(11), 731-739.

Allen, C. K. (1985). *Occupational therapy for psychiatric diseases: Measurement and management of cognitive disabilities.* Boston, MA: Little, Brown and Co.

Allen, C. K. (1987). Activity: Occupational therapy's treatment method. *Am J Occup Ther, 41*(9), 563-575.

Allen, C. K. (1988). Cognitive disabilities. In S. Robertson (Ed.), *Mental health focus: Skills for assessment and treatment* (pp. 3.18-3.33). Rockville, MD: American Occupational Therapy Association.

Allen, C. K. (1991a, July 26). *New developments in cognitive dysfunction theory.* Lecture series, Los Angeles.

Allen, C. K. (1991b). *Why occupational therapists use crafts* [Video]. Colchester, CT: S & S Worldwide.

Allen, C. K. (1994). Creating a need-satisfying, safe environment: Management and maintenance approaches. In C. B. Royeen (Ed.), *AOTA self-study series: Cognitive rehabilitation.* Bethesda, MD: American Occupational Therapy Association.

Allen, C. K. (1996). *Allen Cognitive Test manual.* Colchester, CT: S & S Worldwide.

Allen, C. K. (1999). *Structure of the cognitive performance modes.* (J. Bertrand, Ed.). Ormand Beach, FL: Allen Conferences, Inc.

Allen, C. K., & Allen, R. (1987). Cognitive disabilities: Measuring the social consequences of mental disorders. *J Clin Psychiatry, 48,* 185-190.

Allen, C. K., & Blue, T. (1998). Cognitive disabilities model: How to make clinical judgements. In N. Katz (Ed.), *Cognition and occupation in rehabilitation: Cognitive models for intervention in occupational therapy.* Bethesda, MD: American Occupational Therapy Association.

Allen, C. K., Earhart, C. A., & Blue, T. (1992). *Occupational therapy treatment goals for the physically and cognitively disabled.* Bethesda, MD: American Occupational Therapy Association.

Allen, C. K., Earhart, C. A., & Blue, T. (1993). *Allen Diagnostic Module manual.* Colchester, CT: S & S Worldwide.

Allen, C. K., Earhart, C. A., & Blue, T. (1996). *Understanding the modes of performance.* Ormand Beach, FL: Allen Conferences, Inc.

Allen, C. K., Earhart, C. A., Blue, T., & Therasoft. (1996). *Allen cognitive level documentation* [Computer software]. Colchester, CT: S & S Worldwide.

Anderson, M. (1992). *Intelligence and development: A cognitive theory.* Cambridge, MA: Blackwell.

Averbuck, S., & Katz, N. (1988). Assessment of perceptual cognitive performance: A comparison of psychiatric and brain injured adult patients. *Occupational Therapy in Mental Health, 8,* 57-71.

Burns, T. (1991). *Cognitive performance test (CPT): A measure of cognitive capacity for the performance of routine tasks.* Minneapolis, MN: Author.

Burns, T. (1992). Cognitive Performance Test. In C. K. Allen, C. A. Earhart, & T. Blue (Eds.), *Occupational therapy treatment goals for the physically and cognitively disabled.* Bethesda, MD: American Occupational Therapy Association.

David, S. K., & Riley, W. T. (1990). The relationship of the Allen Cognitive Level test to cognitive abilities and psychopathology. *Am J Occup Ther, 44,* 493-497.

Earhart, C. (1985). Occupational therapy groups. In C. K. Allen (Ed.), *Occupational therapy for psychiatric diseases: Measurement and management of cognitive disabilities* (pp. 235-264). Boston, MA: Little, Brown and Co.

Earhart, C., & Allen, C. (1988). *Cognitive disabilities: Expanded activity analysis.* Pasadena, CA: Author.

Heimann, N. E. (1985). *Investigation of the reliability and validity of the Routine Task Inventory with a sample of adults with chronic mental disorders.* Unpublished master's thesis, University of Southern California, Los Angeles.

Heimann, N., Allen, C. K., & Yerxa, E. (1989). The Routine Task Inventory: A tool for describing the functional behavior of the cognitively disabled. *Occupational Therapy Practice, 1,* 67-74.

Heying, L. (1985). Research with subjects having senile dementia. In C. K. Allen (Ed.), *Occupational therapy for psychiatric diseases: Measurement and management of cognitive disabilities* (pp. 339-365). Boston, MA: Little, Brown and Co.

Josman, N., & Katz, N. (1991). Problem-solving version of the Allen Cognitive Level (ACL) test. *Am J Occup Ther, 45,* 331-338.

Katz, N. (1985). Research on major depression. In C. K. Allen (Ed.), *Occupational therapy for psychiatric diseases: Measurement and management of cognitive disabilities* (pp. 299-313). Boston, MA: Little, Brown and Co.

Katz, N., & Heimann, N. (1990). Review of research conducted in Israel in cognitive disability instrumentation. *Occupational Therapy in Mental Health, 10,* 1-15.

Katz, N., Josman, N., & Steinmetz, N. (1988). Relationship between cognitive disability theory and the Model of Human Occupation in the assessment of psychiatric and non-psychiatric adolescents. *Occupational Therapy in Mental Health, 8,* 31-43.

Kotarbinski, A. (1965). *Praxiology: An induction to the science of efficient action.* New York, NY: Pergammon Press.

Landsmann, L., & Katz, N. (1988). Concrete to formal thinking: Comparison of psychiatric outpatients and a normal control group. *Occupational Therapy in Mental Health, 8,* 73-94.

Lawton, M. P. (1970). Assessment, integration, and the environment of older people. *Gerontologist, 10,* 38-46.

Lawton, M. P. (1971). The functional assessment of elderly people. *J Am Geriatr Soc, 19,* 465-481.

Leontyev, A. (1978). *Activity, consciousness, and personality.* Englewood Cliffs, NJ: Prentice-Hall.

Leontyev, A. (1981). *Problems in the development of the mind.* Moscow: Progress Publishers.

Mayer, M. A. (1988). Analysis of information processing and cognitive disability theory. *Am J Occup Ther, 42,* 176-183.

Moore, D. S. (1978). *An occupational therapy evaluation of sensorimotor cognition: Initial reliability, validity, and descriptive data for hospitalized schizophrenic patients.* Unpublished master's thesis, University of Southern California, Los Angeles.

Mounoud, P. (1982). Revolutionary periods in early development. In T. Bever (Ed.), *Regressions in mental development: Basic phenomena and theories.* Hillsdale, NJ: Lawrence Earlbaum Associates.

Partida, A., & Price, M. (1988). *Chemical dependency: Objective changes in function and treatment modalities.* Paper presented at the American Occupational Therapy Association National Conference, Phoenix, AZ.

Penny, N. H., Musser, K. T., & North, C. T. (1995). The Allen Cognitive Level test and social competence in adult psychiatric patients. *Am J Occup Ther, 49,* 420-427.

Piaget, J. (1952). *The origins of intelligence in children.* (M. Cook, Trans.). New York, NY: International University Press.

Piaget, J. (1971). *Biology and knowledge: An essay on the relations between organic regulations and the cognitive processes.* (B. Walsh, Trans.). Chicago, IL: University of Chicago Press.

Piaget, J. (1972). *The principles of genetic epistemology.* (W. Mays, Trans.). New York, NY: Basic Books.

Piaget, J. (1978). *Behavior and evolution.* (D. Nicholson-Smith, Trans.). New York, NY: Pantheon.

Piaget, J. (1980). *Adaptation and intelligence: Organic selection and phenocopy.* (S. Eames, Trans.). Chicago, IL: University of Chicago Press.

Secrest, L., Wood, E. W., & Tapp, A. (2000). A comparison of the Allen Cognitive Level test and the Wisconsin Card Sorting test in adults with schizophrenia. *Am J Occup Ther, 54,* 129-133.

Shapiro, M. E. (1992). Application of the Allen Cognitive Level test in assessing cognitive level functioning in emotionally disturbed boys. *Am J Occup Ther, 46,* 514-520.

Vygotsky, L. S. (1962). *Thought and language.* Cambridge, MA: M. I. T. Press.

Williams, L. R. (1981). *Development and initial test of an occupational therapy classification test.* Unpublished master's thesis, University of Southern California, Los Angeles.

Wilson, D. S. (1985). *Cognitive disability and routine task behaviors in a community-based population with senile-dementia.* Unpublished master's thesis, San Jose State University, San Jose, CA.

Wilson, D., Allen, C. K., McCormack, G., & Burton, G. (1989). Cognitive disability and routine task behaviors in a community-based population with senile dementia. *Occup Ther Pract, 1,* 58-66.

CHAPTER NINE

Dynamic Interactional Model to Cognitive Rehabilitation—Developing Strategies for Multiple Contexts

KEY POINTS

✧ History and Current Theory
- Traditional Cognitive Model—Cognitive Deficit Focus
- Dynamic Interactional Model—Focus On Cognitive Processing

✧ Theory in Context of Occupational Therapy Practice
- Person/Learner: Metacognition, Awareness, Processing Strategies
- Cognitive Performance—Competence, Self-Efficacy
- Dysfunction—Mismatch Among Person, Task, and Environment
- Task Complexity and Context Influence Cognitive Performance
- Environmental Mismatch Interferes With Competence
- Occupational Therapist: Detective and Collaborator
- Activities: Identify Cognitive Processing Ability, A Vehicle For Learning and Transfer

✧ Theoretical Assumptions Guide Evaluation and Intervention
- Evaluation
  —Dynamic Assessment: Awareness Questions, Strategy Use, Cues, and Task Grading
  —Assessment of Group Behaviors
- Intervention
  —Building Awareness and Metacognitive Strategy Training
  —Strategies to Increase Generalization
  —Person, Task, and Environment Relationships Influence Transfer
  —Group Treatment: Three Group Levels

✧ Contributions and Limitations of the Dynamic Interactional Model

FOCUS QUESTIONS

1. What is the difference between the traditional model and a dynamic interactional model of intervention for cognitive dysfunction?
2. How does the definition of cognition differ in the dynamic interactional model from the traditional description of cognition?
3. According to the dynamic interactional model, what leads to a person's dysfunction?
4. What is the difference between dynamic and static assessment?
5. What three assessment components are identified with the dynamic interactional model?
6. What assessment instruments were developed for the dynamic interactional model?
7. Why is metacognition so important in the dynamic interactional model?
8. What does a client learn from metacognitive training?
9. What strategies are used during metacognitive training?
10. How does one determine if the person is a good candidate for dynamic interactional treatment?
11. How does the therapist use activity analysis in the dynamic interactional model?
12. What is the "zone of proximal development"?
13. What is the primary purpose of treatment in the dynamic interactional model?
14. How can tasks be graded to increase or decrease their complexity?
15. How are groups graded to suit the varying cognitive levels of ability?
16. How does this framework for intervention differ from Allen's cognitive disabilities model?

INTRODUCTION

The occupational therapy literature describes multiple models for understanding cognition and approaching cognitive rehabilitation (Giles & Clark-Wilson, 1999; Katz, 1998). These models provide a structure for addressing cognitive impairments associated with such neurological and psychological conditions as developmental disability, head injury, stroke, Parkinson's disease, and psychiatric disorders such as schizophrenia and depression. Cognitive rehabilitation based upon dynamic interactions can be carried out in health care and community environments, in residential programs, in acute and outpatient rehabilitation, in mental health settings, and in schools. The cognitive interventions can reach across the continuum of care, following the client from the initial intensive care environment to home.

The dynamic interactional model, also referred to as the dynamic interactional approach (DIA), was developed by occupational therapist Joan Toglia and is the model we describe in this chapter. Toglia has said of this approach that it "attempts to integrate the cognitive psychology theories" that describe how people learn and generalize information with rehabilitation principles (Toglia, 1992, p. 104; 1998). She notes that cognitive deficits can result from a variety of conditions but states that the specific assessment and treatment techniques she uses were developed for adults with brain injury (Toglia, 1992, p. 105; 1998, p. 5). One reason that we have selected Toglia for inclusion in our text is because the principles she describes are being applied in intervention with persons who have chronic mental illness, especially those persons who struggle with schizophrenia and who manifest negative symptoms (Fine, 1993; Josman, 1998a; Toglia, 1992, p. 105; 1998, p. 5). Another reason for including Toglia's model is that it pays attention to the psychological and emotional parts of the patient or client as these impact the ability for meaningful participation in occupation.

Toglia distinguishes her approach from other cognitive rehabilitation models, which she believes focus on the specific components of cognition (e.g., attention, perception, knowledge, memory) and that take a deficit-specific approach. She suggests instead that as occupational therapists we are in the position to observe and understand how all the cognitive components work together to enable information processing and functional performance. She, in turn, describes cognition as an "ongoing product of the dynamic interaction between the individual (person), the task (occupation), and the environment (Toglia, 1992, p. 108; 1998, p. 7). Thus, her model is consistent with others that have been identified as person-environment-occupation models (Figure 9-1). With the term "dynamic," she emphasizes that cognition is not "static" but is always in a state of change (Toglia, 1992, p. 108, 1998, p. 7). The occupational therapist who uses this model chooses assessment and intervention that recognize that people need to learn general strategies that will help them cope and adjust to life's changing circumstances.

In the second edition of this text we included Toglia's model within a chapter in which we described a "holistic" approach to working with persons having head injury or having significant cognitive decline. Other theories and approaches for responding to the conditions in this case were discussed as well. In this chapter of our third edition, we address specifically Toglia's model: the dynamic interactional model. This model can be used to develop cognitive and metacognitive strategies and uses learner characteristics to increase occupational performance.

DEFINITION

The **dynamic interactional model** is a restorative cognitive rehabilitation approach used to enhance the functional performance of persons having a cognitive impairment. It begins with the assumption that the person is able to learn,

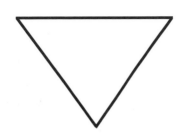

Individual
- Processing strategies and behaviors
- Metacognition
- Individual characteristics (knowledge, motivation, emotions, personal coping style, experience

Task
- Number of items
- Complexity
- Familiarity
- Arrangement
- Movement

Environment
- Social interaction (e.g., cues)
- Physical
- Multiple contexts
- Cultural
- Familiarity/predictability

Figure 9-1. Dynamic interactional model of cognition (reprinted from Toglia, J. [1998]. A dynamic interactional model to cognitive rehabilitation. In N. Katz [Ed.], *Cognition and occupation in rehabilitation* [p. 8]. Bethesda, MD: American Occupational Therapy Association, Inc. © 1998 by the American Occupational Therapy Association, Inc. Reprinted with permission).

but it does not exclude adaptations and compensatory approaches that may improve the client's performance. The dynamic model assumes that there are ongoing interactions between the individual, the task, and the environment that either facilitate or interfere with the cognitive processing required for participation in daily life.

Cognition is broadly defined and is viewed as a dynamic process that includes the components of cognition (memory, attention, etc.); however, rather than trying to isolate these components and address them "one at a time," Toglia focuses on how these components work together to enable the person to do cognitive processing as needed to perform a task. Because it is **dynamic**, a person's cognitive system is constantly changing; it is always responding to what is going on within the person along with what exists within the task and in the environment. Thus, the person is paying attention to many variables, such as one's thoughts, feelings, worries, and anticipations; the challenge of tasks; and the organization or sounds in the environment. Therefore, how well a person is able to process information and function in one setting or situation may be quite different than his or her success in another. Assessment in this model tries to examine the extent to which performance might be improved by determining what attributes of the person, task, or environment could be modified.

The model guides research for theory development in occupational therapy and contributes to our understanding of the importance of the client's learning style and life experience, the relative difficulty and nature of the task, and the

characteristics of the environment on cognitive processing and ultimately functional performance. Toglia and others (Josman, 1993, 1998b; Toglia & Josman, 1994) continue to evaluate the viability of the model in occupational therapy intervention with adults having an acquired brain injury as well as those with psychiatric disorders.

THEORETICAL DEVELOPMENT

Toglia (1998) developed the dynamic interactional model to meet the needs of clients who had a traumatic brain injury or neurological impairment following cerebral vascular accident or acquired brain injury resulting from disease, illness, or the aging process. When Toglia, an occupational therapist, was providing services in the context of a more traditional cognitive rehabilitation model, she noticed that her patients had difficulty in transferring what they had been successful in learning and applying within the rehabilitation setting to other environments (Toglia, 1998, p. 8). Consequently, she began to pay particular attention to those variables that appeared to influence whether or not the individual would be successful outside of the clinical setting. She focused on attributes of the person (e.g., his or her knowledge, emotions, capacity, learning strategies, perceptions of the task and environment, and awareness of one's capabilities), the task (e.g., its physical attributes, its complexity, and familiarity to the person), and the environment or context (physical setting, social components, and cultural attributes) in which the person was functioning. Combining these observations with her study of learning theory, she developed a dynamic interactional model for rehabilitation.

Traditional Cognitive Model—Cognitive Deficit Focus

This model differs from the traditional cognitive rehabilitation model, which emphasizes cognitive components rather than cognitive processing. Citing Trexler (1987), Toglia describes this component-based, deficit-specific approach as "reductionistic" (Toglia, 1992, p. 105; 1998, p. 6). Among the assumptions of the traditional approach are:

- Cognition can be broken down into component subskills
- These subskills are hierarchically arranged (e.g., attention and perception form a basis for higher-order skills such as reasoning)
- Intervention should involve repetition and practice of subskill components, often using paper and pencil or computer tasks

In the traditional approach, one might, for example, begin by trying to determine, "Is there a problem with attention?" "With memory?" Specific assessment instruments would be used to identify the existence of these particular defects. If the patient or client did poorly on a test that measured attention, he or she might be given a graded sequence of paper and pencil or computer "attention" tasks (Toglia, 1992, p. 106; 1998, p. 6). In the same way, the therapist using a traditional model of cognitive rehabilitation assesses each of the cognitive components to identify and remediate deficits in each component. The therapist then uses frequent practice of tasks to improve these component subskills. The focus of intervention is on attention, perception, memory, knowledge, problem solving, or other component deficit and its remediation.

The weakness of the deficit-specific remedial approach, says Toglia, is that it fails to describe how cognitive skills interrelate and ultimately impact task performance (Toglia, 1992, p. 106; 1998, p. 6). While it can improve component function within specific task boundaries, learning may not generalize to multiple or complex tasks; therefore, patients/clients have limited use of their cognitive skills.

Dynamic Interactional Model—Focus on Cognitive Processing

To increase generalized use of cognitive processing skills, the dynamic interactional model integrates person, environment, task perspectives from other disciplines, cognitive rehabilitation (Trexler, 1987), environmental adaptation (Lidz, 1987), learning theory (Bransford, 1979; Brown, Bransford, Ferrara, & Campione, 1983; Feurerstein, 1979; Vygotsky, 1978), and cognitive processing theories (Adamovich, Henderson, & Averbach, 1985; Anderson, 1985; Lidz, 1987) with concepts of occupation to support the client's function-

al performance and overall well-being. There is little attempt made to determine the "absolute level of performance on specific tests of cognitive subskills," and classical hierarchies of function and dysfunction are not used (Toglia, 1992, p. 107; 1998, p. 7). Instead, the therapist acts like a "detective" and tries to uncover clues that will identify those factors that account for the person's ability to function or for failures to perform successfully in numbers of situations and tasks (Toglia, 1992, p. 107; 1998, p. 7). Once these factors have been identified, the therapist can work with the patient/client, family, employer, or other to modify conditions or attributes of the task or performance setting and to teach the client cognitive strategies that he or she can use in multiple situations.

CURRENT PRACTICE IN OCCUPATIONAL THERAPY

Person and Behavior

Toglia's emphasis is on the individual's cognitive processing. This in turn reflects an information processing perspective. To review for the reader, the **information-processing model** (Figure 9-2) conceptualizes a cycle in which the following occurs:

1. Information is taken in from the environment by the individual as "input."
2. This new information is combined with existing information and made sense of; judgments and decisions are made via "throughput" (also called "elaboration").
3. Decisions can be acted upon in the form of "output," which is the person's response or performance.
4. From performance there is generated "feedback," which comes back into the person-system as information and the cycle is perpetuated.

According to Toglia (1998, pp. 8-12), the information-processing cycle is also influenced by what she refers to as the individual's "learner characteristics." Those learner characteristics emphasized by Toglia are his or her:

- Metacognition
- Cognitive processing strategies
- Such personal attributes as beliefs, motivation, emotions, experience, and style of coping

The Learner Characteristic Known as Metacognition

A critical attribute of the person in the dynamic person-occupation-environment triad is the person's ability to judge his or her abilities in relation to a task. This includes knowing one's own cognitive processing abilities and limitations, being able to plan ahead and adjust to changing task demands, and being able to predict the likely consequences of one's actions (Toglia, 1992, p. 109; 1993a, p. 17; 1998, p.

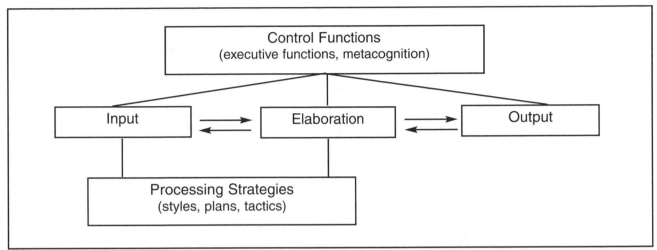

Figure 9-2. This diagram represents information processing or a person's executive function and metacognition (control function). During input, we use our five senses to perceive and attend to information that is elaborated in short- and long-term memory and then organized. The input and elaboration process produces plans or cognitive strategies that result in output (or occupational performance). The three components of input, elaboration, and output produce executive function and metacognition that plan, make decisions, monitor our behavior, and evaluate our performance (adapted from Toglia, J. P. [1992]. A dynamic interactional approach to cognitive rehabilitation. In N. Katz [Ed.], *Cognitive rehabilitation: Models for intervention in occupational therapy* [pp. 104-143]. Boston, MA: Andover Medical Publishers).

11). This is referred to as **metacognition** (Flavell, 1985). According to Toglia, most non-impaired individuals are quite accurate when estimating task difficulty and can adjust their behavior and performance strategies accordingly. To cite her example, if we are having trouble concentrating, we may quite automatically turn down the radio or move to a quieter room (Toglia, 1993a, p. 17). Students typically know when they need to review material before taking an upcoming exam. Part of metacognition is knowing under what conditions we can learn best. Having metacognition is very important because it enables us to make the necessary adjustments that will help us to be successful or improve our performance within our daily life occupation.

As a simple example, if I realize that I have limited short-term memory or get easily sidetracked, I know that I need to create a written list before I go to the grocery store. Without this awareness, I'm liable to go to the store without a list and come home having forgotten much of what I needed to purchase. If you don't recognize that noise keeps you from paying attention, you are less likely to create a quiet nonstimulating environment for yourself at work. If you don't realize that it is a lack of sleep that is impairing your ability to concentrate or enjoy social contacts, you may continue to stay up late watching old movies.

Levels of Awareness

Within this domain of metacognition, Toglia addresses what she refers to as levels of **cognitive awareness**. Citing the work of Crosson et al. (1989), she identifies three types of awareness. **Intellectual awareness** refers to the person's ability to understand at some level that their cognitive function is impaired. **Emergent awareness** refers to the person's ability to recognize that he or she is experiencing a particular performance problem as it is actually occurring. **Anticipatory awareness** is the ability to predict or anticipate when and where one will have difficulty before the problem occurs (Toglia, 1992, p. 129; 1998, p. 11).

We can refer again to the example of one's going to the grocery store. Let's think about our client, "Ida," who has recently had a CVA. Ida is discharged to home following acute inpatient rehabilitation. If she has intellectual awareness, she might tell her family, "I know I'm not the same; I fatigue easily; I get confused; things seem harder for me; I have trouble remembering." If she has emergent awareness, she would know as the problem is unfolding in the grocery store, "Oh my; I can't remember what I came for." If she has anticipatory awareness, she will be able to predict ahead of time, "I'm going grocery shopping this afternoon. I need many things, and I know that I won't be able to remember even half of them unless I do something." It is anticipatory awareness that allows Ida to prepare ahead of time, in this instance, to be dressed and ready when her son comes to take her to the store and to generate and bring along a grocery list. The cognitive performance described in this example can also represent clients who have cognitive impairments that are the outcome of psychiatric disorders (e.g., depression, schizophrenia, etc.) and dementia.

The research suggests that individuals with brain-injury typically overestimate their abilities relative to task demands (Anderson & Tranel, 1989), which in turn would be expected to keep them from learning or employing those cognitive processing strategies that could help them improve their performance. This was consistent with what Toglia found with her own patients (Toglia, 1998, p. 15).

The Person's Use of Processing Strategies

Toglia references Lidz (1987) when defining **processing strategies** and behavior. They are "...defined globally as organized approaches, routines, or tactics that operate to select and guide the processing of information" (Toglia, 1998, p. 8). The person uses these strategies to acquire information and use the information to participate in daily life. A person can process information at two levels. Again referencing others (Anderson, 1985; Lidz, 1987; Nolen, 1988), Toglia describes both levels and gives multiple examples that can increase our understanding of cognitive function. The reader is referred to Cognitive Function Behaviors for sample behaviors and strategies that reflect cognitive function. An extensive list of cognitive function examples, reproduced from Toglia (1998), are in Appendix M.

COGNITIVE FUNCTION BEHAVIORS

- Is aware of the whole task as well as its component parts and necessary details
- Organizes information systematically to achieve a goal
- Initiates and continues action to achieve a goal
- Can adjust behavior in response to the environment
- Can visualize specific detail and abstract concepts
- Has visual perceptual skills that support function
- Can identify significant information to be remembered
- Knows the strategy one uses to remember information
- Can use associations to recall and recognize information
- Can project barriers to performance
- Can find alternative responses to solve or manage problems

Level of Cognitive Processing

The first level of processing is referred to as the **surface level** in which the individual relies on memory and tries to memorize facts and procedures without connecting them to a meaningful context (Nolen, 1988). This approach to processing requires increased time and effort to learn and frequently is not retained over the long-term because it is not meaningful. When people take new information and connect it to current knowledge to improve their ability to effectively participate in daily life, they process information at a deep level. **Deep processing** uses elaboration and organization of information, which increases efficient use of information and usually long-term retention. Thus, the level of processing influences learning and the efficiency of learning (Anderson, 1985; Lidz, 1987; Toglia, 1998, p. 8).

Internal and External Processing Strategies

There are multiple types of cognitive processing strategies. One way that these have been grouped is as internal or external, situational and nonsituational. **Internal strategies** are those mental activities that a person does to remind one's self to do something or to keep on track (e.g., rehearsing something until it becomes automatic or routine, using self-cues and self-questioning). A special type of strategy within those identified as internal is that referred to as **self-monitoring**, wherein the person mentally questions, tracks, and/or evaluates his or her own thoughts or performance (Toglia, 1998, p. 8) (see Self-Monitoring Behaviors and Examples of Self-Monitoring Strategies).

SELF-MONITORING BEHAVIORS

- Assesses task complexity/simplicity and adjusts behavior to meet task need
- Identifies his/her performance boundaries and is aware of one's abilities
- During performance is aware of potential problems and adjusts behavior as needed for success
- Is aware of task context and can adjust performance to meet environmental expectations

---

EXAMPLES OF SELF-MONITORING STRATEGIES

- Self-questioning regarding performance effectiveness
- Checking performance results
- Anticipation of consequences of one's thoughts and actions
- Rate modulation of performance
- Efficient allocation of attention resources (Brown et al. in Toglia & Golisz, 1990)

External strategies make use of external cues, such as when we create and refer to a to-do list or a weekly calendar to help us organize how we will go about meeting responsibilities. **Situational strategies** are, as the term implies, specific to one situation (Toglia, 1998, pp. 8-10) (see Examples of Task Strategies). We may, for example, have strategies that we use to obtain food in a buffet-style restaurant that would not work in a conventional restaurant in which one orders from a menu and is served. A person uses different approaches to communication in a cocktail party situation versus a business meeting. The topics as well as the type of humor in these two environments are very different.

EXAMPLES OF TASK STRATEGIES

- Rehearsal—Use with limited amount of information or situation requiring exact performance

- Grouping information—Use when there is alot of information to recall

- Formulating associations—Use when there is alot of information or multiple procedures to recall

- Visualization—Create an image that assists with recall

- Scanning—Review the task or information and choose key elements to remember (Toglia & Golisz, 1990, p. 7)

Nonsituational strategies are those that the person uses under many or diverse circumstances (Toglia, 1998, p. 10). For example, to hold attention on a task and problem solve, a person may use **self-talk**, saying quietly to the self the steps used in completing a task. After a head injury or when managing a mental disorder or developmental disability, patients or clients may be taught to talk aloud when they are performing kitchen tasks or work activities to increase the quality of their performance and avoid errors of omission (Goldstein, 1973). Researchers in education, psychology, and brain literatures continue to evaluate the effectiveness of specific strategies and may challenge previous views such as those held about self-talk. We encourage the reader to review the literature for recent findings that may influence intervention approaches.

Visualization is another example of a nonsituational strategy that can be used in multiple contexts. Both the actor and sportsman preparing for a "performance" may spend time visualizing his or her role in scenes of the play or within a sport. A client may use visual strategies to prepare for an employment interview. The problem-solving strategies and techniques described within the cognitive-behavioral chapter of this text (Chapter Six) are examples of non-situational strategies.

Use of Cognitive Processing Strategies

These cognitive processing strategies can be used anywhere within the information processing cycle. Knowingly or unknowingly, we all employ strategies that affect the information processing cycle at various points in the cycle—input, elaboration, output, or feedback. Some strategies are selected because they help us at a particular place in the process, as when we turn down the radio or highlight material with a marker in order that we can pay better attention to new information we are reading. However, many strategies help us throughout the process.

For example, I am learning the steps involved in doing a new task at work, so I write down everything my supervisor tells me about the task. The strategy is to write things down. Doing this helps me pay better attention to what she is saying (**input phase**); it helps me organize the information and remember it (**elaboration phase**); and when it comes time to perform the task, referring to my notes helps me stay on task (**output phase**). Whether or not the person will know that he or she needs to employ a cognitive processing strategy or which strategy to select relates directly to the extent of metacognition a person has and the metacognitive strategies that a person uses.

Additionally, the client's life experiences, motivation, personal preferences, and emotions may all impact his or her preferred cognitive processing strategies.

Metacognition and Self-Efficacy

Metacognition is also reflected in the person's sense of **self-efficacy**. As people participate in daily life, they learn about their ability to perform specific tasks and effectively participate in the environment and come to perceive themselves as being capable and in control overall. Ideally, the basis for feelings of self-efficacy is rooted in early life experiences and builds over the lifetime. In this instance, metacognition bolsters one's self-confidence that he or she can meet challenges, such as those imposed by illness and injury.

Nevertheless, with acquired head injury or cognitive impairments that result from disease, the person's ability to use the knowledge that has been learned throughout life or the cognitive strategies that had previously worked so well may be disrupted. Another way to frame this is to say that there may be breakdown or "kinks" in the information processing cycle. The client with head injury or psychosocial disability who recognizes that he or she can no longer do what was easily accomplished before may lose confidence or feel unsure of remaining skills. The job of the therapist is multifaceted and includes:

- Discovering how the client can now best use and process information, including what cognitive processing strategies will enhance performance

- Evaluating the person's extent of metacognition

- Predicting how the client might be best able to do cognitive processing in the future to function in varied situations

The person's interests and life experiences also influence cognitive processing and performance. Understanding and appreciating what is important to the person and those values and beliefs that sustain his or her engagement in the face of challenge and uncertainty is vital to cognitive processing and performance.

Cognitive Performance—Dysfunction and Function

To understand the continuum of function and dysfunction, the person's characteristics, tasks, and environments are evaluated individually and collectively. The clinician looks for the compatible relationships that support function and the mismatch that can exist amongst the three variables.

Dysfunction as a Mismatch

In this model, whether one will be functional or dysfunctional depends on the person's relative success in using cognitive processing to succeed at desired occupations. A person who has **adequate cognitive function** is able to use his or her knowledge and to take in and process information in a manner that enables one to successfully participate in desired tasks of living. As indicated, the person may be more (or less) successful in some situations than in others, and there is no attempt to set absolute parameters on function or dysfunction. The individual with an acquired brain injury or other impairment that has a change in cognitive performance may have difficulty using his or her remaining cognitive abilities in his or her desired occupation. This **impaired performance** is believed to be the outcome of a conflict or "mismatch" between the person, the task, and/or the environment (Toglia, 1998, p. 15). Thus, each of these three variables is evaluated to describe cognitive dysfunction.

Dysfunction is not identified as the impairment of a particular cognitive component or subskill (e.g., poor short-term memory or decreased attention). Rather, dysfunction is based upon a lack of processing and metacognitive strategies and the inability to self-monitor one's performance during varied tasks in multiple environments (Toglia, 1998, p. 15). For example, a person may focus on details that prevent task completion, or socially, clients may not discriminate when to use humor and when it can be offensive. Clients may struggle with when to use assertive and aggressive behavior and are unable to manage the effects of their response when they withdraw or when conflict arises.

Competent cognitive performance is described in terms of the ability for task performance and ability to use information, strategies, and problem-solving behaviors to participate in work, leisure, and social situations and to perform daily living activities. Clients who learn from their experiences and use this knowledge in the future or learn from their mistakes have cognitive function that supports participation in daily life.

For example, the therapist might refer to patients' abilities to efficiently organize and structure a task (e.g., brush one's teeth, make a sandwich, prepare a hot lunch, etc.) and to monitor their own performance and anticipate what to do during activities. The clinician can observe if the client can efficiently access and safely use the knowledge and skills needed to perform tasks and perform these tasks in multiple situations (i.e., in clinic, at home, in the community, with distractions, with assistance, etc.).

Person Factors

There are many factors that may contribute to this mismatch between the person's abilities and task demands. These relate to what is known about cognitive processing, including metacognition and learner characteristics, which have been previously discussed. The individual may exhibit poor performance because he or she lacks or has lost necessary knowledge or is unable to select and use knowledge that one has about an ADL, work, or leisure task. He or she may have limited cognitive problem-solving skills. For example, the person needs to be able to break a big goal into subgoals as required for finding an apartment. The person needs to evaluate if he or she has adequate finances for security deposit and rent, is able to plan a monthly budget to meet expenses, and is able to read in order to search the newspaper or Internet for current listings, etc. If the person has difficulty problem solving, this may result in the patient or client setting unrealistic goals or failing to recognize that in order to meet performance goals he or she will need to employ specific knowledge and special strategies.

Dysfunction can also result when individuals fail to monitor their performance and progress. They do not recognize that they are not keeping pace with what is going on around them or that they are have stopped paying attention. Because of this decrease in metacognitive input, they may not realize that the cognitive strategies that they employ are no longer working successfully. They may not receive or use that feedback about their performance that is coming from inside themselves or from the external environment, and they do not adjust their behavior or change strategies for successful performance in daily living. The previously described changes in self-monitoring and speed of response influence such occupations as driving a car or boat or riding a bicycle.

Individuals may have decreased cognitive performance because they are not sensitive to the whole context of an experience and are unable to see and be sensitive to the perspectives of others. For example, there are different communication expectations in casual situations and work environments. The social protocol in a work environment expects a person to use humor within the boundaries of "political correctness." For example, a man may make frequent comments about "pretty girls," intending to be complimentary, but the people in the environment may interpret it as a sexist statement. Therefore, the client may not have the ability to discriminate social codes and flexibly adapt to the environment to meet the performance expectations of the task setting.

Finally, clients may not have the confidence or motivation to try to use their remaining cognitive abilities, nor to attempt to develop new cognitive strategies. Depression and anxiety as well as too much or too little stimulation may interfere with cognitive processing and thus functional behavior. These changes in a person may make them irritable with others, have low frustration tolerance for tasks, and interfere with interactions with others.

Task Complexity

Task characteristics include those that are easily observed (e.g., the number of items used in the task, how items are arranged, the nature of the stimuli that the task provides, the number of steps or directions given to do the task, and the nature of the posture and physical movements typically used to complete the task). What cannot be directly observed is the type of thinking used to complete the task (Toglia, 1992, p. 112). It seems reasonable to propose that the processing strategies used to accomplish a task be partially determined by the task's complexity. Toglia (1992, p. 112; 1998, p. 13) advises the occupational therapist using this model to analyze the complexity of the task (1992, p. 112), task features, and circumstances (1998, p. 13).

Some of the ways that the cognitive complexity of a task can be graded up or down are by either increasing or decreasing the amount of information one must pay attention to, increasing or decreasing the number of different means by which information is given, increasing or decreasing the speed at which information is given, increasing or decreasing the time allotted to process information and complete the task, or increasing or decreasing the complexity of the information being professed.

In addition to complexity, the therapist can change the **context** of the task (e.g., the client performs the task in the familiar or natural environments of the home or in simulated or therapy situations), or change tasks because of the distractions in the environment. Clinicians may choose to use the same task repeatedly or to vary the tasks used during interventions depending on the clients' needs.

Environmental Mismatch

Toglia does not describe in detail what is encompassed in the environment, although she makes frequent reference to the "social," "cultural," and "physical" nature of the environment. The **physical environment** includes those "physical materials and objects that surround the individual" during task performance; the **cultural environment** refers to "values and expectations accepted by the person's cultural group" (p. 112); the **social environment** "includes the people with whom the individual interacts" (p. 111). Referencing Feuerstein (1979) and Vygotsky (1978), Toglia suggests that "much of learning and higher cognitive skills are mediated

through social interaction" (p. 12). An important attribute of the physical and cultural environments is their familiarity to the client. Toglia (1992) proposes that **familiar environments** provide contextual cues that facilitate the access of previous knowledge and skills in performance and thereby are likely to enhance performance (p. 112).

Environments can support performance, as when they are physically comfortable and provide the just-right amount of stimulation; or, they may detract from performance, as when there is too much commotion going on, or when there is an emotional climate of peer or supervisor disapproval. Because it is not assumed that the patient/client will be able to complete a given task equally well in one environment or context as he or she does in another, the therapist pays careful attention to those attributes of the setting that seem to either support or detract from optimum cognitive processing and ultimately performance.

Bearing in mind that the individual's cognitive processing is believed an outcome of the interaction of person, task, and environment, Toglia reminds the occupational therapist that not only might the client perform better in one setting than another, conversely, his or her behavior may be quite out of skew in one setting as compared to another because he or she fails to recognize that different behaviors are needed in different contexts. Therefore, the client's awareness of setting (awareness of what is available and expected in a setting) and not only awareness of capacity becomes important in this model.

Role of the Occupational Therapist

The roles of the occupational therapist in this model are related and usually occur simultaneously. The clinician can be a detective, a collaborator, and mediator of information processing.

Detective

Toglia describes the occupational therapist as a "**detective**" (Toglia, 1992, p. 107; 1998). The therapist recognizes that every individual is unique, and he or she must try to uncover the cognitive strengths, limitations, and barriers to the client's successful and meaningful participation in everyday life. The occupational therapist uses his or her own knowledge of cognition and cognitive processing, his or her ability to analyze tasks and activities, and careful observation of client performance to identify possible adjustments that can be made to the task, to the occupational setting, or to the approach being taken by the client to the task to establish a better task-environment-person match.

According to Toglia, the therapist-examiner does not just observe behavior, he or she attempts to change behavior (Toglia, 1992, p. 119). Because no two individuals are alike and the therapist is observing a cognitive process as well as a performance outcome, the therapist must use clinical reasoning. This, Toglia says, is "time consuming" and "requires an experienced clinician" (Toglia, 1992, p. 107).

Collaborator

The occupational therapist also has a **collaborative role** that facilitates problem solving. When adjusting the task-environment-person match to solve cognitive performance problems the clinician needs client participation and perspectives in order to adjust the input from the task or the environment. The clinician uses this information and becomes a mediator that can help a client perform by supporting or limiting information processing. The therapist changes the environment, modifies the task, or gives cues to the person to improve the fit between the person-environment-task.

Toglia (1998) sees this role as **mediator** in this collaborative process as analogous to the social learning process, described by Vygotsky (1978), in which children learn from their shared experiences with more knowledgeable peers. The space between what a person can do and what he or she can learn to do with the guidance of a knowledgeable peer in a collaborative relationship is called the "zone of proximal development" (Toglia, 1998, p. 12; Vygotsky, 1978). As a mediator the occupational therapist uses his or her expertise and clinical reasoning to work within the **zone of proximal development** to provide the just right challenge and facilitate the development of cognitive skills and strategies.

Function of Activities

The model suggests that individuals "do" something (be actively engaged in meaningful occupation) in order that the impact of cognitive processing on performance can be assessed and in order that new learning occurs. Toglia (1992, 1993a, 1998) frequently refers to therapeutic occupation as both "activity" and as "task" and seems to use these terms synonymously.

Identify Cognitive Processing Ability

Therapeutic tasks have two important and related functions. The first is that they enable the therapist to identify the relative success or difficulty the patient or client has in doing cognitive processing (e.g., predicting the difficulty of the task, accessing and using knowledge, choosing the correct strategy, maintaining attention and solving problems, monitoring one's performance). Once it has been established that an individual has a cognitive processing impairment and needs to learn new strategies, these will be learned and practiced within the context of both functional activities and what Toglia (1992, 1998) refers to as "remedial tasks" (p. 130).

Functional activities and **tasks**, says Toglia, require the integration of all performance components. **Remedial tasks** can incorporate meaningful stimuli and relate to a client's interests but do not necessarily represent a complete functional activity (Toglia, 1992, p. 130; 1998). Remedial tasks provide an opportunity for the client to learn and practice a specific cognitive strategy. Playing a game of hearts is a functional activity or task, while practicing the process of sorting cards by suit would be a remedial task. Thus, the second function of therapeutic activities and tasks is that they are the vehicles for new learning, practice, and generalization.

Vehicle for Learning and Transfer

By practicing new cognitive skills in both novel and familiar meaningful tasks and activities, the person is also able to enhance **metacognition**. This means that:

- The person is aware of his or her knowledge and what he or she can or cannot do
- The person knows when and how to use his or her knowledge
- The person can monitor his or her performance during tasks and activities (Flavell, 1985; Toglia, 1998, p. 11)

As the person becomes more aware of cognitive processing strengths and limitations, he or she can make adjustments that enhance one's own performance to perform tasks and use or accommodate to the environment.

In addition to increasing metacognition and influencing cognitive processing, tasks also are the vehicle for transfer of learning and generalization. Toglia (1991, 1998, p. 14) describes a continuum of transfer that is influenced by surface and conceptual characteristics of the task. **Surface characteristics** include stimulation provided, the physical use of space for the task, the directions for the task, and the client's physical movements to perform the task (Toglia, 1998, p. 13). Unlike the surface task features, **conceptual characteristics** are not easily seen. They represent the meaning of the task and the individual's strategies, skills, and abilities that influence use of tasks (Toglia, 1991, 1998, p. 13).

To support learning transfer, the therapist helps the client choose tasks that will help the client perform and move along the continuum of transfer (Table 9-1). For example, **near transfer** is facilitated by using similar tasks but changing one to two surface characteristics (e.g., playing a game of cards called hearts and then learning a new card game such as go fish with two people). **Intermediate transfer** uses tasks that have few common surface characteristics. Staying with our card example, teaching a client to play poker with two to four people. **Far transfer** tasks are physically different (e.g., learning to play dominos, bridge, or other strategy games in a social context with two to four people). **Very far transfer** requires the person to perform tasks learned in treatment in one's home or community contexts (Toglia, 1991, 1998, p. 14). For example, in this situation, clients would play one or more of these card games with a church group, in a club, or at home with a group of friends.

Table 9-1

THE TRANSFER CONTINUUM

Same strategy emphasized across different tasks and situations

Near		Intermediate		Far	
Initial task; Instant coffee-jar	Making instant coffee with premeasured packages; different cup, pot; different location of items	Making tea or hot chocolate	Making instant oatmeal or soup, pudding or gelatin per- formed at the counter, table, different kitchens	Making pasta, frozen vege- tables, using different pots	Making toast with butter and jelly, or a peanut butter and jelly sand- wich	Loading and starting the dishwasher or setting a table for two	Making the bed or doing a small load of laundry

Reprinted from Toglia, J. (1998). A dynamic interactional model to cognitive rehabilitation. In N. Katz (Ed.), *Cognition and occupation in rehabilitation* (p. 34). Bethesda, MD: American Occupational Therapy Association, Inc. © 1998 by the American Occupational Therapy Association, Inc. Reprinted with permission.

Table 9-2
DIFFERENT ASSESSMENT METHODS

Static	*Qualitative*	*Dynamic*
Is there a problem?	What is the underlying nature of the problem?	Can performance be facilitated or changed?
What is the problem?	Why is the person having difficulty?	What cues/conditions increase or decrease the symptoms?
What is the severity of the problem?		What is the individual's potential for learning?
Example: Cancellation test The number of items omitted on the right and left side is scored.	*Example: Cancellation test* Different colored pencils are given every 10 seconds to document the pattern of scanning; where it began, how it proceeded.	*Example: Cancellation test* Graded cues are given during or after the task to determine if the client can improve or self-correct performance.

Reprinted from Toglia, J. (1998). A dynamic interactional model to cognitive rehabilitation. In N. Katz (Ed.), *Cognition and occupation in rehabilitation* (p. 17). Bethesda, MD: American Occupational Therapy Association, Inc. Reprinted with permission of Joan Toglia.

THEORETICAL ASSUMPTIONS— GUIDE TO EVALUATION AND INTERVENTION

The theoretical assumptions (see Dynamic Interactional Theoretical Assumptions) are a summary of the basic beliefs about the person, activities or occupations, and the environment or context. These beliefs are adapted from the theory of the dynamic interactional model that is previously described in this chapter. Toglia (1998) provides a comprehensive framework for understanding cognitive processing and its effect on occupational performance. Her theoretical constructs and assumptions reflect a blend of theory from cognitive, behavioral, information processing, and occupational therapy theories and their application. The assumptions about the person-environment-occupation variables and their possible relationships guide evaluation and intervention in occupational therapy.

Evaluation

The dynamic interaction model provides assessment methods that give information about the person's cognitive function within the context of everyday life tasks. Toglia sug-

gests a combination of static, qualitative, and dynamic assessment methods. Static assessment is used to identify problems and their severity. **Qualitative information** describes the process of the person's performance and the source of performance problems. **Dynamic** assessment is used to evaluate if performance can be changed, the possible conditions for managing symptoms, and the person's approach to learning. These methods may be used alone or in combination (Toglia, 1998, pp. 16-17). The qualitative approach is used to observe "where the individual begins and how he proceeds" (1998, p. 16). She contrasts dynamic interactional assessment against what she refers to as "static" (traditional) assessment (Table 9-2).

Static Assessment Methods

Static assessment includes standardized cognitive screening tools and neuropsychological tests. Their objective is to identify and quantify cognitive deficits. According to Toglia, they define "here and now" performance (Toglia, 1992, p. 118). Within static assessment, the person assessed is either able or unable to succeed at the test items. In **standardized static assessment**, the test environment and test conditions are to be the same for each examinee, and the therapist is to remain neutral (i.e., the therapist does not indicate whether

DYNAMIC INTERACTIONAL THEORETICAL ASSUMPTIONS

The following assumptions are drawn from the recent discussion of the dynamic interactional model to cognitive rehabilitation (Toglia, 1998, pp. 5-50).

Concept of Cognition

1. Cognition is a dynamic process that is more than the sum of its multiple components (i.e., attention, visual processing, memory, etc.).

2. The dynamic process of cognition guides assessment and intervention.

3. Cognition is the use of knowledge/information to learn, change, and adapt to one's environment.

4. Cognitive processing is evaluated by using dynamic assessment that looks at the changing relationships among the person, the task, and the environment.

5. The cognitive components emphasized in the dynamic interactional model are information processing; cognitive strategies; metacognition; and individual differences in learning, knowledge, motivation, and problem solving in context.

6. Poor cognitive function represents a mismatch between the task, environment, and person.

7. The dynamic view of cognition differs from the deficits-specific model of cognition, which evaluates the individual components of cognition (attention, memory, perception, etc.), rather than how they work together during cognitive processing.

Person

8. A person may have cognitive impairment as a result of physical, psychological, neurological, or developmental conditions.

9. A person has the ability to receive information from internal and external environments, organize it, assimilate it, and integrate it with previous information.

10. A person has the ability to use information to achieve a goal and change.

11. A person's metacognition is the person's knowledge of what he or she knows and his or her ability to self-monitor his or her behavior and to choose a strategy to learn or modify behavior.

12. A person has different types of awareness: intellectual, emergent, and anticipatory. Awareness is necessary for problem solving and adaptation.

13. A person can improve one's cognitive performance and efficiency by having metacognition— awareness of one's self, the ability to identify a task's relative difficulty and demands that influence performance, and knowledge of when to use specific strategies to optimize performance.

14. A person needs to be able to use feedback (internal and external) to improve cognitive performance.

15. A person needs metacognition to use his or her knowledge in multiple contexts (generalize).

16. A person's life experiences, motivation, personality, and emotions influence learning, strategies used to learn/problem solve, and the goals he or she will try to achieve.

17. A person needs to practice activities in multiple contexts to increase the possibility of generalization.

Task (Occupation)

18. The use of activities and tasks during assessment provides qualitative data for understanding a patient's/client's awareness and his or her use of knowledge and strategies for structuring and completing a task.

19. Tasks are individualized to meet patient/client learning needs and in response to patient's/client's abilities, deficits, and preferences.

20. Activities and tasks can be used to increase a person's awareness and teach strategies to improve use of knowledge to achieve a goal.

21. Tasks are analyzed for their cognitive complexity, to identify criteria that will enable transfer of learning, methods to cue performance, and contexts for modifying task complexity and difficulty.

22. Tasks are used in varied contexts to support generalized use of knowledge, problem solving, and the application of cognitive strategies.

23. Tasks should be meaningful to the person.

24. Novel and familiar tasks are used to facilitate transfer of learning and improved cognitive performance.

Environment and Context of Occupational Therapy

25. The person receives feedback from both internal and external environments.

26. The occupational therapy environment is the "zone of proximal development." The therapist structures the environment with the just right challenge for a person to use his or her knowledge and skills to increase awareness, learn metacognitive strategies, and increase self-efficacy.

27. The environment influences the person's ability to process information and adapt.

28. The physical environment and the therapist's cues provide structure that influences the client's performance.

29. The environment influences the person's performance during the activity or task.

30. The therapist structures the environment to teach strategy use in specific contexts.

31. The structure of the environment can influence the person's control of cognitive symptoms.

32. In occupational therapy, the therapist uses qualitative analysis of task performance to evaluate cognitive components in specific contexts.

33. In occupational therapy, during dynamic assessment of cognition, the occupational therapist evaluates the impact of a task's difficulty, adaptations, and the use of cues on occupational performance.

or not a response is correct, nor change test conditions to accommodate to client performance). This is in sharp contrast to dynamic assessment (Toglia, 1998, p. 16).

Dynamic Interactional Assessment Methods

The goal of **dynamic interactional assessment** is to "identify and specify the conditions that have the greatest influence on performance" (Toglia, 1992, p. 118; 1998, p. 16), both in terms of success and failure. Within a dynamic assessment instrument or procedure, when the client is unable to complete or struggles with a task item, the therapist will indicate that a response is not correct and may alter a test procedure, cue the client, or make other adjustments to see whether these will enable the client to be successful (Toglia, 1992, p. 119; 1998, pp. 16-17).

Dynamic assessment does not refer only or even mostly to the use of formalized assessment tools developed for the model. The therapist doing "dynamic assessment" can do so by observing a patient's/client's performance during occupation in any setting. The overall goals are:

- To determine whether or not the person has adequate knowledge
- Whether he or she can use that knowledge
- What strategies are employed during task performance
- What adjustments (cues, tasks, and environmental modifications initiated by the therapist) might enhance performance
- The extent of the person's awareness of his or her own abilities and limitations

The dynamic assessment process evaluates a client's current performance as well as tries to identify the client's potential to learn and use knowledge in multiple contexts (Toglia, 1998, pp. 16-17).

Components of Dynamic Interactional Assessment

During dynamic interactional assessment three components of assessment are used to estimate the person's potential to learn, his or her approach to solving problems, his or her preference for specific strategies to do tasks, and the effects of the therapist's cues and task changes on the person's performance. Toglia (1993a, 1998, pp. 17-20) cites three assessment components that are integrated during assessment. These are:

1. Awareness questioning
2. Strategy investigation
3. Determining the impact of cuing and task grading (1998, pp. 17-20)

Awareness Questioning

Awareness questioning is used to determine the individual's ability to recognize his or her strengths as well as limitations in regard to cognitive processing and performance. This includes questions that assess the three types of awareness that are described by Crosson et al. (1989) and cited in Chapter Six:

1. **Intellectual awareness** (awareness of one's general capacity, knowledge, and limitations)
2. **Emergent awareness** (the ability to identify that one is having a problem with a particular task within a particular environment, as this unfolds)
3. **Anticipatory awareness** (knowing that one has specific limitations and can expect to have difficulty carrying out a specified cognitive task in a specific environment)

Awareness includes one's ability to reflect back and know that he or she has not performed well, and questions may also probe for this. The questions in Awareness Questions illustrate the kinds of questions the occupational therapist might pose within the assessment process to get a sense of the person's level of awareness.

AWARENESS QUESTIONS

Questions for Intellectual Awareness

- Have you noticed any changes in your memory?
- How well do you think you are able to pay attention now as compared to before your injury/episode/illness?
- How would you rate your concentration now as compared to before the injury (100%, 75%, 50%, 25%, 0%)?
- Roughly how often do you walk away from your job because concentrating on it is overwhelming (very often, several times a day, only infrequently)?
- After the client has completed a task, the therapist can ask, "How do you think you did? How many (items) do you feel you handled correctly? How long do you think you spent on this job?"

Questions for Emergent Awareness

- How difficult is this task for you (very difficult, somewhat difficult, easy, very easy)?
- To the person engaged in a task, "Tell me when you start to have trouble staying focused."
- How do you think you're doing?

Questions for Anticipatory Awareness

- If I asked you to go to the grocery store and come back with three items, how many do you think you would remember?
- How many of these tasks or test items do you think you will be able to do correctly?

Adapted and summarized from Toglia (1993a, 1998).

Table 9-3
SAMPLE GRADED CUE SEQUENCE

Rationale	*Example of Cues*
Check and verify answer	Are you sure you found all the letter As?
General feedback	There are still some left. Can you find them?
Specific feedback	There are still some left on the left side.
Provide alternative approach	Try beginning here. Go slower and use your finger to point to each letter.
Task modification	Change one task parameter (e.g., number of items on the page are reduced; bright red line is placed in the left margin).

Reprinted from Toglia, J. (1998). A dynamic interactional model to cognitive rehabilitation. In N. Katz (Ed.), *Cognition and occupation in rehabilitation* (p. 20). Bethesda, MD: American Occupational Therapy Association, Inc. Reprinted with permission of Joan Toglia.

Having posed these questions, the therapist can compare what the patient or client describes of his or her ability with actual performance, as well as compares it to what others (family members, employers, or other professionals) have said about the client's performance. The client may also make spontaneous comments while performing a task that give the therapist information about the client's awareness of cognitive capacity.

Strategy Investigation

Strategy investigation is the process by which the occupational therapist both observes and asks the person how he or she went about performing the task. The therapist might ask such questions as, "Tell me how you arrived at this answer," or "How did you go about remembering everything you needed to do today?" Toglia refers to this process as **probing**, in part because the therapist pursues questioning in order to clarify exactly what process the person used (Toglia, 1993a, p. 24).

For example, in the Contextual Memory Test (Toglia, 1993b) (described later in this chapter), the examinee is to remember 20 common items depicted on the stimulus card. After recall has been tested, the therapist asks the client, "What strategy did you use to remember these items?" If he or she responds, "I grouped the items," the therapist would probe further and might ask, "How exactly did you group them? How many groups did you have?" or, "What were those groups?" "Did you group them when you were first trying to memorize them, or when you were trying to recall them, or both?"

The person's performance during tasks is believed to be also influenced by his or her remaining abilities, the nature of the task, and the performance setting (physical, social, and cultural elements of the environment). The therapist assesses strategies used by the person to manage task and environ-

ment conditions and use his or her abilities. The therapist might observe, for example, that the client seemed to become distracted by people walking in the hallway.

The therapist would observe what strategies he or she employed to manage or respond to these distractions or how the client set up his or her own work space and organized materials in preparation to begin a task or control the environment. Prior to beginning a task, the clinician asks the client to describe what he or she needs to do to bake a cake, find a job, get a driver's license, etc.

Much of what the therapist learns about the patient's or client's strategies comes from careful observation. Questions can be posed to the client as well, and these can give insight into the person's approach to use remaining abilities to manage one's impairment. Both the therapist and client learn from this investigation. What is discovered through the strategy exploration lays the foundation for the identification or practice of new and familiar strategies in future therapy sessions.

Cuing and Task Grading

The last component of assessment is to determine the client's response to task grading and cuing. When the client has difficulty carrying out a task within the assessment process, the therapist might first provide cues, "hints," or suggestions (typically verbal) that would be expected to improve the client's ability to succeed at the task. When these cues do not appear to improve performance, the therapist changes one or more features of the task to simplify the task. Both verbal cues and changes in task structure are individualized to the specific task and the context of performance. Toglia recommends that "task modifications should be used rather than verbal cues" (1998, p. 18). The assessment instruments developed by Toglia give guides to cuing. Table 9-3 shows an example of cuing during a letter cancellation task.

Summary of Dynamic Interactional Assessment

During occupational therapy assessment and treatment, presuming the absence of sophisticated computer technology, we cannot "see" inside a person's head to observe information processing. Therefore, the occupational therapist depends on the observation of performance plus comments made by the individual relative to his or her information processing and ability to complete desired tasks. Within occupational performance the therapist observes task behavior that entails use of specific cognitive components that must work in concert. Further, the therapist can observe those changes in task performance that result when the therapist provides cues or modifies the task. Thus, evaluation in this model is a **dynamic process**, concerned not just with the outcome of task behavior but with the way that outcome was achieved.

Assessment Instruments

The measurement tools designed by Toglia (1998, pp. 21-26) for the dynamic interactional model were developed through a process that began with a video tape analysis of the performance of persons with acquired brain injuries. Patients performed tasks without standardized cues. Toglia would vary the cues and task structure to see the effect that these changes had on cognitive performance and task outcomes. Toglia then analyzed the tapes to identify the structure of the assessment tasks and the types of cues and questions that influence the client's performance. After the tape analysis, Toglia developed a standardized system of cues, questions, and structuring tasks for the assessment. The test manuals describe how the clients' patterns of responses can be used to plan interventions. The established reliability and validity of the assessments are also in the test manuals.

According to Toglia, the individual and dynamic nature of the assessment process requires the therapist to be trained in the dynamic interactional process in order to gain the expertise needed for interpreting the assessment data. Because the therapist gives cues and may modify the tasks or environment during the dynamic assessment, the assessments are not used to measure change in the person's performance over time. The assessments developed by Toglia and currently available from Psychological Associates are the Contextual Memory Test (CMT) and the Toglia Category Assessment (TCA). The Dynamic Visual Processing Assessment (DVPA) is still in the research process and not available for purchase.

Contextual Memory Test

The CMT (Toglia, 1993a, 1993b, 1998, p. 24) has multiple purposes:

- Identifies the person's awareness of his or her memory capacity
- Identifies the person's ability for free recall
- Identifies the strategies that the client uses to recall the line drawings
- Identifies the person's response to cuing
- Identifies the person's ability to recognize information that he or she is unable to recall

The assessor begins by asking the client several questions to test his or her awareness of memory capacity. The client is then given 90 seconds to study a stimulus card depicting 20 everyday objects that share a common theme. He or she is immediately asked to verbally name as many items as can be remembered. Should the client have difficulty, the therapist gives a cue to assist memory. The second trial, a test of delayed recall, occurs after an interval of 15 to 20 minutes during which time the examinee's attention is directed to another activity. After both the first test of immediate recall and the second test of delayed recall, the assessor asks the client how well he or she believes he or she did.

The test has two statistically equivalent versions: one in which test items relate to a "restaurant" theme, the other in which all items relate to the person's morning routine.

If the client does not perform well on the first administration for immediate and delayed recall, the assessor can recommend memory strategies that the client can use to improve his or her recall, and the client can be tested again with the alternate version of the test. In this way, the assessor can determine if being given a strategy to use improves the client's ability for recall. There are other options in the test to determine whether cues given to the examinee improve his or her ability to recall and to test item recognition. The client's performance and responses provide data that the therapist uses to modify tasks and the environment and plan treatment that includes strategy training, awareness training, and practice in multiple contexts.

The CMT has been normed on several populations: normal adults, adults with chronic mental illness, adults having acquired brain injury, and a small sample of children (Toglia, 1998, p. 22). The reader is referred to the test manual (Toglia, 1993b) and subsequent discussions by Toglia (1998) for details.

Toglia Category Assessment

The TCA (Toglia, 1994; 1998, p. 25) is designed to assess flexibility in categorization and to evaluate deductive reasoning. To assess ability for and flexibility in categorization, the examiner requests the examinee to sort 18 plastic utensils into groups so that items in one group are different in one way from those of other groups. The utensils vary in color (red, yellow, and green), size (small and large), and type (knife, fork, or spoon). Once the examinee has successfully created groups according to one attribute (e.g., he or she has created groups according to color), the person is then instructed to re-group the utensils according to another attribute, and then again according to a third. If the client is unable to identify a way to categorize the items, cannot generate alternative possibilities for grouping, or perseverates (keeps creating the same groups), the therapist provides a sequence of cues.

To evaluate deductive reasoning the clinician uses the TCA to pose questions in the context of a "game." The examiner tells the client that he or she is "thinking of" a particular utensil, and the examinee's task is to determine the utensil the examiner is thinking of without guessing and by asking the least number of "yes/no" questions. The answer can be determined within five questions. As with the categorization portion of the assessment, the examiner may prompt the client who has difficulty solving the problem.

The TCA is available commercially from Psychological Associates. The manual describes reliability and suggests relationships between test responses and possible intervention approaches to problem solving. The test was normed on several populations: normal adults, adults with chronic mental illness, adults having acquired brain injury, and samples of older adults and children are being studied (Toglia, 1998, p. 2).

The Dynamic Visual Processing Assessment

The DVPA (Toglia, 1998, p. 23; Toglia & Finkelstein, 1991) is still in the process of development and is therefore not commercially available. The purpose of the test is to identify those task variables that influence the processing of visual information. The test uses line drawings, presented under different task conditions, to evaluate the client's perception of objects, unilateral inattention, the ability to self-monitor, and the way that visual scanning is organized.

The conditions that influence visual processing are the number of items, the organization of items, the rotation or position of items on the page, and whether the items are familiar to the client. The test can easily modify these conditions to meet the client's need. The therapist usually begins at a moderate level of task difficulty and then either simplifies it or makes it more difficult depending on the client's initial performance.

Because the assessment is not available, Toglia suggests that the therapist collect and use 16 to 25 items (objects) per category and vary their presentation (number, type, and orientation) for client identification. During the assessment, the therapist observes the client's scanning pattern and the ability to self-monitor recognized items. The therapist records the client's performance on a score sheet that identifies correct identifications, omissions, misperceptions, and client comments, and the therapist's observations about the task parameters. Sample task parameters include number of items, types of items, and their position (horizontal, vertical, overlapping, or random placement on the table for viewing) (Table 9-4).

Toglia also suggests guides for cuing (Toglia, 1998, pp. 23-24). In a preliminary study and unpublished dissertation, Kline (1997) found a correlation between the client's performance on the DVPA with IADL (Toglia, 1998, p. 23).

Intervention

Toglia's model evolved from her work with persons having head injury, and she identifies intervention as "treatment." Treatment described as a "multicontextual treatment approach" (1998, p. 28) systematically integrates change. The therapist reacts to the person's performance during a task, evaluates the effectiveness of the person's strategies for successful performance, and may modify the task or adapt the environment while keeping the use of the strategy stable to help the person continue what he or she has started. If dynamic assessment has determined that a person is responsive to cues and task or environmental modification and has the potential for improved metacognitive and strategy development, then he or she may be a good candidate for this kind of treatment. If it is determined that an individual's performance is unlikely to be improved through this kind of intervention, then he or she is a better candidate for functional approaches in which transfer of learning and new learning are not the goals (Toglia, 1992, p. 124).

The therapist who is considering dynamic interactional treatment also takes into account the typical outcomes of the injury or illness, the course of the injury since onset, assessment information from other professionals, the patient's or client's personality, and the person's current knowledge and desire to learn new skills.

Because individuals with head injury or psychosocial disabilities often have a significantly reduced awareness of their own cognitive impairments, dynamic interactional treatment, if it is to occur, often must begin with awareness building. Toglia emphasizes that the person who is unaware that he or she has a problem is unlikely to desire or use strategies to improve his or her own performance.

Building Awareness and Metacognitive Strategy Training

In order to be able to learn and change when a person has a cognitive impairment from chronic illness or brain injury, the person needs to understand what his or her problems are and the circumstances that cause cognitive problems to interfere with the person's performance in daily life. Thus, the person needs to be aware of his or her performance boundaries in order to change one's approach for participating in occupations. Before learning strategies for improving what one can or cannot do, the person needs awareness of one's ability in varied contexts. To increase awareness, Toglia cues the client to answer specific awareness questions prior to task performance. Clients answer questions that identify the following:

- The difficulty of the tasks
- The time needed to complete a task

Table 9-4

DYNAMIC VISUAL PROCESSING ASSESSMENT: SAMPLE ASSESSMENT WORKSHEET

Dynamic Visual Processing Cue Sequence

Omission Cues	Score	*Misperception Cues*
Are you sure you have have seen all the objects on the page? Could there be more?	4	Tell me how you know it is a _____. Could it be anything else?
There are still some that you didn't mention. Can you find them?	3	No, it is not a _____. Look again. or Describe what it looks like.
Look on the right/left/upper/middle of the page. Can you think of a way to help you keep track of the objects? Try it.	2	What category do you think it belongs to (present five choices)?
Try moving your eyes all the way over here (place red line). Try pointing like this to each object you mention in an organized way.	1	Look here (point to specific features).

Reprinted from Toglia, J. (1998). A dynamic interactional model to cognitive rehabilitation. In N. Katz (Ed.), *Cognition and occupation in rehabilitation* (p. 24). Bethesda, MD: American Occupational Therapy Association, Inc. Reprinted with permission of Joan Toglia and Nancy Kline.

- Circumstances that may support or interfere with one's performance
- Strategies they will use to complete the task
- The system for checking one's performance during the task (also referred to as self-monitoring)

Specific strategies used by Toglia are reproduced in Table 9-5.

Initially, the clinician is responsible for giving the awareness questions, and the patient/client answers. The goal is for the client to be able to self-initiate these questions prior to beginning a task in order to estimate the strategies needed to successfully do the task and the system he or she will use to self-monitor how well he or she is doing. These questions are used in conjunction with cognitive process strategies, environmental analysis, and task modifications.

The intent for metacognitive training is to move the client/patient from a system of external cues from the clinician to a self-initiated process in which the client assesses the task requirements and initiates the cognitive strategies that support successful participation and completion of tasks. Possible outcomes of metacognitive training include:

- Client has internalized strategies that he or she uses to self-cue task participation
- Client can identify environmental cues and task variables that support task performance
- Client receives feedback about task performance through self-monitoring strategies
- Client establishes a sense of self through awareness of one's new performance boundaries
- Client has increased self-efficacy and sense of control of performance during tasks and occupations (Toglia, 1998, pp. 32, 36-37)

Strategies to Increase Generalization

The goal of dynamic interactional treatment is to enhance generalization of learning. It is not enough that the client be competent in one specified situation. The aim is that he or she will be able to successfully process information and thereby function in a variety of situations and settings; therefore, the thrust of intervention is to teach the client cognitive processing strategies that can be used in multiple situations. Toglia has referred to this treatment as the "multicontext"

Table 9-5

METACOGNITIVE STRATEGIES AND TRAINING TECHNIQUES

Behavior	Metacognitive Strategy or Technique	Description
Client uses strategies when cued but does not initiate use of a strategy	Anticipation	Client is asked to anticipate any of the following: (a) the types of obstacles that might be encountered prior to performing the task, (b) the possible outcomes or consequences, (c) the need to choose a strategy.
Client overestimates his or her abilities	Self-prediction	Client is asked to predict the general difficulty of the task on a rating scale or predict specific aspects of performance such as accuracy score and time score. Predictions are compared with actual performance.
Client does not spontaneously check work	Self-checking and self-evaluation	After every 5 or 10 minutes, client is asked to self-check his work and fill out a self-evaluation form.
Client does not self-monitor performance during a task	Self-questioning	Client is taught to ask self key questions during a task. The questions may be written on cue cards. External aids such as an alarm or buzzer may be used to remind the individual to read the cue card in the initial stages. Examples of questions include: • Do I understand the problem? • Am I getting sidetracked by irrelevant details? • Do I need more information? • Am I getting stuck?
Unable to monitor time during a task; requires excessive time to perform tasks; performs unnecessary steps; gets caught up in unnecessary details; becomes sidetracked	Time monitoring	Estimate time; set time limits prior to initiation of the task, or compare or evaluate results. Prior to performing the task, visualize one's self performing the task with and without getting sidetracked.

(continued)

Behavior	Metacognitive Strategy or Technique	Description
Client has poor error-monitoring and detection skills	Role reversal	The therapist performs a task and makes errors due to distractibility, impulsivity, etc. The client observes the therapist's performance and gives the therapist feedback (points out errors and states why they may have occurred).

Table 9-5 (Continued)

Reprinted from Togila, J. (1998). A dynamic interactional model to cognitive rehabilitation. In N. Katz (Ed.), *Cognition and occupation in rehabilitation* (p. 37). Bethesda, MD: American Occupational Therapy Association, Inc. © 1998 by the American Occupational Therapy Association, Inc. Reproduced with permission.

approach because the focus is on practicing targeted processing skills in multiple environments (Toglia, 1992, p. 127; 1998, p. 28).

Processing Strategies

Treatment activities focus on areas in which the patient or client has difficulty rather than on strengths (Toglia, 1992, p. 127), and treatment begins where the client's performance breaks down. The therapist identifies one or two cognitive processing strategies that the client is to use to enhance performance. This same strategy is then practiced in multiple situations and settings. Toglia often uses **general strategies** that can enhance generalization and be used in multiple contexts rather than specific situational strategies that are not easily transferred. For example, a general processing strategy is **task segmentation**; the person is taught to analyze a task for its component parts and then work in an organized manner that will prevent or minimize cognitive symptoms.

Clients learn to look for task features that make performance difficult:
- Number of steps and rules to perform a task
- Task details and the supplies needed for the task
- Effects of doing a task in an unpredictable or unfamiliar environment (Toglia, 1998, p. 32)

Other processing strategies are suggested in Table 9-6.

Strategy Example—Chronic Illness

Toglia (1992) describes an example of the application of the dynamic interactional approach. The client she cites is a woman with a diagnosis of chronic schizophrenia having strong negative features. The occupational therapist had noted this woman's difficulty in maintaining attention to tasks. Among her problems were that she frequently looked around the room when she needed to be paying attention to a task, and she often began a task without a clear plan or goal regarding what she was trying to accomplish. She appeared to have particular difficulty coping with more than one or two visual stimuli at a time. The processing strategy that this client was to learn included stopping when she felt herself losing her focus of attention and systematically scanning visual stimuli to determine what should be her focus (p. 133).

Task Analysis and Grading

Once the processing strategy has been identified, the therapist must do a detailed task analysis to determine treatment tasks in which the strategy will be used. The goal is that the client uses the strategy successfully. At first, the task will be as simple as may be needed in order that the patient is able to succeed using the identified strategy. If a patient is unable to do 50% or more of the task correctly or successfully, the task is simplified or down graded. See Task Simplification and Three Levels of Activity on page 289 for guides that assist in grading activities.

When the client performs more than 50% of the task correctly (but not fully correct or accurate), the therapist uses a series of graded cues to improve the client's performance. To give a very simple example, assume a patient, Bill, has attention problems that interfere with everyday performance. He is given the task of sorting playing cards by suit. If Bill, in his first try, sorts less than 50% of the cards correctly, the task could be graded down by having him sort by color only (red or black). If this improves his performance (he now sorts more than 50% of the cards correctly) but he has still made many errors, the

Table 9-6
SAMPLE PROCESSING STRATEGIES

Sample Problem Behaviors/Symptoms	Sample Strategy	Description
Poor planning, attention, self-control	Verbal mediation or self-instructional procedures	Client is taught to say self-cues, task goals, plans, or task instructions out loud or silently before and/or during execution of a task.
Distracted by irrelevant information; difficulty selecting the main point	Underline, circle, or highlight critical details or facts	Client is taught to highlight, circle, or list information most critical to the task or problem.
Tendency to become overwhelmed by the amount of information	Stimuli removal	Client is taught to remove, cover, or visually block out information.
Loses track of steps, performs tasks incompletely; performs unnecessary steps	Visual imagery prior to task performance	Client imagines self performing task in an accurate and smooth manner; vividly imagines achieving the desired outcome or imagines performing task with possible obstacles and effective coping strategies.
Poor visual object recognition	Verbalization of object characteristics	Client is taught to silently verbalize the characteristics of an object prior to determining what the object is.
Difficulty recognizing and locating objects	Visual imagery prior to visual search	Vividly imagines the target item or object before searching for it.
Difficulty finding items; haphazard, disorganized approach	Categorization	Client is taught to rearrange similar items into meaningful clusters or smaller groups (e.g., grocery list, items in a closet or shelf).
Haphazard approach; difficulty focusing on a task; does not know where to begin; appears overwhelmed by the amount of information	Task segmentation	Client is taught to simplify a task by breaking it down into smaller, more manageable components and dealing with one step or component at a time. *(continued)*

Table 9-6 (Continued)		
Sample Problem Behaviors/Symptoms	*Sample Strategy*	*Description*
Difficulty locating and finding items; tendency to omit items or steps during a task	Rearrangement of items	Client is taught to rearrange items prior to starting a task so that they are organized according to the sequence of use, there are spaces between them, they are arranged in a linear rather than scattered arrangement.
Tendency to overfocus on the parts of a visual scene or stimulus	Look all over before responding	Client is taught to gain an impression of the whole before attending to the parts. Look all over; actively scan the entire visual display from different perspectives prior to attending to pieces.
Impulsive; tendency to miss details; disorganized visual scanning	Point or use finger to help focus on details	Client is taught to point to stimuli prior to responding to focus attention on details and/or slow down responses. Finger pointing may also assist in facilitating an organized pattern of visual scanning.

Reprinted from Togila, J. (1998). A dynamic interactional model to cognitive rehabilitation. In N. Katz (Ed.), *Cognition and occupation in rehabilitation* (p. 31). Bethesda, MD: American Occupational Therapy Association, Inc. © 1998 by the American Occupational Therapy Association, Inc. Reprinted with permission.

therapist could cue Bill, "Look carefully. Do you see any in this pile that don't belong? How about this other pile?" Bill could also be given a strategy to follow as he repeats the task: He is to ask himself out loud, "Is this card red or black?" as he turns each card face up. The client then uses this same strategy (ask aloud) in other tasks of equivalent difficulty. Task complexity is not increased until there is evidence that the client can successfully use the strategy in several or more tasks/situations (i.e., he or she has generalized learning).

Transfer of Learning

Toglia applies behavioral learning principles to facilitate **transfer** of knowledge. Behavioral theory tells us that we are more likely to transfer what we have learned to do in one situation to another situation when the two situations or tasks have similar characteristics. By gradually changing the characteristics of a task or setting, we can teach people to repeat the behaviors in multiple and eventually diverse situations. Using this same principle, Toglia recommends having the client who has learned to do a task using a given strategy in one situation to then practice it during another very similar task; gradually, the tasks in which the strategy is to be used become more and more dissimilar.

Respecting Learner Characteristics

The multicontextual approach to treatment uses the person's role as a learner as well as the cognitive, psychosocial, sensory-motor, and physical performance variables that influence the person's participation in daily life. The emphasis, however, is on helping the person use learning and cognitive strategies that are used in multiple situations. The intervention process is influenced by the **characteristics of the learner** such as:

TASK SIMPLIFICATION

One or more of the following can reduce the cognitive processing demands of a task:
- Decreasing the amount of information to which the client must attend
- Decreasing the speed or rate at which the information is given
- Increasing the amount of time the client has to do the task
- Making stimuli in the task more apparent or bolder
- Decreasing or eliminating the number of choices that have to be made within the task, limiting the types of information (e.g., only verbal or only written)
- Decreasing the complexity of the information

Adapted from Toglia, 1993a, pp. 27-31

THREE LEVELS OF ACTIVITY

Toglia recommends a structured system for grading tasks and activities. The system suggests three levels of activity:
- Level One—The activities are used to get a consistent response in a specific context or setting to meet the expectations of that setting. These activities have limited processing demands and depend on the use of many automatic responses.
- Level Two—The activities require the patient to respond to changing demands in the task environment. They require increased ability to monitor and process multiple stimuli and respond with some flexibility.
- Level Three—The third level of activities and tasks emphasizes organization. These tasks require clients to organize new and previously learned experiences to respond to the current challenge or retrieve for later use. This level is the most challenging and requires the client to analyze what is required by an activity.

From Abreu & Toglia, 1987; Luria, 1980

- The individual's previous and current knowledge and awareness
- His or her life experience
- His or her preferred learning style

- The learning strategies that support or interfere with performance in daily life
- The variables that motivate a person to learn and find meaningful task

Integrating these learner characteristics can also influence client satisfaction with the treatment process as the person learns to manage and solve problems unique to his or her disease or disability.

People with an acquired brain injury and mental illness often experience symptoms of anxiety or depression, which bear on the intervention process as well. In addition, every person has individual differences in values, attitudes, and beliefs that influence his or her motivation to learn, choice of meaningful activities, and satisfaction with the treatment process. When the therapist takes the time to listen to and understand what is important to the client, he or she is better able to respond to the client's concerns and to create meaningful experiences for learning and using general cognitive strategies.

Client Knowledge and Expertise

To the extent that the individual can access knowledge and refer to previous experiences (prior to the illness or trauma), he or she brings strengths and resources that are used during treatment. The person's knowledge influences the perception of current experiences and how this new information is used or stored for future use. When individuals create relationships between new experiences and previous knowledge, they are able to process information more quickly. The client's knowledge and experience also influence the treatment tasks and goals that the therapist and client choose. When clients pursue meaningful goals and tasks based on their knowledge and experience, they increase the effectiveness of cognitive processing. The clinician taps into the person's general knowledge and skills from roles such as parent, engineer, physician, businessman, health professional, student, salesman, spouse, athlete, etc. to integrate their performance strengths and learning strategies and style into treatment.

Client Learning Style

Patients and clients also have a preferred way of learning, or **learning style**, that influences problem solving and the outcome of occupational therapy intervention. A person's learning style may reflect a personal preference to learn from "doing" something rather than reading and memorizing information. These clients may prefer trial and error rather than a structured format for acquiring knowledge. Other clients may prefer to learn by observing others and having a model that helps them fulfill roles and learn new strategies. People also learn by interacting with others individually or in a group, or from textbooks and traditional academic structure. Each of us may use any one or more of these styles depending upon our goals and the demands in the environment and tasks. When clients are able to draw upon their previous knowledge and skills and use their preferred learning styles during treatment, they can often decrease the stress of learning and are better able to use their strengths to cope with the cognitive processing challenges imposed by illness or trauma. To increase your understanding of style of learning and preference for learning strategies, think about your own preferences and answer the questions posed in Increase Your Understanding: Learning Style and Strategies.

INCREASE YOUR UNDERSTANDING: LEARNING STYLE AND STRATEGIES

Take a few minutes and reflect on your life experiences in your family, at school, in your neighborhood, or participation in work and community contexts and identify the variables that influence the way you prefer to learn and what strategies you use to learn.

- Do you prefer or choose activities that you do alone or with others? Give you a role within a group? Are done indoors or outside? In the country or city, etc.? Are they quickly mastered or take a lot of practice to learn?

- When learning a new sport, do you want a trainer or coach? Do you learn activities because it allows you to share experiences with friends or be a member of a team? Do you learn on your own from a self-instruction manual and independent practice?

- How do your career goals or interests reflect your personal values and interests? What skills and expertise do you have from your work experiences? What have you learned from being a volunteer, worker, friend, community member, etc.?

- Make a list of general learning strategies you most frequently use to do different kinds of tasks and occupations. What are the variables that support or interfere with your learning?

Specific Treatment Objectives

The dynamic interactional model, a developing intervention model for occupational therapy, is a learning approach that considers the person, the task, and the environment, and how each of these variables can contribute to change. When possible the objective is to change client performance by developing the person's awareness, his or her use of strategies, and through self-monitoring of one's performance. Should a person be unable to learn or change, then the clinician makes changes in the tasks or environments to support the person's use of current knowledge and skills to

achieve the identified learning outcomes. In summary, objectives may include:

- Client will have increased awareness of his or her performance boundaries and the strategies needed for effective participation in tasks, activities, and occupations.

- Client will practice using cognitive strategies during different tasks in order to increase generalization or participation in varied contexts in daily life.

- Client will have the knowledge and skills needed to participate in meaningful activities and various environments.

- Client will use cognitive processing strategies and metacognitive strategies to control or manage his or her symptoms that can interfere with the demands of the task and the environment.

- Client will use task analysis and his or her understanding of the environment to select the cognitive strategies that support normal or compensated performance in daily life.

- Client will use feedback from the task, others, and his or her self-monitoring to change or adapt participation in tasks, activities, and occupations (Toglia, 1998, pp. 28-45).

These objectives may be achieved in individual or group treatment. Toglia's group approaches are described next.

Group Treatment

Toglia recommends a combination of individual and group treatment. Group treatment may be a one-time therapeutic experience with specific goals for that session, or the patient/client may participate in a treatment program that makes consistent use of groups. Group intervention provides opportunities for clients to practice individual task and self-monitoring strategies and to receive and learn from feedback provided by peers as well as the clinician who shares how well group members did on a task and what they contribute to the group experience through cooperation with peers.

The model of group treatment recommended by Toglia & Golisz (1990) is based upon the occupational therapy group theories that were described as early as the 1960s and are also discussed in other chapters in this text. Toglia cites Mosey (1986), Fidler (1969), and Howe and Schwartzberg (1986). The emphasis is on the **process** of the group, not the end product. Examples of the outcome of the process include the following:

- Clients learn from planning and carrying out group tasks and activities.

- Clients manage the requirements for paying attention to and being aware of others' needs.

- Clients learn to respond to unexpected changes, as well as the amount and type of stimuli and distractions that are often quite different in a group activity from those in a solo task.

- Clients have an opportunity to practice and learn about themselves in a group. This is useful information they can use for other social and nonclinical task-group settings.

Group Levels

Toglia identifies three group levels that are graded in much the same way tasks are graded (Toglia & Golisz, 1990, p. 10). The goals for the group at each level are compatible with the participants' ability for cognitive processing. Groups vary according to the complexity of the groups' task, the number of group participants, and the duration of the group. Toglia has integrated recommendations suggested by Adamovich et al. (1985) in her own groups (see Three Group Levels).

Components of Group Structure

Although the number of participants, goals, and length of the group vary, there is a consistent structured format for the three group levels (Toglia & Golisz, 1990). This format reflects that of Howe and Schwartzberg (1986) and has four phases:

1. An introduction of members and a review of previous group meeting (if there is a sequence of group experiences).
2. Identification of the purpose and goals of the group session.
3. A minimum of 20 minutes of active participation in a group task.
4. A discussion of the task experience, goal achievement, and the learning process that occurred.

Variations of Group Structure to Meet Client Needs

The therapist uses his or her clinical reasoning to accommodate specific needs and abilities of group participants and to maintain the client-centeredness of the group experience. An important piece of this reasoning relates to knowing what degree of guidance and structure to provide participants. Thus, no group looks just like any other. Toglia and Golisz (1990, pp. 11-16) discuss guides that can contribute to the therapist's reasoning. Some of these guides are highlighted next.

Opening the Group

To open a lower-level group and help members review what was done previously, the therapist might use a round-robin format in which each participant states his or her name. The therapist asks the clients to relate their names to visual or historical information in order to help group members remember and recall each other's names. In higher-level functioning groups, the therapist might ask each group member to remember an event from a previous group and share his or her perception of the experience.

THREE GROUP LEVELS

Level I—Stimulation Group

A 20-minute group of two to three patients that uses tasks to provide stimulation. Participants may vary in terms of their level of alertness and orientation; they all have severe impairment of attention and recall. Goals for the participants include:
- Increase attention span
- Increase participant awareness of the environment
- Improve orientation
- Decrease mental confusion

Level II—Low-Level Cognitive Group

A 30- to 45-minute group of three patients per staff participant, this group uses tasks, games, and role-play to improve cognitive performance. The goals of the group are:
- Improve attention to the activity
- Contribute to the organization of the experience
- Increase processing of external/environmental stimuli

In the group, clients can increase attention span, practice social skills, and practice individual and group problem solving with assistance.

Level III—High-Level Cognitive Group

The group, which is typically carried out in an outpatient setting, meets for 1 hour or longer. The participants have adequate attention for simple tasks and are ready to improve cognitive performance during complex tasks. Client performance is often impaired by stress and decision-making requirements. The goals of the group are:
- Increase effective and timely decision making
- Increase organized performance and use of strategies during the task and group process
- Improve flexibility for adapting to and interacting in community contexts

Four clients to one practitioner is the recommended group size (Toglia & Golisz, 1990).

Goal Setting

During the goal-setting phase, the therapist may independently or jointly with clients identify the group's goals. Toglia's group goals are of three types:

1. Goals related to group content. For example, in a low performance-level group use activities or games that increase the clients' orientation to time, place, person, etc. In a higher-level group increase the clients' awareness of their rights by orienting the participants to the Americans with a Disability Act, which guides employment with a disability.

2. Process goals that identify social learning. Clients are asked to demonstrate and initiate communication and problem solving or make choices during tasks. They can contribute alternative problem-solving solutions and assume varied roles that contribute to group outcomes.

3. Individual client goals for increasing function in daily life. For example, individual clients may have goals for recall of information from previous groups or may want to assume a leader role in a group, practice giving feedback to other members, or demonstrate their ability to work with a team.

Group Experience and Feedback

During the group's shared task, the therapist observes client participation and analyzes the task and its relationship to the participants' cognitive performance. The therapist uses this analysis to give feedback to participants or facilitate peer feedback, depending on the level of the group. Feedback is more frequently given at the end of higher-level groups, as a "wrap-up." In lower-functioning groups, feedback is given throughout the group's activity in order to help clients become more aware of their performance immediately following a task. Feedback may focus on the relationship between the person–task–environment and how these variables relate and support the person's cognitive performance. They may reinforce the person's choice of strategy and confirm its effectiveness in the group. **Feedback** may focus on the task modifications that are needed to improve a person's performance.

Discussion and Assessment of the Session

In the group's final phase, discussion and assessment of the group session, the therapist helps clients connect the task experience to the goals of the group in order that clients can assess their own learning. The discussion also connects the current experience and the skills learned or used during the group to other contexts. This is done in order to increase the participants' awareness of strategies that they can use in the future. Again, the therapist's feedback and the time devoted to the group summary varies depending on the level of the group.

For example, the lower functioning group summary takes about 5 minutes. The therapist thanks the members for participating and may briefly reiterate the group's purpose. The clinician then gives direct, supportive feedback to participants. The higher-level group summary takes about 15 minutes. During this time, the therapist thanks the participants and then gives the clients time for reflection about the experience. Clients are asked to share their reflections and give feedback to each other. As needed, the therapist helps the group members process the experience by posing questions and providing examples from the groups' process.

Feedback

Citing Kelly (1982), Toglia recommends that the therapist, when working with clients who have cognitive impairment, use direct supportive feedback. **Direct feedback** identifies the patient's or client's behavior and its effectiveness within the group context. Clients learn what they did well and how they can use these skills in the future. If behavior is ineffective, the therapist can suggest alternative responses, which can then be discussed or practiced in future groups. As noted previously, this is the preferred type of feedback for clients in a lower-functioning group. In addition to giving verbal feedback, some therapists videotape the client's performance and review the tape with one or more patients or clients as a means of feedback. Direct verbal feedback and videotapes help the client hear and see what he or she contributes to the task, how he or she works with others, how he or she communicates with others, etc.

Indirect feedback, the use of open-ended questions, is usually not effective with clients who have a head injury, especially those with a recent injury or with chronic mental disorders. Open-ended questions require group participants to monitor their behavior, reflect on their actions, and deduce the relationships among the participants' strategies, their task performance, and its effectiveness within the specific situation. Indirect feedback can be used in higher-level groups and when clients have acclimated to the group experience; however, the therapist must actively facilitate the process and use questions that help clients identify the strategies they used during the group and how these might be used in future situations (Toglia & Golisz, 1990, p. 14). For example, the clinician may ask, "What memory strategies did you use in the group today? When might you use these in the future? Summarize what you contributed to the group today? What was difficult for you in the group today? What would you like to say to the other members of the group about their participation in today's group?"

Activities, Games, and Role Play in Groups

Prior to the group, the therapist plans activities designed to meet the group participants' level of cognitive function. During the group, and based upon the group members' participation, the therapist continues to grade and re-structure activities as needed to help clients interact and learn from each other as well as learn about their skills in a group. To increase member participation in the group, a simple task may be more effective than one that requires use of all performance components. Because participants have limited ability for cognitive processing, they may have difficulty managing a task that demands physical, cognitive, and psychosocial skills. Too great a task challenge is believed to compromise the participant's ability to use his or her group task and communication skills; therefore, the therapist gradually increases task demands in accordance with the patient's or client's increasing cognitive skills (Abreu & Toglia, 1987; Toglia & Golisz, 1990). Toglia suggests that the gradual change in task demands and expectations for group participation are similar to the developmental group structure and expectations described by Mosey (1973). See Appendix N for descriptions of these groups. Toglia's view of there being a parallel between the cognitive groups for clients with brain injury and the continuum of developmental groups is shared by Lundgren and Persechino (1986). These developmental groups also have a history of influencing the groups used in psychosocial interventions.

In addition to tasks and activities, Toglia and Golisz (1990) recommend the use of games in groups with persons having cognitive impairments. Games provide opportunities for participants to learn group task and social skills. They can also challenge the client's cognitive skills. Clients can practice initiation, planning, self-monitoring, and multiple types of attention and problem solving. Participants also have the opportunity to practice roles and learn rules. The reader is referred to Table 9-7 for a summary of elements to consider when analyzing the cognitive demands of a game. This analysis in turn provides a guide for simplifying games.

Considerations for a Group Program for Generalization

When a cognitive rehabilitation program uses groups, the setting must accommodate to the differing needs of clients with low to high level of cognitive functions. Across the continuum, the goal in using activities—whether work, activities of daily living, or games—is to promote the generalization of learning. **Lower-functioning groups** often incorporate a specific focus that structures the weekly routine for clients. Monday might be a cooking group; Tuesday is a group outing; Wednesday group may offer a shared game, and so forth.

The **higher-level functioning groups** are often structured as a series of learning modules. The series of modules fit together to build knowledge and cognitive skills that will help the person re-engage in daily life through work, leisure, and daily occupations (Toglia & Golisz, 1990). For example, in a work readiness group, clients may complete a resume in one session, fill out a job application in another, role play an interview, etc.

Assessment of Group Behaviors

Toglia has created a behavior rating scale that identifies specific behaviors related to two major categories for assessment of group function: assessment of the client's social behavior and assessment of task behaviors. The Behavioral Rating Scale for Group Assessment was adapted by Toglia from the COTE Scale (Brayman, Kirby, Misenheimer, & Short, 1976), the Occupational Therapy Functional Evaluation (Tiffany, 1978), and the Social Interaction Scale of the Bay Area Functional Performance Evaluation (Hemphill, 1982; Klyczek, 1999). The group assessment scale uses a 0 to 4 performance rating scale that is clearly defined for the rater. The form and rating scale can be repro-

duced from the original source (Toglia & Golisz, 1990). Assessment continuums for social behavior and task behavior are highlighted in Group Behavior Rating Scale Continuum on page 295. An assessment form example is in Appendix O.

Summary

The dynamic interactional model provides a foundation for intervention with persons having cognitive dysfunction. Although originally intended for adults with brain injury, principles from this model have been applied with persons having mental illness (Josman, 1998a). The model incorporates what has been learned within information processing and behavioral and cognitive theories and offers an alternative to those cognitive models, which Toglia describes as emphasizing cognitive components and as deficit specific. It focuses instead on the information processing of the person in multiple situations. Dynamic interactional assessment seeks to identify the individual's potential to change and those adaptations or conditions that would enable successful performance in multiple contexts and environments. Treatment emphasizes increasing the client's awareness of his or her own cognitive capacity. It uses strategy training, practice of cognitive strategies in multiple situations to facilitate generalization of knowledge and skills, and ultimately the transfer of learning. It gives guides for task and environment modifications.

CONTRIBUTIONS AND LIMITATIONS OF THE DYNAMIC INTERACTIONAL APPROACH

Contributions

Therapist, researcher, and author Toglia has developed her model through more than a decade of work and study and has contributed to our understanding of the variables that impact cognitive processing and how cognitive processing is evident in occupational performance. Her model represents groundbreaking work in the application of cognitive and behavioral principles as well as task analysis in treatment of the adult with a brain injury and as this specifically applies to occupational therapy.

Describes the Dynamic Nature of Cognition

There is an inherent logic or sensibility in what Toglia proposes: that it is artificial to think of cognitive processing in terms of discrete functions that can be separated; further, that it is through meaningful activity that one can hope to rebuild or enhance cognitive processing. One sees in her descriptive case studies evidence in support of her theories and the dynamic nature of cognition. We also begin to see the roles for metacognitive and cognitive processing strategies during treatment.

Table 9-7
GAME ACTIVITY ANALYSIS AND MODIFICATION

Visual Processing Elements

- Change the game space. You can simplify or eliminate the game board. You can use the environment rather than just the game board. For example, the tabletop space can be painted with a large checker board for playing checkers or chess. You may have seen these in some city parks.
- Change the size of playing pieces and adapt as needed to accommodate to visual impairments or fine motor limitations.
- Use of color rather than small or fine detail pieces increases distinction of the player's marker.

Spatial Features

- Adjust game elements and boundaries of game to accommodate cognitive needs. For example, large plastic soda bottles (empty) can be arranged on the floor in the form of bowling pins in a triangle. A large light-weight ball is used to knock them down.

Social Opportunities

- Use rules of the game to develop social skills.
- Use the structure of games for developing team roles and skills.
- Use role-play or partner experiences for practice of desired social skills.

Cognitive Variables

- Vary the client's rate of response for performing within time constraints. For example, you can shorten the length of the game to meet client ability.
- Build client attention by using the game process to focus attention. The length and type of game can be structured to use client abilities or develop new cognitive skills through the time required for the game, the use of rules, and process of the game (e.g., taking turns, monitoring whose turn it is, and paying attention to previous moves or actions by other players).
- Consider the complex and abstract nature of the game and if it is familiar to client. Game questions and performance expectations can be simple or complex; adjust them as needed.

Movement

- Vary the amount of stress on cognitive processing through the gross and fine movements required to participate in the game. Vary also the process of the game to change the expected or spontaneous movement required.

Adapted from Toglia, J. P., & Golisz, K. (1990). *Cognitive rehabilitation: Group games and activities* (p. 20). Tucson, AZ: Therapy Skill Builders. (*Note*: The authors of this text contributed the examples.)

Alternative to Deficit-Specific Models

This model offers an alternative to the prevailing deficit-specific approaches that have been used not only in occupational therapy but overall in cognitive rehabilitation. It is holistic insofar as it is concerned with knowing "Who is this person with a brain injury, and what does he or she bring to the therapeutic experience?" as well as paying judicious attention to those attributes of the task and setting that either enhance or impede successful cognitive processing and function. Rather than promoting mere repetition of a partic-

ular task or task-component and approaching all patients with something of a cookie-cutter approach, the therapist in this model adapts tasks and uses cues and learning strategies to best meet each client's unique characteristics.

In this regard, principles in the dynamic interactional approach are consistent with those of client-centered intervention. In teaching clients new strategies that they can use in multiple settings, the model strives to give the individual tools to function more normally and independently within a broader life sphere. Although Toglia doesn't speak as directly

GROUP BEHAVIOR RATING SCALE CONTINUUM

Social and task behaviors have a continuum with multiple points of performance. The following represent the two ends of the continuum or performance boundaries for function and dysfunction. The reader is referred to the original source for scaling and format of client performance documentation. See Appendix O for completed sample ratings.

General Social Behavior

- Attendance: Voluntary participation in group to refusal to attend.

- Initiation: Actively involved in group experience to no initiative and passive participation.

- Affect: Effective response to group context to not in control of one's emotions during the group.

- Social interaction: Effective in multiple group roles to unable to respond when approached to contributes during group.

- Team behavior: Helps and encourages others to participate in the group experience to being self-centered during the group.

- Response to feedback: Aware of errors and uses constructive feedback given regarding group participation to unaware of errors and is angered by feedback or withdraws from the group experience.

- Communication: Organizes and expresses thoughts related to group situation to tangential and incomplete thoughts about the current group focus.

Task Behavior

- Track task events: Effectively monitors task process to being too detailed and inability to monitor essential aspects of the task.

- Goal orientation: Attends to task goal in structured or unstructured context to not interested in the task.

- Modulates speed of response: Timely/efficient response to task demands to slow or impulsive response that interferes with task process.

- Frustration tolerance: Manages tasks and demands independently to unable to participate in group tasks even with adaptations and staff support.

- Decision making: Can make independent or support group decision as needed to achieve goal to unable to make decision and expects others to do so.

- Memory (names, activity, rules, monitor process, etc.): Spontaneous recall of information needed to participate in group task to requires verbal cues to retrieve information or unable to participate.

- Orientation (self, place, time, etc.): Intact awareness and orientation to unable to provide information.

Adapted from Toglia, J. P., & Golisz, K. (1990). *Cognitive rehabilitation: Group games and activities* (pp. 59-60). Tucson, AZ: Therapy Skill Builders.

---

to this issue as do the proponents of the cognitive behavioral model, her approach would also be expected to enhance feelings of control and efficacy in the adult with a brain injury.

A Continuum for Transfer of Learning

Toglia does not minimize the many problems posed by brain injury, and she writes that this approach might not be for everyone. Not all people with a brain injury are capable of the learning that this model tries to promote. As she says, the "level of severity, stage of recovery, and type of cognitive dysfunction" will all influence what will prove to be the most effective approach (Toglia, 1992, p. 138; 1998, p. 46). One cannot minimize the complexity of what Toglia is proposing that we do. The advantage of reductionistic approaches, while also their drawback, is that they break cognition into manageable pieces. When we do what Toglia suggests and try to look at how all the pieces come together, our job would appear to be much more complicated or at least difficult to manage. There are so many variables to consider within even the seemingly simplest task that it is no wonder Toglia states that the demand is high for clinical reasoning. That is not necessarily a limitation of the model but does speak to the complexity of what it encompasses. It will be a challenge to

compare the results of so-called deficit specific approaches with that of dynamic interactional model considering the multiple variables that need to be controlled. Toglia herself uses compensatory strategies with her patients within the umbrella of this model, so one might look at this model as on a continuum with those models in which minimal transfer of knowledge is expected.

Occupation is Central

Occupation is of central importance in this model as both a vehicle for assessment and for new learning, and Toglia speaks especially to the importance of functional performance in context. One could suppose, therefore, that the patient or client would find it easier to recognize the relevance of what they are being asked to do in therapy, even where disorientation and confusion are common sequela to brain injury.

Limitations

Awareness training and self-monitoring are cornerstones for intervention in this model. But, as Toglia states, self-monitoring and the efficacy of teaching self-monitoring strategies to adults with a brain injury has been minimally studied. It is difficult, therefore, to point to hard evidence that says strategy training will in fact improve an individual's performance in multiple environments; however, there are some case studies (Cicerone & Giacino, 1992; Deelman, Berg, & Koning-Haanstra, 1990; Nelson & Lenharat, 1996; Soderback, Bengtsson, Ginsburg, & Ekholm, 1992; Toglia, 1989a, 1989b; Von Cramon, Matthes-Von Cramon, & Mai, 1991) that suggest the benefits of strategy training and self-monitoring (Toglia, 1998, p. 44). This, however, is just a beginning.

There are no studies or writings by Toglia that support our hypothesis that this approach is more satisfying to clients. The conditions that promote transfer of learning have been studied in normal adults and children, and again there are a few case studies of clients with brain injuries. The important outcome of these studies is that "generalization is only achieved when it is built into the training program" (Toglia, 1998, p. 44). Toglia also cites Mateer, Sohlberg, and Youngman (1990) who "found that those studies reporting positive outcomes used a wider variety of training tasks…" (p. 45). In a Neistadt (1994) study, she also reports the benefits of a variety of tasks in order to achieve transfer.

Unanswered Questions

Toglia poses questions that remain to be answered: Can the adult with a brain injury be taught to use processing strategies efficiently? If so, which type of brain injury is most amenable, and what strategies might be expected to be easier or more difficult to learn and use (Toglia, 1992, p. 139; 1998)? Who is likely to profit the most? Can this model be effectively used with other populations, such as developmental disability? Since the model relies heavily on verbal mediation, can it be adapted for persons with language impairment? Given the individual nature of the approach, can populations of patients be compared to evaluate outcomes of the model (Toglia, 1998, p. 46)?

Limited Application in Mental Health

Toglia reminds us that the model has been minimally applied with persons having schizophrenia, and although the results have been promising, this too remains an area that needs considerable further study. Allen (1994) and Allen & Blue (1998) (Chapter Eight) say that to expect persons with debilitating chronic mental illnesses like schizophrenia to do more than minimal new learning is to expect more of them than they can produce. How then does the therapist determine which is the better approach? Given the constraints on treatment and the pressure to contain costs, this raises important practical concerns as well. How many tries at new learning would be considered a fair implementation of this approach? When does one conclude that new learning or transfer of learning is not possible for persons with chronic mental disorders or cognitive disorders?

Expertise of the Occupational Therapist

The therapist wanting to duplicate Toglia's approach has guidelines in what she has published thus far, but there is more to know. When the therapist's job is to be a "detective," we can expect that some will be better at this function than others. Further, task and activity analysis specific to cognitive parameters would appear to require expertise in the area of cognition. How the interested therapist might gain the skills necessary to carry out dynamic interactional treatment is not directly addressed, but one could envision, in part, therapist mentorship by those occupational therapists who have become experts in the application of Toglia's model.

In summary, Toglia has begun a complex challenge to develop a model that responds to the dynamic relationships among the person, task and occupations, and the environment. In this process she has contributed a dynamic form of assessment and a multicontextual approach to intervention. From her work we can see the evolution of theory, and she herself reminds us that the model is in its "initial stages of development" and needs to be "systematically tested and compared" (Toglia, 1998, p. 46). Like the other models in occupational therapy that focus on the person, environment, and occupation, the dynamic interactional model needs to be studied and tested. We look forward to this next stage of theory development and its process of discovery that will contribute to our literature and the efficacy of practice of occupational therapy.

REFERENCES

Abreu, G. C., & Toglia, J. P. (1987). Cognitive rehabilitation: A model for occupational therapy. *Am J Occup Ther, 41*, 439-448.

Adamovich, B., Henderson, J., & Averbach, S. (1985). *Rehabilitation of closed head-injury clients.* San Diego, CA: College Hill Press.

Allen, C. K. (1994). Creating a need-satisfying, safe environment: Management and maintenance approaches. In C. B. Royeen (Ed.), *AOTA self-study series: Cognitive rehabilitation.* Bethesda, MD: American Occupational Therapy Association.

Allen, C. K., & Blue, T. (1998). Cognitive disabilities model: How to make clinical judgments. In N. Katz (Ed.), *Cognition and occupation in rehabilitation* (pp. 225-280). Bethesda, MD: American Occupational Therapy Association.

Anderson, J. (1985). *Cognitive psychology and its implications.* New York, NY: Freeman.

Anderson, S. W., & Tranel, D. (1989). Awareness of disease states following cerebral infarction, dementia, and head trauma: Standardized assessment. *Clinical Neuropsychologist, 3*, 327-339.

Bransford, J. (1979). *Human cognition: Learning, understanding, and remembering.* Belmont, CA: Wadsworth.

Brayman, S., Kirby, T., Misenheimer, A., & Short, M. J. (1976). Comprehensive occupational therapy evaluation scale. *Am J Occup Ther, 30*, 94-104.

Brown, A., Bransford, J., Ferrara, R., & Campione, J. (1983). Learning, remembering, and understanding. In J. Flavell & E. Markman (Eds.), *Handbook of child psychology* (Vol. 3, pp. 77-158). New York, NY: Wiley.

Cicerone, K. D., & Giacino, T. J. (1992). Remediation of executive function deficits after traumatic brain injury. *Neurorehabilitation, 2,* 12-22.

Crosson, C., Barco, P. P., Velozo, C., Bolesta, M., Cooper, P. V., Werts, D., & Brobeck, T. C. (1989). Awareness and compensation in postacute head injury rehabilitation. *J Head Trauma Rehabil, 4,* 46-54.

Deelman, B. G., Berg, I. J., & Koning-Haanstra, M. (1990). Memory strategies for closed head-injured patients. Do lessons in cognitive psychology help? In R. Wood & I. Fussy (Eds.), *Cognitive rehabilitation in perspective.* London: Taylor Frances.

Feuerstein, R. (1979). *The dynamic assessment of retarded performers: The learning potential device, theory, instruments, and techniques.* Baltimore, MD: University Park Press.

Fidler, G. (1969). The task-oriented group as a context for treatment. *Am J Occup Ther, 23,* 148-153.

Fine, S. (1993). Interaction between psychological variables and cognitive function. In C. Royeen (Ed.), *AOTA self-study series: Cognitive rehabilitation.* Rockville, MD: American Occupational Therapy Association.

Flavell, J. H. (1985). *Cognitive development.* Englewood Cliffs, NJ: Prentice Hall.

Giles, G. M., & Clark-Wilson, J. (Eds.). (1999). *Rehabilitation of the severely brain-injured adult* (2nd ed.). Cheltenham, United Kingdom: Stanley Thornes (Publishers) Ltd.

Goldstein, A. (1973). *Structured learning therapy: Toward a psychotherapy for the poor.* New York, NY: Academic Press.

Hemphill, B. (1982). *The evaluative process in psychiatric occupational therapy.* Thorofare, NJ: SLACK Incorporated.

Howe, M., & Schwartzberg, S. (1986). *A functional approach to group work in occupational therapy.* Philadelphia, PA: J. B. Lippincott.

Josman, N. (1993). *Assessment of categorization skills in brain injured and schizophrenic persons: Validation of the Toglia Category Assessment (TCA).* Doctoral dissertation, New York University, NY.

Josman, N. (1998a). The dynamic interactional model in schizophrenia. In N. Katz (Ed.), *Cognition and occupation in rehabilitation.* Bethesda, MD: American Occupational Therapy Association.

Josman, N. (1998b). Reliability and validity of the Toglia Category Assessment Test. *Can J Occup Ther, 66,* 33-42.

Katz, N. (Ed.). (1998). *Cognition and occupation in rehabilitation.* Bethesda, MD: The American Occupational Therapy Association.

Kelly, M. (1982). *Social-skills training: A practical guide for interventions.* New York, NY: Springer Publishing Co.

Kline, N. F. (1997). *The Modified Dynamic Visual Processing Assessment (Modified DVPA): Its relationship to function.* Doctoral dissertation, New York University.

Klyczek, J. P. (1999). The Bay Area Functional Performance Evaluation. In B. Hemphill-Pearson (Ed.), *Assessments in occupational therapy mental health: An integrative approach* (pp. 87-108). Thorofare, NJ: SLACK Incorporated.

Lidz, C. S. (1987). Cognitive deficiencies revisited. In C. S. Lidz (Ed.), *Dynamic assessment.* New York, NY: Guilford Press.

Lundgren, C. C., & Persechino, E. L. (1986). Cognitive group: A treatment for head-injury adults. *Am J Occup Ther, 40,* 397-401.

Luria, A. R. (1980). *Higher cortical functions in man* (2nd ed., B. Haigh, Trans.). New York, NY: Basic Books.

Mateer, C., Sohlberg, M., & Youngman, P. (1990). The management of acquired attention and memory deficits. In R. Wood & I. Fussey (Eds.), *Cognitive rehabilitation in perspective.* London: Taylor & Francis.

Mosey, A. (1973). *Activities therapy.* New York, NY: Raven Press.

Mosey, A. (1986). *Psychosocial components of occupational therapy.* New York, NY: Raven Press.

Neistadt, M. E. (1994). Perceptual retraining for adults with diffuse brain injury. *Am J Occup Ther, 48,* 225-233.

Nelson, D. L., & Lenharat, D. A. (1996). Resumption of outpatient occupational therapy for a young woman five years after traumatic brain injury. *Am J Occup Ther, 50,* 223-228.

Nolen, S. B. (1988). Reasons for studying: Motivational orientations and study strategies. *Cognition and Instruction, 5,* 269-287.

Soderback, I., Bengtsson, I., Ginsburg, E., & Ekholm, J. (1992). Video feedback in occupational therapy: Its effect in patients with neglect syndromes. *Arch Phys Med Rehabil, 73,* 1140-1146.

Tiffany, E. G. (1978). Psychiatry and mental health. Section 4: Contexts or settings for treatment. In H. L. Hopkins & H. D. Smith (Eds.), *Willard and Spackman's occupational therapy* (5th ed., pp. 322-325). Philadelphia, PA: J. B. Lippincott.

Toglia, J. (1989). Approaches to cognitive assessment of the brain-injured adult: Traditional methods and dynamic investigation. *Occupational Therapy Practice, 1,* 36-57.

Toglia, J. (1991). Generalization of treatment: A multicontext approach to cognitive perceptual impairment in the brain injured adult. *Am J Occup Ther, 45*(6), 505-516.

Toglia, J. (1992). A dynamic interactional approach to cognitive rehabilitation. In N. Katz (Ed.), *Cognitive rehabilitation: Models for intervention in occupational therapy.* Boston, MA: Andover Medical Publishers.

Toglia, J. (1993a). Attention and memory. In C. Royeen (Ed.), *AOTA self-study series: Cognitive rehabilitation.* Rockville, MD: American Occupational Therapy Association.

Toglia, J. (1993b). *The Contextual Memory Test: Manual.* Tucson, AZ: Therapy Skill Builders.

Toglia, J. (1994). *Dynamic assessment of categorization skills: The Toglia Category Assessment.* Pequannock, NJ: Maddock.

Toglia, J. P. (1998). The dynamic interactional model to cognitive rehabilitation. In N. Katz (Ed.), *Cognition and occupation in rehabilitation.* Bethesda, MD: American Occupational Therapy Association.

Toglia, J., & Finkelstein, N. (1991). *Test protocol: The Dynamic Visual Processing Assessment.* New York, NY: New York Hospital-Cornell Medical Center.

Toglia, J. P., & Golisz, K. (1990). *Cognitive rehabilitation: Group games and activities.* Tucson, AZ: Therapy Skill Builders.

Toglia, J. P., & Josman, N. (1994). Preliminary reliability and validity studies of the TCA. In J. P. Toglia (Ed.), *Dynamic assessment of categorization: TCA—The Toglia Category Assessment.* Pequannock, NJ: Maddock.

Trexler, L. (1987). Neuropsychological rehabilitation in the United States. In M. Meier, A. Benton, & L. Diller (Eds.), *Neuropsychological rehabilitation* (pp. 437-460). New York, NY: Guilford Press.

Von Cramon, D. Y., Matthes-Von Cramon, G., & Mai, N. (1991). Problem-solving deficits in brain injured patients: A therapeutic approach. *Neuropsychological Rehabilitation, 1,* 45-64.

Vygotsky, L. S. (1978). *Mind in society: The development of higher psychological processes.* Cambridge, MA: Harvard University Press.

CHAPTER TEN

Sensory Motor Model— Physiological Basis for Improved Function

KEY POINTS

✧ History and Current Theory
- Ayers and Sensory Integration
- King and Intervention for Adults with Schizophrenia
- Ross and Burdick Expand to Movement Activities

✧ Theory in Context of Occupational Therapy Practice
- Adaptation and the Developmental Process
- Characteristics of Sensory-Motor Dysfunction
- Occupational Therapist—Active Group Participant
- Sensory Input Controls the Environment to Support Performance
- Activity Gives Sensory Input, Elicits an Adaptive Response, and Normalizes Movement
- Activity Facilitates Socialization and Cognitive Skill Building

✧ Theoretical Assumptions Guide Evaluation and Intervention
- Evaluation
  —Assessment of Sensory, Motor, Cognitive, and Psychosocial Performance
- Intervention
  —Functional Goals For an Adaptive Response Through Sensory-Motor Activity
  —Control and Monitor the Environment
  —Group Interventions: The Five-Stage Group
  —Ready Approach For Clients with Developmental Disability

✧ Contributions and Limitations of Sensory-Motor Approaches

FOCUS QUESTIONS

1. What characterizes the special population for whom this framework is intended?

2. How are central nervous system (CNS) impairments in processing sensation believed to impact the ability for motor performance? For functional performance?

3. What is meant by the phrase "central nervous system plasticity," and why is the assumption of plasticity important to this framework?

4. How is adaptation defined in this frame of reference, and what is an adaptive response?

5. What sensory systems are viewed as particularly critical and most often dysfunctional in the population described?

6. By what criteria are activities chosen?

7. What is the therapist's role? How is this similar to and different from the role as described in other frameworks?

8. Describe how a therapist might control sensory input.

9. How do King's treatment goals differ from those of Ross?

10. What does the term "ready" refer to in the Ready Approach?

11. What do King, Ross, and the Ready Approach have in common?

12. How are these sensory-motor approaches believed to improve functional performance?

HISTORICAL UPDATE

In the first edition of this text, sensory-integrative therapy was identified as a special instance of developmentally based treatment: one that emphasizes sensory input, movement, and non-cortical activity. At that time, occupational therapists Lorna Jean King (1974a, 1974b, 1978) and Mildred Ross (Ross & Burdick, 1981) were cited as proponents of sensory integrative methods to be used with an adult psychiatric population. Subsequently, several important changes in emphasis in the area of adult sensory integrative treatment led us to devote a separate chapter to this area of study and to describe it somewhat differently than was done in 1987 (Bruce & Borg, 1993). In part to differentiate this frame of reference from sensory-integration used in pediatric care and also because some have found the term "sensory integration" to be a misleading descriptor for what is achieved in treatment, we chose the descriptor "movement-centered frame of reference" to suggest that Ross and King were proposing a model that would mobilize clients.

In this third revision of the text, we find a model of practice that has continued to evolve in its emphasis. In hindsight

and looking at the use of the model with persons having schizophrenia, an important contribution appears to have been that work in this sensory-integrative or movement area has reminded occupational therapists to pay attention to physical features (e.g., sensory, motor, neurophysiological) of the environments and tasks in which their clients are engaged. Therapists recognize, for example, that persons with schizophrenia, persons regressed or depressed, or persons having developmental disabilities may need a period of initial sensory alerting or calming in order to pay attention to a therapeutic activity.

Ultimately, this idea of a movement-centered framework has become one of diverse applications in which the shift appears to be toward emphasis on sensory input along with movement. For this reason, and looking at this framework as having many applications in practice we refer to these here collectively as **sensorimotor models**. Note these models differ from the models that are predominately used in physical medicine, which may be termed "neuromotor," "motor learning," or "sensorimotor."

Sensory integration with children is a specialty rich in its literature, and not primarily what is being addressed here. Nevertheless, there is considerable sharing of principles with sensory integration, and the interested reader may wish to pursue the citations in the chapter. In this chapter we look primarily at the use of sensory and motor principles with an adult population, with some reference given to work with children. By adult, we refer to persons in their teenage years and beyond.

As we turn to these models, we see that they are developmental in their basic premise, holistic, and at home with many principles of neurophysiology. Collectively, they represent an avenue for therapeutic intervention that has shown promise for working with clients with chronic, often severe behavior problems and whose ability to engage in meaningful, functional activity has been significantly impaired.

DEFINITION

The sensorimotor models described in this chapter are directed toward an adolescent or adult population identified as having CNS dysfunction, typically having behavior and performance problems, and often having psychiatric diagnoses. This population is believed to have problems with processing sensation into normal, fluid movement, which in turn relates to impoverished body image, confidence, and task and social behavior. Therapeutic occupation is selected according to its neurophysiological properties and its ability to enhance the opportunity for an integrated, organized response. Sensory-motor applications represent a restorative approach in which it is expected that something in the **person** will change as a consequence of therapeutic intervention.

THEORETICAL DEVELOPMENT

Occupational therapists practicing in the area of physical dysfunction have long been concerned with motor performance and the contributory roles of sensation, muscle and joint action, and, of course, nerve activity. Approaches developed by Rood and described by Stockmeyer (1967, 1972); work by Ayres (1969, 1972a, 1972b, 1972c, 1973, 1975, 1977, 1978, 1979, 1980, 1989), Ayres & Heskett (1972), Bobath (1975, 1978, 1980), Brunnstrom (1961, 1970), Knott and Voss (1968), Voss (1972), and Voss, Ionta, and Myers (1985), and more recently such sensory-motor techniques as myofascial release (Barnes, 1990a, 1990b; Travell, 1983), therapeutic touch (McCormack, 1991; McCormack & Galantino, 1997), and the Feldenkrais method (Jackson-Wyatt, 1997) have been used by occupational therapists to prepare the person for participation in functional activity. The principles applied in these neurophysiological approaches used in physical medicine, however, had little impact on mental health care until the early 1970s. Although earlier occupational therapists may have recognized that when psychiatric patients engaged in hard physical labor and exercise their symptoms often improved, why and how this came about was not clear.

Ayres and Children with Learning Disabilities

The work of psychologist and occupational therapist Dr. A. Jean Ayres appears to have been a key impetus in bringing motor and sensory skills to the attention of therapists working in psychiatry.

Sensory Integration

Sensory integration refers to the ability of the CNS to take in sensation from multiple sources at the same time, to filter and organize this sensory information in order to discern its meaning, and then to use this information to generate an adaptive response. Addressing what she referred to as the problem of poor sensory integration in children with a learning disability, Ayres proposed that many children have difficulty moving, learning, and behaving normally because their CNS cannot adequately organize sensation (Ayres, 1972b, 1973). Describing a developmental scheme, Ayres wrote that higher cortical organization such as that used for conscious reasoning depends on sensory organization at lower levels. She illustrated how input from the vestibular system (i.e., inner ear), muscles and joints, and simple touch played especially significant roles in literally grounding the person and giving him or her the necessary information needed to orient the self to the environment and prepare for an adaptive response. The vestibular system, she wrote, is the "...unifying system. It forms the basic relationship of a person to gravity and the physical world. All other sensations are processed in reference to this vestibular information" (Ayres, 1979).

Adaptive Response

First, says Ayres, the brain organizes incoming sensory information. As part of this process, the brain **inhibits** (stops or slows) or **facilitates** (increases or enhances) the flow of messages across nerve junctions or synapses. This self-adjusting process, called **modulation**, may be faulty in some individuals who exhibit sensory integration problems. Having sorted out information, the brain can respond adaptively. One characteristic of an adaptive response is that it is in itself organizing (i.e., it helps the brain organize sensation and movement and in so doing leads to a more complex state or organization). The repeated use of nerve pathways, including their synapses, in a specific sensorimotor function creates a kind of neural memory or map of that function. The brain can then recreate that movement easily in subsequent attempts (Ayres, 1979).

Development

Ayres describes the first 7 years of life as primarily devoted to organizing sensations. Neural connections continue to be established until around 10 years of age. New connections can be established at later ages, but the process becomes much more difficult. The child who cannot adequately take in or organize sensory information fails to build nerve pathways that permit free and confident movement (Ayres, 1972b, 1973, 1979).

Assessment

Ayres studied children of many ages but worked primarily with 4- to 8-year-olds. She designed and eventually standardized assessments to identify the extent and nature of sensory integrative dysfunction. What began as individual tests in the 1960s were later combined and published as the Southern California Sensory Integration Tests (SCSIT) (Ayres, 1972c, 1980) and the Southern California Postrotary Nystagmus Test (SCPNT) (Ayres, 1975; Mailloux, 1990). Since the publication of the SCSIT in 1972, this assessment has been refined and is currently available as the Sensory Integration and Praxis Test (SIPT) (Ayres, 1989).

Therapeutic Intervention

Therapy based on the sensory-integrative model strives to improve the ability for integrating sensory information and therefore remediating the sensory-integrative problem.

Ayres believed that because a child's CNS undergoes much development through age 10, sensory integrative skills not developed at the earlier or typical developmental period might still be developed during childhood given appropriate therapeutic intervention (Ayres, 1979). The goal of sensory integrative therapy is to provide controlled sensory input in a manner that the child can effectively integrate, thereby enabling the development of an adaptive response (Ayres, 1979). An **adaptive response** is one that is developmentally on-target and meaningful to the child. If the child is older, therapy may help him or her "learn how to facilitate certain messages and inhibit others, to direct information to the proper places in his or her brain and body, and to put all the messages together into useful perceptions and behaviors" (Ayres, 1979).

The goal of sensory integrative intervention is an improvement in CNS processing, specifically the production of an adaptive response and not toward isolated skill development. Therapeutic occupation is often playful and occurs within an environment in which the therapist can modulate the type and intensity of sensory input. This is especially vital because children with sensory-integrative processing problems may have strong physiological reactions when they cannot regulate incoming sensation.

Typically, the therapy setting has ample space; large floor mats; scooter boards; blocks; large therapy balls; an overhead suspension system for trapezes, swings, and inner tubes; and an assortment of toys—all of which allow for safe exploration and physical play by the child.

Sensory integrative intervention may also include specific techniques to supply sensory input (e.g., compression to the joints or pressure brushing or physical positioning of the child to enhance proprioceptive, vestibular, or other input, and to enhance adaptive motor responses). The therapist engaged in sensory integrative intervention is exhorted to play with the child and have fun—something that we shall see is reflected in sensorimotor work with adults. The reader is referred to Fisher, Murray, and Bundy (1991), Bundy (1997), and Wilbarger and Wilbarger (1991) for definitive work in this area.

Although Ayres devoted the bulk of her study to children with learning disabilities, she observed:

> It always comes as a surprise to me when the theory of sensory integrative dysfunction... is identified primarily with learning disorders. Most of the concepts derive from basic research on the vertebrate brain, a science that knows virtually nothing of educational handicaps... (As cited by King, 1988, p. 3.54, but not otherwise documented for source)

When a child has sensory-integration impairments, his or her ability to interact socially, to perform academically, and/or to play may be impaired and often results in behavior problems and/or erosion of the child's self-esteem. Simply stated, he or she cannot successfully do what age-mates are doing easily. The therapist, therefore, may determine that the child with an identified psychosocial problem (e.g., acting out behavior, depression, or withdrawal) would profit from sensory-integrative intervention. This is the same principle that has been applied to adults.

King and Adult Schizophrenia

Occupational therapist Lorna Jean King, like Ayres, viewed sensory integration as the ability of the human organism to perceive, process, and use sensory data in a way that permits fluid, purposeful movement. The integrative process depends on the constant interaction of all systems within the organism and is thought to be governed by the CNS, especially the noncortical or subcortical portions of the CNS—those housed in the cerebellum and brain stem. You can easily illustrate subcortical movement to yourself. Think for a moment of arising from a chair to get your favorite snack. You are (most likely) able to do this without having to think about how to get up, nor do you experience a loss of balance. Perhaps you daydreamed about an earlier phone call or what to have for dinner. Because you did not have to concentrate on the process of moving or keeping your balance, one could say that your actions were accomplished subcortically. For adequate subcortical regulation to occur, the necessary input must occur from all of the senses, plus proper arousal (i.e., the person cannot be overstimulated or understimulated).

Characteristics of Chronic Schizophrenia

L. J. King treated psychiatric patients with chronic disability; many had a diagnosis of schizophrenia (see Schizophrenia). King observed that in addition to experiencing sensory distortions (e.g., loss of visual form and size constancy) many of these individuals exhibited physical characteristics similar to those described by Ayres. These included poor muscle tone, a dislike of movement, and a lack of response to vestibular input. Generally, this pattern included the following:

- Limited mobility of the head
- "S" curvature of the spine (lordosis)
- Shuffling gait
- Tendency to hold arms and legs in a flexed, adducted, and internally rotated position
- Dominance confusion
- Atrophy of the thenar eminence and weak grip strength
- Poor balance

SCHIZOPHRENIA

King (1974a) uses the categories discussed by Sullivan (1947) regarding schizophrenia. **Process schizophrenia** was the term he used to describe the development of schizophrenia early in childhood, necessitating treatment. This he contrasted with **reactive schizophrenia**, which suggests that the individual functioned at least marginally well until a breakdown occurred during a period of recognizable stress. This classification of process versus reactive schizophrenia is not used in the current nomenclature, and it can be noted that by definition in the *Diagnostic and Statistical Manual of Mental Disorders* (DSM-IV-TR), the label schizophrenia implies some degree of chronicity.

- Lessened responsiveness to vestibular stimulation (e.g., lack of nystagmus with spinning) (King, 1974a, 1974b)

Underactive Vestibular System

King postulated that persons with chronic schizophrenia, like learning-disabled children, are unable to move fluidly because they have an ineffective proprioceptive feedback mechanism, the most important component of which is an underactive or under-reactive vestibular regulating system (King, 1974a) (i.e., the person with chronic schizophrenia cannot, at a subcortical level, effectively use sensory information regarding his or her own position in space). This inability leads to restrictive, protective movement. By limiting movement, the individual tends to exacerbate the problem by decreasing vestibular and proprioceptive input. Having to think about moving slows the person, and movement loses its fluidity. This tends to interfere with the individual's ability to engage in normal physical activity, ultimately lessens his or her comfort in social situations, and increases withdrawal.

Decreased Sense of Pleasure

In what may be a related characteristic, many persons with chronic schizophrenia have difficulty experiencing events as pleasurable: a symptom referred to as **anhedonia**. King wanted to reverse what she described as a downward spiral of decreased movement and decreased social involvement. Citing Ayres' work and describing her approach as "sensory integration" (King, 1974a), she introduced activities that would increase proprioceptive and especially vestibular sensory input and encourage movement regulated subcortically. Interestingly, King observed that patients with anhedonia seemed to enjoy vestibular input. Once her patients began to enjoy moving, motivation became less of a problem, and patients' interaction with each other became more spontaneous.

Noncortical Activities

Therapeutic activities, said King (1974a), were to be first and foremost noncortical and pleasurable. This is contrasted, for example, with exercise and dance routines in which the participant's attention is brought to his or her own movement patterns. Activities were also chosen for their ability to normalize movement patterns, strengthen upper trunk stability, and increase flexibility. It was believed that these motor changes would improve body image and self-confidence, improve attentional and social response, and lay the necessary foundation for building skills related to cognition and daily tasks.

Intervention with the Adult Population

Following King's 1974 publications, interest grew in sensory integration treatment for an adult population. Studies were developed to better demonstrate physical characteristics specific to process or chronic schizophrenia (Blakeney, Strickland, & Wilkinson, 1983; Endler & Eiman, 1978; Huddleston, 1978; Levy, Holzman, & Proctor, 1978; Lindquist, 1981). A link between sensory integration treatment and patient improvement was studied in relation to changes in verbalization (Bailey, 1978), ward behavior (Reisman & Blakeney, 1993; Rider, 1978), physical changes (King, 1977; Reisman & Blakeney, 1993; Rider, 1978), and changes in body image (Crist, 1979; Levine, O'Connor, & Stacey, 1977; Rider, 1978). One problem that became evident in these early studies was that there were no standardized assessments to evaluate sensory integration in adults; therefore, researchers used tests such as the SCSIT to evaluate adult function (Falk-Kessler, Quittman, & Moore, 1988). Another problem was that the group studies used to evaluate the effectiveness of sensory-integrative principles with adults had small samples and lacked control groups (Hixson & Mathews, 1984; Reisman & Blakeney, 1993). This idea of a "sensory integrative" model for adults was criticized because it applied an approach that had been developed with and for children with learning disabilities. Further, it did so with persons in whom sensory integrative processing problems had not been clearly identified (Fisher et al., 1991).

In the midst of this criticism, King responded. She first emphasized that evidence increasingly pointed to the origin of psychiatric disorder as being primarily neurological, not social. She reviewed the studies that had been done to verify the findings described in her earlier publication and found them inconclusive. She suggested, however, that as the profession of occupational therapy became better at research, the efficacy of sensory integration techniques would be more evident (King, 1983, pp. 3.52-3.59). Work has been done to standardize portions or adaptations of the SCSIT for use with adults (Falk-Kessler et al., 1988; Hsu & Nelson, 1981; Jongbloed, Collins, & Jones, 1986; Petersen, Goar, & Van Deusen, 1985; Petersen & Wikoff, 1983). Perhaps King's pivotal point was that persons with chronic schizophrenia traditionally have shown limited improvement, even with advances in medications; therefore, anything that could bring about improved function would be worth exploring.

Ross, Burdick, and Expansion Beyond Sensory Integration

In 1981, Mildred Ross, an occupational therapist, and Dona Burdick, a recreation therapist, collaborated to write *Sensory Integration: A Training Manual for Therapists and Teachers for Regressed, Psychiatric, and Geriatric Patient Groups* (1981). They saw in their long-term and regressed patients some postures and movement patterns similar, but not necessarily identical, to those identified with chronic schizophrenia, as well as similar problems with motivation, short attention span, and disorganized behavior.

Movement Activities

Believing that these patients, too, had sensory integration deficits, Ross and Burdick articulated an approach that could be used in therapeutic groups. Activities that would involve full body movement for a total body adaptive response were selected (Ross & Burdick, 1981). As with King's approach, activities were chosen for their neurophysiological properties, and many either gave strong sensory input (especially vestibular or proprioceptive) or required participants to physically move.

In addition, these therapists envisioned a developmental sequence within the therapy group. The first stages of the group were designed to alert and evoke interest, provide sensory input, and demand a motor response. These activities were judged to be organizing and believed to pave the way for activity more cognitive in nature. Later, group stages were designed to elicit a response that involved verbalization, reflection, or reasoning.

Ross' More Recent Contributions

In 1991, 1997, and 1998, Ross enhanced what was presented in the Ross and Burdick publication (1981). Her subsequent work (1991, 1997; Ross & Bachner, 1998) reflects a modified content. Ross identifies the sensory integrative theories of Ayres and King as only an incomplete part of the rationale for what she refers to as "motor rehabilitation" (Ross, 1991, p. 47). The work of Dr. Karol Bobath and physiotherapist Berta Bobath (Bobath, 1978, 1980; Bobath & Bobath, 1975), known as neurodevelopmental theory (NDT), is credited for its usefulness in helping the therapist look at movement; for its emphasis on balance, posture, and movement patterns; and for the permission it gives the therapist to handle and guide the patient (Ross, 1991, pp. 56-58).

Ross recommends the study of other neurodevelopmental approaches so that therapists might expand their knowledge of movement. Those cited included spatiotemporal adaptation (Gilfoyle, Grady, & Moore, 1980), proprioceptive neuromuscular facilitation (PNF) (Knott & Voss, 1968; Voss, 1972), and the functional integration of Feldenkrais (1966, 1977 [see the brief description and resources for Feldenkrais Method]). Ross emphasizes the preparatory role played by appropriately modulated sensory stimulation and proposes that movement produces "immediate and profound physiological changes that can influence behavior" (Ross, 1991, 1997).

Expanding to Include Cognitive Goals and Social Goals

In contrast to King's focus on non-cortical treatment activities, Ross includes therapeutic activities that expect a cognitive response. She proposes that activity be used to "organize behavior" (Ross, 1998a, p. 330). The organization achieved by the sensory and motor phases of treatment paves the way for the group participant to then think about what was accomplished, to give feedback to other group members, and

FELDENKRAIS METHOD

Moshe Feldenkrais integrated principles from anatomy, physics, psychology, learning, and human development to develop the Feldenkrais method. This method can be used with children and adults of all ages to increase their awareness of how they move and to integrate their movements for efficient function. The methods are used with persons who are healthy and want to be more physically fit and have a greater sense of well-being. They also help a person with a disability, chronic disease, chronic pain, or injury increase his or her awareness of how position and use of one's body influences one's stress, balance, coordination, mobility, and participation in daily life. Feldenkrais advocates believe that a person's awareness of how we use our body and learning to use one's body efficiently can improve physical and emotional well-being. The methods are process-oriented and assume that everyone can learn to use his or her abilities to learn strategies that improve one's performance in the environment. The methods are learned in group and individual contexts.

The Feldenkrais method continues to develop through the efforts of the Feldenkrais Guild and the practitioners trained in accredited programs. Clients as well as persons with other professional training can participate in training programs. Training does not include medical training.

The Guild has a quarterly newsletter, *SenseAbility*, that describes methodology and case stories that represent populations of varied age and ability and include application in many environments (e.g., work, classroom, home, athletic performance, etc.)

Additional Resources

Alon, R. (1996). *Mindful spontaneity*. Berkeley, CA: North Atlantic Books.

Feldenkrais Guild, P. O. Box 489, Albany, OR 97321. Phone: 800-775-2118.

Feldenkrais, M. (1991). *Awareness through movement: Easy exercises to improve personal growth*. New York, NY: Harper.

Shafarman, S. (1997). *Awareness health: The Feldenkrais Method for dynamic health*. Cambridge, MA: Perseus Publishing.

to learn or modify problem-solving strategies. Toward this end, the author discusses the application of Abreu and Toglia's cognitive rehabilitation model (Abreu & Toglia, 1984, 1987). The literature to which Ross refers describes intervention with persons having traumatic brain injury. In their manual, Abreu and Toglia use a holistic approach in which they assume that the individual with a brain injury is still capable of learning but needs assistance with maximizing existing problem-solving strategies and learning new cognitive strategies that will better compensate for existing limitations.

Identifying an Appropriate Population

Ross describes her patients/clients as part of a special population or "those groups of individuals who require more than the usual amount of cues and assists for their CNS to become organized sufficiently to make an appropriate and sustained response. Their nervous systems require assistance from the environment and their caretakers to perform adaptively" (Ross, 1991, p. 2). Such special populations might include individuals in geriatric centers, those with developmental disability (from mild to severe retardation), or chronic psychiatric problems, plus any others who are judged to have neurological impairment.

Picking Up Threads Laid by King

Ross' population is broader than that discussed by King, and her theoretical base goes beyond that of sensory integration to include several sensory integrative and motor rehabilitation theories traditionally associated with treatment in the area of physical dysfunction. Ross also expands her therapeutic goals to include cognitive or cortical activity, in contrast to King's emphasis on the non-cortical; however, several similar themes exist in both therapists' writing, including an emphasis on appropriate movement and sensory stimulation, with special attention afforded the proprioceptive and vestibular systems. Both hold the following similar beliefs:

- A belief in the need for sensory information to be given in a controlled manner by the therapist
- A belief in the organizing role of movement
- A focus on the pleasurable nature of activity
- A developmental view of the way motor patterns evolve
- A strong belief in and reliance on the body-mind relationship
- A belief and understanding that many, if not all, psychiatric processes are neurological at their base

This final emphasis is consistent with the position taken by Claudia Allen and discussed in Chapter Eight. In contrast to Allen, however, King and Ross express the view that neurologically compromised persons can learn and improve as a result of therapeutic intervention.

CURRENT PRACTICE IN OCCUPATIONAL THERAPY

The Person and Behavior

The perspective of the person in this frame of reference is the whole person and how he or she adapts in everyday environments. It emphasizes the physiological aspects of occupational performance and the role of sensory input to facilitate an adaptive response throughout one's life.

Normal Human Function

The person is, above all, a single, unified organism or whole; anything that affects the body will influence thinking, emotion, and ultimately behavior. This view is consistent with other holistic models detailed in this book, but the emphasis in intervention in this framework is on the physiological side of a person's being.

Adaptation

It is the nature of the person to organize, adapt, and thereby become more complex. **Adaptation** is an active process by which the person meets the challenges of his or her environment, while at the same time fulfilling personal needs and desires. The adaptive process is in itself self-satisfying and self-perpetuating. Adaptation is often accomplished most efficiently when it is organized subcortically or unconsciously (King, 1978). Stated another way, a great deal of what each person does daily is accomplished without special attention. This frees people's attention and energy to be focused on more cognitively demanding tasks. When a person perceives him- or herself adapting successfully, he or she feels a sense of mastery, which acts as a powerful internal motivator for future adaptation.

Developmental Process

Adaptation is a developmental process within the organism; one that is governed by the laws of growth and development evident within the phylogenetic history of the species. Activity governed by phylogenetically older parts of the CNS (e.g., the brain stem) forms the foundation for adaptive activity governed by phylogenetically newer portions (e.g., the cerebral cortex). Likewise, sensory and motor skills developed in early childhood do so in an invariant order and form the basis for skills that will emerge in later childhood and adulthood. The CNS retains some plasticity; changes can occur within the CNS in late childhood and adulthood, but these are more difficult to bring about than would be expected in early life.

The brain is "primarily a sensory processing machine," and sensory input is the raw material upon which all adaptation is based at any age (Ayres, 1979). In other words, the brain needs information before it can direct the person how to act. Sensation and its accurate perception also lays the foundation for an accurate and positive body concept. Good movement promotes body scheme, stimulates better posture, and is organizing to the CNS.

Dysfunction

Dysfunction is an impairment in the ability for successful adaptation. As defined in this frame of reference, the person who has inadequate function for adaptation is one who has neurological or CNS deficit. This damage may result from trauma or disease processes evident from birth (e.g., mental retardation and developmental disability), from those evolving later in life (Alzheimer's disease), from such mental illnesses as schizophrenia and depression, or when aging, neglect, or social factors have created a living environment devoid of adequate sensory stimulation. Those children who have untreated sensory integration problems may adapt relatively well and exhibit only minor impairments as adults, or they may, at the extreme, go on to develop severe perceptual disturbances, very low self-esteem, and disorganized behavior as is seen in schizophrenia (King, 1978; Ross, 1991).

Characteristics of Dysfunction

Whatever the origin of the sensory and motor deficits, characteristics often shared in common by persons with sensorimotor dysfunction include mood disorders (agitation, confusion, or apathy), poor social and communication skills, a dislike of movement or a need to increase movement, an inability to sustain interest and attention, a rigid or flexed body posture, a lessened ability to ignore unpleasant sensation, poor body image, and low self-esteem. This population also has limitations of higher cognitive function.

Role of Stress

The contributory role of stress in psychiatric dysfunction is referred to by proponents of sensory-motor therapy. Because of the reciprocity between physical and emotional states, psychological stress—the stress of everyday life—can be expected to exact a physical toll. In this respect, states of disease are often conceptualized as ones in which the body or mind has decompensated from stress overload. Many individuals with schizophrenia, for example, describe an increase in hallucinations and distortions in time perception during periods of increased stress (Hatfield, 1989).

Stress as an etiological component of dysfunction is cited here because physically demanding activity such as that used in motor approaches has also been used as a means to reduce stress. It has been postulated that movement contributes to the normalization of function in persons with schizophrenia because of its ability to reduce their stress (King, 1983).

Role of the Occupational Therapist

As in other frames of reference, the occupational therapist has multiple roles that are assumed to meet the needs of the clients, effectively respond to the expectations of the environment, and manage sensory input from the environment.

Group Facilitator

Both King and Ross describe the application of sensorimotor principles in a group context. Within this context the occupational therapist has an important role as group leader. As group facilitator the therapist is responsible for creating a climate of respect and the expectation that each participant has something to contribute to the group.

Spontaneity

King's work and Ross' 1981 and 1991 texts emphasize the role of the occupational therapist as an active participant engaged with his or her clients.

Picture therapists providing sensory input for participants through individual or group activities, perhaps giving them vestibular stimulation through spinning them in a desk chair, playing Simon Says, or tossing a ball, and you get an image for the very active role King and Ross recommend. King describes the role of the therapist as having fun and being spontaneous (King, 1974a). The therapist's enthusiasm and active participation not only serve as a model for everyone in the group but become a part of the sensory environment, acting to alert and energize. In a similar vein, Ross describes the therapist's role in group intervention as being "an interactive facilitator and part of the environment who must move about, provide appropriate touching, use a calm voice, and make eye contact to obtain member involvement" (Ross, 1991, p. 4). Doing this also contributes to what Ross refers to as the therapist's "special role in making members feel wanted, safe, and expectant" (Ross, 1991, p. 5).

Controlling Sensory Input

As with sensory-integrative work with children, the therapist has an equally vital role in controlling the environment, not just creating excitement and stimulation. Because many adults for whom this intervention is appropriate have difficulty modulating sensory input, the therapist creates an environment in which sensory messages are neither too intense, too rapid, nor too subdued to be effectively integrated, and an environment that provides an opportunity for a motor response at the level at which the individual can succeed. Ross writes that the therapist's goal is to introduce a "rhythm to the group to maintain a sense of balance or to promote the return to homeostasis" (Ross, 1998b, p. 316). This is done by increasing or decreasing the level of excitement, judiciously selecting activities that require a motor response by participants, and incorporating reflection through discussion.

Praising and Supporting Engagement

The therapist also recognizes the importance of his or her role in bringing the participant's attention to successes. Many persons with poor function have been reluctant to be involved with activity or with each other and may tend to see themselves as failures. Frequent, clear, and sincere praise for involvement acts not only as a reward but may be necessary if the person is to recognize his or her own accomplishments or improvement.

While the limited abilities of persons with whom this approach is used require that the therapist create an initial structure and provide clear expectations and guidelines for participation, Ross encourages the therapist to fade into the background and allow group members to express their concerns and assume leadership within the group as they are able. When participants can appropriately assert their wishes and their needs within the group, they build important social and communication skills.

In describing her work with persons with developmental disability, Ross reminds the therapist to use a language (vocabulary) that is meaningful to the participants, both in terms of their cognitive understanding and their cultural experiences. For example, many persons with developmental disability have been taught that they need to behave as adults. Describing an activity as a "game" may be less comfortable for these people than identifying a game as an "activity" (Ross, 1998b, p. 322).

Sensory Input Through Touch

Of all the therapeutic frames of reference discussed in this text, this sensory-motor application most emphasizes the value of acceptable touch (i.e., in his or her touch the occupational therapist has a means to supply proprioceptive and tactile input, to calm, to alert, to reassure, and to recognize). If we recall the patients/clients described by Ross—often older or tending to regress and withdraw—we realize this population is frequently left alone and may receive little appropriate touch from others. A hug for a job well done, an arm around the shoulder, or taking a person's hands and guiding them through the process of mixing a cake batter are examples of positive and appropriate touch. Not incidentally, this touch can communicate caring and support. (Note: In some intervention environments there may also be written or unwritten guides for client-therapist interactions and the role of touch within therapy contexts. For example, a handshake may be preferred to a hug to acknowledge achievement.)

Ongoing Assessment

As a specialist in the area of motor development, the occupational therapist working with clients/residents who are being treated with psychotropic medications (especially antipsychotics) is in a position to assess any physical changes that indicate adverse reactions to these medications. These observations would need to be brought to the immediate attention of the person prescribing medications.

The physical posturing and movement described by King in relation to long-standing schizophrenia is similar to the extrapyramidal or parkinsonian-like effects that can follow the prolonged use of antipsychotic medications called **tardive dyskinesia** (Smith, 1993; Van Schroeder & Chung, 1993). While it has been difficult to determine the extent to which medication may be responsible for physical sequelae in schizophrenia, study in this area has alerted clinicians to pay special attention to physical changes in their clients.

Responsibilities of the Client

Because many of the persons participating in sensory-motor approaches perform at a lower level of function, at least initially, there is not the expectation that they will enter into a formal contract with the therapist. This does not mean, however, that the responsibility for therapy is the therapist's alone. As Ross writes, the therapist must hold two fundamental beliefs:

1. That each participant can learn
2. That each participant has some wisdom that needs to be shared

According to Ross, "Even though the group is composed of people who find it difficult to express their needs in an organized manner; even when they are enslaved to emotions that they cannot effectively harness... they know something others do not know..." (Ross, 1991, pp. 41-42).

The Function of Activity

In this frame of reference, activities serve multiple purposes. Activities provide sensory input that can facilitate movement, elicit pleasure, and provide opportunities for socialization and skill development. All of these functions of activity can support the person's adaptive response in an environment.

Elicit an Adaptive Response

Activity is used to organize behavior (Ross, 1998a, p. 330). Activities used in sensory-motor approaches are analyzed and selected primarily for their physiological properties and their ability to elicit an adaptive response (i.e., the activity involves the participant in enjoyable, goal-directed behavior). The individual does not come to occupational therapy to engage in aimless, repetitive reaching or bending but will reach for blocks in a relay game, bend to plant a garden, or verbally share his concerns with the participants in a group. Thus, the **activities** used in occupational therapy will be parts of life that, when accomplished, can help the individual feel that he or she is a more effective person within his or her own world.

Activities Provide Sensory Input

Ross proposes two guiding principles when working with persons having chronic disabilities. The first principle is to "consider when and how the planned activities are to be introduced" (Ross, 1998b, p. 310). First, the therapist is especially interested in the ability of the activity to alert or calm the CNS. Vestibular input given slowly, as occurs in gentle rocking, and heavy proprioceptive pressure are calming and may be used, for example, with an agitated individual. Softer touch can be stimulating, as are cold temperatures, strong odors, and so on. Tables 10-1 and 10-2 provide other examples of alerting and soothing stimuli. Ross summarizes this area when she writes of activities, "Some operational principles may be stated simply:

- Whatever is novel alerts.
- Whatever is fast excites.
- Whatever is routine or familiar soothes and composes.
- Whatever is slow relaxes" (Ross, 1998b, p. 310).

Table 10-1

ALERTING AND CALMING THROUGH SENSORY STIMULATION

Senses	*Methods Used to Stimulate*	*Behaviors*
Touch		
Protopathic	Rubbing/different textures, self-touch	Alerting
Epicritic	Self-touch	Calming
Vestibular	Rotation	
	—Fast	Alerting
	—Slow	Calming
Proprioception	Pressure	
	—Light	Alerting
	—Moderate	Calming
Vision	Bright colors—Light	Alerting
	Pastels—Low intensity	Calming
Hearing	Contrast sounds—Loud	Alerting
	Repetitive changes—Slow	Calming
	Melodious and soft sounds	Calming
Smell	Pungent smells	Alerting
	Potpourri of sweet smells	Calming
Taste	Strong flowers—Crunchy	Alerting
	Smooth texture—Tepid temperatures	Calming

Reprinted from Ross, M. (1997). Alerting and calming through sensory stimulation. In: *Integrative group therapy: Mobilizing coping abilities with five stage group* (p. 177). Bethesda, MD: American Occupational Therapy Association. © 1997 by the American Occupational Therapy Association, Inc. Reprinted with permission.

The second principle is that a "moderate approach to arousal achieves longer lasting results" (Ross, 1998b, p. 310). Ross advises that the goal of using sensory input be to strive for moderate, longer-lasting control, appropriate arousal, and balance. The idea is not to overexcite, nor to lull. If one uses novelty too soon or overexcites group members, they tend to become flooded and disorganized.

It is not only the ability of the sensation to calm or alert but also the very fact that sensory information is entering the CNS that provides the patient/client with an invitation for an adaptive response. Using activities that will stimulate one or more senses is encouraged; however, it is often preferable to introduce one kind of sensory input at a time in order to not overstimulate the group participants (Iwasaki & Holm, 1989). Because many clients demonstrate problems related to the vestibular and proprioceptive systems, activity is chosen especially for its incorporation of vestibular stimulation (e.g., movement of the head through many planes), its incorporation of deep pressure touch, and its ability to give proprioceptive feedback to joints and tendons (e.g., clapping and jumping) (King, 1974a, 1974b).

Normalize Movement

King, Ross, and Ayres all pay particular attention to the posture and movement patterns used in the therapeutic

Table 10-2
ALERTING AND CALMING THROUGH MUSIC AND MOVEMENT

Alerting	*Calming*
Increased muscle activity with increased muscle tension	Decreased motor activity, relaxed muscle fibers
Head up, chest out, general extension pattern	Head down, torso bent (forward flexion), deep breathing
Light touch, patting, whisking, brushing movements	Heavy pressure touch, massage
Percusive movements	Swinging or sustained movements
Nonrepetitive or uneven rhythmic patterns	Slow, repetitive movements, axial or locomotor
Uneven locomotor movements (skip, gallop, slide)	
Fast, loud music of variable intensity, sharp sounds	Slow, dreamy, lyrical music: Adagio
Linear acceleration and deceleration in loco-motor patterns	Linear movement consistency
Defy gravity, up and down	Give in to gravity, body hanging, collapse or rag doll movements
Fast spinning or twirling	Slow turning

Reprinted from Ross, M. (1997). Alerting and calming through music and movement. In: *Integrative Group therapy: Mobilizing coping abilities with five stage group* (p. 178). Bethesda, MD: American Occupational Therapy Association. © 1997 by the American Occupational Therapy Association, Inc. Reprinted with permission.

activity. Ross refers to her desire to ultimately reach a level of full-body movement and stimulate many senses during the course of her five stages (Ross, 1991, pp. 2-3).

In response to the dysfunctional posture and movement that King identified as characteristic of process schizophrenia, she proposed that therapeutic activity could counter abnormal movement or normalize patterns of excessive body flexion, adduction, and internal rotation, as well as increase joint range of motion (King, 1974a). Playing volleyball would exemplify this kind of activity. In an effort to normalize tone, activity should include the bilateral use of tonic muscles against resistance, as occurs in digging a garden or playing tug-of-war. These embody the heavy work patterns to which Rood refers (Stockmeyer, 1972).

Citing the work of Bobath and Bobath, Ross also discusses the importance of proper positioning in seated activities and the use of activities that demand shifting, reaching, and bending; stimulate balance responses; and counter the collapse into flexion and extension (Ross, 1991, p. 56).

Provide a Vehicle for Pleasant Experiences

Ayres, King, and Ross all emphasize that activities experienced as pleasurable by the individual are more likely to be repeated and, therefore, more likely to lead to a habituated, adaptive response. As Ross says, "whatever is pleasurable" to the person can be a potential treatment activity. She adds that when therapists get too concerned about the age appropriateness of tasks, they might be confusing their personal values with the patient's or client's own preferences (Ross, 1991). In addition to emphasizing that the activity be pleasant (pleasure of course being subjective), King (1974a) proposes that activity be non-cortical or that patients/clients focus on the fun that they are having and not on how their bodies are moving. Perhaps slightly different in tone, King suggests, too, that if the activity does not "induce smiles and pleasure" as from recreation, it should bring about a feeling of mastery, as from a work-oriented task. In either case, the participant feels a sense of satisfaction.

Provide a Vehicle for Socialization

As noted, sensory-motor approaches can be used individually, but they often occur in a group context. Activities are then selected in part for their ability to engage patients with each other. Not only does the therapist provide sensory stimulation, but participants may be asked to pass materials to each other, pat each other, apply textured materials to each other's arms, sing together, stamp their feet in unison, or give each other verbal feedback. In this way, the adaptive response(s) being built include those of normal social behavior. As group members become less physically withdrawn and more at ease, they often become more willing to risk social spontaneity. The adaptive response spiral then moves forward as success and satisfying social engagement lead to further engagement and self-confidence.

Facilitate Cognitive Skill Building

As discussed, King proposes staying with non-cortical activities, whereas Ross uses a sensory-motor base to prepare for eventual development of cognitive strategies. Activities are evaluated and selected in relation to their cognitive demands, such as that for sustained attention or memory. In the example of group treatment that follows later in this chapter, both cognitive and non-cortical activities are used in one group session.

Theoretical Assumptions—Guide Evaluation and Intervention

The theoretical assumptions (See Sensory-Motor Theoretical Assumptions) are a summary of the basic beliefs about the person, activities or occupations, and the environment or context. These beliefs are adapted from the theories of Ayres, Ross, & King that contribute to the sensory motor models previously described in this chapter. The assumptions about the person-environment-occupation variables and their possible relationships guide evaluation and intervention in occupational therapy

Evaluation

An accurate assessment of the person's functional abilities, especially as related to movement and body scheme, serves several related purposes:

- It suggests the activities at which the individual can succeed and helps the occupational therapist know where to begin.
- It may shed light on the reason(s) for poor function.
- It allows the therapist to establish a baseline of function, state goals, and subsequently measure progress.
- It may give useful information about the cues and environment structure that help the patient/client to succeed and can point to a need for future testing (Smaga & Ross, 1991).

Assessment instruments are selected for their utility in screening for neurological deficits, often those identified as **neurological soft signs**, which do not localize within the CNS but lead to problems with learning, motor, sensory, and integration functions (Falk-Kessler et al., 1988).

Assessment Instruments

Southern California Sensory Integration Tests and the Sensory Integration and Praxis Tests

Although these tests have been standardized for children aged 4 to 10, selected subtests have been used with adults, and some work has established normative test scores for adults (Ayres, 1972c, 1989). Table 10-3 on page 314 lists the subtests within the SIPT, which is available from Western Psychological Services, Los Angeles, CA.

Schroeder-Block-Campbell Adult Psychiatric Sensory Integration Evaluation

The SBC (Schroeder, Block, Trottier, & Stowell, 1983) was developed to provide a standardized, comprehensive evaluation tool for use by occupational therapists working with an adult psychiatric population. It consists of three subscales and takes about 75 minutes to complete, but it does not have to be completed at one sitting. The physical assessment subscale evaluates neurophysical abilities needed for everyday tasks (e.g., those related to balance, coordination, and hand function). The abnormal movements subscale measures abnormal movements such as hypokinetic and hyperkinetic movement, in addition to such extrapyramidal symptoms as akathisia and tardive dyskinesia. The childhood history section asks the patient about early growth and development and looks for indications of developmental delays or other neurological soft signs. A non-standardized use of the person-drawing elicits information pertaining to body image (Hamada & Schroeder, 1988; Schroeder et al., 1983).

Parachek Geriatric Behavior Rating Scale

This quick screening tool (Miller & Parachek, 1989) consists of 10 multiple-choice items: three related to physical condition, four to self-care, and three to social behavior. Scores are designed in part to help designate functional levels (level one through three); the lowest level indicating a need for substantial nursing care, and the person rated at the highest level capable of most self-care. A manual has been designed for use with the Parachek scale and suggests possible occupational therapy intervention strategies (Miller & Parachek, 1989; Parachek & King, 1986).

Smaga and Ross Integrated Battery

Said to be based on clinical experience, the SARIB (Ross, 1991) "evaluate[s] clients with low functional ability for placement in similar ability groups" (Smaga & Ross, 1991, p. 107). An extensive test, this battery could conceivably be performed over several sessions. Its subtests include the Llorens-Rubin Motor Control Test, the Elizur Test of Psycho-Organicity (in itself a standardized test available from Western Psychological Services), Schilder's Arm Extension

SENSORY-MOTOR THEORETICAL ASSUMPTIONS

The following theoretical assumptions are based on the theoretical views of Ayres, Ross, and King:

Person

1. The person is best viewed as a "single organism, highly complex and completely unified" (King, 1974a).
2. Anything that affects the body will inexorably affect the mind and vice versa (King, 1974a).
3. The same principles of neurophysiology are applicable and adaptable to persons of all ages (Ross & Burdick, 1981).
4. It is the nature of the person to organize through adaptive response.
5. It is self-satisfying for the person to engage in purposeful, goal-directed activity.
6. Higher cortical organization depends on organization at lower levels.
7. The CNS becomes more complex in a sequential manner.
8. The CNS is "plastic" and remains capable of change even in adulthood.
9. The person (child and adult) often selects just the activity that he or she needs for healthy development.
10. The vestibular system is the unifying system, as it forms the framework for organizing experience.
11. Good movement promotes body scheme and is organizing.
12. Movement produces "immediate and profound physiological changes that can influence behavior" (Ross, 1991).
13. Much so-called "mental" illness is physiological in origin.
14. Persons with CNS damage have more difficulty integrating relevant sensation and ignoring irrelevant stimuli.
15. Persons with CNS problems are capable of learning.
16. There is an optimal amount of sensory input that the individual can successfully process. Sensory input must be provided at the level at which the CNS can manage; the aim is to provide neither too little, nor too much.

Activity/Occupation

17. Activities/stimulation have properties that affect the CNS.
18. Select sensory attributes of an activity promote the brain's ability to organize an adaptive response.
19. Activities that are experienced as pleasurable can motivate a person to interact with others and to participate in his or her environment.
20. Activities/stimuli that are aversive can bring about a fearful response, anger, or withdrawal by an individual.
21. Activities can be analyzed according to their neurophysiologic properties and their social-emotional connotations and requirements, and can be graded accordingly.
22. It is important that activities used in occupational therapy are those in which the participant can succeed.
23. Treatment that provides controlled sensory input within the context of meaningful activity and results in an adaptive response (or behavior) will enhance sensory integration and improve behavior (Ross & Burdick, 1981; Sensory Integration International, 1988).

Environment/Context

24. The environment in which activity occurs provides stimulation and a context that affects the person's CNS. For example, this stimulation can be calming or arousing, frightening, or be ignored, and it can either facilitate or detract from an organized and adaptive response by the person.
25. The occupational therapist is an important part of the therapeutic environment.
26. Environments need to be carefully controlled and monitored by occupational therapists who are treating individuals with sensory processing problems.

Test, and a request for a person-drawing (Llorens, 1967). Overall, test items relate to range of motion, posture, gait, balance, strength, visual performance, coordination, motor planning, sensory perception, stereognosis, proprioception, judgment, memory, and "other behaviors that influence performance." The test is described in detail, with scoring sheets, in Ross' *Integrative Group Therapy: The Structured Five-Stage Approach* (1991). Evidence in support of its use is based upon its' authors clinical experience, and research evidence is not available.

Let's Do Lunch

Let's Do Lunch (Bachner, 1998) is a non-standardized assessment tool based on mealtime activities. It was designed specifically for adults with developmental disabilities. Unlike the other instruments described, it assesses the client's ability to bring together multiple performance components in a meaningful, real-life situation. It is administered during mealtime and was "developed to deal with the challenges of combining quality of care, client satisfaction, and payer acceptance" (Bachner, 1998, p. 270). Let's Do Lunch is a

---

Table 10-3
AREAS OF FUNCTION

1. Space visualization
2. Figure-ground perception
3. Manual form perception
4. Kinesthesia
5. Finger identification
6. Graphesthesia
7. Localization of tactile stimuli
8. Praxis on verbal command
9. Design copying
10. Constructional praxis
11. Postural praxis
12. Oral praxis
13. Sequencing praxis
14. Bilateral motor coordination
15. Standing and walking balance
16. Motor accuracy
17. Post-rotary nystagmus

Areas of function summarized from the Sensory and Integration and Praxis Tests (Ayres, 1989).

---

structured observation of the client from his or her first entering the dining room until his or her departure and includes selecting and obtaining food, sitting and positioning one's self at the table, socializing with others, properly using utensils and meal accoutrements, consuming food, and putting away one's tray and used utensils. Performance is scored from 0 (independent) to 3 (total assist) in the areas of sensory, perceptual, neuromuscular, motor, cognitive, and psychosocial function.

Many other standardized and non-standardized tests have been cited in the literature for use with this sensory-motor approach. These tests include portions of the Frostig and Purdue perceptual tests, various versions of the human figure drawing, the Nurses Observation Scale for Inpatient Evaluation (NOSIE) (Honigfield & Gillis, 1966), and the Allen Cognitive Level Test (Allen, 1996).

Intervention

The psychodynamic frame of reference assumes that if the person feels differently and perceives his or her problem solving as having improved, one could expect this individual's appearance to reflect this in a brighter affect. In contrast, a sensory-motor framework believes that if one can effectively process sensation and move with more confidence, his or her feelings about the self can be expected to improve. The stage is concurrently set for social skill building and for tackling cognitive problems. Thus, it is prudent to remind ourselves that while therapeutic intervention is sensory- or motor-based, goals become those of enhanced occupational performance.

Functional Goals

The ultimate aim of treatment is to bring about an organized, adaptive whole-person response. Intervention goals are written as changes in functional, demonstrable behaviors in the areas of movement, sensorimotor skill acquisition, posture, affect, social interaction (including verbalization), body-image, self-esteem, and cognition. More specifically, these goals might begin with one or more of the following. The individual exhibits:

- Increased awareness or use of both sides of body
- Normalized whole-body flexor-extensor tone
- Improved balance and posture during activity
- Increased voluntary movement of the head through more than one plane during activity
- Improved motor planning
- Increased range of motion during activity

- Normalized gait
- Normalized patterns of adduction and internal rotation
- Increased spontaneous movement during activity
- Increased tolerance of touch

Subsequent to, or at times along with, these motor goals, goals might include those related to normalized affect, clarity of thinking, and socialization. Typifying these goals, but not to be considered inclusive, are the following. The individual exhibits:

- Signs of increased spontaneity (e.g., smiling, initiating conversation)
- Lengthened attention to a task
- Appropriate assertive behavior (e.g., asking for assistance)
- Signs of increased confidence and improved self-image (e.g., improved hygiene, willingness to take appropriate risks)
- Ability to share materials, space, and ideas with others during activity
- Increased ability to stay calm, alert, and effectively in control

Intervention Process

King limits her description of the actual process of treatment to a somewhat general discussion of the characteristics of activities to be used and the exhortation to the therapist to keep the treatment session fun. Ross goes into much greater detail, but her application of this model is exclusively with groups and, as noted, includes a strongly cognitive component. The therapist planning intervention, therefore, needs to use clinical judgment when planning a program to be used with an individual or group of clients.

Both King and Ross believe there is an advantage to using groups, in part because a group enhances the fun and available energy, provides opportunities for participants to support each other and opportunities to learn social and communication skills, and is more efficient. This does not mean that sensory-motor intervention has to be carried out within a group. In fact, the therapist may use a one-to-one format with the person who cannot yet tolerate the group, as we shall discuss (Hanschu, 1998).

Beginning Therapy

The stage is set when the occupational therapist takes control of the therapeutic environment. The therapist pays special attention to the sensory stimulation within the setting, striving to maintain the optimum necessary level of arousal and creating a sense of safety. King writes that, in general, activities are either recreation or games. They are selected according to the physical demands that they make. Task-oriented activities, states King, "will usually be effective after a patient's level of functioning has been raised to a certain level" (King, 1974a). This relates to the need to begin by alerting the participant and selecting an activity at a level at which the person can succeed. The goal is to alert pleasure centers and build confidence.

Proprioceptive and Tactile Stimulation

When a participant is agitated, apathetic, or confused, Ross advises the therapist to give proprioceptive input (Ross, 1991). One way to supply this input is through the use of a hand-held vibrator. Ross writes, "Persons who may reject other kinds of touch or are suffering from sensory deprivation for any reason can demonstrate immediate pleasure after the vibrator is offered, often resulting in a relaxing effect that can last from minutes to a few hours" (Ross, 1991, p. 83). It is recommended "not as a treatment tool in itself," but as a tool that encourages participation in treatment.

The kind of vibrator to which Ross refers is one with low amplitude and a frequency range (Hz) of 100 or higher. It is used only if the individual indicates his or her desire and only for 2 or 3 minutes. Used in this way the vibrator may be moved along the chin, on the back, arms, or other areas as described by Ross.

Other ways that appropriate initial touch can be supplied include massaging creams or lotions into the client's hands, arms, or feet, if tolerated.

Using Motor Activity

The literature describes intervention sessions lasting from 30 minutes to 1 hour, typically, having one or more gross motor activities that are introduced following sensory input, as indicated. These motor activities in themselves continue to supply heightened, controlled sensory stimulation. For example, a typical session might begin with a brief hand massage. Then an individual (or group participants) might be asked to stand against a piece of large paper on the wall, while the therapist traces around his or her arms and upper torso. Finally, the therapist and participant(s) might toss a beach ball or use some other activity in which individuals have to reach above their head.

Throughout therapy, persons are encouraged to explore and enjoy the media offered, and the therapist remains flexible, observing each person's reactions to activity and modifying intervention as needed.

The Five Stage Group

By far, the most extensive development of a sensory-motor group is found in Ross's work (1991, 1997, 1998a, 1998b). Ross describes her five-stage group as a systematic and sequential method for organizing the presentation of activities within a group format (Ross, 1998a, p. 329). The persons for whom the five-stage group has been identified include persons with chronic schizophrenia, older adults, individuals who have regressed, are severely depressed, and especially developmentally disabled. Ross goes on to state that the presentation of therapeutic activity is **developmental** insofar as each group stage is dependent on the stage before it to enhance its acceptance, and it is "**hierarchical**" in that each stage incrementally makes more demands on or increases the challenge to the participant. Following a five-stage model, Ross uses neurodevelopmental principles to sequence the presentation of motor, perceptual, and cognitive activities, as well as to establish guidelines for therapist intervention and expected participant behavior. Each of these stages occurs within the individual group session. Outlined very briefly, these five stages are as follows.

Stage 1. Orientation

In Stage 1, members are acknowledged and the purpose of the group is stated. The goal is to get participants' attention and to help them feel "wanted, safe, and expectant" (Ross, 1991, p. 5). The therapist tries to arouse the members' alerting and pleasure centers through the use of activity involving sensory input and by encouraging touching and handling of interesting media. For example, clients can choose a simple musical instrument from those that are passed around and experiment with the sounds. The therapist or clients can use textured items to rub against their arms and faces to increase sensation. Scented soaps or fresh herbs are passed around the group for each person to smell and identify the fragrance.

Stage 2. Movement

In this stage, movement is emphasized. Movement activities can be arousing (e.g., blowing and chasing soap bubbles, ripping newspaper in preparation for later use during papier mâché projects) or calming (e.g., rolling a group member in a parachute). Whatever the movement selected, the therapist is careful to choose activities at the level at which members can succeed.

Stage 3. Visual Motor Perceptual Activities

In this stage, tasks that require "less physical and more thoughtful action" are offered (Ross, 1991, p. 23). Having been able to attend and succeed at a task, the participant has more available energy and ability to perform. Games, including those that are competitive, might be introduced to emphasize perceptual motor accuracy. These games include safe darts, identifying and naming objects in the room, touch-discrimination activities, Simon Says, the hokey-pokey, and games of pantomime.

Stage 4. Cognition

Members are asked to focus on a cognitive task. They are encouraged to be thoughtful and creative and to share verbally with each other. For example, participants might be asked to share how they feel about themselves or the activity in which they participated. Poetry, creative storytelling, reminiscence, show and tell, and brief slide presentations could be used to stimulate dialogue with each other.

Stage 5. Closure

This stage closes the day's session. The occupational therapist informs the group before closing, so that they might mentally prepare. The therapist determines an appropriate closure, given the group's mood and the session theme. The goal is to achieve a sense of accomplishment and an inner sense of calm. For example, the day's activities may be reviewed, refreshments could be provided, and/or affirmations given (Ross, 1998a, p. 337).

An Alternative Sensory-Motor Application: The Ready Approach

Another application using a sensory orientation with adults having developmental disability that is similar in principle to that described by Ross and King is identified as the Ready Approach (see Case Example: The Ready Approach). Being "**ready**" to respond means "the (individual's) brain is able to catch on to what is happening, generate adaptive responses, and keep up with new situational demands" (Hanschu, 1998, p. 203).

CASE EXAMPLE: THE READY APPROACH

Hanschu (1998, p. 166) cites an example presented by Reisman (1993) in which dramatic improvement is attributed to use of the Ready Approach.

The client was a 41-year-old institutionalized woman. Since childhood, she had been persistently "picking at" herself, which created oozing sores requiring medical treatment. A variety of behavioral techniques, including aversives and restraints, had failed to reduce either the frequency or intensity of this behavior. This behavior alone kept the woman from living in a less restrictive environment.

A program of intensified sensory input was started. At first the woman was given doses of proprioception and pressure touch for about 10 minutes of each of her waking hours. Following this, she participated with a helper in an activity that she enjoyed. Within 6 months, her picking behavior was significantly reduced, from approximately "one pick per minute" to only a few picks per several hours. With this change in behavior, she was able to be successfully placed in a "homelike" foster care setting, where she lived with a couple and their dog. The foster couple continued to provide doses of sensory input, gradually fading the frequency of these doses to use only during stressful times. Six months following her discharge to this setting, the placement was judged as a success by everyone involved, and the picking behavior had not returned.

The Ready Approach is described by Hanschu (1998) as a "frame of reference," sensory in its orientation, that was developed at an institution that was a "placement of last resort for adults with severe developmental disabilities" (p. 169). (See also Reisman, 1993; Reisman & Hanschu, 1992, 1993.) The residents in this facility all displayed significant behavior disorders, especially aggression, defensiveness, and self-stimulation. Citing the sensory integration principles articulated by Ayres (1972b, 1979) and Fisher et al. (1991), the proponents of this model, ultimately determined that they could not rely solely on sensory integration theory to explain the needs of nor plan intervention for the residents they served (p. 180). They determined that the problems they were seeing were better conceived as problems with sensory processing. Under this head of sensory processing, Hanschu identifies four distinct processing problems:

1. Sensory defensiveness
2. Disordered sensory modulation
3. Inadequate sensory registration
4. Sensory integrative dysfunction (Hanschu, 1998, p. 192)

Sensory integration is identified as the most "sophisticated" level of sensory processing. In adults with severe processing problems, states Hanschu, needs that must be addressed first would be those related to sensory defensiveness, modulation, and impaired registration.

Staff at the facility adapted sensory integrative and neurodevelopmental principles to create individualized programs that emphasized strong sensory input for each resident (see Case Example: The Ready Approach on p. 316). The types of sensory input given were primarily tactile (touch), proprioceptive (joint sensations), and vestibular (movement). This was supplied through the use of **heavy work** (physical exertion that uses the large muscles of the body), direct joint compression or stretch at joints, pressure touch to backs, arms, and legs, and movement of the head through space (p. 175). The sensory input was provided through what is referred to as **enriched sensory diets** (Wilbarger & Wilbarger, 1991), in which staff structured the residents' day so that they had periodic natural opportunities for helpful sensation as well as providing up to two 45- minute sessions of sensory input per day for some individuals (Hanschu, 1998, p. 191). The rationale for using sensory input of this type is that it is processed primarily at the brainstem level. As Hanschu writes, brain stem sensations "wake up the nervous system and help it to become **ready** to support increased neural activity associated with our being alert and doing something" (p. 181).

The aim in the Ready Approach is not just to enhance sensory input, however. The goal is to "improve the effectiveness and efficiency of sensory processing." This might require increasing doses of direct, strong sensory input (like touch, proprioception, or vestibular input) or modifying the environment so that the sensation that comes in can be better handled by a "struggling CNS," for example, by creating an environment in which there are fewer distractions and interruptions (pp. 190-191).

Positive changes observed in residents with whom the Ready Approach has been used include:

- Improved alertness
- Increased ability for appropriate self-regulation of arousal
- Improved interest and attention
- Better sleep-related behavior, eating habits, and mealtime behavior
- Improved behavior related to dressing and staying dressed
- Appropriate initiation of interaction with others (Hanschu, 1998, p. 186)

Proponents describe other behavior changes as often quite remarkable; some residents perform complex skills not previously believed to be in their skill repertoire. The interested reader is referred to the sources cited.

Summary

It seems reasonable to suggest that every mental health condition brings with it some physical, often observable behavior or concern. Whether the downcast eyes of the depressed person, the determined face of the compulsively preoccupied, the nail-biting of the anxious, or the rapid speech of the person in a manic phase, we often see in the dysfunctional population, as well as ourselves, signs of what is experienced internally. For some individuals, this physical evidence is particularly striking. It is to this group of persons, many with symptoms and non-adaptive behaviors that have been unresponsive to traditional intervention, that sensory-motor oriented therapy is directed.

In the multiple applications of this frame of reference, the occupational therapist chooses activities based on their neurophysiological properties. Input is provided through activities and therapist touch and is designed to alert or calm the CNS. Therapeutic activities that encourage an appropriate motor response and normalize posture or movement patterns are also selected. Ultimately, this sensory and motor work physically prepares the person to engage in more adaptive self-care, social and cognitive tasks, and occupations.

Proponents use theories of growth and development to support the contention that in making contact and moving the body, adaptation occurs first at the non-cortical level within the CNS. The conscious decision to act then becomes more a viable option, and learning is facilitated. Sensory-motor approaches stand out as an instance in occupational therapy in which sensation and movement, not the psyche, emotions, or cognitive processes, are the focus in a holistic framework.

CONTRIBUTIONS AND LIMITATIONS OF SENSORY-MOTOR APPROACHES

Contributions

Resource for Persons with Long-Term Limitations

A significant contribution of this frame of reference lies in its outreach to a heterogeneous population of persons with significant limitations in function. These people have often been managed in residential settings, frequently exhibiting behaviors that compromise their quality of life; many have been heavily medicated. King, Ross, Hanschu, and Reisman all assert that in their experience, individuals receiving this kind of intervention do improve and that improvements carry over even after intervention has been terminated. This framework identifies a classical use of occupational therapy wherein activity is used to elicit a total-person adaptive response, and daily life activities are the therapeutic occupation.

Respect for Clients

Although holistic in its ideology, intervention in this framework is quite focused on controlled sensory input and enhanced motor function and does not attempt to be all things to all persons, as holism is sometimes accused. While one should not confuse writing style with content, King, Ross, and proponents of the Ready Approach are upbeat in their writing, which fits with the optimistic tenor of these sensory-motor applications overall. It is not that all problematic behavior is eliminated, but one is given a way of looking at dysfunction and remediation that recognizes health, even in persons who are very disturbed, and the literature describes significant improvements in function. In a recent personal communication (January, 2001) Ross, now retired, states that she hopes that "young clinicians will continue to use and develop these approaches," most important, that they will continue to hold an optimistic attitude toward those persons who live with chronic disabilities.

Practical Intervention

The nature of the intervention described is practical and invites participation by persons in clients' natural environments. In a climate in which the occupational therapist is increasingly a consultant, much of the therapeutic touch and enriched sensory diet described could be provided by careproviders carefully educated by the occupational therapist. The inclusion of these persons and the expansion of therapeutic physical contact outside of the traditional therapy session would be expected to enhance the impact of intervention and becomes a win-win situation for third-party payers, caregivers, and clients.

It is perhaps ironic that professionals need permission to touch their patients, but with the abuse of touch that has come to light in our society it is helpful to be reminded of the healing quality of appropriate and caring touch. This permission fits with the overall exhortation for occupational therapists' engagement with their clients within the intervention process.

Limitations

Limited Understanding of Theory

There is still much to be learned as one looks at these sensorimotor approaches collectively. These are well articulated by King when she writes,

> The first question to ask about any treatment for any condition is, "Does it work?" If the answer is negative, one needs go no further. If the answer is positive, then one needs to narrow the question to, "For which patients is it most successful?" The answer to that question, by helping to define the characteristics of a certain group, will assist with answering the third question, "Why does it work?" (King, 1983, p. 3.57).

Limited Research

Although some limited research was conducted in an effort to support King's initial findings, the results were, in King's own words, "meager" and inconclusive (King, 1983, p. 3.57). Ross' approach goes far beyond sensory integration practice and draws from a broad theoretical base. If we take King's, Ross', and the Ready Approach collectively, we see that they are really three different approaches, and with each one can raise King's questions, Does it work? For whom? and Why? King's reference to the suitability of this framework to persons with chronic (non-paranoid) schizophrenia raises the question, How chronic in terms of years need one be to be considered a suitable candidate for treatment? Is it the chronicity in years or the presence of a particular neurological profile that identifies appropriate candidates for these approaches? What is this neurological profile, and how is it evidenced in daily behavior? If, as both Ross and King propose, this framework is suited to many geriatric patients, what are the criteria for its use with these individuals? Schizophrenia is a medical diagnosis; old age is not.

Medication's role in producing and remediating the physical symptoms in many of those persons with whom sensorimotor approaches have been used has not been clearly distinguished from other influences in CNS dysfunction and on behavior. It may not be possible to determine this role because it is difficult to find a population in long-term care that is not receiving medication.

Limited Intervention Guides

In terms of very practical questions and reflecting back on anecdotal information given by King, Ross, Reisman, and Hanschu, it is not evident exactly how best to carry out a sensory-motor approach with a specific individual or group of persons. In describing her work with individuals having developmental disabilities, Hanschu refers to the need to make "situational judgments related to what sensation is needed, how much, and how to provide it." She goes on to suggest that one of the best ways to gain the knowledge necessary to make these kinds of decisions is to be mentored by someone already skilled in using sensory approaches (Hanschu, 1998, p. 205).

Similar questions that require clinical judgment and an acquired expertise in use of sensory-motor methods include those related to how long sensory-motor approaches are best carried out with an individual—days? weeks? months? Is there a point of diminishing return, and to what time frame do sensory-motor advocates refer when they write that improvement persists even after intervention is terminated? How do we know it continues? What steps, if any, are needed to keep participants from regressing if they function within an environment in which there is ordinarily little activity or stimulation? Might sensory-motor approaches act as prevention to problems?

As with other frames of reference discussed in this text, there are caveats specific to this framework. Hanschu underscores Ross' suggestion to her readers that they become well-informed in the area of neurophysiological approaches. The basis for such understanding is provided in the coursework required for occupational therapy certification. Additional coursework and/or training may be necessary if handling or physical-motor techniques are to be mastered.

Bearing in mind the questions posed, with the return emphasis in psychiatry on neurological function and the expanded ability to see how the CNS really works, it is an exciting time to further explore sensory-motor approaches, especially if these approaches offer hope for improving persons' quality of life.

REFERENCES

Abreu, B., & Toglia, J. (1984). *Cognitive rehabilitation manual.* New York, NY: Author.

Abreu, B., & Toglia, J. (1987). Cognitive rehabilitation: A model for occupational therapy. *Am J Occup Ther, 41,* 439-448.

Allen, C. K. (1996). *Allen cognitive test manual.* Colchester, CT: S & S Worldwide.

Ayres, A. J. (1969). Deficits in sensory integration in educationally handicapped children. *J Learn Disabil, 2,* 68-71.

Ayres, A. J. (1972a). Improving academic scores through sensory integration. *J Learn Disabil, 5,* 24-28.

Ayres, A. J. (1972b). *Sensory integration and learning disorders.* Los Angeles, CA: Western Psychological Services.

Ayres, A. J. (1972c). *Southern California Sensory Integration Tests: Manual.* Los Angeles, CA: Western Psychological Services.

Ayres, A. J. (1973). An interpretation of the role of the brain-stem in intersensory integration. In H. Cottrell (Ed.), *The body senses and perceptual deficit.* Boston, MA: Boston University Press.

Ayres, A. J. (1975). *Southern California Postrotary and Nystagmus Test Manual.* Los Angeles, CA: Western Psychological Services.

Ayres, A. J. (1977). Cluster analyses of measure of sensory integration. *Am J Occup Ther, 31,* 362-366.

Ayres, A. J. (1978). Learning disabilities and the vestibular system. *J Learn Disabil, 11,* 30-41.

Ayres, A. J. (1979). *Sensory integration and the child.* Los Angeles, CA: Western Psychological Services.

Ayres, A. J. (1980). *Southern California Sensory Integration Test: Manual* (Rev. ed.). Los Angeles, CA: Western Psychological Services.

Ayres, A. J. (1989). *Sensory Integration and Praxis Tests.* Los Angeles, CA: Western Psychological Services.

Ayres, A. J., & Heskett, W. M. (1972). Sensory integrative dysfunction in a young schizophrenic girl. *Journal of Autism and Childhood Schizophrenia, 2,* 174-181.

Bachner, S. (1998). Let's Do Lunch: A comprehensive nonstandardized assessment tool. In M. Ross & S. Bachner (Eds.), *Adults with developmental disabilities: Current approaches in occupational therapy.* Rockville, MD: American Occupational Therapy Association.

Bailey, D. (1978). The effects of vestibular stimulation on verbalization in chronic schizophrenics. *Am J Occup Ther, 32*(7), 445-450.

Barnes, J. F. (1990a). Myofascial release: The missing link in traditional treatment. In C. Davis (Ed.), *Complementary therapies in rehabilitation.* Thorofare, NJ: SLACK Incorporated.

Barnes, J. F. (1990b). *Myofascial release: The search for excellence.* Palo Alto, CA: MFR Seminars.

Blakeney, A. B., Strickland, L. R., & Wilkinson, J. H. (1983). Exploring sensory integrative dysfunction in process schizophrenia. *Am J Occup Ther, 37,* 399-406.

Bobath, B. (1978). *Adult hemiplegia: Evaluation and treatment* (2nd ed.). London: W. Heinemann Medical Books.

Bobath, K. (1980). *A neurophysiological basis for the treatment of cerebral palsy* (2nd ed.). London: Heinemann Medical Books Ltd.

Bobath, B., & Bobath, K. (1975). *Motor development in the different types of cerebral palsy.* London: W. Heinemann Medical Books.

Bruce, M. A., & Borg, B. (1993). *Psychosocial occupational therapy: Frames of reference for intervention* (2nd ed.). Thorofare, NJ: SLACK Incorporated.

Brunnstrom, S. (1961). Motor behavior of adult hemiplegic patients. *Am J Occup Ther, 25,* 6-12.

Brunnstrom, S. (1970). *Movement therapy in hemiplegia: A neurophysiological approach.* New York, NY: Harper and Row.

Bundy, A. (1997). Play and playfulness: What to look for. In L. D. Parham & L. S. Fazio (Eds.), *Play in occupational therapy for children* (pp. 52-66). St. Louis, MO: Mosby.

Crist, P. (1979). Body image changes in chronic non-paranoid schizophrenics. *Can J Occup Ther, 46*(2), 61-65.

Endler, P., & Eiman, M. (1978). Postural and reflex integration in schizophrenic patients. *Am J Occup Ther, 32*(7), 456-459.

Falk-Kessler, J., Quittman, M., & Moore, R. (1988). The SCSIT: A potential tool for assessing neurological impairment in adult psychiatric outpatients. *Occupational Therapy Journal of Research, 8*(3), 131-146.

Feldenkrais, M. (1966). *Body and mature behavior-anxiety, sex, gravitation, and learning.* New York, NY: International Universities Press.

Feldenkrais, M. (1977). *Awareness through movement: Health exercises for personal growth.* New York, NY: Harper and Row.

Fisher, A., Murray, E., & Bundy, A. (Eds.). (1991). *Sensory integration theory and practice.* Philadelphia, PA: F. A. Davis.

Gilfoyle, E. M., Grady, A. P., & Moore, J. C. (1980). *Children adapt* (2nd ed.). Thorofare, NJ: SLACK Incorporated.

Hamada, R., & Schroeder, C. (1988). Schroeder-Block-Campbell Adult Psychiatric Sensory Integration Evaluation: Concurrent validity and clinical utility. *Occupational Therapy Journal of Research, 8*(2), 75-88.

Hanschu, B. (1998). Using a sensory approach to serve adults who have developmental disabilities. In M. Ross & S. Bachner (Eds.), *Adults with developmental disabilities: Current approaches in occupational therapy.* Rockville, MD: American Occupational Therapy Association.

Hatfield, A. (1989). Patients' accounts of stress and coping in schizophrenia. *Hospital and Community Psychiatry, 40*(11), 1141-1145.

Hixson, V. J., & Mathews, A. W. (1984). Sensory integration and chronic schizophrenia: Past, present, future. *Can J Occup Ther, 51*, 19-24.

Honigfield, G., & Gillis, R. (1966). NOSIE-30, a treatment-sensitive ward behavior scale. *Psychol Rep, 19*, 180-182.

Hsu, Y., & Nelson, D. (1981). Adult performance on the Southern California Kinesthetic and Tactile Perceptual Tests. *Am J Occup Ther, 35*, 788-791.

Huddleston, C. (1978). Differentiation between process and reactive schizophrenia based on vestibular reactivity, grasp strength, and posture. *Am J Occup Ther, 32*(7), 438-444.

Iwasaki, K., & Holm, M. (1989). Sensory treatment for the reduction of stereotypic behaviors in persons with severe multiple disabilities. *Occupational Therapy Journal of Research, 9*, 170-183.

Jackson-Wyatt, O. (1997). Feldenkrais method and rehabilitation. In C. Davis (Ed.), *Complementary therapies in rehabilitation: Holistic approaches for prevention and wellness.* Thorofare, NJ: SLACK Incorporated.

Jongbloed, L., Collins, J., & Jones, W. (1986). A sensorimotor integration test battery for CVA clients: Preliminary evidence of reliability and validity. *Occupational Therapy Journal of Research, 6*(3), 131-150.

King, L. J. (1974a). A sensory integrative approach to schizophrenia. *Am J Occup Ther, 28*(9), 529-536.

King, L. J. (1974b). Information from author's notes taken during a workshop given by Ms. King at Colorado State University, Ft. Collins, CO, May 19.

King, L. J. (1977). *The objects manipulation Test.* Scottsdale, AZ: Greenroom Publications.

King, L. J. (1978). Toward a science of adaptive responses. *Am J Occup Ther, 32*(7), 429-437.

King, L. J. (1983). Occupational therapy and neuropsychiatry. *Occupational Therapy in Mental Health, 3*(1), 1-12.

King, L. J. (1988). Occupational therapy and neuropsychiatry. In S. Robertson (Ed.), *Mental health focus: Skills for assessment and treatment* (pp. 3.52-3.59). Rockville, MD: American Occupational Therapy Association.

Knott, M., & Voss, D. E. (1968). *Proprioceptive neuromuscular facilitation* (2nd ed.). New York, NY: Harper and Row.

Levine, I., O'Connor, H., & Stacey, B. (1977). Sensory integration with chronic schizophrenics: A pilot study. *Can J Occup Ther, 44*, 17-21.

Levy, D., Holzman, P., & Proctor, L. (1978). Vestibular responses in schizophrenia. *Arch Gen Psychiatry, 35*, 972-981.

Lindquist, J. (1981). Activity and vestibular function in chronic schizophrenia. *Occupational Therapy Journal of Research, 1*(1), 56-78.

Llorens, L. (1967). An evaluation procedure for children 6-10 years of age. *Am J Occup Ther, 21*(2), 64-67.

Mailloux, Z. (1990). An overview of the Sensory Integration and Praxis Tests. *Am J Occup Ther, 44*(7), 589-594.

McCormack, G. (1991). *Therapeutic use of touch for the health professional.* Tuscon, AZ: Therapy Skill Builders.

McCormack, G., & Galantino, M. L. (1997). Non-contact therapeutic touch. In C. Davis (Ed.), *Complementary therapies in rehabilitation: Holistic approaches for prevention and wellness.* Thorofare, NJ: SLACK Incorporated.

Miller, E., & Parachek, J. (1989). *Parachek Geriatric Behavior Rating Scale: Revised and expanded treatment manual.* Phoenix, AZ: Center for Neurodevelopmental Studies, Inc.

Parachek, J., & King, L. J. (1986). *Parachek Geriatric Rating Scale and treatment manual.* Phoenix, AZ: Center for Neurodevelopmental Studies, Inc.

Petersen, P., Goar, D., & Van Deusen, J. (1985). Performance of female adults on the Southern California Figure-Ground Visual Perception test. *Am J Occup Ther, 37*, 525-530.

Petersen, P., & Wikoff, R. (1983). The performance of adult males on the Southern California Figure-Ground Visual Perception test. *Am J Occup Ther, 37*, 554-560.

Reisman, J. (1993). Using a sensory integrative approach to treat self-injurious behavior in an adult with profound mental retardation. *Am J Occup Ther, 47*(5), 403-411.

Reisman, J. E., & Blakeney, A. B. (1993). Exploring sensory integrative treatment in chronic schizophrenia. In R. Cottrell (Ed.), *Psychiatric occupational therapy: Proactive approaches.* Rockville, MD: American Occupational Therapy Association.

Reisman, J., & Hanschu, B. (1992). *Sensory integration inventory—Revised for individuals with developmental disabilities: User's guide.* Hugo, MN: PDP Press.

Reisman, J., & Hanschu, B. (1993). Using the consultative model introduce sensory integration services for adults with developmental disabilities. *Occupational Therapy Practice, 47*(4), 38-46.

Rider, B. (1978). Sensorimotor treatment of chronic schizophrenia. *Am J Occup Ther, 32*(7), 451-455.

Ross, M. (1991). *Integrative group therapy: The structured five-stage approach* (2nd ed.). Thorofare, NJ: SLACK Incorporated.

Ross, M. (1997). *Integrative group therapy: Mobilizing coping abilities with five-stage group.* Bethesda, MD: American Occupational Therapy Association.

Ross, M. (1998a). A five-stage model for adults with developmental disabilities. In M. Ross & S. Bachner (Eds.), *Adults with developmental disabilities: Current approaches in occupational therapy.* Rockville, MD: American Occupational Therapy Association.

Ross, M. (1998b). Groups are physical, social, and emotional therapy. In M. Ross & S. Bachner (Eds.), *Adults with developmental disabilities: Current approaches in occupational therapy.* Rockville, MD: American Occupational Therapy Association.

Ross, M., & Bachner, S. (Eds.). (1998). *Adults with developmental disabilities: Current approaches in occupational therapy.* Rockville, MD: American Occupational Therapy Association.

Ross, M., & Burdick, D. (1981). *Sensory integration: A training manual for therapists and teachers for regressed, psychiatric, and geriatric patient groups.* Thorofare, NJ: SLACK Incorporated.

Schroeder, C., Block, M., Trottier, E., & Stowell, M. S. (1983). *SBC Adult Psychiatric Sensory Integration Evaluation* (3rd ed.). Kailua, HI: Schroeder.

Sensory Integration International. (1988, September). *Neurobiological foundation for sensory integration.* Document, seminar presented at Boston University.

Smaga, B., & Ross, M. (1991). Assessment: The Smaga and Ross Integrated Battery (SARIB) assessment. In M. Ross (Ed.), *Integrative group therapy: The structural five-stage approach* (2nd ed., pp. 107-142). Thorofare, NJ: SLACK Incorporated.

Smith, D. (1993). Effects of psychotropic drugs on the occupational therapy process. In R. F. Cottrell (Ed.), *Psychosocial occupational therapy: Proactive approaches* (pp. 385-388). Rockville, MD: American Occupational Therapy Association.

Stockmeyer, S. (1967). An interpretation of the approach of Rood to the treatment of neuromuscular dysfunction. *Am J Phys Med Rehabil, 46*, 900-956.

Stockmeyer, S. (1972). A sensorimotor approach to treatment. In P. Pearson & C. Williams (Eds.), *Physical therapy services in the developmental disabilities.* Springfield, IL: Charles C. Thomas.

Sullivan, H. (1947). *The conceptions of modern psychiatry.* Washington, DC: William Allen White Foundation.

Travell, J. (1983). *Myofascial pain and dysfunction.* Baltimore, MD: Williams & Wilkins.

Van Schroeder, C., & Chung, R. (1993). Occupational therapy impacts the care of patients at risk for tardive dyskinesia. In R. Cottrell (Ed.), *Psychosocial occupational therapy: Proactive approaches.* Rockville, MD: American Occupational Therapy Association.

Voss, D. E. (1972). Proprioceptive neuromuscular facilitation: The PNF method. In P. Pearson & C. Williams (Eds.), *Physical therapy services in developmental disabilities* (pp. 223-281). Springfield, IL: Charles C. Thomas.

Voss, D. E., Ionta, M., & Myers, B. (1985). *Proprioceptive neuromuscular facilitation: Patterns and techniques* (3rd ed.). New York, NY: Harper and Row.

Wilbarger, P., & Wilbarger, J. (1991). *Sensory defensiveness in children 2-12: An intervention guide for parents and other caretakers.* Santa Barbara, CA: Avanti Education Programs.

CHAPTER ELEVEN

Suicidal Behavior—Critical Information for Clinical Reasoning

KEY POINTS

✧ Current and Past Perspectives of Suicide

✧ Orienting to Suicide Prevention

✧ Seeing Beyond the Demography of Suicide

✧ Characteristic Emotion and Cognition of Suicide

✧ Crisis Model within Broader Intervention

✧ Key Aims in Prevention

✧ Psychoeducational Model for Occupational Therapy Intervention

✧ Maintaining the Therapeutic Relationship

✧ Guidelines for Intervention with Adults, Adolescents, and Children

✧ Occupational Therapy Intervention Using a Skill-Building Model

✧ Cognitive, Affective, and Behavioral Strategies and Family Education

✧ Response to Suicide as a Lifestyle

FOCUS QUESTIONS

1. What is the significance of ambiguity in the suicide wish and in intervention?

2. How does intervention during the acute suicide phase (during crisis) differ from intervention during the long-term phase, after the crisis has passed?

3. What factors would be expected to diminish the person's ability to exercise sound judgment when suicidal?

4. How do mild, moderate, and severe depression look different in regard to the person's participation in everyday occupation?

5. How can having high performance standards contribute to a person's suicide crisis?

6. What special strains are placed on the therapeutic relationship when a client is suicidal?

7. What would you do if a client hinted that he or she was feeling suicidal?

8. Why is structuring for success especially important in intervention with suicidal or depressed persons?

9. What characteristics of children and adolescents put them at a greater risk for suicide should they become suicidal?

10. What does occupational therapy provide that is especially important to older children and adolescents who are depressed and/or suicidal?

11. What is meant by the term **activity scheduling**, and why is it used with depressed children?

INTRODUCTION

The problems associated with suicide cannot be understood apart from the theoretical frameworks that have been summarized in this text. Depending on one's theoretical orientation, suicide will be understood in terms of given compatible assumptions regarding the etiology of dysfunction, the general nature of the person, the role of occupation, and beliefs about intervention. The additional information that follows, however, is provided to help the reader become more familiar with some of the general knowledge that has been gained across the social sciences regarding suicide as a special problem.

We include the following information because we have found, in our work with students, that the new therapist often responds to the suicidal patient or client with much anxiety. In truth, we are probably all anxious when we work with a client whom we know to be suicidal. The information provided here may help the reader appraise and use his or her own intervention assumptions and to assist the therapist to understand and respond to the needs of the individual who is suicidal. We hope this information will be useful, regardless of the theoretical framework favored. We recognize that

not every intervention guideline proposed in the ensuing discussion is equally compatible with all intervention frameworks. Where we create disagreement, we encourage the reader to engage in dialogue with colleagues.

Much of the information we present in this chapter reiterates what has been in previous editions of this text. In addition, in this newest edition, we have paid special attention to the problem of suicide among older children and adolescents. Many of the demographics upon which earlier chapters depended have changed in number but not in direction; however, one significant change has been in the method most often employed in the act of suicide. As reported in 1998 by the American Foundation for Suicide Prevention, firearms are now the most frequent method of suicide for men and woman of all ages and for boys and girls aged 10 through 14.

The Need for Information

At some point, the occupational therapist is likely to engage with a patient or client who is considering suicide. These individuals may be psychiatric patients or persons who are coping with physical loss or limitations, as well as with family concerns. The therapist may be the first to recognize the suicide wish, or the person may be in treatment because the severity of his or her depression is recognized. It is imperative that all individuals in health fields have core information regarding suicide—information that includes suicide theory, suicide predictors, and basic concepts in suicide prevention. Even if health professionals are not directly providing treatment to suicidal individuals, they need to know the resources available in their own communities; resources that can respond to the needs of the individual during the crisis phase, as well as be available later for support. The student who has not already done so is encouraged to participate in courses or seminars designed to enhance his or her understanding and skills in the area of suicide prevention.

CURRENT UNDERSTANDING OF SUICIDE

Suicide is the deliberate self-inflicted termination of one's life. It is regarded as existing on one end of a broad continuum of what are termed self-destructive or life-threatening behaviors (Victoroff, 1983; Worden, 1976). Many individuals who eventually attempt suicide have a prior history of self-destructive behavior. While taking a gun to one's head is clearly self-destructive, it follows that one also can discern the self-destructive potential of forgetting to take one's insulin, if diabetic, or drinking alcohol to excess; and many individuals who ultimately die of disease may, in retrospect, be viewed as having taken quite active steps to hasten their own death. Although the discussion of suicide theory and prevention in this text focuses on the more obvious suicide behaviors and expressed plans to take one's own life, the therapist will undoubtedly encounter equally troubling instances of less clear, yet very self-destructive behavior in the patients or clients for whom he or she cares.

Suicide No Longer Seen as an Indicator of Mental Illness

While it was once generally believed that individuals did not try to take their own life unless they were mentally ill, that theme is no longer evident in contemporary suicide literature. Today, the wish to die, even if a transient desire that is not well developed, is conceived as experienced by most persons at some time in their lives. A suicide wish, even if well developed, is not perceived as a sign of mental illness as such. Stress, mental illness (especially depressive disorders, schizophrenia, dementia, and alcohol abuse), physical illness (especially serious or terminal illness), and older age, however, have all been identified as significantly increasing the risk of suicide (American Foundation for Suicide Prevention, 1996; Kaplan & Sadock, 1998, pp. 864-869; Kaplan, Sadock, & Grebb, 1994, pp. 804-805).

Past Perspectives on Suicide

Suicide has been correlated to many emotional states: depression, anger, guilt, hopelessness, and apathy. Suicide and suicide attempts have been conceived as a wish to sleep, a wish for psychological rebirth, a way to become immortal, and a way to escape the unbearable.

For a long time, the traditional Freudian psychoanalytical posture regarding suicide dominated the literature and generally dictated the treatment response. Briefly stated, Freud believed that depression is a response to the loss of a significant love object. Object loss may be actual separation from the object or, at a lesser level, the inability to be as dependent on the loved person as one wishes; it elicits conscious or unconscious rage. This anger is turned inward against the self in an act of self-destruction (Freud, 1949; Hendin, 1961; Shneidman, 1976). Currently, less emphasis is placed on the role of hostility, whereas hopelessness and loss of self-esteem are given more attention. Further, as behavioral theory, existential-humanism, and social and cognitive psychology continue to affect suicide theory as well as general psychosocial intervention, they have significantly modified the view of health, stress, distress, and helping in response to suicide. Overall, there has been more emphasis given to the relationship of the suicidal individual within the whole social milieu, the individual's patterns of coping in all areas of his or her life, and the conscious and cognitive components of the individual's actions (Helig, 1984; Kaplan & Sadock, 1998, pp. 868-869; Kaplan et al., 1994; Maris, 1981; Pretzel, 1984; Tripodes, 1976; Valente & Hatton, 1984; Victoroff, 1983).

Physiological States and Suicide

Although not conclusive, much recent study has been done to better understand the relationship of depression and stress on biochemical changes in the body. Those substances of special interest have been the neurotransmitter substances in the CNS, especially the catecholamines (norepinephrine and dopamine) and the indolamine serotonin (de Catanzaro, 1986; Guttmacher, 1988; Kaplan & Sadock, 1998, p. 869; Kaplan et al., 1994; Maris, 1981, p. 283).

Note: Specifically, a serotonin deficiency has been identified in some depressed patients who have attempted suicide; animal and human studies have suggested an association between deficiency of serotonin and impulsive behavior as well (Kaplan & Sadock, 1998, p. 869; Kaplan et al., 1994, p. 808). The focus on the biochemical or physiologic manifestations of suicidal depression goes along with the strong re-emergence in psychiatry of interest in the brain, as we have discussed previously in our text.

Orienting to Suicide Prevention

Above and beyond the personality of the suicidal individual, three contextual dimensions of suicide bear directly on the understanding and prevention of suicide:

1. **Suicide crisis** is an acute, not chronic, state usually measured in hours or days, not months or years. Although many individuals have a life history of self-destructive behavior or make many suicide threats or attempts during a lifetime, the actual crisis that occurs when one seriously contemplates decisive action is either alleviated or the person makes an attempt in a short period of time. This perspective on suicide as a crisis problem has significantly affected the current approach to suicide across a variety of theoretical treatment frameworks. This is not to say that all suicidal individuals receive only brief crisis treatment, as many suicidal individuals experience a suicide crisis in the context of general stress, physical or psychological, that dictates long-term intervention. The acute phase of intervention will focus on the person's present experiencing of crisis. The alleviation of intense symptoms is sought, success is nurtured, and the therapist often becomes more directive and parental.

2. Virtually all students of human nature view the death wish as ambivalent. The paradigm of suicide is not merely a matter of wanting to die or not wanting to die but rather one in which there often appears to be both a desire to die and a wish to live. A young person may view suicide as a solution to end the pain he or she is experiencing, rather than a final act to end one's life.

3. Most suicidal events are **dyadic** (i.e., there is often a significant other person about whom the individual is

thinking when he or she considers dying). The significant other may be someone whom the person wishes to make take notice or punish, or someone whose burden he or she wishes to lessen. The significant other may be someone already dead whom the individual wishes to join (Shneidman, 1976).

DEMOGRAPHY OF SUICIDE

Suicidologists have attempted to correlate statistical or demographic data in an attempt to identify high-risk individuals (American Foundation for Suicide Prevention, 1998; Diggory, 1976; Dorpat & Ripley, 1960; Kaplan & Sadock, 1998, p. 871; Kaplan et al., 1994; Linden & Breed, 1976; Litman & Wold, 1976; Swanson & Breed, 1976; Wise & Rundell, 1988; Worden, 1976). Authors in this field emphasize that such demographic information may be misleading because 1) it does not accurately reflect failed suicide attempts, and 2) many deaths that were in fact suicide are not identified as such. For example, such deaths may be covered up by family members or members of the community because of the stigma attached to suicide and because of the punitive laws and insurance disclaimers pertaining to suicide.

The following data are frequently cited:

- Gender: The most statistically significant and consistent differential in suicide rates is between men and women. The rate is from two to seven times greater for men than for women (American Foundation for Suicide Prevention, 1998; Kaplan & Sadock, 1998, p. 864; Kaplan et al., 1994; Linden & Breed, 1976; Resnik, 1980).
- Age: The second most significant, relatively consistent factor relates to age. The suicide rate of white males tends to increase consistently with age; the highest rate of suicide is among the eldest males. The suicide rate of white females peaks between the ages of 40 to 54 and does so again after age 75 (American Foundation for Prevention of Suicide, 1996; Kaplan & Sadock, 1998, p. 864). It should be noted that although the rate among young people is still low in comparison to other previously mentioned groups, it has become one of the leading causes of death in this age group. Suicide has been reported to be the second leading cause of death among college students, third leading cause among those age 15 to 24, and fourth leading cause for those age 10 to 14 (American Foundation for Prevention of Suicide, 1998).
- Race: The suicide rate for caucasians is nearly twice that of non-caucasians, but the suicide rate among African-Americans is increasing, as it has among certain Native Americans and recently immigrated groups. Whereas suicide rates for caucasians increase with age, the rate for African-Americans increases through ages 25 to 29 and then declines (Kaplan & Sadock, 1998, p. 865; Swanson & Breed, 1976).

- Social involvement: Any factors that lessen social contact tend to increase suicide risk. These factors include death of spouse, separation or divorce, living alone, emotional isolation within a marriage, unemployment, and low participation in social groups (Kaplan & Sadock, 1998, p. 865; Kaplan et al., 1994, p. 804; Resnik, 1980; Worden, 1976).
- Previous attempt: While the statistics vary, it is believed that between one-fourth to one-half of those persons who eventually kill themselves have previously attempted suicide (American Foundation for Suicide Prevention, 1996); and statistically, a history of having attempted suicide has been cited as the strongest single predictor of suicide (American Foundation for Suicide Prevention, 1996; Kaplan & Sadock, 1998, p. 867).
- Health factors: Poor physical or emotional health is correlated to an increased rate of suicide (Kaplan & Sadock, 1998). Poor health includes chronic or acute health problems, a history of emotional or mental disorder, and substance abuse. Alcohol abuse (25% of all suicides have been related to alcohol dependence) and manic depressive episodes have been especially implicated (American Foundation for Suicide Prevention, 1996; Dorpat & Ripley, 1960; Kaplan & Sadock, 1998, p. 865; Murphy, 1986; Robins, 1981; Worden, 1976). According to the American Foundation for Suicide Prevention, one out of every five people with manic-depressive illness will die by suicide.
- Judgment: Anything known to decrease the ability of an individual to exert sound judgment increases the risk of suicide. Judgment may be diminished by high emotionality, impulsivity, cognitive dysfunction, mental disorder, physical disorders (especially those affecting the CNS), intoxication, and sleep or food deprivation (Resnik, 1980).
- Other factors known to correlate statistically with suicide include a family history of suicide and early parent loss (American Foundation for Suicide Prevention, 1996; Kaplan & Sadock, 1998; Roy, 1983).

Seeing Beyond Statistics

Although the preceding factors may be of special significance to those attempting to identify high-risk individuals, these findings cannot be construed as a means for deciding whether or not an individual will attempt or succeed at suicide. When working with individuals in one's own practice, statistics may not bear out. Certainly, the emotional character of the individual is of critical importance; however, no past profiles or statistics can assure us that our client will be safe from his or her own self-destruction. When an individual's hopelessness is great enough by his or her own measures, suicide looms as a possibility.

CHARACTERISTIC EMOTION AND COGNITION OF SUICIDE

Although there is much variability in the person's potential for suicide, the health professional should be sensitive to general characteristics that suggest depression. These characteristics may be expressed through the person's behavior, feelings, and thoughts. A sample of these characteristics is described below.

Depression

Depression is frequently referred to as the key emotion of suicide. Although most people who are depressed are not suicidal, most suicidal people are depressed. According to recent statistics, over 60% of persons who commit suicide are identified as having major depression (American Foundation for Suicide Prevention, 1998).

All helping professionals need to be able to recognize the signs of depression in children and adults. Cognitive psychologist Aaron Beck (Beck, Rush, Shaw, & Emery, 1979) has stair-stepped depression into three levels of severity. In **mild depression**, the depression fluctuates; the person may indicate that some of the joy or "snap" has gone out of his or her life, but he or she can function and overcome the feelings of depression through some or much of the day. There may be an increased tendency to cry.

In **moderate depression**, the depression is more persistent, and fewer and fewer things are enjoyed. The decreased enjoyment of normal activities or gratification within activities is cited by Beck as the single most consistent symptom overall of depression. Often the person who is moderately depressed describes him- or herself as feeling "bored" most of the time. In both mild and moderate depression, the person may experience feelings of self-doubt and self-reproach (e.g., the feeling that one has failed and let others down. Increasingly, he or she expects to fail). With moderate depression, there may be a pervasive sense of being "sad" or "blue," and the person cries easily or much of the time. As depression increases, the person tends to become more indecisive until it becomes difficult or impossible to make decisions about the seemingly simplest of things. Likewise, motivation flags, and it becomes increasingly difficult to mobilize the energy needed for basics tasks, school, and work. This person who is mildly or moderately depressed may experience the wish to be more dependent on others and often becomes angry when others do not foster this dependence.

In **severe depression**, the person may be totally immobilized by his or her depression. Sometimes this severe depression is referred to as vegetative depression. The person may stop eating and engaging in normal self-care; he or she may withdraw to bed and refuse to leave his or her room. The person with severe depression often needs immediate medical attention because this immobility can lead to death. He or she is often unable to cry and has, instead, what are referred to as "dry tears." What had earlier been feelings of self-reproach are now feelings of self-loathing and may include delusions of worthlessness, of unpardonable sin, or of one's body deteriorating.

Depression alone, however, may be a misleading indicator for suicide. The person with moderate to severe depression may not have the energy needed to carry out a suicide wish. Suicide may be attempted after depression has lifted and energy returns.

There are other emotional and cognitive factors that create an emotional profile for depression discussed in the literature (Beck et al., 1979; James, 1984; Kaplan & Sadock, 1998, pp. 533–538; Neuringer, 1976; Shneidman, 1976; Swanson & Breed, 1976; Victoroff, 1983). These are described next.

Hopelessness

A diminished self-esteem most often leads to hopelessness. Not only is the individual in a situation that seems unredeemable, as may occur with chronic illness, he or she frequently feels shame, disgrace, and impoverishment of life itself (Shneidman, 1976). Especially significant is the impact of loss—loss of a loved one, a part of the self, or self-esteem. A person who loses the ability to walk and holds no hope that this function will return may see suicide as a way out of a hopeless situation. When a loved one will not come back, suicide may be a means to escape that reality or to try to force the other to realize how much pain he or she has caused.

Closely related to hopelessness is a disturbance in motivation. Although the dynamics of motivation are subject to interpretation according to theoretical framework, it is evident that many suicidal patients are able to produce actions on their own behalf, but they no longer experience the desire to do so. Suicide preoccupation is thereby an immobilizing influence.

Rigidity

Frequently, others regard the individual committing suicide as relatively inflexible and unable to shift roles. He or she is unable to perceive alternatives, keeping the self in a mold that others are blamed for creating.

Rigidity is often demonstrated in the thinking of the suicidal individual. There is a tendency toward polar or **dichotomous thinking** (i.e., the individual tends to think in terms of right or wrong, moral-immoral, always or never [Neuringer, 1976]). When involved in activity, the person may be able to only see occupational engagement as resulting in success or failure, not in terms of enjoying the process or the opportunities for socialization that it affords. Rigid thinking reduces the ability for effective problem solving and especially for compromise.

Commitment

Many suicidal individuals have high goals or aspirations, whether occupational or relational. These expectations cannot be moderated, and when they are not met, a sense of failure develops.

Failure

The individual feels that he or she has failed to live up to personal, often high expectations and can perceive no other standards as viable. Failure may be occupation-related (e.g., being unable to hold down the right kind of job or get into the college of one's choice). Failure in a simple task (e.g., being unable to complete an occupational therapy task) may be viewed as a blow to the esteem as much as failure in a life task (e.g., gaining employment) when the individual uses idiosyncratic logic. Failure may also be relationship oriented (e.g., failure to be a good mother, inability to sustain the interest and attention of a spouse, or inability to engage with friends comfortably). Guilt is a frequent adjunct to failure. For example, the individual feels guilty because he or she thinks that personal behavior has disappointed others or perceives the self as a burden to others.

Shame

Individuals experience shame when their failures are made public. When one loses a job or fails in school, the failure is no longer private. A loss of self-esteem and a loss of pride develop. This sense of shame may be a distorted response because the individual may assume that others have a negative opinion of him or her when they may not.

Isolation

Isolation can precede or become an integral part of the suicide picture. The person with few significant others in life is already at greater risk. Additionally, with the loss of self-esteem and hope, the individual emphasizes the relative strength and success of others and his or her lack of significance. There is also a kind of cognitive isolation in which the individual, even if with others, feels increasingly that, "No one can know how I really feel, and I am really different from everyone else." Increased withdrawal from others develops, which lessens the potential support others might give and reduces the opportunity for positive experiencing.

Anger

Although anger does not necessarily cause suicide, it is often present in the person who attempts suicide. Anger may appear as overt, acting out behavior or may seem to be hidden. Sometimes anger increases shame, as when the individual concludes, "Because I am angry, I am not worth being cared about."

Perception of Time

Several authors have noted that the suicidal individual is more present-oriented (Binswanger, 1958; Brockopp & Lester, 1970; Greaves, 1971; Neuringer, 1976). These individuals find it difficult to project themselves into the future and imagine what would happen "if." In addition, Neuringer (1976) found evidence that time, in the present, is perceived as moving very quickly. The self-destructive person feels that life is moving by quickly, yet it is difficult to picture one's self in the future.

Idiosyncratic Logic

The lack of logic or what might be better conceived as idiosyncratic logic has been frequently noted (Alvarez, 1970; Beck et al., 1979; James, 1984; Neuringer, 1976; Tripodes, 1976). What often occurs is that the decision to act is made, then the individual interprets all subsequent events as pointing to the validity of the decision. Tripodes (1976) emphasized that suicide notes frequently dwell on issues or incidents, or cite as obvious concern, events that others would regard as irrelevant (Dorpat & Ripley, 1960). The individual writing the note describes him- or herself as different from others and, therefore, not to be evaluated according to common beliefs. The individual inaccurately perceives a cause-effect relationship when two events occur together. He or she cannot decenter or see how personal perceptions and opinions are different from others and tends to think in terms of absolutes or tends to perceive all circumstances as having equal importance (Tripodes, 1976 [see Example that Illustrates the Emotional Profile of Suicide]).

Alvarez (1970) also speaks about what he calls the private logic of suicide. Suicide may come to represent to the person an act of success where before there had been indecisiveness and powerlessness. It may seem an act of great power and control, despite the fact that it leads to an extinction of power. Suicide may be most difficult to accept by those who are left behind when it is the choice of an individual whose life, by external measures, seems to be successful. The person may have an internal belief that he or she does not deserve success or happiness; or success, as culturally defined, may seem empty and pointless. When there is no major obvious loss, yet there is a diminution of self and purpose in the eyes of the self, to the outsider the reason for suicide is beyond reason.

CRISIS MODEL WITHIN BROADER INTERVENTION

The crisis model of intervention has a dual focus: 1) to respond to the high anxiety and tension that is overwhelming the client and may produce a suicide response; 2) to help the client problem solve to manage the symptoms and cur-

EXAMPLE THAT ILLUSTRATES THE EMOTIONAL PROFILE OF SUICIDE

" ...Ever since I can remember I've been different than everyone else, which really sucks."

"...me too. The school system is set up for everyone to feel like a moron. I am branded gifted and currently in grade 12. I just got a mid-80 on an exam and cried my eyes out. Pathetic? I know it is, but I can't help it. I am so competitive that it isn't funny. The worst part is knowing that I'm completely off base in my reactions to things, but I just can't help it. I can't deal with failure. And this makes me want to die because I can't live up to my impossibly high expectations (or anyone else's), and when someone tries to tell me that an 80 is at least a pass I just want to punch them. I want to be left alone, and I also want help. It's just so complicated and at times stupid that I don't know where to begin."

Dialogue from Kids Helpline, Bell Online; Sponsored by Bell & Sympatico, World Wide Web, October, 1999.

---

rent situation that produced the current crisis. The goal of problem solving during crisis is to facilitate healthy adaptation, help the client find strengths and abilities to cope with the current situation, and prevent future crisis. Intervention may include a combination of one or more of the following: (1) medication, (2) environmental adaptation, (3) education, (4) brief hospitalization, or (5) therapy sessions that vary from one or two crisis meetings to a series of sessions over a 1- to 2-month period (Kaplan & Sadock, 1998, p. 896).

Life Out of Balance

In general, the wish to commit suicide or the act of suicide is seen as a response to a crisis in which the individual's perceptions about what is wrong with the self and one's own life are not countered by a belief that he or she can somehow change the experience or change his or her feelings.

We might think of living as a balancing act. On the one hand are life's demands as exemplified by personal and role expectations, losses, and disappointments. On the other hand are life's rewards or plusses as provided by social contact and interpersonal sharing, personal satisfaction, accomplishments at work and play, increases in status and joys. Balancing these two is the individual's coping capacity. This includes, but is not limited to, his or her capacity for self-observation, insight, and judgment; the ability for perseverance; the person's beliefs about purpose; his or her values; and the repertoire of life skills (Figure 11-1).

In a time of exceptional stress, coping capacity may be diminished or may be perceived as inadequate to manage all that life demands. When there is loss of a loved one, of wage-

earning capability, or of self-esteem, then not only do demands become greater, but personal resources may dwindle. How often and unfortunate that when we experience the loss of someone we love, it is he or she we identify as the one person who could help us. Added to this is a loss of coping capacity, perhaps due to fatigue or emotional burn-out, or perhaps due to a recent questioning of values and purpose. The part of the person that normally restores equilibrium—the mediator—is ineffective.

The suicidal person is frequently an individual who has had or is currently identified as having psychiatric problems (see Mental Disorders Related to Suicide). As a result, many suicidal crises occur in the context of broader intervention. The individual's coping capacity has already been shown to be less effective, and his or her demands and rewards are in precarious balance.

MENTAL DISORDERS RELATED TO SUICIDE

In two often-cited studies, Dorpat and Ripley (1960) and Robins (1981) investigated large groups of completed suicides. Using hospital records and talking to family members, associates and physicians concluded that 95% to 100% of the individuals were psychiatrically ill. Both studies especially implicated alcoholism and manic depression (bipolar depression). More recent descriptions of practice have also identified schizophrenia as a primary psychiatric problem correlated with suicide.

It is becoming increasingly clear to health professionals that the now familiar crisis model is not sufficient to deal with suicide. Much more attention is being given to less intensive but longer-term follow-up within the community to assist the individual to improve quality of life, to increase his or her awareness regarding avenues of support, and to help the individual avert future crises.

INTERVENTION

First, we address intervention specific to adults. We then direct our attention to specific concerns and strategies when responding to the needs of suicidal children and adolescents.

Levels of Intervention

The occupational therapist may become involved in intervention at several levels. When the suicide crisis occurs with an adult who is already in a treatment program (e.g., in an inpatient or community mental health setting), the occupational therapist would likely be engaged as a member of

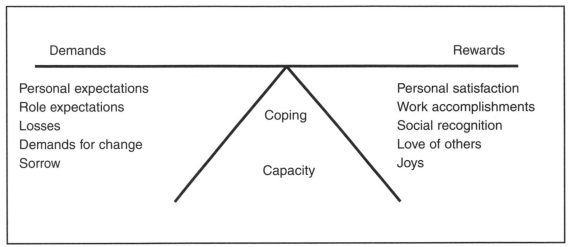

Figure 11-1. Suicide (reprinted with permission from Bruce, M., & Borg, B. [1993]. *Psychosocial occupational therapy: Frames of reference for intervention* [2nd ed.]. Thorofare, NJ: SLACK Incorporated).

the treatment team. This involvement would also occur when the individual is brought into a short- or long-term treatment program at a mental health facility, as a response not only to the crisis but to what is envisioned as more generalized dysfunction.

When the individual is a patient or client of the occupational therapist but not within a psychosocial setting (as with home health care or physical rehabilitation settings), the clinician's primary role in intervention is to be alert to suicidal messages, to assist in clarifying that a suicide threat exists, and to guide the individual to intervention that responds to the client's needs for medication, education, therapy, or environmental change.

When the individual receives crisis treatment only, as may occur through a crisis mental health program, the occupational therapist may or may not be involved. Those who are (e.g., case managers) should have additional training in crisis management (Cottrell, 1999). Many crisis centers, for example, provide crisis intervention in a limited number of sessions (e.g., from one to six individual psychotherapeutic sessions with a staff counselor). More recently, attention has been given to the usefulness of offering community support groups and activities for the individual after the crisis has abated. Although the literature has few descriptions of the occupational therapist's role in this regard, wellness education (Swarbrick, 1997), community follow-up, and other psychoeducational programs are viable avenues for occupational therapy (Greenberg et al., 1988).

Key Aims in Prevention

Attempts to prevent suicide are aimed at picking up suicide messages, providing protection when necessary, helping the individual more realistically assess his or her demands and alternatives, rebuilding self-esteem through successful experiences, rebuilding a supportive social network, increasing the individual's self-reliance, and increasing the individual's ability to identify and respond effectively to stress situations that trigger suicidal thoughts.

Ambivalence

One important ingredient in prevention is the existence of ambivalence. An individual will almost always be personally ambivalent, even when the wish for death or relief is strong. Most persons have a powerful contradictory instinct for survival. Suicide is not conceived as an easy act to accomplish. Perhaps that is why many individuals contemplating suicide will talk about it or drop hints, knowing that this behavior increases the likelihood of rescue. Although it is generally believed that most persons who commit suicide want to die, the study of attempted suicides does not support this premise (Stengel, 1964; Worden, 1976). Many suicide attempts and actual suicides are carried out with the thought, "I don't care whether I live or die." Often, the emotional stress of the suicide attempt adds to the mental muddling that may well have existed before the attempt (Stengel, 1964). The result is ambivalence that is compounded by confusion. This ambivalence buys time for would-be helpers. How much time is not always clear; however, the helping community must make contact during this period, establish some trust and rapport, and make an impact on the individual, so that he or she decides to postpone any definitive self-destructive action and to wait and see what happens. This paradigm may be changing, however, as firearms become the most frequent tool of completed suicides. With the increased availability of guns in the home, it has been reported that 83% of gun-related deaths in the home are the result of suicide, often by someone other than the gun owner (American Foundation for Suicide Prevention, 1998). Suicide attempts with guns are most always immediately fatal, with less opportunity for pre-attempt intervention and minimal opportunity for post-attempt rescue.

Mental Health Intervention

Within the mental health community, intervention is frequently aimed at reducing the person's depression. In that instance, medication is typically prescribed. These medications include lithium carbonate (for bipolar disorder); Prozac (Disata Products/Eli Lilly and Company, Indianapolis, IN) or other serotonin-re-uptake inhibitors (classified as anti-depressants), or other anti-depressant medications. We suggest that the reader check any one of the medical/pharmacology resources for details that describe specific medications, their effects, and reactions. With severe depression and where medications have not been successful, electroconvulsive therapy and, more recently, transcranial magnetic stimulation may be used.

While many managed care providers reimburse for medication only, studies suggest that in the treatment of depression a combination of medication and psychotherapy works best (Kaplan & Sadock, 1998; Kaplan et al., 1994; Murphy et al., 1995). Psychoeducational or cognitive therapies aimed at cognitive restructuring have been especially popular in recent years.

Other avenues and strategies traditionally identified for managing depressive disorders include increased exercise, participation in support groups, relaxation therapy, pursuit of leisure and personal interests, increased education and career exploration, stress management, lifestyle changes to improve overall health, and participation in creative outlets.

Hospitalization

Whether or not a suicidal individual will be hospitalized depends on many factors, including the presence of a support network, whether or not the person is able to make a commitment to not kill him- or herself, the severity of the depression, the existence of confusion or cognitive impairment, and whether or not the person has attempted suicide and/or has a specific plan. Being a danger to one's self is currently an acceptable condition in all states for involuntary hospitalization (Kaplan & Sadock, 1998, p. 870; Kaplan et al., 1994, p. 810).

Psychoeducational Model for OT Intervention

Although not describing an occupational therapy program, Kiev (1976) offers a model of therapy for suicidal adults that is consonant with principles of occupational therapy across a variety of intervention settings and frameworks. As Kiev writes, regarding persons with chronic problems,

> Personality changes do not come about in therapy sessions but in real life situations when patients are able to experiment with new ways of being and behaving. ...(and) patients can focus on concrete problems in work, at home, or in interpersonal relationships. (Kiev, 1976)

Occupational therapy is not a panacea for suicide, but by providing an opportunity for active engagement it offers the individual a chance to experience the self more successfully and renegotiate some of his or her cognitive distortions. It must be reiterated that many persons who are suicidally depressed have an apparent problem with motivation. These individuals often avoid occupational therapy as well as other kinds of participation because, as they say, they are too tired or no longer interested in accomplishing anything. If the individual is in attendance within the occupational therapy setting, Kiev's guidelines, which he termed a **psychoeducational frame** (and which exemplify an application of the cognitive behavioral model discussed in Chapter Six), may be useful. In Kiev's model, the individual is helped to accomplish the following:

- Concretize goals
- Ascertain what is standing in the way of goal attainment
- Look realistically at the feasibility of goals, including a realistic evaluation of personal skills and abilities and the availability of others
- Assess what can and cannot be changed
- Determine what assumptions and patterns of behaving are standing in the way of positive change
- Establish feasible strategies for achieving goals based on one's own strengths
- Be certain that goals suit the self and are not tailored to imitate others
- Check that goals are kept to a reasonable number (Kiev, 1976)

Judging the Self by Personal Standards

Once intervention goals have been established, the individual is encouraged in pursuing these goals to achieve the following:

- Focus on present and daily events
- Look to the self, not others, for approval
- Avoid preoccupation with detail and over-attention to mistakes; such preoccupation tends to create tension or tedium
- Avoid comparing one's own performance to that of others
- Become increasingly self-reliant; self-reliance is seen as essential to self-esteem
- Look realistically at failure and rejection. Tolerance for mistakes will be sought, and both success and failure will be judged by personal standards, not the expectations of others. Relatedness to others will be encouraged, but the individual must see that others have needs and demands that do not include him or her (Kiev, 1976)

Stress-Management Strategies

Stress is a symptom that is identified with multiple disorders, such as those related to adjustment, anxiety, mood, post-trauma, and some medical conditions. The stress comes from the person's thoughts and behaviors. For example, the person may think that he or she has inadequate personal and environmental resources to meet the demands of the situation or environment expectation. The person may not have the available defenses and coping behaviors for managing personal or environmental stresses. Some clients with minimal clinical assistance can learn to manage stress symptoms and reactions. Others are overwhelmed by the stress and may become suicidal. These people require medication and more assistance.

Anticipating Problems: Cuing into Internal Signals

As therapy proceeds and the crisis subsides, the patient or client may need help to identify and monitor those visceral changes and situational events that tend to signal that he or she is in a situation that feels overwhelming. Consistent with cognitive-behavioral principles, the individual might be assisted in identifying:

- Bodily changes that signify stress (e.g., muscles feel tight and the person feels tired)
- Problem situations that make him or her feel especially vulnerable (e.g., arguments with a spouse, loss of employment, multiple exams at the semester's end, or frustration during tasks)
- Personal responses that indicate that he or she is overwhelmed (e.g., the person begins to avoid normal social discourse, avoids calling friends, starts drinking, or calls in sick to work)

Having done this, the person can be taught to employ specific stress-management strategies. Those that might be taught as part of an occupational therapy educationally-oriented intervention program include organizational strategies (e.g., breaking tasks down into manageable pieces), deep/meditative breathing, alternative relaxation techniques such as Tai ch'i and yoga, taking time-out from stressful situations, physical exercise, journaling, and the use of other creative outlets and healthful lifestyle education.

Exercise as a Strategy for Combating Depression

Regular physical activity can decrease stress. It is frequently recommended for managing anxiety and depression. It also can contribute to the treatment of obesity, heart disease, diabetes, and high blood pressure (Bowen, 1999; Buning, 1999; Kaplan & Sadock, 1998). Adults (Robinson & Avallone, 2000) and children (Brollier, Hamrick, & Jacobson, 1994) benefit from exercise interventions with individualized goals and strategies to accommodate to the person's needs. See group treatment examples associated with the cognitive-behavioral frame of reference, Chapter Six and Appendix L of this text.

Exercise is defined as "...any physical activity that is planned, structured, repetitive, and purposeful" (McArdle,

Katch, & Katch, 1996, p. 698). Particularly cited have been the benefits of aerobic exercise, which can include walking, jogging, cycling, swimming, and lifting weights. Exercise has been shown to increase body levels of serotonin and endorphins (chemicals known to increase a sense of well-being). In addition, exercise often has a positive effect on self-concept, feelings of control and mastery, and body image, and contributes to increased cardiovascular and overall health. Evidence suggests that physical exercise may reduce the psychophysiological stress response and helps the body recover from the effects of stress (Cotton, 1990; Fillingim & Blumenthal, 1993; Scott, 1999).

People who fit the "classic" personality profile for suicide may approach exercise as they do other tasks. It becomes something that they feel that they must do exceptionally well and without exception. Therapists who work with individuals who tend toward perfectionism will often need to help these persons examine their own expectations and not create in their approach to exercise the same unrealistic or rigid standards that have set them up for stress in the past.

MAINTAINING THE THERAPEUTIC RELATIONSHIP

An integral piece of the intervention process concerns the therapeutic relationship. The therapeutic relationship is not different when working with the individual who is suicidal. The relationship is based on collaboration and client-centered principles. Extra demands, however, may be placed on the clinician to respond to dependency and control issues.

Responding to Dependency

Suicidal individuals often wish to have a relationship in which they can be dependent on another person. They frequently look to others for approval and nurture. They tend to see others as having high expectations for them and are frequently angry when others do not allow them the closeness and dependency they seek. With severe depression, this may not be apparent at first, as the person may withdraw from others; however, the dynamics will often emerge later in the therapy process. It may be quite natural to encourage dependency when an individual is in great distress. In fact, when the individual is in severe crisis, appears out of control, or has a limited ability for sound judgment, many professionals across disciplines take a parental, protective stance. Over any extended period, however, such dependency does not serve the best interests of the patient or client and tends to wear out helping staff. Being too dependent keeps an individual from realizing his or her own strengths, from accepting personal responsibility for his or her own well-being, and in a very vulnerable position. The staff tend to become drained and frustrated, feeling that they have given all that they can. The therapist needs to realize that in fostering dependency, the ultimate message is not, as we might believe, "I care for you," (though we may) but rather, "I don't believe that you can take care of yourself."

Staff Feeling Controlled

The individual wanting to be taken care of may intentionally or unintentionally use suicide as a way to mobilize others around him or her. The patient or client can further keep them there by suggesting, "If you don't take care of me as I have asked, I will kill myself," with the implied, "and it will be your fault." At times, the staff will become angry, feeling controlled or manipulated. In response, they may push away an individual who has a genuine need for contact. For this reason, the intervention staff needs to work with the suicidal individual to help increase his or her own sense of strength and resourcefulness, to communicate a belief in his or her abilities, and to help the individual look more realistically at the extent to which others can meet the person's needs. Clearly, a suicidal individual may place excess demands on helping staff, and many suicidal persons will choose to maintain a needy and helpless posture in regard to others. It can be an advantage to work along with other staff in a team approach to provide staff with support and a broadened perspective through their interaction with each other.

When Clinicians Avoid the Subject of Suicide

Another impediment to therapeutic relationships may arise when the clinician is particularly uncomfortable with thinking or talking about death. For example, the therapist may cut off any dialogue in this area. Although in particular instances some therapists refuse to talk about suicide with their clients or patients, many believe that the suicidal individual needs to consider the ramifications of taking his or her life, as one would weigh any important decision. What is essential is that the person look realistically at the decision and not with a lot of distortions and fantasies about what would be accomplished.

When the therapist's response to the individual's suicide talk is, "Oh, let's not dwell on this; let's think about the positive," the therapist may unwittingly increase the patient's sense of isolation and strengthen the cognitive distortion he or she experiences. The extent to which the therapist believes the suicidal or depressed individual should be allowed or encouraged to talk about personal feelings will also depend in part on the theoretical treatment base.

Although this text does not delve into the ethics of suicide, there are differing views regarding the morality of suicide, some of which have received considerable attention in the popular media. Readers wishing to discuss this issue might want to address the following:

- Can the decision to commit suicide ever be a healthy decision?
- Should an individual ever be allowed to take his or her life, if the decision seems well thought through?
- How far should one go to protect one from one's self?
- What if the individual is terminally ill? Chronically miserable?
- If the individual does not have the final word about his or her own life, who should?
- Who and what determine competence? Incompetence?
- What if you, with a clear head, decided you had had enough of life?

Taking a Break From Introspection

Most therapists agree that for an individual to experience the self in a more positive way, the person needs to experience him- or herself through active engagement. Further, most realize that the patient or client often profits from a break in thinking about issues that are not going to be quickly resolved. The occupational therapist will need to balance this recognition with the realization that the exhortation to participate in activity may be misinterpreted as a demand to perform, not entirely unlike the demands the individual already puts upon him- or herself or perceives as coming from others. In addition, many individuals who are suicidal are not used to talking about their feelings, whether about suicide or any other kind of feeling. Rather, the individual, as part of his or her increasing disengagement and isolation, may be very uncommunicative. The therapist must be particularly sensitive with this person so as not to inadvertently shut out the person.

Inadvertently Isolating the Patient/Client

A third difficulty can arise in the therapeutic relationship that is often quite particular to occupational therapy. When the therapist fears the patient's or client's suicide potential, the therapist may be reluctant to allow the person to participate in occupational therapy, the domain in which the therapist has primary responsibility. Fearing that the individual might use occupational therapy materials to harm him- or herself or that the person cannot be adequately supervised in the occupational therapy setting, the therapist suggests that the individual not be allowed to come with the other patients or clients to the therapy setting. The therapist might offer instead to work with the patient individually or indicate that the person can participate in occupational therapy after he or she has stopped feeling suicidal. The result can be that the individual is more isolated and has less opportunity to experience the self in a positive way. The therapist also has communicated the belief, "I believe you are out of control," or "I am frightened of being with you."

Maintaining Safety Precautions

Certainly, occupational therapy settings tend to offer a myriad of potentially lethal materials: from machinery to toxic glues, from kitchen knives to potential ropes. It can be very frightening to think that a patient or client might use something acquired in occupational therapy to take his or her own life, and the instinct might be to prohibit the person's participation. This decision, however, needs to be considered carefully. Occupational therapy offers an opportunity for the individual to begin to regain a sense of worth and mastery. Monitoring materials by making certain that all items are accounted for before the person leaves the occupational therapy setting may be preferred. It often makes sense to ask a staff member to stay with the individual while he or she is in the occupational therapy setting, not just to watch the patient/client but to provide support and encouragement during this stressful time. One may see this as a way of communicating, "I know you are having difficulty with self-control. I respect this, and I will help you with setting limits." In allowing the patient/client to participate in occupational therapy, the message is given that the therapist sees coping skills and positive potential that the individual may not see in him- or herself. The individual is also given the chance to re-establish social contact and healthy re-engagement when the tendency may have been toward disengagement. Although a severe suicide crisis can, in some instances, be judged as necessitating strong protective measures by treatment staff, when such protection lasts for weeks and months, the situation may need reappraisal.

OTHER THERAPEUTIC GUIDELINES FOR INTERVENTION WITH ADULTS

The following guidelines may be useful when working with the individual who is suicidal in a variety of intervention settings:

- **A patient/client may select indirect ways to tell you about his or her suicidal thoughts.** It is difficult for many individuals to admit, even to themselves, that they are contemplating suicide. They may fear that if they tell you, you will think badly of them, reject them, or try to stop them. As discussed earlier, however, ambivalence often comes into play. This ambivalence may be acted out as hints (e.g., the individual communicates that he or she is finishing up family business or the patient refuses to set any new occupational therapy goals). He or she may tell you "good-bye" when you are unaware that treatment was to be terminated. A person-drawing may show the patient fading into non-existence or engaged in a self-destructive act. A direct question such as, "Are you thinking

about taking your own life?" is considered better than beating around the bush and may help alleviate the person's anxiety as he or she wrestles with keeping these thoughts a secret (American Foundation for Suicide Prevention, 1998; MacKinnon & Michels, 1971). We do not give the person the idea of committing suicide by asking such a question. The person may deny being suicidal and have other explanations for his or her behavior, but we have communicated our willingness to continue to work with him or her in occupational therapy or to assist the individual to gain access to other resources for treatment.

- **If a patient/client tells you, even offhandedly, that he or she is considering suicide, take the remark seriously.** The information needs to be shared with all involved health professionals. Again, the indirect or casual mentioning of the suicidal wish may be a reflection of ambivalence. Do not assume that the individual has told everyone his or her thoughts. The individual may have chosen to share this information with you only.

- **Determine whether the individual has a specific plan to accomplish the suicide.** It is believed that the person who has a specific plan is more lethal. If the person tells you his or her plans, however, at some future time, this information may help you or others intervene. For example, if a patient suddenly disappears from the treatment setting, you may have information about where he or she would go. If the person tells you that he or she plans to drive a car into oncoming traffic, the treatment team may act to prevent the patient's access to vehicles.

- **Know your community resources well and know the steps to make a referral.** For referrals outside your agency, see Table 11-1.

- **Play for time.** Recognizing the ambivalence, try to arouse the person's curiosity and interest so that he or she continues to postpone any definitive action while waiting to see where therapy might lead. Make provocative references to the next session or the next person whom the patient/client will be seeing; the references are designed to not be coy but to stimulate his or her curiosity and to concretize the image of self as projected into the future (Beck et al., 1979).

- **Facilitate the expression and clarification of concerns.** People who are very depressed often lack the energy to talk about their feelings and concerns, and they may need much support and encouragement from others to help identify them. It is not just feelings about suicide that may need to be expressed, but concerns about all areas of the individual's functioning. For example, if a patient or client can talk about fears of failure, confusion about values, or concerns about finding a job or paying bills, there is more opportunity for the individ-

Table 11-1
MAKING A CRISIS REFERRAL

1. Know community mental health resources specific to crisis intervention (e.g., public facilities, clinics; emergency rooms; private therapists or physicians).
2. Describe to the individual the reason for your referral and your choice of referral.
3. Determine if the person is able to follow through with referral; if not, contact the crisis agency and make an appointment; identify yourself, your relationship to the patient/client, and describe his or her needs.
4. If the person is in acute crisis, do not leave the individual alone until help has been arranged.
5. Arrange for the patient/client to follow through with the referral; the therapist may need to arrange for someone to accompany the patient/client to the agency.
6. If the patient/client is uncooperative, call 911 or your local emergency number.
7. Consider the person's needs and the policies of your institution and follow-up on the referral.

Adapted from Hatton, C. L., & Valente, S. M. (1984). *Suicide: Assessment and intervention* (2nd ed., p. 10). Norwalk, CT: Appleton-Century-Crofts and Guidelines provided by the American Foundation for Suicide Prevention, 1998. Reprinted with permission from Bruce, M., & Borg, B. (1993). *Psychosocial occupational therapy: Frames of reference for intervention* (2nd ed.). Thorofare, NJ: SLACK Incorporated.

ual to clarify his or her own needs and to renegotiate distortions. In occupational therapy, as patients and clients re-enter into active engagement, the clinician may find it helpful to assist patients/clients in recognizing their own feelings about "**doing**." The individual does not need to examine every one of his or her actions, but he or she does need the opportunity to talk about and learn from experiences.

- **Expressing feelings may help alleviate stress and may provide an opportunity to reduce feelings of isolation.** It may allow you and others to provide emotional support and physical limits if needed and then begin the process by which the patient can start becoming aware of alternatives for coping.

- **Remain alert to the existence of or changes in behavior related to lethal danger signals** (Table 11-2). These factors are considered indicative of increased suicide danger, for they decrease the ability of the individual to judge a situation accurately, lessen internal constraints, or indicate that a choice to act has been made and accepted by the individual.

- **Let the individual know what you intend to do.** Although confidentiality is respected, the individual needs to know that you will not keep anything secret that he or she has told you if it is toward the end of aiding the suicide. The person may get angry with you, but you must emphasize that his or her welfare is the most important issue. If you intend to limit access to tools or materials, you need to let the individual know your reasons.

- **Help the intervention team and the individual assess his or her strengths and personal and community resources.** Think in terms of preventing future crises.

- **Communicate your belief that there is hope but don't negate the individual's feelings nor the gravity of the problem.** Communicate that you see the patient/client as worthwhile and that you believe that viable options exist.

- **Be aware that the person who is depressed and suicidal may be acutely sensitive to any perceived criticisms from you or any perceived task failures.** Try to keep the channels of communication and expression of feeling very open. Structuring for success is appropriate. Learning to deal with failure may need to be saved for the time when equilibrium has been restored.

- **Identify how coping skills gained in occupational therapy are the same skills that will assist the person in functioning in the everyday world.** Be aware that the person's pessimism and low esteem tend to block him or her from perceiving alternatives. Do not allow yourself to be put off by this attitude.

- **Be aware of the influence and interaction of other patients or clients.** A misguided patient or client may be talked into helping the suicidal patient/client gain access to restricted materials or into helping the person cover his or her tracks. In addition, when one patient or client becomes suicidal, it may stir the suicidal thoughts of others in the milieu and provide a type of permission for them to pursue their wishes. When there is a community approach to intervention, the

---

Table 11-2
SUICIDE DANGER SIGNALS IN ADULTS

---

1. Distrust and withdrawal from significant others
2. Mental confusion
3. Substance abuse (e.g., drugs, alcohol, over-use of medication)
4. Extreme hopelessness
5. A history of impulsiveness or current impulsive behavior
6. Family history of suicide
7. Paradoxical calm or sudden uplift in mood, indicating the decision to act has been made
8. The existence of a specific plan

Adapted from Valente, S. M., & Hatton, C. L. (1984). *Suicide: Assessment and intervention* (2nd ed., p. 110). Norwalk, CT: Appleton-Century-Crofts. Reprinted with permission from Bruce, M., & Borg, B. (1993). *Psychosocial occupational therapy: Frames of reference for intervention* (2nd ed.). Thorofare, NJ: SLACK Incorporated.

---

issue of suicide becomes everyone's issue. Priorities may rearrange themselves to allow everyone a chance to explore their own feelings around this issue.

- **Be aware of your own boundaries and communicate them clearly to the patient/client.** Patients/clients need to know when you are and are not available to them. If an individual or individuals are designated as contact persons to be called on (e.g., by phone) after hours, encourage the person to use the appropriate channels.
- **If a patient or client seems reluctant to end his or her therapy sessions with you, it may be helpful to alert the person 10 to 15 minutes before time is up and ask if there are any issues he or she wishes to raise.** It may also be helpful in establishing a sense of completion if you talk with the individual at the end of each session and summarize what has been accomplished.

Suicide Intervention with Older Children and Adolescents

Although there are some common problems and intervention strategies for young people and adults who are suicidal, young clients have special needs and developmental issues that are considered by the clinicians who work with young clients and their families. The following summaries related to child and adolescent suicide contribute to the clinical reasoning that occupational therapists use in hospital and community environments.

Demography

Child suicide is very uncommon. In 1993, 230 boys and 85 girls between 10 and 14 committed suicide in the United States, and only six children under the age of 10 were reported to have committed suicide. (*Note:* Data of this type often has a 2-year lag in publication, and these figures do not represent the most recent statistics; however, the data provided are believed broadly representative of the current situation [American Foundation for Suicide Prevention, 1998]).

Adolescent suicide among older adolescents is more common. In the United States in 1993, 1,560 boys and 323 adolescent girls aged 15- to 19-years-old committed suicide, representing a suicide mortality rate of 10.9 per 100,000. Suicide is the third leading cause of death among those aged 15 to 24 (American Academy of Child and Adolescent Psychiatry, 1997). Between three and four times as many boys committed suicide as did girls (American Foundation for Suicide Prevention, 1998). As indicated, guns were the most frequently used method of suicide, with 64% of suicides in the 10- to 24-year age group attributed to the use of firearms (American Foundation for Suicide Prevention, 1998). Figures are less clear, but it is estimated that roughly one in 10 adolescents attempts suicide. Experts seem to agree that adolescent suicide and suicide attempts are probably underreported, and that as many as an additional million attempts may be made that are not reported.

Among youth, suicide and suicide attempts often occur following a stressful event, most commonly a disciplinary crisis, divorce or separation of parents, disappointment or rejections (e.g., fight with girlfriend or boyfriend), failing an exam at school, or failing to obtain a desired job. As with adults, older children and adolescents are more likely to attempt suicide if they are significantly depressed or have a mental disorder or other cognitive impairments. Especially implicated are depressive disorder, substance abuse, and conduct disorder. A high proportion of suicide completers and attempters has had a close family member or friend who attempted or committed suicide. Like their adult counterparts, older adolescents who have attempted suicide have been found to have an abnormally low level of active serotonin, but this finding has not been identified in younger teens (American Foundation for Suicide Prevention, 1998).

What Will I See?

Depression

Like adults, older children and adolescents who attempt suicide are more likely to be significantly depressed. In this age group, depression is believed closely associated with loss of self-worth or self-esteem (Kaplan & Sadock, 1998; Wenar, 1994). Common symptoms of depression in children and adolescents include fatigue; flat affect; boredom/low energy; decreased initiative; poor school performance; sadness; being easily frustrated, irritable, or argumentative; social withdrawal; fearfulness; eating and sleep disturbances; decreased attention and memory; and extreme sensitivity to rejection and failure. The beliefs associated with depression in older children are similar to those present in adults. Wenar (1994) describes these as the low esteem triad:

- "I am no good" (worthlessness)
- "There's nothing I can do about it" (helplessness)
- "I will always feels this way" (hopelessness)

One by-product is that depressed children frequently cannot tolerate praise or rewards.

Behavior Changes

Recent changes in a young person's behavior that may indicate his or her increased likelihood to attempt suicide include more frequent accidents, risky or dangerous behavior (e.g., running away from home, sexual promiscuity, substance abuse, reckless driving), preoccupation with death or morbid themes, and giving away important personal possessions (Francis & Hart, 1992; Reynolds & Mazza, 1994). Other behavior changes reflecting depression include changes in sleep or eating habits, withdrawal from friends or family, drug or alcohol use, neglect of personal appearance, increased somatic complaints (stomachache, headache), expressions of chronic worry, and suicidal thoughts or plans (Kaplan & Sadock, 1998; McWhirter, Hunt, & Shepard, 1999).

Telling

Some adolescents who have attempted suicide report that they have told no one, including their peers, while other studies suggest that a high percent of suicide completers tell someone within 1 week prior to their suicide (Reynolds & Mazza, 1994).

Family Problems

Family problems including recent separation of parents, quarrels, and a history of family discord are all associated with an increased risk for adolescent suicide attempt and completion (American Foundation for Suicide Prevention, 1996, 1997; Kaplan & Sadock, 1998; Kaplan et al., 1994; Vernon, 1999).

Unique Characteristics of Children and Adolescents

Although adolescents and older children share many characteristics with adults who attempt and complete suicide, they have characteristics that make them unique. One of these is that children and adolescents are generally viewed as being more impulsive; therefore, while they too are believed to be ambivalent in their suicide wish, they are more likely to act impulsively. Another difference is that children and adolescents have less life experience and less practice with problem solving. They may, therefore, have more difficulty imagining how a difficult problem could ever be resolved. Children and adolescents differ from adults in their perception of time and their recognition that undesirable events can and do change. Overall, children have less say or influence over major decisions and often feel they cannot control important events. Finally, it has been shown that adolescents are more often influenced by peers and are more likely to attempt suicide when someone in their peer group has attempted or completed suicide (Kaplan & Sadock, 1998, p. 1251; Kaplan et al., 1994; Reynolds & Mazza, 1994; Vernon, 1999).

Intervention with Children and Adolescents

Active Listening

Whatever the context in which the occupational therapist encounters children and adolescents, the critical first step in suicide prevention is active listening. The young person who talks about feeling overwhelmed, depressed, or "rotten," or gives hints that he or she may not "be around much longer" needs to be listened to and taken very seriously. As when working with adults, the therapist may encounter such an individual within a mental health setting in which there will often be a team approach. The child or adolescent may be seen in the context of school, physical rehabilitation, or other setting in which instance the therapist may need to make a referral to another professional or agency. Children and adolescents are often quite selective about who they trust and will talk to. It is critical that the clinician be honest with the young client and let him or her know that the therapist cannot keep secrets that would be conceivably harmful to the client.

Intervention with Children and Adolescents in Mental Health Settings

Psychiatric Hospitalization

The decision of whether or not to hospitalize a child or adolescent who is suicidal will be made in accordance with many factors: whether an attempt has been made; the potential lethality of his or her attempt; the extent of his or her depression and extent of hopelessness; if there is diagnosable mental illness; the presence of complicating other issues such as the co-occurrence of pregnancy in females or of substance abuse; and the confidence placed in the child/adolescent's family and their ability to structure a safe and supportive home environment. Children and adolescents who are depressed may be administered the same anti-depressive medications as adults. Prior to discharge, adolescents may be asked to sign a written contract or agreement to not commit suicide. They also have a follow-up program, and the young client and his or her family are given a suicide hotline number (Kaplan & Sadock, 1998, p. 1252; Kaplan et al., 1994).

Psychological Intervention and Family Therapy

Inpatient therapy with children and adolescents who have attempted suicide usually begins with an assessment of the child's/adolescent's mental state, the family situation, and any special problems that may co-exist. Intervention with parents or family therapy is recommended. With young people who are suicidal and/or depressed, a cognitive behavioral orientation is frequently used. The patient/client is taught to re-examine and reframe negative beliefs and, as with adults, to recognize when he or she is becoming stressed. Role playing and group discussions may be used to help the individual learn and practice alternative problem solving as well. The problem-solving strategies described in Chapter Six (cognitive-behavior) are taught to the young client and help him or her manage current problem-situations and also increase confidence that he or she will be able to manage in the future. Social skills training, including assertiveness training, is used as many of these young people lack confidence in their ability to manage social problems (American Foundation for Suicide Prevention, 1998; Francis & Hart, 1992; Kaplan & Sadock, 1998, p. 1249; Kaplan et al., 1994; Stark, Rouse, & Kurowski, 1994; Vernon, 1999).

Prevention

The American Foundation for Suicide Prevention and the World Health Organization are among the many public agencies that advocate for greater gun control and decreased availability of firearms as an important step in suicide prevention for all age groups. In recent years, screening for depression among older children and adolescents has become a cornerstone in suicide prevention (McWhirter et al., 1999; Reynolds & Mazza, 1994). Among the suicide screening tools for this age group are the Suicidal Ideation Questionnaire and the Reasons for Living Inventory (Reynolds & Mazza, 1994). Screening often occurs in middle or high schools, with follow-up one-to-one interviews with adolescents whose screening questionnaire indicates a high risk. Many school systems bring in extra counselors to offer comprehensive counseling to all students within a school where one student has committed suicide. Suicide hotlines—made available through local hospitals, colleges, and community agencies and support lines, including those over the Internet—have grown but have not been proven to be effective in suicide prevention (Reynolds & Mazza, 1994).

OT Intervention Using a Skills-Building Model

When the occupational therapist works with children or adolescents who are suicidal within a mental health setting, the first therapeutic task is to maintain a safe environment. When the client is cognitively clear, it is not unusual for the intervention team to contract with the client around not harming him- or herself or agreeing to inform staff when he or she feels they may lose control. Staff supervision generally is reduced as the client becomes more capable of self-control. Within a mental health setting, OT intervention goals are often aimed at teaching skills that will help the client to combat depression, manage stress, and improve problem solving. Intervention strategies can be grouped around those designed to increase activity, utilize peer groups, provide practice in problem solving, and challenge beliefs (Stark et al., 1994). All of this is designed to address what is believed to be a central issue in depression in children and adolescents: low self-esteem. Psychologists suggest that low self-esteem results from the existence of a large discrepancy between the idealized self (what one wants to be) and the perceived self (how one really is, in one's own eyes) (McWhirter et al., 1999; Pope, McHale, & Craighead, 1988; Stark et al., 1994).

The strategies used with children are based upon cognitive theories that originated with the study of adults (Beck et al., 1979; Rehm, Kaslow, & Rabin, 1987) and have been adapted for use with younger people. It is recognized that children and adolescents are developmentally different than adults. Children and young adolescents, for example, tend to be more concrete in their thinking and may need more concrete examples. They too, tend to become bored with "talking" therapy and respond better to stories, games, projects, and social activities. Hence, occupational therapy can serve a very strategic role in intervention with depressed and suicidal children and adolescents.

Increasing Activity

The child or adolescent who is depressed and suicidal has typically withdrawn from family, friends, and normal activities. The goal is to increase normal participation in activities of interest including arts and crafts, games, and outdoor play. Activities provide opportunities for positive social feedback, are a potential source of mastery and pleasure, a way to increase the sense of control, and a diversion from negative preoccupation. Stark et al. (1994) recommend **activity scheduling**, the purposeful incorporation of enjoyable and goal-directed activities into the young client's day (p. 287). The child/adolescent not only identifies what he or she likes to do, but actually schedules times each day and week in which these activities will be carried out. With children, family cooperation will often be needed to support follow-up at home. Such activity scheduling is one example of "homework" that is frequently assigned in using this cognitive-behavioral model.

Scheduling Mastery Activities and Teaching the Client to Give Self-Reinforcement

Another important part of scheduling is around that for completing school assignments, volunteer projects, or household chores. These too can be recorded on a daily calendar. Because the depressed client is often overwhelmed at the prospect of having to tackle projects, it becomes important for the therapist to help the child/adolescent break these tasks down into manageable units.

When the young client completes the task (or task component) he or she is taught to reward him- or herself. Giving rewards to one's self increases the likelihood that rewards will occur and increases one's sense of self-control. The therapist might begin by helping the child identify what he or she enjoys, including favorite snacks, activities, objects, and so on. The therapist needs to determine if the reward is available within the young person's environment and whether it can serve as a self-reward (see Stark et al., 1994 for a more thorough discussion of these strategies with children). The youngster then selects the reward. For example, when the client completes a project or homework assignment, he or she might reward him- or herself with a ride on a bike, drawing, or playing a favorite video game.

Improving Social Skills

Many depressed children and adolescents feel inadequate when relating with peers in social situations. Occupational therapy task groups provide an opportunity for the child/adolescent to learn and practice skills around expressing one's needs, cooperating, handling disappointment, and sharing in accomplishment, to name just a few. While role-playing is frequently identified as a tool for building social skills, the occupational therapy task group provides real experiences in which social skills can be practiced.

Cognitive Strategies

Cognitive strategies for adolescent and childhood interventions integrate games and activities to increase the young client's awareness of what they feel and think and then evaluate what they do. During cognitive interventions clients learn to use cognitive strategies to problem solve and effectively participate in daily life.

Effective Education

A cognitive approach is often used with even young children who are depressed. The goal is to help both children and adolescents recognize the relationship between feelings, thoughts, and actions (Stark et al., 1994). It is believed that younger children are able to recognize inner feelings and concerns, but they may need help learning words to describe these feelings (Stark et al., 1994). Games such as emotional charades, emotional password, and other pantomime games or drawings can be used to help the child learn words for feelings (Stark et al., 1994, p. 285). Being able to talk about feelings may help a child who is anxious, fearful, sad, or worried about illnesses, family, or school problems, and is viewed as a preventative strategy for maintaining emotional health. There are many resources available that describe awareness and esteem-building activities for young and older children. We have referenced several of these at the chapter's end.

Teaching Children and Adolescents to Re-Examine Beliefs

Children and adolescents, like adults, can be taught to re-examine beliefs, especially those maladaptive cognitions that exacerbate stress, lower self-esteem, and build feelings of defeat. Stark et al. (1994) suggest that children age 6 or 7 and older can be taught to be "thought detectives." If a child/adolescent fails an exam at school or isn't invited to a social event, he or she might conclude that, "I can't do anything right," "I'm not going to get into the best college," or "No one likes me." The same kind of thinking is evident when the child in an occupational therapy task group concludes that his or her contribution to a mural isn't as good as someone else's, or that peers who disapprove of his behavior think he is "stupid" or worthless. The clinician helps the child/adolescent first become alert to the thoughts he or she has and then to question:

- What is the evidence that this belief is true?
- What is another way of understanding the event?
- Even if the belief is true, how bad is it?

Younger children may need the help of the therapist or other adult to intercept these negative beliefs (Stark et al., 1994, p. 293).

Other Cognitive Strategies

Other cognitive strategies that can be used with children and adolescents within the context of their engagement in occupational therapy activities include self-monitoring, thought stopping, helping children to re-examine their standards and systems for evaluating their own performance and expectations, and teaching specific methods of problem solving (Kendall, 1977; Lewin & Reed, 1998; Stark, 1990; Stark et al., 1994). Problem-solving strategies were described in our discussion of the cognitive-behavioral framework (Chapter Six).

Family Education

It is important that gains made in the therapeutic setting are carried over within the home. One strategy a clinician can use is to briefly inform parents of what the child has been working on within the occupational therapy setting and encourage the parents to notice and praise similar accomplishments at home. Parents may also be asked to make sure that "homework" assignments are done, to be empathic listeners, and to be liberal in their praise.

Research indicates that families of depressed children are often families who don't engage in recreational activities (Stark, Rouse, & Livingston, 1991). Occupational therapists can assist parents by providing them with ideas for inexpensive resources and activities that parent and child might be able to enjoy together; and where the intervention setting permits, the therapist may arrange to meet with parent and child together and help parents learn to play and have fun with their children.

Teaching Relaxation Skills

Children and adolescents who have learned to identify that they feel stressed or upset can learn means to manage their stress. Among these are deep muscle (progressive) relaxation, diaphragmatic breathing, and brief on-the-spot exercises. Progressive relaxation, in which the various muscle groups of the body are tensed and then relaxed, is taught to children much as it is to adults, with the important difference of using the child's vocabulary. The child engaged in tasks who feels he or she is becoming stressed can be taught to take a time out to stretch, stand up, and "shake out" the tension with a silly dance or similar techniques (see Relaxation Exercises for Children). Deep or diaphragmatic breathing used for relaxation is similar to that taught to children who have asthma or obstructed breathing.

Teaching Life Skills

One of the central premises in the understanding of suicide is that the person, in this case the child or adolescent, believes that he or she has more to cope with than he or she can handle. An important contribution that can be made by occupational therapy either through direct service or through consultation is in the creation of programming directed at teaching the young client necessary life skills. We have already referred to social skills, problem solving, and emotion management; however, other skills may be needed by the young client who is soon to be mother or father, or the young client who has dropped out of school and has minimal employment skills or little of the know-how needed to live on his or her own. Occupational therapists may be able to provide these services through alternative school or after-school programs, through community mental health centers, or in other settings.

RELAXATION EXERCISES FOR CHILDREN

Children can be taught to stop and take a "time-out" from stress. Sometimes that means having fun and looking silly! The following are examples of 1-minute exercises an individual child or group of younger children can be taught to do when their participation in a task or activity is getting too intense:

Shake, Rattle, and Roll
1. Stand with your arms hanging at your sides. Shake your fingers, both hands, wrists, and both arms all the way up to your shoulders. Continue shaking until your arms feel warm and tingly (15 to 20 seconds).
2. Pick up your left foot and shake your foot, ankle, then your whole left leg until it feels tired (15 to 20 seconds).
3. Do the same thing with your right leg.
4. Now, shake your whole trunk and body—arms, legs, everything!
5. Sit down and relax!

The Big Yawn
1. Stop whatever you're doing and open your mouth wide until you feel a big yawn coming on.
2. Make a big sound as you exhale.
3. Yawn again, making a noise as you yawn if you'd like.
4. By now you might feel like yawning a few more times.
5. When you're ready, inhale quietly through your nose then let all the air out in a long, noisy breath.
6. Go back to what you were doing.

Pretend Your Nose is a Crayon (adapted from Greenberg, C. (1991). *Pretend your nose is a crayon, and other strategies for staying younger longer.* Boston, MA: Houghton-Mifflin)
1. Stop what you're doing.
2. Very slowly, pretend your nose is a crayon, and write your name in the air in BIG, BIG letters.
3. Now, very slowly, draw three circles around your name, going in the same direction as the hands on a clock.
4. Next draw three circles around your name, going in the opposite direction. Remember, go slowly!
5. Relax and go back to what you were doing.

Exercise

Aerobic exercise has been shown to have the same positive effects in children as it does in adults. Brollier, Harmick, and Jacobson (1994) studied the effects of aerobic exercise on depression in adolescents and found it particularly effective with adolescent boys. Other studies have supported these findings.

SUMMARY

The occupational therapist may interact with suicidal persons of all ages. What we have provided in this chapter represents an overview of current thinking and professional intervention strategies. The reader should be aware that in addition to professional support and intervention there is a growing support base available via the World Wide Web. Use of such search words as "suicide" and "child and adolescent depression" opens the web to extensive resource material and support groups specific to older children/adolescents and adults, and for friends and family of persons who are depressed and suicidal. The use of this peer network is consistent with professional findings that emphasize the importance of ongoing support for individuals who are depressed and suicidal and their families.

Responding to Suicide as a Lifestyle

In a study of clients at the Los Angeles Suicide Prevention Center, approximately one-half of those who attempted suicide were chronically suicidal, tending to be needy, dependent, chronically depressed, and often chronic abusers of drugs and alcohol (Litman & Wold, 1976). These individuals made frequent demands on treatment staff and eventually wore out staff who found them to be incessantly demanding. In response, the center developed an outreach service that they called "Continuing Relationship Maintenance." Paraprofessionals and professional staff supervised the volunteers who conducted this program, which was not considered therapy. The individuals, post-crisis, were taught to use community resources and met both individually and in groups to engage in supportive activities. Activities included both social activities and active listening by an attentive volunteer. This experimental program, in a manner consistent with the recommendation of the Center for Studies of Suicide Prevention, National Institute of Mental Health, emphasized the importance of the gradual "amelioration of self-destructive lifestyles" with less emphasis on "active intervention to ensure temporary safety of the patients" (Litman & Wold, 1976).

Although occupational therapy and other possible ancillary services were not discussed in this preventive program, similar programming would seem an ideal place for occupational therapists to contribute their expertise.

REFERENCES

Alvarez, A. (1970). *The savage God: A study of suicide.* New York, NY: Bantam Books, Random House.

American Academy of Child and Adolescent Psychiatry. (1997). Available: www.aacap.org.

American Foundation for Suicide Prevention. (1996). Available: www.afsp.org.

American Foundation for Suicide Prevention. (1997). Available: www.afsp.org.

American Foundation for Suicide Prevention. (1998). Available: www.afsp.org.

Beck, A. T., Rush, A. J., Shaw, B. F., & Emery, G. (1979). *Cognitive therapy for depression.* New York, NY: Guilford Press.

Binswanger, L. (1958). The case of Ellen West. In R. May, E. Angel, & H. Ellenberger (Eds.), *Existence.* New York, NY: Basic Books.

Bowen, J. E. (1999). Health promotion in the new millenium—Opening the lens—Adjusting the focus. *Occupational Therapy Practice, 4,* 14-18.

Brockopp, G., & Lester, D. (1970). Time perception in suicidal and nonsuicidal individuals. *Crisis Intervention, 2,* 98-100.

Brollier, C., Hamrick, N., & Jacobson, B. (1994). Aerobic exercise: A potential occupational therapy modality for adolescents with depression. *Occupational Therapy in Mental Health, 12,* 19-29.

Buning, M. E. (1999). Fitness for persons with disabilities—A call to action. *Occupational Therapy Practice, 4,* 27-31.

Cotton, D. H. (1990). *Stress management: Integrated approach to therapy.* New York, NY: Brunner/Mazel.

Cottrell, R. F. (1999). *Psychosocial occupational therapy: Proactive approaches* (2nd ed.). Rockville, MD: American Occupational Therapy Association.

de Catanzaro, D. (1986). *Suicide and self-damaging behavior.* New York, NY: Academic Press, Inc.

Diggory, J. (1976). United States suicide rates, 1933-1968: An analysis of some trends. In E. Shneidman (Ed.), *Suicidology: Contemporary developments.* New York, NY: Grune and Stratton.

Dorpat, T., & Ripley, H. (1960). A study of suicide in the Seattle area. *Compr Psychiatry, 1,* 349-359.

Fillingim, R. B., & Blumenthal, J. A. (1993). The use of aerobic exercise as a method of stress management. In P. M. Lehrer & R. L. Woolfold (Eds.), *Principles and practice of stress management* (2nd ed., pp. 443-462). New York, NY: Guilford Press.

Francis, G., & Hart, K. (1992). Depression and suicide. In V. B. Van Hasselt & D. Kolko (Eds.), *Inpatient behavior therapy for children and adolescents.* New York, NY: Plenum Press.

Freud, S. (1949). *Mourning and melancholia.* London: Hogarth Press Limited.

Greaves, G. (1971). Temporal orientation in suicidal patients. *Percep Mot Skills, 33,* 10-20.

Greenberg, L., Fine, S. B., Cohen, C., Larson, K., Michaelson-Baily, A., Rubinton, P., & Glick, I. D. (1988). An interdisciplinary psychoeducation program for schizophrenic patients and their families in an acute care setting. *Hospital and Community Psychiatry, 39,* 277-282.

Guttmacher, L. (1988). *A concise guide to somatic therapies in psychiatry.* Washington, DC: American Psychiatric Press, Inc.

Helig, S. (1984). A personal statement. In C. L. Hatton & S. M. Valente (Eds.), *Suicide: Assessment and intervention* (2nd ed., pp. 256-261). Norwalk, CT: Appleton-Century-Crofts.

Hendin, H. (1961). Suicide: Psychoanalytic point of view. In N. Farberow & E. Shneidman (Eds.), *The cry for help* (pp. 181-192). New York, NY: McGraw-Hill Book Co.

James, N. (1984). Psychology of suicide. In C. L. Hatton & S. M. Valente (Eds.), *Suicide assessment and intervention* (2nd ed., pp. 33-53). Norwalk, CT: Appleton-Century-Crofts.

Kaplan, H., & Sadock, B. (1998). *Synopsis of psychiatry* (8th ed.). Philadelphia, PA: Lippincott, Williams & Wilkins.

Kaplan, H., Sadock, B., & Grebb, J. (1994). *Synopsis of psychiatry* (7th ed.). Baltimore, MD: Williams & Wilkins.

Kendall, P. C. (1977). On the efficacious use of verbal self-instructional procedures with children. *Cognitive Therapy and Research, 1,* 311-341.

Kids Helpline, Bell Online, Bell & Sympatico. (1999). kidshelp.sympatico.ca/talk/talk-index.html.

Kiev, A. (1976). Crisis intervention and suicide prevention. In E. Shneidman (Ed.), *Suicidology: Contemporary developments* (pp. 445-478). New York, NY: Grune and Stratton.

Lewin, J., & Reed, C. (1998). *Creative problem-solving in occupational therapy.* Philadelphia, PA: Lippincott, Williams & Wilkins.

Linden, L., & Breed, W. (1976). The demographic epidemiology of suicide. In E. Shneidman (Ed.), *Suicidology: Contemporary developments* (pp. 71-98). New York, NY: Grune and Stratton.

Litman, R., & Wold, C. (1976). Beyond crisis intervention. In E. Shneidman (Ed.), *Suicidology: Contemporary developments* (pp. 525-546). New York, NY: Grune and Stratton.

MacKinnon, R., & Michels, R. (1971). *The psychiatric interview in clinical practice* (p. 208). Philadelphia, PA: W. B. Saunders Co.

Maris, R. W. (1981). *Pathways to suicide: A survey of self-destructive behaviors.* Baltimore, MD: Johns Hopkins Press.

McArdle, W. D., Katch, F. I., & Katch, V. L. (1996). *Exercise physiology: Energy, nutrition, and human performance* (4th ed.). Philadelphia, PA: Lea and Febriger.

McWhirter, E. H., Hunt, M., & Shepard, R. (1999). Counseling children and adolescents at risk. In A. Vernon (Ed.), *Counseling children and adolescents* (2nd ed.). Denver, CO: Love Publishing Co.

Murphy, G. (1986). Suicide and attempted suicide. In G. Winokur & P. Clayton (Eds.), *The medical basis of psychiatry.* Philadelphia, PA: W. B. Saunders Co.

Murphy, G. E., Carney, R. M., Knesevich, M. A., Wetzel, R. D., & Whitworth, P. (1995). Cognitive-behavior therapy, relaxation training, and tricyclic antidepressant medication in the treatment of depression. *Psychol Rep, 77,* 403-420.

Neuringer, C. (1976). Current developments in the study of suicidal thinking. In E. Shneidman (Ed.), *Suicidology: Contemporary developments* (pp. 229-252). New York, NY: Grune and Stratton.

Pope, A. W., McHale, S. M., & Craighead, W. E. (1988). *Self-esteem enhancement with children and adolescents.* New York, NY: Plenum Press.

Pretzel, P. (1984). A personal statement. In C. L. Hatton & S. M. Valente (Eds.), *Suicide: Assessment and intervention* (2nd ed., pp. 249-255). Norwalk, CT: Appleton-Century-Crofts.

Rehm, L. P., Kaslow, N. J., & Rabin, A. (1987). Cognitive and behavioral targets in a self-control therapy program for depression. *J Consult Clin Psychol, 55,* 60-67.

Resnik, H. (1980). Suicide. In H. Kaplan, A. Freedman, & B. Sadock (Eds.), *Comprehensive textbook of psychiatry.* Baltimore, MD: Williams and Wilkins.

Reynolds, W. M., & Mazza, J. (1994). Suicide and suicidal behaviors in children and adolescents. In W. M. Reynolds & H. F. Johnston (Eds.), *Handbook of depression in children and adolescents.* New York, NY: Plenum Press.

Robins, E. (1981). *The final months: A study of the lives of 134 persons who committed suicide.* New York, NY: Oxford University Press.

Robinson, A. M., & Avallone, J. (2000). Occupational therapy in acute in-patient psychiatry: An activities health approach. In R. P. Fleming Cottrell (Ed.), *Proactive approaches in psychosocial occupational therapy.* Thorofare, NJ: SLACK Incorporated.

Roy, A. (1983). A family history of suicide. *Arch Gen Psychiatry, 40,* 971-978.

Scott, A. H. (1999). Wellness works: Community service health promotion groups led by occupational therapy students. *Am J Occup Ther, 53,* 566-574.

Shneidman, E. (1976). Current overview of suicide. In E. Shneidman (Ed.), *Suicidology: Contemporary developments* (pp. 1-22). New York, NY: Grune and Stratton.

Stark, K. D. (1990). *Childhood depression: School-based intervention.* New York, NY: Guilford Press.

Stark, K. D., Rouse, L. W., & Kurowski, C. (1994). Psychological treatment approaches for depression in children. In W. M. Reynolds & H. F. Johnston (Eds.), *Handbook of depression in children and adolescents.* New York, NY: Plenum Press.

Stark, K. D., Rouse, L. W., & Livingston, R. (1991). Treatment of depression during childhood and adolescence: Cognitive-behavioral procedures for the individual and family. In P. C. Kendall (Ed.), *Childhood and adolescent therapy: Cognitive-behavioral procedures.* New York, NY: Plenum Press.

Stengel, E. (1964). *Suicide and attempted suicide.* Baltimore, MD: Penguin Books.

Swanson, W., & Breed, W. (1976). Black suicide in New Orleans. In E. Shneidman (Ed.), *Suicidology: Contemporary developments* (pp. 99-128). New York, NY: Grune and Stratton.

Swarbrick, P. (1997). A wellness model for an acute psychiatric setting. *Mental Health Special Interest Section Quarterly, 20,* 7-14.

Tripodes, P. (1976). Reasoning patterns in suicide notes. In E. Shneidman (Ed.), *Suicidology: Contemporary developments* (pp. 203-233). New York, NY: Grune and Stratton.

Valente, S. M., & Hatton, C. L. (1984). Intervention. In C. L. Hatton & S. M. Valente (Eds.), *Suicide: Assessment and intervention* (2nd ed., pp. 83-148). Norwalk, CT: Appleton-Century-Crofts.

Vernon, A. (1999). *Counseling children and adolescents* (2nd ed.). Denver, CO: Love Publishing Co.

Victoroff, V. (1983). *The suicidal patient: Recognition, intervention, management.* Oradell, NJ: Medical Economics Co.

Wenar, C. (1994). *Developmental psychology: From infancy through adolescence.* New York, NY: McGraw-Hill, Inc.

Wise, M. G., & Rundell, J. (1988). *Concise guide to consultation psychiatry.* Washington, DC: American Psychiatric Press, Inc.

Worden, J. (1976). Lethality factors and the suicide attempt. In E. Shneidman (Ed.), *Suicidology: Contemporary developments* (pp. 131-162). New York, NY: Grune and Stratton.

RECOMMENDED READING

American Association of Suicidology. Available: www.suicidology.org.

Carlson, T. (1995). *The suicide of my son: A story of childhood depression.* Duluth, MN: Benline Press.

Center for Disease Control and Prevention (CDC) National Center for Injury Control and Prevention. Available: www.cdc.gov/ncipc.

Gaylin, W. (Ed.). (1968). *The meaning of despair.* New York, NY: Science House.

Redfield, J. (1999). *Night falls fast.* New York, NY: Alfred Knopf.

Wrobleski, A. (1994). *Suicide: Survivors guide for those left behind.* Minneapolis, MN: Wrobleski.

RESOURCES FOR SELF-AWARENESS GAMES AND ACTIVITIES FOR CHILDREN AND ADOLESCENTS

Cleghorn, P. (1996). *The secrets of self-esteem.* Shaftesbury, Dorset: Element Books Limited.

Ellison, S., & Gray, J. (1995). *365 afterschool activities: TV-free fun anytime for kids ages 7-12.* Naperville, IL: Sourcebooks, Inc.

http://ashland.com/education/lesson_plans.

Landgarten, H. (1981). *Clinical art therapy: A comprehensive guide.* New York, NY: Brunder/Mazel, Inc.

Morris, L. R., & Schulz, L. (1986). *Creative play activities for children with disabilities.* Champaign, IL: Human Kinetics Books.

Murdock, M. (1987). *Spinning inward: Using guided imagery with children for learning, creativity, and relaxation.* Boston, MA: Shambhala Publications.

Parham, L. D., & Fazio, L. S. (1997). *Play in occupational therapy for children.* St. Louis, MO Mosby.

Sher, B. (1995). *Popular games for positive play: Activities for self-awareness.* Tucson, AZ: Therapy Skills Builders.

Sher, B. (1998). *Self-esteem games: 300 fun activities that make children feel good about themselves.* New York, NY: John Wiley & Sons.

American Occupational Therapy Association Psychosocial Core of Occupational Therapy

Central to the study and practice of occupational therapy are those concepts and principles that attest to the inexorable union of body and mind and to the inherent significance of purposeful activity in the quest for health, self-actualization, and social efficacy (AOTA, 1979; Christiansen, 1991). Occupational therapy has historically viewed human performance from a broad, holistic perspective. The doctrine of Moral Treatment in the late 17th and early 18th centuries employed many of the beliefs and concepts that became the foundation of occupational therapy. This philosophy of humane treatment was built on a set of beliefs attesting to the value of human relationships, the importance of a pleasant, humane environment, and the value of daily purposeful activity.

From its inception, occupational therapy has viewed the human being as a complex mix of internal physical, psychologic, social, and cultural variables living within an equally dynamic environmental mixture of social, cultural, interpersonal, economic, and political variables (Kielhofner, 1985). Human performance, the ability "to do," has come to be understood from the perspective of the dynamic interrelationship of the person and the environmental context. Any intervention, any restorative or rehabilitative effort acknowledged as occupational therapy, must address and skillfully accommodate the interrelatedness of these internal and external variables for each unique individual (Fidler, 1996; Fidler & Fidler, 1983).

The profession has continued to develop from a deeply rooted belief in the critical importance of "doing," of active engagement in purposeful activity as a catalyst in the development of self, and in fulfillment of social membership. This conviction is supported by the concept that the innate human drive to explore and master the environment is essential to human existence and adaptation, not only to ensure survival, but to enable the process of humanization. Such a process can be understood as motivation toward achieving a sense of competence, self-reliance, social role learning, and societal contribution.

Occupational therapy seeks to engage an individual's motivation to undertake those activities that minimize disability, encourage compensating behaviors, and/or establish a new activity repertoire to fulfill basic personal needs and meet social role requirements. A fundamental principle that underlies this goal is that an individual's motivation is triggered and sustained when there is a congruence between the characteristics of an activity and the biopsychosocial characteristics of the person (Fidler, 1996; Fidler, 1981).

Seen from these perspectives, the psychosocial dimensions of the discipline become clearly evident. To speak of independence, competency, self-development, motivation, social membership, and the like, is to accept and respond to the construct that says what touches the body touches the mind, and what touches the mind affects the body. The efficacy of occupational therapy intervention is measured by its considered inclusion of these principles and beliefs, regardless of the nature or acuteness of a disability (Yerxa, 1967).

These psychosocial concepts and postulates are addressed in the developing science on which occupational therapy is based. This evolving body of knowledge seeks to explain how purposeful activity relates to physical integrity, psychologic structure, social relatedness, and the cultural meanings of activities (Fidler, 1988). Such study also investigates how these interrelationships may generate and sustain the motivation and ability to cope with and manage relevant roles and activities of living in ways that are more satisfying than not to self and significant others (Fidler, 1981).

Any injury, illness, or disability elicits a variety of psychosocial responses on the part of the individual and that person's family. Such reactions may be characterized, for example, by a hindering lack of motivation, refusal to participate, an expressed sense of hopelessness, anger, overconcern or protectiveness, or denial. Although such psychologic reactions are not the primary diagnosis, they must be understood and dealt with by the occupational therapy practitioner if intervention goals are to be achieved. An appreciation for and accommodation to the impact of the family's expectations and reactions is a significant aspect that must shape any occupational therapy intervention. Understanding the complex psychosocial dimensions of human performance, knowing which activities can best be expected to elicit the desired adaptive response, and possessing the artful skill of enabling trusting, reciprocal relationships, are integral aspects of all occupational therapy practice.

The therapeutic use of self characterizes the interpersonal dynamic of a helping relationship and is therefore an essential feature of a professional skills repertoire (Mosey, 1986; Peloquin, 1989). The importance of this skill extends well beyond the parameters of the therapeutic dyad. The development and display of an interpersonal competence is a significant component in team membership, collaboration, collegial engagement, family relationships, supervision, teaching, and mentoring. Interpersonal competence is a crucial variable in the occupational therapy practitioner's role of agent for growth and change in self and others.

The psychosocial dimensions of human performance are acknowledged as fundamental in all aspects of occupational therapy, whether practice occurs in settings such as the classroom, rehabilitation center, hospital, nursing home, or community. Such perspectives comprise the context within which occupational therapy practitioners view and address the dynamics of individual performance. These are the psychologic and sociologic foundations from which all occupational therapy specialization develops and-matures.

There is a difference between the psychosocial foundations of occupational therapy and the specialty of mental health practice. Like other areas of specialization, mental health practice is grounded in the psychosocial core concepts of the profession; but, like other specialties in occupational therapy, it reaches beyond this core to develop a specialized knowledge and expertise that is applicable to a particular population or disability.

Thus, mental health as a specialty practice in occupational therapy is the application of both core and specialized knowledge to those individuals with a diagnosis of mental illness. This area of expertise encompasses knowledge of how psychopathologies (e.g., faulty perceptions, aversions to interpersonal encounters, cognitive dysfunctions, pathologic affective states, or aberrant social behavior) impact the ability to cope with and manage daily living roles and activities. It includes the skillful application of occupational therapy principles, procedures, and interpersonal processes to assess, remediate, and/or compensate for the disabilities of a mental illness and to enable a more satisfying level of performance (Mosey, 1986). These processes call upon a specialized knowledge and skill of engaging the individual with a mental illness in selected individual and group activities that can be expect-

ed to have a remedial effect on given psychopathologies and at the same time be congruent with those activities of daily living that are relevant to that person's lifestyle.

Occupational therapy is a profession committed to making it possible for individuals to attain a way of living that gains for them and for those with whom they share living, a mutual sense of satisfaction, achievement, and contribution. This mission requires vigorous pursuit of an educational process and research endeavors focused on the development and refinement of knowledge about the multidimensional aspects of human occupation, the crucial meanings and roles of purposeful activity, and the skillful application of such knowledge. This endeavor thus includes a continuing incentive to reach a sophisticated appreciation of the psychodynamics of human performance and an artful skill in interpersonal engagement.

It is such study and learning that shapes and enables internalization of an identity of a professional self. These goals can be realized to the extent of our abiding commitment to demonstrate in our education and daily practice, a profound understanding of the unity of mind and body.

References

American Occupational Therapy Association. (1979). The philosophical base of occupational therapy. *Am J Occup Ther, 11*, 785.

Christiansen, C. (1991). Occupational therapy: Intervention for life performance. In C. Christiansen & C. Baum (Eds.), *Occupational therapy: Overcoming human performance deficits* (pp. 1-43). Thorofare, NJ: SLACK Incorporated.

Fidler, G. (1981). From crafts to competence. *Am J Occup Ther, 35*, 567-573.

Fidler, G. (1988). Examining the knowledge base of occupational therapy. (Unpublished paper.)

Fidler, G. S. (1996). Lifestyle performance: From profile to conceptual model. *Am J Occup Ther, 50*, 139-147.

Fidler, G., & Fidler, J. (1983). Doing and becoming: The occupational therapy experience. In G. Kielhofner (Ed.), *Health through occupation* (pp. 267-280). Philadelphia, PA: F. A. Davis.

Kielhofner, G. (1985). *A model of human occupation: Theory and application.* Baltimore, MD: Williams & Wilkins.

Mosey, A. (1986). *Psychosocial components of occupational therapy.* New York, NY: Raven.

Peloquin, S. (1989). Sustaining the art of practice in occupational therapy. *Am J Occup Ther, 43*, 219-226.

Yerxa, E. (1967). 1966 Eleanor Clarke Slagle lecture: Authentic occupational therapy. *Am J Occup Ther, 21*, 1-9.

Author:

Gail S. Fidler, OTR, FAOTA for
The Commission on Practice
Linda Kohlman Thomson, MOT, OT(C), FAOTA—
Chairperson

Adopted by the Representative Assembly 4/95 A)
Edited 1997

This material was previously published by the American Occupational Therapy Association in 1997 in the *Am J Occup Ther, 51*, 868-9.

Reprinted from American Occupational Therapy Association. (1998). *Reference manual of the official documents of the American Occupational Therapy Association, Inc.* (7th ed.). Bethesda, MD: American Occupational Therapy Association. © 1998 by the American Occupational Therapy Association, Inc. Reprinted with permission.

Uniform Terminology for Occupational Therapy—Third Edition

This is an official document of The American Occupational Therapy Association. This document is intended to provide a generic outline of the domain of concern of occupational therapy and is designed to create common terminology for the profession and to capture the essence of occupational therapy succinctly for others.

It is recognized that the phenomena that constitute the profession's domain of concern can be categorized, and labeled, in a number of different ways. This document is not meant to limit those in the field, formulating theories or frames of reference, who may wish to combine or refine particular constructs. It is also not meant to limit those who would like to conceptualize the profession's domain of concern in a different manner.

Introduction

The first edition of Uniform Terminology was approved and published in 1979 (AOTA, 1979). In 1989, *Uniform Terminology for Occupational Therapy—Second Edition* (AOTA, 1989) was approved and published. The second document presented an organized structure for understanding the areas of practice for the profession of occupational therapy. The document outlined two domains. *Performance areas* (activities of daily living [ADL], work and productive activities, and play or leisure) include activities that the occupational therapy practitioner emphasizes when determining functional abilities (occupational therapy practitioner refers to both registered occupational therapists and certified occupational therapy assistants). *Performance components* (sensorimotor, cognitive, psychosocial, and psychological aspects) are the elements of performance that occupational therapists assess and, when needed, in which they intervene for improved performance.

This third edition has been further expanded to reflect current practice and to incorporate contextual aspects of performance. *Performance areas, performance components,* and *performance contexts* are the parameters of occupational therapy's domain of concern. *Performance areas* are broad categories of human activity that are typically part of daily life. They are activities of daily living, work and productive activities, and play or leisure activities. *Performance components* are fundamental human abilities that—to varying degrees and in differing combinations—are required for successful engagement in performance areas. These components are sensorimotor, cognitive, psychosocial, and psychological. *Performance contexts* are situations or factors that influence an individual's engagement in desired and/or required performance areas.

Performance contexts consist of *temporal* aspects (chronological age, developmental age, place in the life cycle, and health status) and *environmental* aspects (physical, social, and cultural considerations). There is an interactive relationship among performance areas, performance components, and performance contexts. Function in performance areas is the ultimate concern of occupational therapy, with performance components considered as they relate to participation in performance areas. Performance areas and performance components are always viewed within performance contexts. Performance contexts are taken into consideration when determining function and dysfunction relative to performance areas and performance components, and in planning intervention. For example, the occupational therapist does not evaluate strength (a performance component) in isolation. Strength is considered as it affects necessary or desired tasks (performance areas). If the individual is interested in homemaking, the occupational therapy practitioner would consider the interaction of strength with homemaking tasks. Strengthening could be addressed through kitchen activities, such as cooking and putting groceries away. In some cases, the practitioner would employ an adaptive approach and recommend that the family switch from heavy stoneware to lighter-weight dishes, or use lighter-weight pots on the stove to enable the individual to make dinner safely without becoming fatigued or compromising safety.

Occupational therapy assessment involves examining performance areas, performance components, and performance contexts. Intervention may be directed toward elements of performance areas (e.g., dressing, vocational exploration), performance components (e.g., endurance, problem solving), or the environmental aspects of performance contexts. In the latter case, the physical and/or social environment may be altered or augmented to improve and/or maintain function. After identifying the performance areas the individual wishes or needs to address, the occupational therapist assesses the features of the environments in which the tasks will be performed. If an individual's job requires cooking in a restaurant as opposed to leisure cooking at home, the occupational therapy practitioner faces several challenges to enable the individual's success in different environments. Therefore, the third critical aspect of performance is the performance context, the features of the environment that affect the person's ability to engage in functional activities.

This document categorizes specific activities in each of the performance areas (ADL, work and productive activities, play or leisure). This categorization is based on what is considered "typical," and is not meant to imply that a particular individual characterizes personal activities in the same manner as someone else. Occupational therapy practitioners embrace individual differences, and so would document the unique pattern of the individual being served, rather than forcing the "typical" pattern on him or her and family. For example, because of experience or culture, a particular individual might think of home management as an ADL task rather than "work and productive activities" (current listing). Socialization might be considered part of a play or leisure activity instead of its current listing as part of "activities of daily living," because of life experience or cultural heritage.

Examples of Use in Practice

Uniform Terminology—Third Edition defines occupational therapy's domain of concern, which includes performance areas, performance components, and performance contexts. While this document may be used by occupational therapy practitioners in a number of different areas (e.g., practice, documentation, charge systems, education, program development, marketing, research, disability classifications, and regulations), it focuses on the use of uniform terminology in practice. This document is not intended to define specific occupational therapy programs or specific occupational therapy interventions. Examples of how performance areas, performance components, and performance contexts translate into practice are provided below.

- An individual who is injured on the job may have the potential to return to work and productive activities, which is a performance area. In order to achieve the outcome of returning to work and productive activities, the individual may need to address specific performance components, such as strength, endurance,

soft tissue integrity, time management, and the physical features of performance contexts, like structures and objects in his or her environment. The occupational therapy practitioner, in collaboration with the individual and other members of the vocational team, uses planned interventions to achieve the desired outcome. These interventions may include activities such as an exercise program, body mechanics instruction, and job site modifications, all of which may be provided in a work-hardening program.

- An elderly individual recovering from a cerebrovascular accident may wish to live in a community setting, which combines the performance areas of ADL with work and productive activities. In order to achieve the outcome of community living, the individual may need to address specific performance components, such as muscle tone, gross motor coordination, postural control, and self-management. It is also necessary to consider the sociocultural and physical features of performance contexts, such as support available from other persons, and adaptations of structures and objects within the environment. The occupational therapy practitioner, in cooperation with the team, utilizes planned interventions to achieve the desired outcome. Interventions may include neuromuscular facilitation, practice of object manipulation, and instruction in the use of adaptive equipment and home safety equipment. The practitioner and individual also pursue the selection and training of a personal assistant to ensure the completion of ADL tasks. These interventions may be provided in a comprehensive inpatient rehabilitation unit.

- A child with learning disabilities is required to perform educational activities within a public school setting. Engaging in educational activities is considered the performance area of work and productive activities for this child. To achieve the educational outcome of efficient and effective completion of written classroom work, the child may need to address specific performance components. These include sensory processing, perceptual skills, postural control, motor skills, and the physical features of performance contexts, such as objects (e.g., desk, chair) in the environment. In cooperation with the team, occupational therapy interventions may include activities like adapting the student's seating in the classroom to improve postural control and stability and practicing motor control and coordination. This program could be developed by an occupational therapist and supported by school district personnel.

- The parents of an infant with cerebral palsy may ask to facilitate the child's involvement in the performance areas of activities of daily living and play. Subsequent to assessment, the therapist identifies specific performance components, such as sensory awareness and neuromuscular control. The practitioner also addresses the physical and cultural features of performance contexts. In collaboration with the parents, occupational therapy interventions may include activities such as seating and positioning for play, neuromuscular facilitation techniques to enable eating, facilitating parent skills in caring for and playing with their infant, and modifying the play space for accessibility. These interventions may be provided in a home-based occupational therapy program.

- An adult with schizophrenia may need and want to live independently in the community, which represents the performance areas of activities of daily living, work and productive activities, and leisure activities. The specific performance categories may be medication routine, functional mobility, home management, vocational exploration, play or leisure performance, and social interaction. In order to achieve the outcome of living independently, the individual may need to address specific performance components, such as topographical orientation; memory; categorization; problem solving; interests; social conduct; time management; and sociocultural features of performance contexts, such as social factors (e.g., influence of family and friends) and roles. The occupational therapy practitioner, in cooperation with the team, utilizes planned interventions to achieve the desired outcome. Interventions may include activities such as training in the use of public transportation, instruction in budgeting skills, selection and participation in social activities, instruction in social conduct, and participation in community reintegration activities. These interventions may be provided in a community-based mental health program.

- An individual with a history of substance abuse may need to reestablish family roles and responsibilities, which represent the performance areas of activities of daily living, work and productive activities, and leisure activities. In order to achieve the outcome of family participation, the individual may need to address the performance components of roles; values; social conduct; self-expression; coping skills; self-control; and the sociocultural features of performance contexts, such as custom, behavior, rules, and rituals. The occupational therapy practitioner, in cooperation with the team, utilizes planned interventions to achieve the desired outcomes. Interventions may include roles and values exercises, instruction in stress management techniques, identification of family roles and activities, and support to develop family leisure routines. These interventions may be provided in an inpatient acute care unit.

Person-Activity-Environment Fit

Person-activity-environment fit refers to the match among the skills and abilities of the individual; the demands of the activity; and the characteristics of the physical, social, and cultural environments. It is the interaction among the performance areas, performance components, and performance contexts that is important and determines the success of the performance. When occupational therapy practitioners provide services, they attend to all of these aspects of performance and the interaction among them. They also attend to each individual's unique personal history. The personal history includes one's skills and abilities (performance components), the past performance of specific life tasks (performance areas), and experience within particular environments (performance contexts). In addition to personal history, anticipated life tasks and role demands influence performance.

When considering the person-activity-environment fit, variables such as novelty, importance, motivation, activity tolerance, and quality are salient. Situations range from those that are completely familiar to those that are novel and have never been experienced. Both the novelty and familiarity within a situation contribute to the overall task performance. In each situation, there is an optimal level of novelty that engages the individual sufficiently and provides enough information to perform the task. When too little novelty is present, the individual may miss cues and opportunities to perform. When too much novelty is present, the individual may become confused and distracted, inhibiting effective task performance.

Humans determine that some stimuli and situations are more meaningful than others. Individuals perform tasks they deem important. It is critical to identify what the individual wants or needs to do when planning interventions.

The level of motivation an individual demonstrates to perform a particular task is determined by both internal and external factors. An individual's biobehavioral state (e.g., amount of rest, arousal, tension) contributes to the potential to be responsive. The features of the social and physical environments (e.g., persons in the room, noise level) provide information that is either adequate or inadequate to produce a motivated state.

Activity tolerance is the individual's ability to sustain a purposeful activity over time. Individuals must not only select, initiate, and terminate activities, but they must also attend to a task for the needed length of time to complete the task and accomplish their goals.

The quality of performance is measured by standards generated by both the individual and others in the social and cultural environments in which the performance occurs. Quality is a continuum of expectations set within particular activities and contexts.

I. Performance Areas	II. Performance Components	III. Performance Contexts

A. Activities of Daily Living
  1. Grooming
  2. Oral Hygiene
  3. Bathing/Showering
  4. Toilet Hygiene
  5. Personal Device Care
  6. Dressing
  7. Feeding and Eating
  8. Medication Routine
  9. Health Maintenance
  10. Socialization
  11. Functional Communication
  12. Functional Mobility
  13. Community Mobility
  14. Emergency Response
  15. Sexual Expression
B. Work and Productive Activities
  1. Home Management
    a. Clothing Care
    b. Cleaning
    c. Meal Preparation/Cleanup
    d. Shopping
    e. Money Management
    f. Household Maintenance
    g. Safety Procedures
  2. Care of Others
  3. Educational Activities
  4. Vocational Activities
    a. Vocational Exploration
    b. Job Acquisition
    c. Work or Job Performance
    d. Retirement Planning
    e. Volunteer Participation
C. Play or Leisure Activities
  1. Play/Leisure Exploration
  2. Play/Leisure Performance
	A. Sensorimotor Component
	  1. Sensory
	    a. Sensory Awareness
	    b. Sensory Processing
	      (1) Tactile
	      (2) Proprioceptive
	      (3) Vestibular
	      (4) Visual
	      (5) Auditory
	      (6) Gustatory
	      (7) Olfactory
	    c. Perceptual Processing
	      (1) Stereognosis
	      (2) Kinesthesia
	      (3) Pain Response
	      (4) Body Scheme
	      (5) Right-Left Discrimination
	      (6) Form Constancy
	      (7) Position in Space
	      (8) Visual-Closure
	      (9) Figure Ground
	      (10) Depth Perception
	      (11) Spatial Relations
	      (12) Topographical Orientation
	  2. Neuromusculoskeletal
	    a. Reflex
	    b. Range of Motion
	    c. Muscle Tone
	    d. Strength
	    e. Endurance
	    f. Postural Control
	    g. Postural Alignment
	    h. Soft Tissue Integrity
	  3. Motor
	    a. Gross Coordination
	    b. Crossing the Midline
	    c. Laterality
	    d. Bilateral Integration
	    e. Motor Control
	    f. Praxis
	    g. Fine Coordination/Dexterity
	    h. Visual-Motor Integration
	    i. Oral-Motor Control
	B. Cognitive Integration and Cognitive Components
	  1. Level of Arousal
	  2. Orientation
	  3. Recognition
	  4. Attention Span
	  5. Initiation of Activity
	  6. Termination of Activity
	  7. Memory
	  8. Sequencing
	  9. Categorization
	  10. Concept Formation
	  11. Spatial Operations
	  12. Problem Solving13. Learning
	  14. Generalization
	C. Psychosocial Skills and Psychological Components
	  1. Psychological
	    a. Values
	    b. Interests
	    c. Self-Concept
	  2. Social
	    a. Role Performance
	    b. Social Conduct
	    c. Interpersonal Skills
	    d. Self-Expression
	  3. Self-Management
	    a. Coping Skills
	    b. Time Management
	    c. Self-Control
		A. Temporal Aspects
		  1. Chronological
		  2. Developmental
		  3. Life Cycle
		  4. Disability Status
		B. Environmental Aspects
		  1. Physical
		  2. Social
		  3. Cultural

Uniform Terminology for Occupational Therapy—Third Edition

Occupational therapy is the use of purposeful activity or interventions to promote health and achieve functional outcomes. Achieving functional outcomes means to develop, improve, or restore the highest possible level of independence of any individual who is limited by a physical injury or illness, a dysfunctional condition, a cognitive impairment, a psychosocial dysfunction, a mental illness, a developmental or learning disability, or an adverse environmental condition. *Assessment* means the use of skilled observation or evaluation by the administration and interpretation of standardized or nonstandardized tests and measurements to identify areas for occupational therapy services.

Occupational therapy services include, but are not limited to:

1. the assessment, treatment, and education of or consultation with the individual, family, or other persons; or

2. interventions directed toward developing, improving, or restoring daily living skills, work readiness or work performance, play skills or leisure capacities, or enhancing educational performance skills;

3. providing for the development, improvement, or restoration of sensorimotor, oral-motor, perceptual or neuromuscular functioning; or emotional, motivational, cognitive, or psychosocial components of performance.

These services may require assessment of the need for and use of interventions such as the design, development, adaptation, application, or training in the use of assistive technology devices; the design, fabrication, or application of rehabilitative technology such as selected orthotic devices; training in the use of assistive technology, orthotic or prosthetic devices; the application of physical agent modalities as an adjunct to or in preparation for purposeful activity; the use of ergonomic principles; the adaptation of environments and processes to enhance functional performance; or the promotion of health and wellness (AOTA, 1993, p. 1117).

I. Performance Areas

Throughout this document, activities have been described as if individuals performed the tasks themselves. Occupational therapy also recognizes that individuals arrange for tasks to be done through others. The profession views independence as the ability to self-determine activity performance, regardless of who actually performs the activity.

A. *Activities of Daily Living*—Self-maintenance tasks.

1. *Grooming*—Obtaining and using supplies; removing body hair (use of razors, tweezers, lotions, etc.); applying and removing cosmetics; washing, drying, combing, styling, and brushing hair; caring for nails (hands and feet); caring for skin, ears, and eyes; and applying deodorant.

2. *Oral Hygiene*—Obtaining and using supplies; cleaning mouth; brushing and flossing teeth; or removing, cleaning, and reinserting dental orthotics and prosthetics.

3. *Bathing/Showering*—Obtaining and using supplies; soaping, rinsing, and drying body parts; maintaining bathing position; and transferring to and from bathing positions.

4. *Toilet Hygiene*—Obtaining and using supplies; clothing management; maintaining toileting position; transferring to and from toileting position; cleaning body; and caring for menstrual and continence needs (including catheters, colostomies, and suppository management).

5. *Personal Device Care*—Cleaning and maintaining personal care items, such as hearing aids, contact lenses, glasses, orthotics, prosthetics, adaptive equipment, and contraceptive and sexual devices.

6. *Dressing*—Selecting clothing and accessories appropriate to time of day, weather, and occasion; obtaining clothing from storage area; dressing and undressing in a sequential fashion; fastening and adjusting clothing and shoes; and applying and removing personal devices, prostheses, or orthoses.

7. *Feeding and Eating*—Setting up food; selecting and using appropriate utensils and tableware; bringing food or drink to mouth; cleaning face, hands, and clothing; sucking, masticating, coughing, and swallowing; and management of alternative methods of nourishment.

8. *Medication Routine*—Obtaining medication, opening and closing containers, following prescribed schedules, taking correct quantities, reporting problems and adverse effects, and administering correct quantities by using prescribed methods.

9. *Health Maintenance*—Developing and maintaining routines for illness prevention and wellness promotion, such as physical fitness, nutrition, and decreasing health risk behaviors.

10. *Socialization*—Accessing opportunities and interacting with other people in appropriate contextual and cultural ways to meet emotional and physical needs.

11. *Functional Communication*—Using equipment or systems to send and receive information, such as writing equipment, telephones, typewriters, computers, communication boards, call lights, emergency systems, Braille writers, telecommunication devices for the deaf, and augmentative communication systems.

12. *Functional Mobility*—Moving from one position or place to another, such as in-bed mobility, wheelchair mobility, transfers (wheelchair, bed, car, tub, toilet, tub/shower, chair, floor). Performing functional ambulation and transporting objects.

13. *Community Mobility*—Moving self in the community and using public or private transportation, such as driving, or accessing buses, taxi cabs, or other public transportation systems.

14. *Emergency Response*—Recognizing sudden, unexpected hazardous situations, and initiating action to reduce the threat to health and safety.

15. *Sexual Expression*—Engaging in desired sexual and intimate activities.

B. *Work and Productive Activities*—Purposeful activities for self-development, social contribution, and livelihood.

1. *Home Management*—Obtaining and maintaining personal and household possessions and environment.

   a. *Clothing Care*—Obtaining and using supplies; sorting, laundering (hand, machine, and dry clean); folding; ironing; storing; and mending.

   b. *Cleaning*—Obtaining and using supplies; picking up; putting away; vacuuming; sweeping and mopping floors; dusting; polishing; scrubbing; washing windows; cleaning mirrors; making beds; and removing trash and recyclables.

   c. *Meal Preparation and Cleanup*—Planning nutritious meals; preparing and serving food; opening and closing containers, cabinets and drawers; using kitchen utensils and appliances; cleaning up and storing food safely.

   d. *Shopping*—Preparing shopping lists (grocery and other); selecting and purchasing items; selecting method of payment; and completing money transactions.

   e. *Money Management*—Budgeting, paying bills, and using bank systems.

   f. *Household Maintenance*—Maintaining home, yard, garden, appliances, vehicles, and household items.

   g. *Safety Procedures*—Knowing and performing preventive and emergency procedures to maintain a safe environment and to prevent injuries.

2. *Care of Others*—Providing for children, spouse, parents, pets, or others, such as giving physical care, nurturing, communicating, and using age-appropriate activities.

3. *Educational Activities*—Participating in a learning environment through school, community, or work-sponsored activities, such as exploring educational interests, attending to instruction, managing assignments, and contributing to group experiences.

4. *Vocational Activities*—Participating in work-related activities.

   a. *Vocational Exploration*—Determining aptitudes; developing interests and skills, and selecting appropriate vocational pursuits.

   b. *Job Acquisition*—Identifying and selecting work opportunities, and completing application and interview processes.

   c. *Work or Job Performance*—Performing job tasks in a timely and effective manner; incorporating necessary work behaviors.

   d. *Retirement Planning*—Determining aptitudes; developing interests and skills; and selecting appropriate avocational pursuits.

   e. *Volunteer Participation*—Performing unpaid activities for the benefit of selected individuals, groups, or causes.

C. *Play or Leisure Activities*—Intrinsically motivating activities for amusement, relaxation, spontaneous enjoyment, or self-expression.

1. *Play or Leisure Exploration*—Identifying interests, skills, opportunities, and appropriate play or leisure activities.

2. *Play or Leisure Performance*—Planning and participating in play or leisure activities. Maintaining a balance of play or leisure activities with work and productive activities, and activities of daily living. Obtaining, utilizing, and maintaining equipment and supplies.

II. Performance Components

A. *Sensorimotor Component*—The ability to receive input, process information, and produce output.

1. *Sensory*

   a. *Sensory Awareness*—Receiving and differentiating sensory stimuli.

   b. *Sensory Processing*—Interpreting sensory stimuli:

   (1) *Tactile*—Interpreting light touch, pressure, temperature, pain, and vibration through skin contact/receptors.

   (2) *Proprioceptive*—Interpreting stimuli originating in muscles, joints, and other internal tissues that give information about the position of one body part in relation to another.

   (3) *Vestibular*—Interpreting stimuli from the inner ear receptors regarding head position and movement.

   (4) *Visual*—Interpreting stimuli through the eyes, including peripheral vision and acuity, and awareness of color and pattern.

   (5) *Auditory*—Interpreting and localizing sounds, and discriminating background sounds.

   (6) *Gustatory*—Interpreting tastes.

   (7) *Olfactory*—Interpreting odors.

   c. *Perceptual Processing*—Organizing sensory input into meaningful patterns.

   (1) *Stereognosis*—Identifying objects through proprioception, cognition, and the sense of touch.

(2) *Kinesthesia*—Identifying the excursion and direction of joint movement.

(3) *Pain Response*—Interpreting noxious stimuli.

(4) *Body Scheme*—Acquiring an internal awareness of the body and the relationship of body parts to each other.

(5) *Right-Left Discrimination*—Differentiating one side from the other

(6) *Form Constancy*—Recognizing forms and objects as the same in various environments, positions, and sizes.

(7) *Position in Space*—Determining the spatial relationship of figures and objects to self or other forms and objects.

(8) *Visual-Closure*—Identifying forms or objects from incomplete presentations.

(9) *Figure Ground*—Differentiating between foreground and background forms and objects.

(10) *Depth Perception*—Determining the relative distance between objects, figures, or land marks and the observer, and changes in planes of surfaces.

(11) *Spatial Relations*—Determining the position of objects relative to each other.

(12) *Topographical Orientation*—Determining the location of objects and settings and the route to the location.

2. *Neuromusculoskeletal*

a. *Reflex*—Eliciting an involuntary muscle response by sensory input.

b. *Range of Motion*—Moving body parts through an arc.

c. *Muscle Tone*—Demonstrating a degree of tension or resistance in a muscle at rest and in response to stretch.

d. *Strength*—Demonstrating a degree of muscle power when movement is resisted, as with objects or gravity.

e. *Endurance*—Sustaining cardiac, pulmonary, and musculoskeletal exertion over time.

f. *Postural Control*—Using righting and equilibrium adjustments to maintain balance during functional movements.

g. *Postural Alignment*—Maintaining biomechanical integrity among body parts.

h. *Soft Tissue Integrity*—Maintaining anatomical and physiological condition of interstitial tissue and skin.

3. *Motor*

a. *Gross Coordination*—Using large muscle groups for controlled, goal-directed movements.

b. *Crossing the Midline*—Moving limbs and eyes across the midsagittal plane of the body.

c. *Laterality*—Using a preferred unilateral body part for activities requiring a high level of skill.

d. *Bilateral Integration*—Coordinating both body sides during activity.

e. *Motor Control*—Using the body in functional and versatile movement patterns.

f. *Praxis*—Conceiving and planning a new motor act in response to an environmental demand.

g. *Fine Coordination/Dexterity*—Using small muscle groups for controlled movements, particularly in object manipulation.

h. *Visual-Motor Integration*—Coordinating the interaction of information from the eyes with body movement during activity.

i. *Oral-Motor Control*—Coordinating oropharyngeal musculature for controlled movements.

B. *Cognitive Integration and Cognitive Components*—The ability to use higher brain functions.

1. *Level of Arousal*—Demonstrating alertness and responsiveness to environmental stimuli.

2. *Orientation*—Identifying person, place, time, and situation.

3. *Recognition*—Identifying familiar faces, objects, and other previously presented materials.

4. *Attention Span*—Focusing on a task over time.

5. *Initiation of Activity*—Starting a physical or mental activity.

6. *Termination of Activity*—Stopping an activity at an appropriate time.

7. *Memory*—Recalling information after brief or long periods of time.

8. *Sequencing*—Placing information, concepts, and actions in order.

9. *Categorization*—Identifying similarities of and differences among pieces of environmental information.

10. *Concept Formation*—Organizing a variety of information to form thoughts and ideas.

11. *Spatial Operations*—Mentally manipulating the position of objects in various relationships.

12. *Problem Solving*—Recognizing a problem, defining a problem, identifying alternative plans, selecting a plan, organizing steps in a plan, implementing a plan, and evaluating the outcome.

13. *Learning*—Acquiring new concepts and behaviors.

14. *Generalization*—Applying previously learned concepts and behaviors to a variety of new situations.

C. *Psychosocial Skills and Psychological Components*—The ability to interact in society and to process emotions.

1. *Psychological*

a. *Values*—Identifying ideas or beliefs that are important to self and others.

b. *Interests*—Identifying mental or physical activities that create pleasure and maintain attention.

c. *Self-Concept*—Developing the value of the physical, emotional, and sexual self.

2. *Social*

a. *Role Performance*—Identifying, maintaining, and balancing functions one assumes or acquires in society (e.g., worker, student, parent, friend, religious participant).

b. *Social Conduct*—Interacting using manners, personal space, eye contact, gestures, active listening, and self-expression appropriate to one's environment.

c. *Interpersonal Skills*—Using verbal and nonverbal communication to interact in a variety of settings.

d. *Self-Expression*—Using a variety of styles and skills to express thoughts, feelings, and needs.

3. *Self-Management*

a. *Coping Skills*—Identifying and managing stress and related reactors.

b. *Time Management*—Planning and participating in a balance of self-care, work, leisure, and rest activities to promote satisfaction and health.

c. *Self-Control*—Modifying one's own behavior in response to environmental needs, demands, constraints, personal aspirations, and feedback from others.

III. Performance Contexts

Assessment of function in performance areas is greatly influenced by the contexts in which the individual must perform. Occupational therapy practitioners consider performance contexts when determining feasibility and appropriateness of interventions.

Occupational therapy practitioners may choose interventions based on an understanding of contexts, or may choose interventions directly aimed at altering the contexts to improve performance.

A. *Temporal Aspects*

1. *Chronological*—Individual's age.

2. *Developmental*—Stage or phase of maturation.

3. *Life Cycle*—Place in important life phases, such as career cycle, parenting cycle, or educational process.

4. *Disability Status*—Place in continuum of disability, such as acuteness of injury, chronicity of disability, or terminal nature of illness.

B. *Environmental Aspects*

1. *Physical*—Nonhuman aspects of contexts. Includes the accessibility to and performance within environments having natural terrain, plants, animals, buildings, furniture, objects, tools, or devices.

2. *Social*—Availability and expectations of significant individuals, such as spouse, friends, and caregivers. Also includes larger social groups which are influential in establishing norms, role expectations, and social routines.

3. *Cultural*—Customs, beliefs, activity patterns, behavior standards, and expectations accepted by the society of which the individual is a member. Includes political aspects, such as laws that affect access to resources and affirm personal rights. Also includes opportunities for education, employment, and economic support.

REFERENCES

American Occupational Therapy Association. (1979). *Occupational therapy output reporting system and uniform terminology for reporting occupational therapy services.* Rockville, MD: Author.

American Occupational Therapy Association. (1989). Uniform Terminology for occupational therapy (2nd ed.). *Am J Occup Ther, 43*, 808-815.

American Occupational Therapy Association. (1993). Definition of occupational therapy practice for state regulation (Policy 5.3.1). *Am J Occup Ther, 47*, 1117-1121.

Authors

The Terminology Task Force:
Winifred Dunn, PhD, OTR, FAOTA—Chairperson
Mary Foto, OTR, FAOTA
Jim Hinojosa, PhD, OTR, FAOTA
Barbara A. Boyt Schell, PhD, OTR/L, FAOTA
Linda Kohlman Thomson, MOT, OTR, OT(C), FAOTA
Sarah D. Hertfelder, MEd, MOT, OTR/L—Staff
  Liason for the Commission on Practice
Jim Hinojosa, PhD, OTR, FAOTA—Chairperson

Adopted by the Representative Assembly July 1994.

Note: This document replaces the following documents, all of which were rescinded by the 1994 Representative Assembly:

Occupational Therapy Product Output Reporting System (1979)

Uniform Terminology for Reporting Occupational Therapy Services—First Edition (1979)

Uniform Occupational Therapy Evaluation Checklist (1981)

Uniform Terminology for Occupational Therapy—Second Edition (1989)

Life Developmental Tasks

Life Stage Process	Developmental Tasks	Psychosocial Crisis	Central Process
Infancy (birth to 2 years)	1. Social attachment 2. Sensorimotor primitive intelligence causality 3. Object permanence 4. Maturation of motor functions	Trust versus mistrust	Mutuality with the caregiver
Toddlerhood (2 to 4 yrs)	1. Self-control 2. Language development 3. Fantasy and play 4. Elaboration of locomotion	Autonomy versus shame and doubt	Imitation
Early school age (5 to 7 yrs)	1. Sex role identification 2. Early moral development 3. Concrete operations 4. Group play	Initiative versus guilt	Identification
Middle school age (8 to 12 yrs)	1. Social cooperation 2. Self-evaluation 3. Skill learning 4. Team play	Industry versus inferiority	Education
Early adolescence (13 to 17 yrs)	1. Physical maturation 2. Formal operations 3. Membership in the peer group 4. Heterosexual relationships	Group identity versus alienation	Peer pressure

Life Stage Process	*Developmental Tasks*	*Psychosocial Crisis*	*Central Process*
Later adolescence (18 to 22 yrs)	1. Autonomy from parents 2. Sex role identity 3. Internalized morality 4. Career choice	Individual identity versus role diffusion	Role experimentation
Early adulthood (23 to 30 yrs)	1. Marriage 2. Childbearing 3. Work 4. Lifestyle	Intimacy versus isolation	Mutuality among peers
Middle adulthood (31 to 50 yrs)	1. Management of the houselhold 2. Childrearing 3. Management of a career	Generativity versus stagnation	Person environment fit and creativity
Later adulthood (51 and older)	1. Redirection of energy to new roles 2. Acceptance of one's life 3. Developing a point of view about death	Integrity versus despair	Introspection

Adapted from Newman and Newman. (1979). *Development through life: A psychosocial approach* (pp. 30-31). Homewood, IL: The Dorsey Press. Reprinted with permission from Bruce, M., & Borg, B. (1993). *Psychosocial occupational therapy: Frames of reference for intervention* (2nd ed.). Thorofare, NJ: SLACK Incorporated.

Key Elements of Person-Environment Models

Theorist	How Is the Person Conceptualized?	How Is the Environment Conceived?	Person-Environment Interaction (Adaptation)	OT Application
Baker and Intagliata	Individual: • physical status • mental status • needs • knowledge	The individual's perceived or experienced environment and the actual environment	The individual responds as: • active participant or instinctive responder	• Focus on client perceptions of environment and quality of life • Clients with mental health problems
Bronfenbrenner	Individual: • as a social agent seeks and creates meaning in social environment	Social and cultural milieu of the individual	Interdependence: • change in one domain of social environment effects change in another domain	Emphasis on client's social environment (e.g., family interventions, pediatric practice, social development)
Bandura	Individual: • six basic cognitive capacities	The individual's perceptions of the environment are key	Perceived self-efficacy: • person's perceptions of his or her ability to be successful in an activity in a particular environment	• Focus on environmental perceptions • Encourages consultation with clients

Theorist	How Is the Person Conceptualized?	How Is the Environment Conceived?	Person-Environment Interaction (Adaptation)	OT Application
Gibson and Gibson	Individual: • as a developing curious, motivated learner • task oriented • perception	• The context or surroundings of the individual • Supportive or constraining (affordance)	Interdependence: • personal activities matched to affordable environment	Child development in the context of his or her surroundings
Mandala of Health	Community: • distinctive needs of community • social policy	biological physical cultural economic	Social and political implications of health Need to change environment not people	Community health advocacy
Kahana	Individual: • needs • preferences	The social characteristics of the residential setting	Congruence: • the well-being and function of the individual • individual choice of environment	• Discharge planning, particularly with older adults • Social environments
Kaplan	Individual: • the internal organization of incoming information about the enviromnent	Individual: • opportunities • choices	Temporal flexibility: • to each experience one brings memories of past experiences whlch affect perception and anticipation	• General practice • Psychiatric environments
Lawton	Individual: • the person possesses a set of abilities, which constitute competence	Environmental press: • the forces in the environment in terms of their demand character-istics	Two possible responses: • adaptive behavior whether + or - • affective response	Gerontology and frail individuals

Theorist	How Is the Person Conceptualized?	How Is the Environment Conceived?	Person-Environment Interaction (Adaptation)	OT Application
Moos	Group of persons: • residing in an institutional setting • sociodemographics • self-concept • health factors • functional abilities	Environmental system consisting of: • physical factors • policy factors • suprapersonal factors • social climate factors	Stability and change within the institution for well-being of residents and staff	Assessing institutions and sheltered-care environments
Weisman	Employees	Physical setting: • properties • components Organizations: • policy • objective	Congruence: • manipulation of the physical environment to ensure that the policies and objectives of the organization are met	Work environments

Reprinted with permission from Christiansen, C., & Baum, C. (1997). *Occupational therapy: Enabling function and well-being* (2nd ed., pp. 77-78). Thorofare, NJ: SLACK Incorporated.
Note: See Chapter 2 for sources and references.

Occupational Therapy Code of Ethics

Preamble

The American Occupational Therapy Association's Code of Ethics is a public statement of the common set of values and principles used to promote and maintain high standards of behavior in occupational therapy. The American Occupational Therapy Association and its members are committed to furthering the ability of individuals, groups, and systems to function within their total environment. To this end, occupational therapy personnel (including all staff and personnel who work and assist in providing occupational therapy services [e.g., aides, orderlies, secretaries, technicians]) have a responsibility to provide services to recipients in any stage of health and illness who are individuals, research participants, institutions and businesses, other professionals and colleagues, students, and to the general public.

The *Occupational Therapy Code of Ethics* is a set of principles that applies to occupational therapy personnel at all levels. These principles to which occupational therapists and occupational therapy assistants aspire are part of a lifelong effort to act in an ethical manner. The various roles of practitioner (occupational therapist and occupational therapy assistant), educator, fieldwork educator, clinical supervisor, manager, administrator, consultant, fieldwork coordinator, faculty program director, researcher/scholar, private practice owner, entrepreneur, and student are assumed.

Any action in violation of the spirit and purpose of this Code shall be considered unethical. To ensure compliance with the Code, the Commission on Standards and Ethics (SEC) establishes and maintains the enforcement procedures. Acceptance of membership in the American Occupational Therapy Association commits members to adherence to the Code of Ethics and its enforcement procedures. The *Code of Ethics, Core Values and Attitudes of Occupational Therapy Practice* (AOTA, 1993), and the *Guidelines to the Occupational Therapy Code of Ethics* (AOTA, 1998) are aspirational documents designed to be used together to guide occupational therapy personnel.

Principle 1. Occupational therapy personnel shall demonstrate a concern for the well being of the recipients of their services. (beneficence)

A. Occupational therapy personnel shall provide services in a fair and equitable manner. They shall recognize and appreciate the cultural components of economics, geography, race, ethnicity, religious and political factors, marital status, sexual orientation, and disability of all recipients of their services.

B. Occupational therapy practitioners shall strive to ensure that fees are fair and reasonable and commensurate with services performed. When occupational therapy practitioners set fees, they shall set fees considering institutional, local, state, and federal requirements, and with due regard for the service recipient's ability to pay.

C. Occupational therapy personnel shall make every effort to advocate for recipients to obtain needed services through available means.

Principle 2. Occupational therapy personnel shall take reasonable precautions to avoid imposing or inflicting harm upon the recipient of services or to his or her property. (non-maleficence)

A. Occupational therapy personnel shall maintain relationships that do not exploit the recipient of services sexually, physically, emotionally, financially, socially, or in any other manner.

B. Occupational therapy practitioners shall avoid relationships or activities that interfere with professional judgment and objectivity.

Principle 3. Occupational therapy personnel shall respect the recipient and/or their surrogate(s) as well as the recipient's rights. (autonomy, privacy, confidentiality)

A. Occupational therapy practitioners shall collaborate with service recipients or their surrogate(s) in setting goals and priorities throughout the intervention process.

B. Occupational therapy practitioners shall fully inform the service recipients of the nature, risks, and potential outcomes of any interventions.

C. Occupational therapy practitioners shall obtain informed consent from participants involved in research activities and indicate that they have fully informed and advised the participants of potential risks and outcomes. Occupational therapy practitioners shall endeavor to ensure that the participant(s) comprehend these risks and outcomes.

D. Occupational therapy personnel shall respect the individual's right to refuse professional services or involvement in research or educational activities.

E. Occupational therapy personnel shall protect all privileged confidential forms of written, verbal, and electronic communication gained from educational, practice, research, and investigational activities unless otherwise mandated by local, state, or federal regulations.

Principle 4. Occupational therapy personnel shall achieve and continually maintain high standards of competence. (duties)

A. Occupational therapy practitioners shall hold the appropriate national and state credentials for the services they provide.

B. Occupational therapy practitioners shall use procedures that conform to the standards of practice and other appropriate AOTA documents relevant to practice.

C. Occupational therapy practitioners shall take responsibility for maintaining and documenting competence by participating in professional development and educational activities.

D. Occupational therapy practitioners shall critically examine and keep current with emerging knowledge relevant to their practice so they may perform their duties on the basis of accurate information.

E. Occupational therapy practitioners shall protect service recipients by ensuring that duties assumed by or assigned to other occupational therapy personnel match credentials, qualifications, experience, and scope of practice.

F. Occupational therapy practitioners shall provide appropriate supervision to individuals for whom the practitioners have supervisory responsibility in accor-

dance with Association policies, local, state and federal laws, and institutional values.

G. Occupational therapy practitioners shall refer to or consult with other service providers whenever such a referral or consultation would be helpful to the care of the recipient of service. The referral or consultation process should be done in collaboration with the recipient of service.

Principle 5. Occupational therapy personnel shall comply with laws and Association policies guiding the profession of occupational therapy. (justice)

A. Occupational therapy personnel shall familiarize themselves with and seek to understand and abide by applicable Association policies; local, state, and federal laws; and institutional rules.

B. Occupational therapy practitioners shall remain abreast of revisions in those laws and Association policies that apply to the profession of occupational therapy and shall inform employers, employees, and colleagues of those changes.

C. Occupational therapy practitioners shall require those they supervise in occupational therapy-related activities to adhere to the Code of Ethics.

D. Occupational therapy practitioners shall take reasonable steps to ensure employers are aware of occupational therapy's ethical obligations, as set forth in this Code of Ethics, and of the implications of those obligations for occupational therapy practice, education, and research.

E. Occupational therapy practitioners shall record and report in an accurate and timely manner all information related to professional activities.

Principle 6. Occupational therapy personnel shall provide accurate information about occupational therapy services. (veracity)

A. Occupational therapy personnel shall accurately represent their credentials, qualifications, education, experience, training, and competence. This is of particular importance for those to whom occupational therapy personnel provide their services or with whom occupational therapy practitioners have a professional relationship.

B. Occupational therapy personnel shall disclose any professional, personal, financial, business, or volunteer affiliations that may pose a conflict of interest to those with whom they may establish a professional, contractual, or other working relationship.

C. Occupational therapy personnel shall refrain from using or participating in the use of any form of communication that contains false, fraudulent, deceptive, or unfair statements or claims.

D. Occupational therapy practitioners shall accept the responsibility for their professional actions which reduce the public's trust in occupational therapy services and those that perform those services.

Principle 7. Occupational therapy personnel shall treat colleagues and other professionals with fairness, discretion, and integrity. (fidelity)

A. Occupational therapy personnel shall preserve, respect, and safeguard confidential information about colleagues and staff, unless otherwise mandated by national, state, or local laws.

B. Occupational therapy practitioners shall accurately represent the qualifications, views, contributions, and findings of colleagues.

C. Occupational therapy personnel shall take adequate measures to discourage, prevent, expose, and correct any breaches of the Code of Ethics and report any breaches of the Code of Ethics to the appropriate authority.

D. Occupational therapy personnel shall familiarize themselves with established policies and procedures for handling concerns about this Code of Ethics, including familiarity with national, state, local, district, and territorial procedures for handling ethics complaints. These include policies and procedures created by the American Occupational Therapy Association, licensing and regulatory bodies, employers, agencies, certification boards, and other organizations who have jurisdiction over occupational therapy practice.

REFERENCES

American Occupational Therapy Association. (1993). Core values and attitudes of occupational therapy practice. *Am J Occup Ther, 47*, 1085-1086.

American Occupational Therapy Association. (1998). Guidelines to the occupational therapy code of ethics. *Am J Occup Ther, 52*, 881-884.

Authors:

The Commission on Standards and Ethics (SEC):
 Barbara L. Kornblau, JD, OTR, FAOTA—Chairperson
 Melba Arnold, MS, OTR/L
 Nancy Nashiro, PhD, OTR, FAOTA
 Diane Hill, COTA/L, AP
 Deborah Y. Slater, MS, OTR/L
 John Morris, PhD
 Linda Withers, CNHA, FACHCA
 Penny Kyler, MA, OTR/L, FAOTA—Staff Liaison

April 2000
Adopted by the Representative Assembly 2000M15

Note: This document replaces the 1994 document, Occupational Therapy Code of Ethics (*Am J Occup Ther, 48*, 1037-1038).

Prepared 4/7/2000

Occupational Therapy Process— The Guide to Occupational Therapy Practice: Quick Reference

STAGE ONE

Site of Intervention

Institutional Settings

- Inpatient hospitals
- Inpatient rehabilitation
- Inpatient mental health
- Subacute units/transitional care
- Nursing facilities
- Prisons

Outpatient Settings

- Hospital outpatient
- Outpatient clinics
- Outpatient office
- Outpatient rehabilitation
- Partial hospitalization

Home and Community Settings

- Home care
- Halfway houses
- Group homes
- Assisted living
- Sheltered workshops
- Industry and business
- Schools
- Early intervention centers
- Daycare centers
- Community mental health centers
- Hospice
- Wellness and fitness centers

Referral

Referral Sources

- Physician
- Non-physician practitioners
- Teachers and school administrators
- Family or caregivers
- Self
- Insurance companies
- Industries and businesses
- State and local agencies

Screening

Obtaining data to determine the need for evaluation and intervention

Evaluation

Through interview, skilled observation, and testing, evaluate:

- History, prior functional level in ADL, work and other productive activities, and play/leisure
- Occupations, tasks, and activities that can and cannot be performed
- Needs, plans, and goals of the client, family, or caregiver
- Participation in meaningful and purposeful occupations
- Rehabilitation potential
- Underlying performance components causing the functional performance limitations
- Contextual factors affecting performance in occupations (including environment, age, and general health)

Stage Two

Intervention Plan

Developed with the client, family, caregiver, or referral source to determine the functional outcomes.

- Short-term:
  updated weekly or biweekly
- Long term:
  achieved by discharge

Note: Rate of improvement varies by the client and the situation

Intervention/Re-Evaluation

- Remediation/restoration
  Changing the biological, physiological, psychological, or neurological process
  Teaching/training skills, habits, and behaviors
- Compensation/adaptation
  Adapting the task objects
  Changing the task methods
  Modifying the environment
  Training the family or caregiver
- Disability prevention
- Health promotion

Re-evaluation

Evaluate progress on goals
Modify intervention goals
Change the intervention methods

Discharge/Follow-Up

Intervention is discontinued when one or more of the following occurs:

- Functional goals/outcomes have been achieved
- A plateau in progress has been reached
- Participation in intervention is restricted because of complications
- Prescribed occupational therapy maintenance program is followed independently or with assistance
- Discharge is requested

At discharge, indicators for potential follow-up are identified.

Follow-Up

The need for additional occupational therapy may result from changes in functional status, living situation, workplace, caregiver, technology, development, personal interest, or age.

Reprinted from Moyers, P. A., & The Commission on Practice. (1999). The guide to occupational therapy practice. *Quick Reference*. Bethesda, MD: American Occupational Therapy Association, Inc. © 1999 by the American Occupational Therapy Association, Inc. Reprinted with permission.

Mood Disorders— Occupational Therapy Practice Guidelines: Quick Reference

Selected DSM-IV Diagnoses

296.xx Major depression disorder
300.4   Dysthymic disorder
296.xx Bipolar I disorder

296.89 Bipolar II disorder
301.13 Cyclothymic disorder

Referral

Referral Sources

- Physician
- Non-physician practitioners
- Family members
- Self

Referral Basis

Impairments that impede the client's ability to function safely in activities of daily living (ADL), work, and other productive or leisure activities.

Underlying Referral Premise

Occupational therapy treatment will improve the client's performance in one or more areas (see Referral Basis) within a reasonable time period.

Evaluation

Through interview, observation, and clinical testing, evaluate:

- Client's history and prior functional level in ADL, work, and other productive activities
- Functional activities that the client can and cannot perform
- Client's and family members' needs, plans, and goals
- Client's rehabilitation potential
- Underlying components causing the functional performance deficits
- Contextual factors affecting the client's functional performance (e.g., environmental, age, general health

Care Plan

Developed with the client and family members to determine treatment goals and outcomes:

- Short-term: updated weekly or biweekly
- Long-term: functional outcomes

Note: Rate of improvement varies by person

Treatment Intensity, Frequency, and Duration

Acute care hospital**
Individual or group treatment, 15- to 60-minute sessions, one to two times a day, 7 to 14 days (may extend to 30 days)

Long-term residential treatment setting**
Individual or group treatment, 30- to 90-minute sessions, one to four times a week

Partial hospitalization programs**
Individual or group treatment, 30- to 90-minute sessions, three to five times a week, 2 to 8 weeks

Community mental health centers/outpatient centers**
Individual or group treatment, 30- to 90-minute sessions, one to four times a week

Home care (by home health agency or private practitioner)***
Individual treatment, 30- to 90-minute sessions, one to three times a week

Note: Frequency and duration may vary depending on the individual needs of the client, severity of the illness, and the role of the occupational therapy practitioner in that setting.

**Client must demonstrate measurable functional improvement weekly.

***Client must demonstrate measurable functional improvement every 2 weeks.

Discharge/Follow-Up

Discharge

Therapy will be discontinued when one of the following criteria is met:

- Client has achieved functional goals and outcomes
- Client has reached a plateau in progress
- Client is unable to participate in treatment because of medical, psychological, or social complications
- Client no longer needs skilled occupational therapy services
- Client does not desire continued occupational therapy services

At discharge, occupational therapist will identify indicators for potential follow-up care.

Follow-Up

Readmittance to occupational therapy may result from changes in functional status, living situation, workplace, caregiver, or personal interests.

Evaluation

Evaluation Method

Interviews
Self-assessment questionnaires
Checklists and rankings
Occupational histories
Occupational narratives
Skilled observation
Skill ratings
Task simulations
Standardized tests
Non-standardized tests

Data Obtained

Premorbid functioning in ADL, work and productive activities, and play or leisure
Interests and values regarding roles and occupations
Occupational engagement patterns
Disability experience
Potential therapeutic occupations, tasks, and activities
Abilities and limitations in occupational performance
Possible goals for future occupational performance
Performance context that supports or interferes with occupational performance
Performance components skills and impairments
Functioning in performance areas or performance components according to population norms

Procedural Terminology for Evaluation

Performance Areas
Occupational therapy evaluation
Occupational therapy reevaluation
Occupational therapy check-out of orthotic/prosthetic use
Physical performance measurement
Performance Components
Swallowing/oral function
Manual muscle testing
Range of motion measurements
Neuromuscular evaluation
Developmental testing
Cognitive evaluation

Intervention

Types of Intervention and Procedural Terminology

	Focus of Intervention
Remediation/Restoration	
• Changing the biological, physiological, psychological, or neurological processes	Restoring or remediating impairments in performance components
Procedural terminology	Splinting and strapping, biofeedback training, swallowing and oral function, physical agent modalities, therapeutic exercises, aquatic therapy, neuromuscular reeducation, sensory integrative activities, manual techniques, work hardening/conditioning, therapeutic activities
• Teaching/training	Establishing new skills in performance components, habits, or behaviors
Procedural terminology	Therapeutic activities, self-care/home management training, community/work reintegration training, wheelchair management/propulsion training, work hardening/conditioning, development of cognitive skills
Compensation/Adaptation	
• Changing the task	Adapting the task requirements, procedures, task objects
• Changing the context	Modifying or adapting the task, environments
Procedural terminology	Self-care/home management, community work/integration
Disability Prevention	
• Primary prevention	Occupations that prevent health problems
• Secondary prevention	Safe task methods and task objects
• Tertiary prevention	Safe occupational performance
Health promotion	
• Lifestyle redesign	Purposeful and meaningful occupations
	Balance of rest, work, play/leisure
	Healthy interaction with the environment

Outcome	Uniform Terminology for Occupational Therapy

Outcome

Occupational performance

- Independence in ADL, work, and productive activities, play/leisure
- Performance component function

Prevention of Injury or Disability

General Health

- Symptom status improvement
- Enhanced development

Satisfaction

- Client
- Family
- Caregiver
- Referral source

Quality of Life

- Purposeful participation as a member of a community
- Emotional well-being
- Sleep and rest
- Energy and vitality
- Life satisfaction

Uniform Terminology for Occupational Therapy

Performance Areas

A. Activities of Daily Living
1. Grooming
2. Oral hygiene
3. Bathing/showering
4. Toilet hygiene
5. Personal care device
6. Dressing
7. Feeding and eating
8. Medication routine
9. Health maintenance
10. Socialization
11. Functional communication
12. Functional mobility
13. Community mobility
14. Emergency response
15. Sexual expression

B. Work and Productive Activities
1. Home management
   a. Clothing care
   b. Cleaning
   c. Meal preparation/cleanup
   d. Shopping
   e. Money management
   f. Household maintenance
   g. Safety procedures
2. Care of others
3. Educational activities
4. Vocational activities
   a. Vocational exploration
   b. Job acquisition
   c. Work or job performance
   d. Retirement planning
   e. Volunteer participation

C. Leisure Activities
1. Leisure exploration
2. Leisure performance

Performance Components

(Underlying factors—Refer to reference for complete listing)
A. Sensorimotor
B. Cognitive
C. Psychosocial/psychological

Performance Contexts

A. Temporal Aspects
1. Age
2. Stage of development
3. Life cycle
4. Disability status

B. Environmental Aspects
1. Physical
2. Social
3. Cultural

Reprinted from American Occupational Therapy Association. (1994). Uniform Terminology for occupational therapy—Third edition. *Am J Occup Ther, 48*, 1047-1059.

Inpatient and Outpatient Levels of Evaluation

Level 1—Client Focused

Client Characteristics
- Usually involving one or two performance area deficits
- One or more functional problems of minimal to moderate severity

Average Time: 30 to 45 minutes face-to-face with the client and family members

Example: Evaluation of a client:
- Client has supportive family or social environment
- May have exacerbation of a chronic condition
- Able to cooperate and fully engage in treatment process (e.g., a man 55 years of age who is unemployed and recovering from acute manic episode is now an outpatient and requires assistance for medications and money management; his thinking has cleared, and he wants to seek employment with assistance from the community mental health center)

Level 2—Detailed

Client Characteristics
- Usually involving two to four performance area deficits
- Illness of moderate complexity

Average Time: 45 minutes face-to-face with the client and family members

Example: Evaluation of a client:
- Presence of co-existing conditions (medical condition such as diabetes, high blood pressure, aging issues)
- There are questions whether the client is safe in current living situation (e.g., a woman 79 years of age with dysthymic disorder lives with husband; since she has had chronic obstructive pulmonary disease, she has not left the house; when discharged home after a hip fracture, she remains dependent on her husband for self-care and all home management activities, and her husband is not sure he can continue to care for her)

Level 3—Comprehensive

Client Characteristics
- Usually involving five to more performance area deficits
- Recent acute illness

Average Time: 60 minutes face-to-face with the client and family members

Example: Evaluation of a client:
- Unable to work
- Unable to care for self and family members
- Suicide attempt
- Unsafe in current living situation (e.g., a single mother 35 years of age with major depressive disorder who was recently fired from her job; sleeps 15 hours a day; is unable to care for her child, prepare meals, or maintain the household; is unable to concentrate or initiate activities and has no attention to safety issues related to self or the child)

Special Evaluation

(Complex, requiring separate written paper)
- Work readiness
- Driving
- Work or work site evaluation
- Home or environmental modifications

Examples of Treatment Techniques	Suggested CPT Codes
• Occupational therapy evaluation	97003
• Occupational therapy re-evaluation	97004
• Neuromuscular re-education of movement, balance, coordination, kinesthetic sense, posture, and proprioception	97112
• Therapeutic procedure(s), group (two or more individuals)	97150
• Therapeutic activities (dynamic activities to improve functional performance)	97530
• Self-care/home management training and compensatory training, meal preparation, safety procedures	97535
• Community/work reintegration training (e.g., shopping, transportation, money management, avocational activities, and/or work environment/modification analysis, work task analysis)	97537
• Development of cognitive skills to improve attention, memory, problem solving, includes compensatory training and/or sensory integrative activities	97770
• Unlisted service or procedure	97799
• Neurobehavioral status exam (clinical assessment of thinking, reasoning, and judgment, e.g., acquired knowledge, attention, memory, visual spatial abilities, language functions, planning)	96115

Note: CPT is a trademark of the American Medical Association. CPT five-digit codes, nomenclature, and other data are copyright 1999 by the American Medical Association. All rights reserved. Reprinted with permission. No fee schedules, basic units, relative values, or related listings are included in the CPT. The AMA assumes no liability for the data contained herein.

Codes shown refer to CPT 2000. CPT codes are updated annually. New and revised codes become effective January 1. Always refer to annual updated CPT publication for most current codes.

Allowable codes vary by locale, site of service, and payer policy. Payer policy may recognize CPT E & M (99201-99215) to code occupational therapy evaluations.

Styles of Defense

Defense mechanisms or defenses are used unconsciously by the person's ego in order to keep anxiety-producing thoughts, information, or wishes out of consciousness. These processes are used by everyone to some degree and are the ego's way of managing thoughts or feelings that would otherwise be unmanageable. Their use can characterize the person's way of relating, or what one would call the personality.

Vaillant (1993) characterized the defenses on a continuum from "psychotic" to "mature," based upon their utility in promoting mature, adult function. Defenses other than those identified as "mature" (see below) tend to distort reality and often impair the person's ability to sustain satisfying interpersonal relationships, make it more difficult for one to successfully resolve real conflicts, and may impede satisfying engagement in occupation.

PSYCHOTIC DEFENSES

Psychotic defenses are primitive and based upon the perceptions of an immature or defective central nervous system. They ignore reality and may be used by persons who are psychotically disturbed. They are also used in one's childhood, and in dreams and imagination.

1. *Delusional projection:* unacceptable inner conflicts or impulses are perceived and acted upon as if they were outside the self; for example, the person may have delusions of persecution.
2. *Distortion:* what is perceived as external reality is grossly reframed to suit inner needs; this may, for example, enable feelings of grandeur or wish-fulfilling delusions.
3. *Psychotic denial:* ignores the existence or reality of painful external information; for example, the person fully insists on and believes a death or loss has not occurred.

IMMATURE DEFENSES

Persons who have personality disorders often use immature defenses. The term "immature" is not meant to be critical but suggests that the ego develops through adulthood. They are distinguished from the psychotic defenses in that external reality testing is not grossly impaired.

4. *Projection:* the person attributes to another person unacceptable thoughts and feelings he/she is having. For example, I am unconsciously angry with you, but I believe that you are angry with me.
5. *Fantasy:* ignores real people and events and allows the person to indulge in "autistic retreat" (into imagination) to gratify unmet needs. Fantasies are a way to avoid the overt expression of aggressive, dependent, sexual, or other unacceptable impulses. The person does not fully believe the fantasies nor insist on acting them out.
6. *Hypochondriasis:* the magnification or exaggeration of physical symptoms (pain, somatic illness) in order to ward off bereavement, loneliness, or unacceptable impulses toward others; it is not an effort to obtain gratification and secondary gain from having the sick role. For example, a mourner complains of symptoms identical to those of the heart condition that just killed a loved one.
7. *Passive aggression:* unacceptable aggressive feelings toward others are expressed through passivity, masochism, or fuming against the self. For example, the individual may procrastinate, intentionally fail, or "drag one's feet" in order to stall a project.
8. *Acting out:* the direct expression of an unconscious wish or impulse that serves to avoid the conscious experiencing of painful or unacceptable feelings; may include impulsive, delinquent acts or temper tantrums. Acting out may, for example, mask the grief of children. People who are acting out are not without a conscience, but are not consciously aware of what is driving their behavior.

NEUROTIC DEFENSES

Neurotic defenses are less intrusive to others than are immature defenses and employ relatively less self-deception; persons who are under stress often use them:

9. *Displacement:* the person shifts his/her feelings about one person to another that resembles the former in some way; this new object (person) is less daunting or significant. For example, a male client quarrels with his wife, then shouts at the female therapist when she enters the room.

10. *Isolation of affect (intellectualization):* the excessive use of intellectual processes to avoid experiencing uncomfortable feelings; the person may pay excessive attention to external or irrelevant details in order to avoid perceiving the whole or to avoid one's feelings. Use of this defense, for example, allows one to perform bloody, surgical procedures or organize funerals without being overwhelmed by feelings.

11. *Repression:* the process by which the ego pushes painful or anxiety-producing information (thoughts or feelings) out of consciousness. This defense is at the root of many of the other defenses.

12. *Reaction formation:* the process by which the conscious thought and feelings are the polar opposite of unfelt, unconscious thoughts and wishes. For example, a person who is highly pious might be responding to unconscious wishes to engage in immoral behavior.

MATURE DEFENSES

13. *Altruism:* the process of doing for others (e.g., through public service or charity) thereby also gratifying the self.

14. *Sublimation:* feelings and impulses are not camouflaged or denied but instead are channeled into a socially acceptable outlet. For example, aggressive impulses might be channeled into a game of handball; these or other feelings might be expressed through the arts.

15. *Suppression:* one makes the conscious or semi-conscious decision to put a thought, idea, or wish "on the back burner" and not pay attention to it at the present.

16. *Anticipation:* planning for emotionally painful events in smaller "doses"; anticipation spreads anxiety over time. In anticipatory grief, for example, the person starts preparing for the expected loss.

17. *Humor:* permits one to directly face painful thoughts/events without discomfort; it does not deny the seriousness or painfulness of the event.

Adapted from Vaillant, G. E. (1993). *Wisdom of the ego.* Cambridge, MA: Harvard University Press.

The reader is also referred to Kaplan, H. I., & Sadock, B. J. (1998). *Synopsis of psychiatry* (8th ed., pp. 219-221). Philadelphia, PA: Lippincott, Williams & Wilkins.

Person Drawings

The pictures in this appendix are presented to exemplify the patient's expression of his or her image and concerns as they are presented in figure drawings. These drawings were used as tools for interaction and were not interpreted by the occupational therapist. They facilitated a shared discussion of self-image, roles, interests, likes and dislikes, and patient concerns.

THE PATIENT AND HIS ENVIRONMENT

Patients may depict their environment or objects within the environment that represent a conflict, concern, or problem that they are experiencing.

Figure I-1. The patient (a 15-year-old girl) depicts her dilemma as being between continuing her lifestyle as a runaway and staying at home following the rules of her parents. She drew the "welcome" mat, and stated that she wished there was such a mat at her home.

Figure I-2. The patient (a 15-year-old girl) reflects her attitude about her "hold and treat" status (hospital commitment). Her primary concern was her loss of "freedom," rather than the reasons for her hospitalization—drug and alcohol abuse, promiscuity, being overweight, and her parents' refusal to have her return home to live.

Figure I-3. The patient (a 20-year-old male) identified himself as a "biker." (A biker is a person who owns a motorcycle and may belong to a particular motorcycle gang or identify with a special group of people. He may choose a transient lifestyle, have an antisocial attitude, and seek power.) This patient was in the hospital for an inability to control his aggression.

Figure I-4. The patient (a 30-year-old female) is hospitalized for depression. She states that the chair in her drawing is her only support and that she needs something to lean on. She expressed feelings of being overwhelmed by the demands of her husband, the responsibilities of her job, and that she had multiple financial concerns.

THE PATIENT AND PHYSICAL FUNCTION

The patient's physical well-being may be seen in patient drawings.

Figure I-5. The patient, a 69-year-old male with organic brain syndrome, was hospitalized because of agitation and paranoia. His drawing is typical of one drawn by a patient with organic problems.

Figure I-6. The patient (an 18-year-old female) was hospitalized for depression and a suicide attempt. She is hemiplegic due to surgery for removal of a benign tumor. After completing the drawing, she shared her feelings regarding her disability and the hopelessness she felt. Physically, she was more capable than her drawing suggests and than her discussion indicated.

Figure I-7. The patient (a 19-year-old female) was hospitalized for anorexia. Her weight at the time of this drawing was 85 pounds. During the discussion that followed this drawing, she verbalized many angry feelings.

THE PATIENT AND SYMBOLIC DRAWINGS

The drawings presented in this section are symbolic. Patients who may or may not be reality oriented may choose to express their feelings, concerns, or problems symbolically. Patients who are diagnosed as "psychotic" may have lucid periods. Thus, the patient may be asked to do a self-portrait during the evaluation process, or the drawing may be requested after the patient is stabilized on medications. The occupational therapist may limit the discussion of symbolism if the discussion increases the patient's confusion, promotes agitation, or is otherwise to the detriment of the patient.

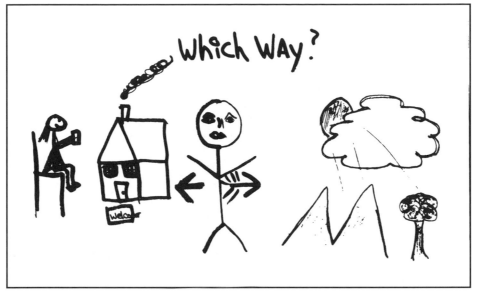

Figure I-1. Dilemma (reprinted with permission from Bruce, M., & Borg, B. [1993]. *Psychosocial occupational therapy: Frames of reference for intervention* [2nd ed.]. Thorofare, NJ: SLACK Incorporated).

Figure I-2. Hold and treat (reprinted with permission from Bruce, M., & Borg, B. [1993]. *Psychosocial occupational therapy: Frames of reference for intervention* [2nd ed.]. Thorofare, NJ: SLACK Incorporated).

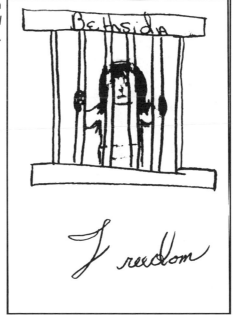

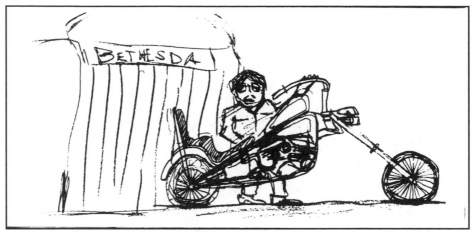

Figure I-3. Biker (reprinted with permission from Bruce, M., & Borg, B. [1993]. *Psychosocial occupational therapy: Frames of reference for intervention* [2nd ed.]. Thorofare, NJ: SLACK Incorporated).

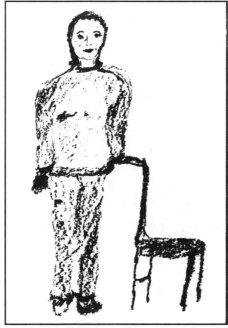

Figure I-4. Chair (reprinted with permission from Bruce, M., & Borg, B. [1993]. *Psychosocial occupational therapy: Frames of reference for intervention* [2nd ed.]. Thorofare, NJ: SLACK Incorporated).

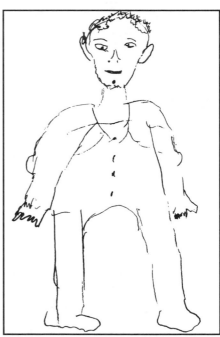

Figure I-5. Organic brain syndrome (reprinted with permission from Bruce, M., & Borg, B. [1993]. *Psychosocial occupational therapy: Frames of reference for intervention* [2nd ed.]. Thorofare, NJ: SLACK Incorporated).

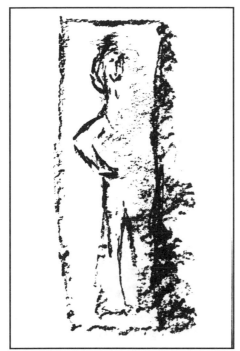

Figure I-6. Hemiplegia (reprinted with permission from Bruce, M., & Borg, B. [1993]. *Psychosocial occupational therapy: Frames of reference for intervention* [2nd ed.]. Thorofare, NJ: SLACK Incorporated).

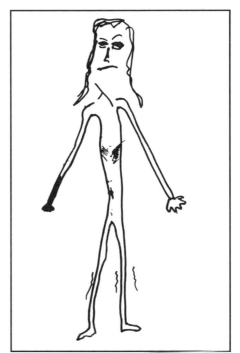

Figure I-7. Anorexia (reprinted with permission from Bruce, M., & Borg, B. [1993]. *Psychosocial occupational therapy: Frames of reference for intervention* [2nd ed.]. Thorofare, NJ: SLACK Incorporated).

Figure I-8. The patient (a 30-year-old male) was diagnosed as "psychotic," or not reality oriented. He drew himself as a tree and expressed the dichotomy of his conflict in the angel-devil drawings. His discussion focused on issues of right and wrong, good and evil, and God and the devil. The therapist chose to limit the discussion of religious issues and helped him to verbalize his conflicts regarding "right" or "wrong" choices that were affecting his job performance and daily function at home.

Figure I-9. The patient (a 19-year-old male) was hospitalized for depression and psychotic episodes due to drug abuse. Through his symbolic self-portrait, he expressed his feelings and identity through his concerns, which related to political and social movements.

Figures I-1OA and I-1OB. The patients (ages 20 and 30 years old, respectively) were psychotic at the time of the drawings. Each drew herself symbolically and wished to discuss, at length, the symbolism. When this occurs, the therapist must determine the benefits of the discussion to the patient and its usefulness to treatment planning. The therapist may limit the discussion.

Figure I-11. The patient (an 18-year-old male) depicted his concerns through symbols that he added to his person drawing. He drew a light bulb and shared his concern with "thoughts that go on in my head"; he described himself as "always getting into trouble," as expressed through "horns" and the "halo" in the drawing.

THE PATIENT AND DRAWING EMPHASES

Patients also express concerns and problems through emphases in drawings that may be represented by accentuating body parts, colors used, and pressure of the lines drawn.

Figure I-12. The patient (an 18-year-old male) drew body parts to express his concern regarding his male identity and to express "if I'm alive I have a heart."

Figure I-13. The patient (a 28-year-old male) drew his heart and expressed his fear that "something was wrong with his heart." Anxiety was his chief complaint.

Figure I-14. The patient (a 16-year-old male) was hospitalized for bipolar depression, manic phase, and verbalized his multiple concerns regarding homosexuality. Note the spontaneous elaboration of the drawing to the right of the main figure.

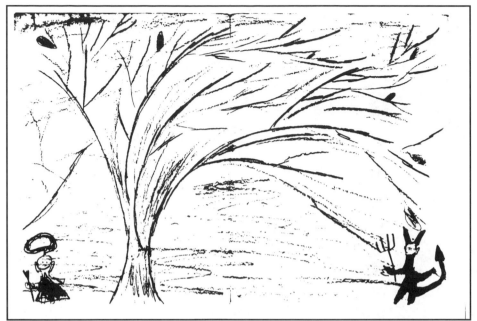

Figure I-8. Tree (reprinted with permission from Bruce, M., & Borg, B. [1993]. *Psychosocial occupational therapy: Frames of reference for intervention* [2nd ed.]. Thorofare, NJ: SLACK Incorporated).

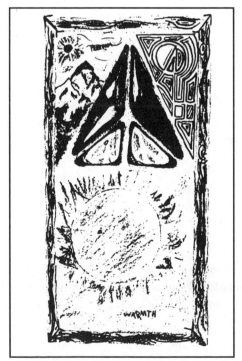

Figure I-9. Symbolic rectangle (reprinted with permission from Bruce, M., & Borg, B. [1993]. *Psychosocial occupational therapy: Frames of reference for intervention* [2nd ed.]. Thorofare, NJ: SLACK Incorporated).

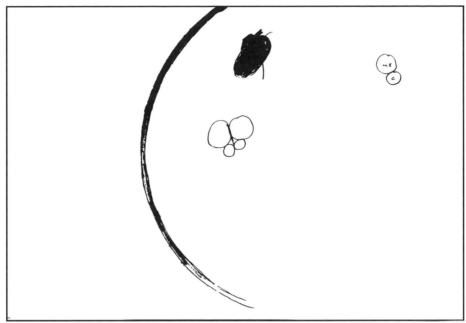

Figure I-10A. Symbolism (reprinted with permission from Bruce, M., & Borg, B. [1993]. *Psychosocial occupational therapy: Frames of reference for intervention* [2nd ed.]. Thorofare, NJ: SLACK Incorporated).

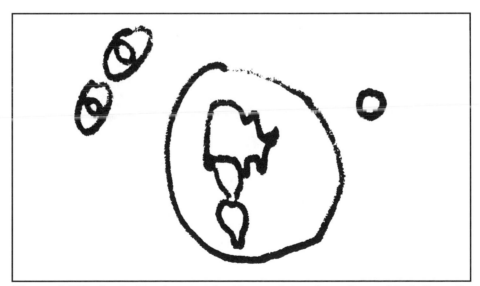

Figure I-10B. Symbolism (reprinted with permission from Bruce, M., & Borg, B. [1993]. *Psychosocial occupational therapy: Frames of reference for intervention* [2nd ed.]. Thorofare, NJ: SLACK Incorporated).

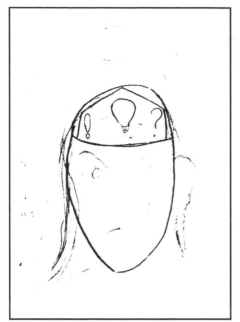

Figure I-11. Light bulb (reprinted with permission from Bruce, M., & Borg, B. [1993]. *Psychosocial occupational therapy: Frames of reference for intervention* [2nd ed.]. Thorofare, NJ: SLACK Incorporated).

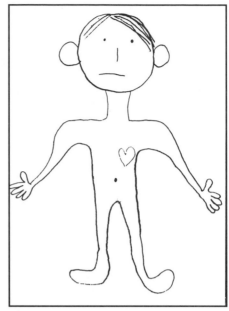

Figure I-12. Heart and male organ (reprinted with permission from Bruce, M., & Borg, B. [1993]. *Psychosocial occupational therapy: Frames of reference for intervention* [2nd ed.]. Thorofare, NJ: SLACK Incorporated).

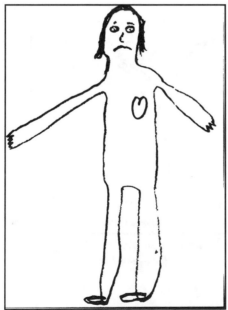

Figure I-13. Heart—anxiety (reprinted with permission from Bruce, M., & Borg, B. [1993]. *Psychosocial occupational therapy: Frames of reference for intervention* [2nd ed.]. Thorofare, NJ: SLACK Incorporated).

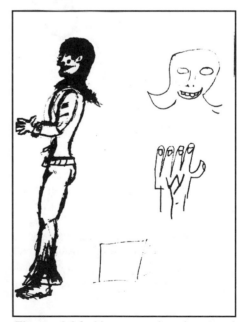

Figure I-14. Homosexuality (reprinted with permission from Bruce, M., & Borg, B. [1993]. *Psychosocial occupational therapy: Frames of reference for intervention* [2nd ed.]. Thorofare, NJ: SLACK Incorporated).

THE PATIENT AND SIMILARITY DRAWINGS

Figures I-15A and I-15B. These two drawings were made by two women of triplets (both 19 years old). The women were not in treatment at the same time but were both hospitalized within the same 1 1/2-year time period. Both were experiencing the adjustment problems of young adulthood.

THE PATIENT AND DRAWING ABILITY

The patient need not have artistic ability in order to represent him- or herself and information that promotes understanding of his or her problems. Sometimes the patients have creativity that produces a drawing, but they may be unable or unwilling to share views of themselves.

Figure I-16. The patient (a 21-year-old man) was hospitalized for depression. He drew a stick figure and verbalized his concerns about "no job and no plans for the future."

Figure I-17. The patient (a young woman) was hospitalized for depression and has artistic ability, as depicted in her sketch of a girl. She later committed suicide.

Figures I-18A and I-18B. The patient (a 15-year-old female) was hospitalized for drug abuse, psychotic episodes, running away from home, and school truancy. She has artistic ability, which is demonstrated in both of her drawings. The symbolic picture was completed shortly after admission to the hospital, and the picture of the young girl was done after 6 months of treatment. Through symbolism, she discussed wanting to be "like the virgin to crush out all evil... like Robin Hood to be able to give to the poor... give freedom to men and women."

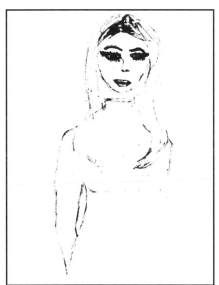

Figure I-15A. Triplets (reprinted with permission from Bruce, M., & Borg, B. [1993]. *Psychosocial occupational therapy: Frames of reference for intervention* [2nd ed.]. Thorofare, NJ: SLACK Incorporated).

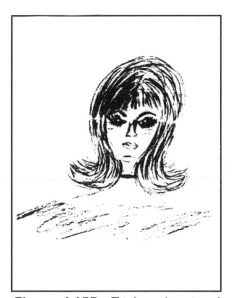

Figure I-15B. Triplets (reprinted with permission from Bruce, M., & Borg, B. [1993]. *Psychosocial occupational therapy: Frames of reference for intervention* [2nd ed.]. Thorofare, NJ: SLACK Incorporated).

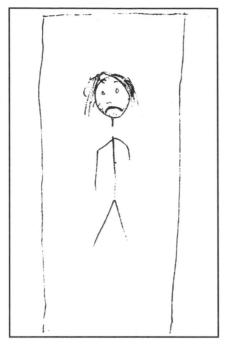

Figure I-16. Depression (reprinted with permission from Bruce, M., & Borg, B. [1993]. *Psychosocial occupational therapy: Frames of reference for intervention* [2nd ed.]. Thorofare, NJ: SLACK Incorporated).

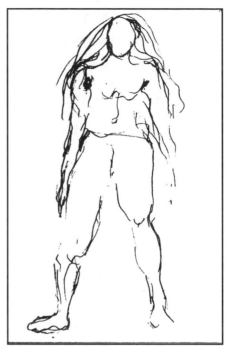

Figure I-17. Suicide (reprinted with permission from Bruce, M., & Borg, B. [1993]. *Psychosocial occupational therapy: Frames of reference for intervention* [2nd ed.]. Thorofare, NJ: SLACK Incorporated).

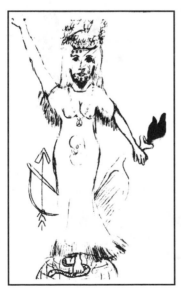

Figure I-18A. Girl at admission (reprinted with permission from Bruce, M., & Borg, B. [1993]. *Psychosocial occupational therapy: Frames of reference for intervention* [2nd ed.]. Thorofare, NJ: SLACK Incorporated).

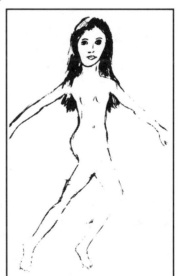

Figure I-18A. Girl after 6 months (reprinted with permission from Bruce, M., & Borg, B. [1993]. *Psychosocial occupational therapy: Frames of reference for intervention* [2nd ed.]. Thorofare, NJ: SLACK Incorporated).

Intensive Outpatient Program Example—Application of Cognitive-Behavior Frame of Reference

Throughout this text, we have referred to the changes in mental health programming and the changes of occupational therapist roles to respond to these changes and the needs of the clients. The following program example is a sample of an outpatient mental health program that responds to client needs and the use of cognitive-behavioral principles for an educational program in occupational therapy intervention in contemporary practice.

Admission Criteria: Person with Global Assessment of Function Score of 45 to 60
Person able to contract for safety
Persons age 18 to 90 years

Purpose: Provide biopsychosocial treatment
Assist persons with depression and anxiety
Provide a multidisciplinary team approach
Provide a program that is compatible with work, home, and education responsibilities
A client-centered, goal-oriented and solution-focused program

Theoretical Model: Cognitive-behavioral focus on the person's locus of control; things one can change; changing one's thoughts, behavior, and feelings
Focus on the role of one's beliefs and the changing dynamics of daily life

Reading and Resource: Covey, S. (1989). *The seven habits of highly effective people.* New York: Simon and Schuster. Use for client homework assignments.

Format: Meet three times per week, 3 days a week.

Services Provided: Psychiatric assessment, psychosocial assessment, medication management, psychological testing, group therapy, psychoeducational classes, family education, and support.

Outcome Measure: Symptom Checklist (SCL-90-R)
Global Assessment of Function (GAF)
Beck Depression Inventory

Psychoeducational Classes:
Class size—4 to 6 people, maximum 10

Course Topics for Classes:
Assertive communication
Relationships
Wellness
Stress management
Relaxation
Goal-setting and coping skills
Time management
Anger management
Problem solving and decision making
Self-esteem
Community resources
Relapse prevention
Spirituality

The reader is referred to Chapter Six for details. This format can be used in various contexts and with multiple populations.

Task Check List

Directions: Circle number in appropriate column and add for total.	Rarely Sometimes Often		Circle rater/student familiarity − 1 2 3 4 5 +	Rarely Sometimes Often		Name _____ Rater _____ Date _____	Rarely Sometimes Often	
I. ENTRY LEVEL			**IV. RELATIONSHIP LEVEL**			**VII. ACHIEVEMENT LEVEL**		
States desire to attend	0 1	2	Seeks approval	0 1	2	Assumes self-responsibility	0 1	2
Stays through classes	0 1	2	Accepts feedback	0 1	2	Completes tasks	0 1	2
Hallucinates/delusional	2 1	0	Is outgoing and friendly	0 1	2	Manages stress	0 1	2
Is easily distracted	2 1	0	Interacts with peers	0 1	2	Is able to abstract	0 1	2
Stays on topic/coherent	0 1	2	Seeks reinforcement	0 1	2	Is self-motivated	0 1	2
Is disruptive/combative	2 1	0	Works productively 1-1	0 1	2	Generalizes	0 1	2
Speaks & acts at normal pace	0 1	2	Gives compliments	0 1	2	Competent in ADL skills	0 1	2
Observes limits	0 1	2	Receives compliments	0 1	2	Makes discharge plans	0 1	2
Affect is appropriate	0 1	2	Uses staff appropriately	0 1	2	Seeks independence	0 1	2
Threatens suicide	2 1	0	Shares feelings with others	0 1	2	Generates + self-statements	0 1	2
TOTAL	2	0	TOTAL	1	9	TOTAL	1	0
II. ACCEPTANCE LEVEL			**V. EXPLORATORY LEVEL**					
Attentive	0 1	2	Asks questions	0 1	2			
Suspicious, guarded	2 1	0	Seeks new situations	0 1	2			
Answers questions	0 1	2	Makes suggestions	0 1	2			
Engages others	0 1	2	Tries new behaviors	0 1	2			
Is rude or indifferent	2 1	0	Requests feedback	0 1	2			
Keeps appointments	0 1	2	Initiates activities	0 1	2			
Withdraws/lacks trust	2 1	0	Reveals feelings	0 1	2			
Refuses feedback	2 1	0	Considers goals	0 1	2			
Denies problems	2 1	0	Role plays	0 1	2			
Accepts contacts with staff	2 1	0	Expresses concern for others	0 1	2			
TOTAL	2	0	TOTAL	1	8			
III. ORDER LEVEL			**VI. MASTERY LEVEL**					
Appears neat and orderly	0 1	2	Makes decisions	0 1	2			
Follows rules	0 1	2	Problem solves	0 1	2			
Adheres to schedule	0 1	2	Exercises good judgment	0 1	2			
Acts impulsively	2 1	0	Sets treatment goals	0 1	2			
Organizes tasks	0 1	2	Self-reinforces	0 1	2			
Is rigid or compulsive	2 1	0	Generates alternatives	0 1	2			
Follows directions	0 1	2	Verbalizes spontaneously	0 1	2			
Complies with treatment	0 1	2	Is able to relax	0 1	2			
Is punctual	0 1	2	Exerts self-control	0 1	2			
Attends regularly	0 1	2	Takes notes/completes assignments	0 1	2			
TOTAL	2	0	TOTAL	1	4			

SUMMARY GRAPH

	I	II	III	IV	V	VI	VII
20							
19							
18							
17							
16							
15							
14							
13							
12							
11							
10							
9							
8							
7							
6							
5							
4							
3							
2							
1							
0							

Sample Cognitive-Behavior Group Descriptions

The group descriptions in this appendix are sample skills development groups that can be used in multiple contexts and integrated with different activities for improving occupational performance. The clients can learn and practice skills in one or a series of sessions. It is preferable to have a series of four to six groups to provide an opportunity for skill mastery and practice in multiple contexts.

SOCIAL SKILLS GROUP
(COREY, 2000; ROSE, 1986)

Description

A group for clients to learn and practice social behaviors. The leader facilitates client participation through a group structure that supports participation and decision-making by all members. Sample activities include a diary of social situations, group problem solving, role play, and homework tasks related to specific group goals.

Goals

Clients work together to do the following:
1. Identify problem situations that require skills training
2. Learn social behavior from each other
3. Practice skills in varied contexts (e.g., role-plays or in the community)
4. Give or receive feedback
5. Learn from homework assignments
6. Achieve other specific behavior goals

Protocol

Group Introduction
The session begins with the leader reviewing the group's purpose and procedures, and perhaps providing examples of those skills the group has been working to improve.

Client Skill Demonstration
Experienced group members may demonstrate role-play to new members and describe how this method is used in the group.

Identifying the Group Agenda
The leader uses questions to solicit concerns that have emerged since the last group meeting.

Group Experience, Problem Solving, and Skill Practice
Clients have been asked to keep a diary of social events and dilemmas they experienced. Using a round robin format, each group member describes a difficult personal situation that was noted in his or her diary this past week. Before the group is over, each member will have identified a problem and problem-solved with group members to identify alternative solutions. The client chooses the alternative that feels like the best choice. A group member models this response and then the client practices the skill during a role-play.

Feedback and Closure
Group members then give the client feedback regarding his or her performance, its effectiveness, and/or need for practice. Clients may then assign themselves homework to be completed before the next meeting (Corey, 2000, p. 374).

For details and examples of the group protocol and process, the reader is referred to Rose (1986).

ASSERTIVENESS TRAINING
(ALBERTI & EMMONS, 1995; COREY, 2000)

Description

A group in which members learn to effectively express themselves in situations that require them to express opinions, interests, feelings, and "rights." Clients learn to respond without violating the rights of others and without anxiety.

Clients learn a variety of communication strategies that can be used in multiple contexts.

Goals

Clients work together to learn the following:
1. Effectively express feelings (e.g., approval, anger, disagreement, appreciation.)
2. Recognize that it is acceptable to express their feelings, thoughts, and attitudes
3. Identify the variables that impede communication
4. Decrease their anxiety about expressing opinions to others
5. Initiate skills for self-expression

Protocol

Group Introduction

The first session of the sequence begins with a description of the group and its purpose. Group members then introduce themselves.

Identify Group Series Goals

The leader identifies what is meant by assertive, aggressive, and non-assertive behaviors, and models sample assertive responses to demonstrate the behaviors that will be practiced in the group.

Didactic Information

The leader then provides a brief description of the relationship between the person's thoughts and one's behavior. The didactic information includes examples of rational and irrational beliefs, and their effect on assertiveness as well as other behavior. The leader then describes how a log can be used for self-monitoring regarding situations in which anxiety (or other emotion) impedes effective assertive behavior.

Homework

Following the description of the self-monitoring, the leader then gives the clients a homework assignment to use the log each day. The session is closed with a relaxation exercise.

Subsequent Group Sessions

The subsequent sessions have a similar format.

Group Introduction

The session begins with a welcome, the introduction of new members, and review of homework.

Behavior Demonstration and Discussion

Next the trainer demonstrates assertive, non-assertive, and aggressive behaviors. Members evaluate the behaviors demonstrated and give each other feedback based on their perspectives of the scenario.

Education, Problem Solving, and Awareness

Each session has a brief didactic presentation designed to increase client awareness of the relationship between thoughts and behavior, and subsequent discussions that relate an identified strategy to specific situations.

Homework

New homework is assigned, and the session closes with an exercise for managing anxiety, stress, etc. (Corey, 2000, pp. 375-377).

The reader who anticipates conducting an assertiveness group or serving as a resource to others who will conduct these groups is referred to Alberti and Emmons (1995).

COPING SKILLS GROUP— A MULTIMODAL APPROACH

The previous two sample groups we have described have a single primary focus for skill development. Lazarus (1989, 1995) believes that the therapist should have a repertoire of strategies for skill development and use them within a social learning model of therapy to produce the desired change as identified by the client. This approach he calls "multimodal group therapy." In a sense, this group approach is a generic group format that can be used by the therapist to build a variety of skills within a social learning model.

Description

Multimodal group learning occurs in a homogeneous group and begins with an assessment Lazarus calls "BASIC I.D." This anagram represents each of the seven variables that influence the client's function in daily life: behavior, affect, sensations, imagery, cognition, interpersonal relationships, and drugs/biology (Lazarus, 1989, 1995). Within daily function, all of the variables are believed to interact in a manner that results in competence or some type of difficulty. It is these difficulties that will become the focus of the group. In order to establish what will be the group's focus, each prospective group member completes a life history or life function questionnaire. This information identifies how the seven variables interact and what specific problems are shared by group participants.

Goals

Clients change their behavior and develop coping skills as they meet a broad spectrum of group objectives. These can include:
1. Identify conflicts and feelings
2. Learn strategies to change maladaptive behaviors and acquire desired skills
3. Acquire correct information for problem solving
4. Learn to build and improve interpersonal relationships
5. Manage the daily stresses in life

6. Recover from traumatic events
7. Treat or manage their biological problems

Procedures

Group Framework

The clinician works within a social cognitive learning framework and explores the client preferences and priorities for learning in each of the seven BASIC I.D. areas.

Leader Roles

During group sessions the leader assumes varied roles depending on the learning strategies applied, the clients' response to the group interactions, and the learning focus. The therapist may be an educator, a consultant, a facilitator, a role model, or a trainer.

Group Experiences

Learning strategies used in the group can include role-play, relaxation exercises, behavior rehearsal, cognitive restructuring, or evaluating one's thoughts to gain a different perspective, modeling, assertive training, and various methods of feedback and reinforcement.

The reader is referred to the original sources for a more detailed description (Lazarus, 1989, 1993, 1995, 1996a, 1996b, 1997a, 1997b).

MEICHENBAUM'S STRESS INOCULATION TRAINING

Stress inoculation training occurs in a series of sessions. The number depends on the needs and skills of the clients. It is assumed that clients can benefit from periodic return to training to refine one's skills, maintain the skills learned, and get support for managing disease symptoms or the situations that require stress management. Three phases of treatment are identified. The amount of practice in each phase depends on the needs of the individual client. It is best to have a series of four to six groups if possible. Therapists may also include each phase within one group.

Description

The training involves three stages of implementation. The client should experience all three stages: (1) identify personal beliefs about stress, (2) practice coping skills to develop a coping repertoire, and (3) apply coping skills in context.

Group Experiences

During each of these three stages clinicians may provide *didactic information* about stress, facilitate Socratic discussion, and help restructure cognitive perspectives on stress. Clients have *learning experiences* that give opportunities for problem solving, relaxation, and social skill and coping skill training. The leader teaches members to self-monitor, and use self-instruction and self-reinforcement methods. The leader may suggest environmental modifications or help group members identify their own.

Goals—Stage One

During the groups in stage one of training the client:
1. Identifies the meaning of stress and forms a concept of it as a transaction between the person (himself/herself) and the environment
2. Identifies his or her role in causing and maintaining stress
3. Keeps a diary to record stressful events, his or her reactions, and the variables that contribute to stress
4. Learns such coping strategies as time management, self instruction, lifestyle re-design, social skills, and relaxation. Clients are encouraged to integrate daily activities into their stress-management program (e.g., walking, gardening, knitting, yoga, medication, or exercise)

Goals—Stage Two

During the group experiences in stage two the client:
1. Identifies thoughts and feelings related to the stressful event
2. Presents evidence to support or challenge one's interpretation of the event
3. Plans homework to test one's stress-management skills and to gather data for evaluation of one's performance in varied contexts
4. Uses self-instruction methods to contradict negative self-statements and establish constructive management of stress

Goals—Stage Three

During the group experiences in stage three the client practices using the knowledge and skills he or she acquired in stages one and two to:
1. Master coping skills and transfer them to many situations in daily life
2. Create homework assignments to test effective stress management
3. Evaluate and record one's performance to evaluate transfer of skills and development of maintenance skills for stress management (Corey, 2000, pp. 377-379)

The reader is referred to Meichenbaum (1977, 1985, 1986) or Corey (2000) for detailed group protocols and sample experiences.

HEALTH AND FITNESS GROUP

In their publication *Healthy People 2000* (1995) and *Healthy People 2010* (2000), the U.S. Department of Health and Human Services recommended that everyone evaluate their own fitness and consider what they could do to contribute to their own as well as the fitness of others. The occupational therapy profession has a strong philosophical basis in support of wellness and a healthy lifestyle. Current literature further supports this philosophy and describes innovative roles for occupational therapists in health and wellness (Bowen, 1999; Buning, 1999; Chen, Neufeld, Feely, & Skinner, 1999; Minor, 1997). The following are guides that occupational therapists can consider when collaborating with clients and team members to develop fitness programs.

Description

A group in which participants are educated regarding the value of physical activity and its psychological benefits as well as its physical and health contributions to well being. This can be done through an educational group format, with hand-outs or other literature that highlights key points of information. Participants are encouraged to plan daily activities to integrate exercise (e.g,. use stairs at work, walk or ride a bike to school, form walking groups, and fitness programs that prepare clients for adaptive skiing and other modified sport programs). It is important for the clinician to consider the client's lifestyle and collaborate on a plan of activities that supports fitness and the person's interests.

Behavioral Intervention and Skill Development

To develop and maintain fitness skills the therapist designs a program that helps the clients establish a physical fitness and healthy exercise routine as well as identifies general behaviors that support health and wellness. Behavioral intervention should include the following:

- Establish a system for client self-monitoring in regard to his or her fitness program and updating goals.
- Identify fitness changes that the client wishes to make, such as those related to endurance, cardiac fitness, appearance, weight loss or gain, and participation in activities.
- Recommend a balance of daily self-care, work, and leisure activities that integrate fitness and other personal goals.

Maintenance of Fitness and Relapse Prevention

The philosophy behind cognitive-behavioral fitness groups is to motivate and maintain participation through programs that meet the individual needs of the client and avoid more traditional rigid program structures. The following guides can be used to support client motivation and sense of control, and meet the person's fitness needs:

- Avoid rigid expectations and help the clients build flexibility into the fitness goals and plans for the population and individuals in the group.

- Help the participants identify the barriers that can interfere with adherence to the plan (e.g., too much to do or fatigue).
- Discuss strategies for responding to the barriers that decrease adherence and collaborate with clients to choose their strategies.
- Identify and discuss the strategies that promote the client's feeling in control of personal fitness and physical mastery.
- Use daily activities whenever possible to achieve the client's goals.
- Discuss the difference between missing the routine once in awhile (**lapse**) versus failure or quitting a program. Emphasize that programs need periodic revision and that it is natural to miss one's routine once in awhile.
- When necessary, establish clinician, family, or phone support through a system of contact monitoring. However, it is best if a client feels personal responsibility for a self-monitoring system (Brownell & Fairburn, 1995, p. 476).

REFERENCES

Alberti, R. E., & Emmons, M. L. (1995). *Your perfect right: A manual for assertiveness trainers* (7th ed.). San Luis Obispo, CA: Impact.

Bowen, J. E. (1999). Health promotion in the new millennium. *OT Practice, 4,* 14-18.

Brownell, K. D., & Fairburn, C. G. (1995). *Eating disorders and obesity.* New York, NY: The Guilford Press.

Buning, M. E. (1999). Fitness for persons with disabilities—A call to action. *OT Practice, 4,* 27-31.

Chen, C. Y., Neufeld, P. S., Feely, A. A., & Skinner, C. S. (1999). Factors influencing compliance with home exercise programs among patients with upper-extremity impairment. *Am J Occup Ther, 53,* 171-180.

Corey, G. (2000). *Theory and practice of group counseling* (5th ed.). Bellmont, CA: Wadsworth/Thomas Learning.

Healthy People 2000. (1995). Available: www.odphp.osophs.dhhs.gov/pubs/hp2000.

Healthy People 2010. (2000). Available: www.health.gov/healthypeople.

Lazarus, A. A. (1989). *The practice of multimodal therapy.* Baltimore, MD: John Hopkins University.

Lazarus, A. A. (1993). Tailoring the therapeutic relationship or being an authentic chameleon. *Psychotherapy, 30,* 404-407.

Lazarus, A. A. (1995). Multimodal therapy. In R. J. Corsini & D. Wedding (Eds.), *Current psychotherapies* (5th ed., pp. 322-335). Tasca, IL: F. E. Peacock.

Lazarus, A. A. (1996a). Some reflections after 40 years of trying to be an effective psychotherapist. *Psychotherapy, 33,* 142-145.

Lazarus, A. A. (1996b). The utility and futility of combining treatment in psychotherapy. *Clinical Psychology: Science and Practice, 3,* 59-68.

Lazarus, A. A. (1997a). *Brief but comprehensive psychotherapy: The multimodal way.* New York, NY: Springer.

Lazarus, A. A. (1997b). Can psychotherapy be brief, focused, solution-oriented, and yet comprehensive? A personal evolutionary perspective. In J. K. Zieg (Ed.), *The evolution of psychotherapy: The third conference* (pp. 83-94). New York, NY: Brunner/Mazel.

Meichenbaum, D. (1977). *Cognitive behavior modification.* New York, NY: Plenum Press.

Meichenbaum, D. (1985). *Stress inoculation training.* New York, NY: Pergamon Press.

Meichenbaum, D. (1986). Cognitive behavior modification. In F. H. Kanfer & A. P. Goldstein (Eds.), *Helping people change: A textbook of methods* (3rd ed.). New York, NY: Pergamon Press.

Minor, M. (1997). Promoting health and physical fitness. In C. Christiansen & C. Baum (Eds.), *Occupational therapy— Enabling function and well-being* (2nd ed.). Thorofare, NJ: SLACK Incorporated.

Rose, S. D. (1986). Group methods. In F. H. Kanfer & A. P. Goldstein (Eds.), *Helping people change: A textbook of methods* (3rd ed., pp. 437-469). New York, NY: Pergamon Press.

Processing Strategies and Behaviors— Dynamic Interactional Model

Structure	Strategies and Behaviors
Attention	

- Reacts to gross change in the environment
- Detects subtle changes in task conditions
- Initiates exploration (search of the environment)
- Searches for information in a planned, systematic manner
- Inhibits automatic responses
- Maintains goal-directed behavior
- Is unhindered by internal or external distractions peripheral to the task
- Sustains focus of attention on task (eye contact)
- Persists with a repetitive activity over time
- Paces and monitors speed of response
- Reduces stimuli/Identifies irrelevant information (cross out, sort, remove what is unneccessary)
- Identifies relevant information (highlights, distinguishes critical details spontaneously, compares stimuli, and chooses important facts)
- Simultaneously attends to overall stimulus as well as details
- Keeps track of rules, facts, pieces of information (external vs. internal methods)
- Allocates resources by placing greater effort and concentration on more critical aspects of the task
- Easily disengages focus of attention when necessary
- Follows changes in task, stimuli, or rules without error, withdrawal, or resistance

Visual Processing

- Initiates active visual search
- Plans and systematically explores the visual display
- Sustains visual fixation on stimuli for appropriate length of time
- Distinguishes critical features of the object or picture
- Detects and compares subtle visual details
- Attends to the overall configuration
- Shifts scanning approach with different stimuli arrangements
- Localizes information in space
- Pays equal attention to all parts of the visual field or stimulus figure
- Paces and monitors speed or response to visual information
- Simultaneously keeps track of what is seen
- Looks at the whole and divides it into parts

Structure	*Strategies and Behaviors*
Visual Processing	• Recognizes the stimulus from different perspectives (involves identifying critical attributes, visual imagery, and abstract thinking) • Can use visual imagery to describe objects or pictures that are not present • Simultaneously attends to the parts and whole
Memory	• Recognizes overall context • Recognizes most important details or information • Focuses, fixates on stimulus to be recalled • Sustains focus of attention on material to be remembered • Spontaneously shifts focus of attention to the different stimuli to be remembered • Uses stimuli-reduction methods (e.g., studies only a limited portion at one time and breaks the large amount into smaller, more manageable units) • Summarizes or identifies the main points or theme • Uses rehearsal (requires sustained repetitive activity) • Uses association (requires ability to recognize similarities and differences between stimuli and organize information into concept categories) • Uses elaboration (the ability to link meaningless with meaningful information) • Has the ability to access previous knowledge and relate new information to old information • Uses visual imagery • Initiates use of memory strategy (e.g., if unable to spontaneously recall, does not give up but persists in trying to use active retrieval strategies to trigger memory) • Spontaneously uses external aids to assist in recall
Problem Solving	• Recognizes that an obstacle or problem exists • Predicts the consequences of an obstacle or action • Analyzes the conditions of the problem • Recognizes when information is incomplete and actively searches for needed information • Attends to relevant details; highlights or lists critical information • Prioritizes information • Distinguishes critical facts, assumptions, and irrelevant information • Summarizes the main issues • Simultaneously keeps track of all the relevant information; uses external aids when appropriate • Narrows down range of possibilities • Has ability to hypothesize (goes beyond "here and now" and anticipates events or plans future goals) • When problem is large, breaks problem up into two or more manageable subproblems • When stuck, re-examines the problem in a different way, reorganizes information diferently, asks questions for clarification, talks aloud through each step, or brainstorms • Is able to view situation or problem from different vantage points • Formulates a plan (sequence of action) • Shifts to alternative strategies, plans when needed • Classifies or groups related information together • Initiates the plan of action

Structure	*Strategies and Behaviors*
Problem Solving	• Shows flexibility and reversibility in thinking • Simultaneously holds in mind all the qualites of a situation, object, or experience • Monitors speed or pace as carrying out the task • Persists with the task in searching for a solution • Spontaneously checks work

Reprinted from Toglia, J. (1998). A dynamic interactional model to cognitive rehabilitation. In N. Katz (Ed.), *Cognition and occupation in rehabilitation* (pp. 9-10). Bethesda, MD: American Occupational Therapy Association, Inc. © 1998 by American Occupational Therapy Association, Inc. Reprinted with permission.

Developmental Groups

PARALLEL GROUP

This is a group composed of participants who have the ability to trust others enough to tolerate being with more than one person at a time. They can acknowledge the presence of other group members through eye contact or casual conversation. The occupational therapist is the leader of the group and thus provides the group boundaries, explains the purpose of the group, the expectations for behavior in the group, and is responsible for giving feedback to the participants regarding their performance during the group. He or she provides an occupational therapy environment, which is a safe place to work and where the patient can feel accepted and valued. The goal of the group is to have each person work on his or her own chosen task while sharing space with other participants. For example, a craft group may be started in which each person is working on a craft project of his or her choice.

PROJECT GROUP

This is a group experience in which the participants are expected to come together to interact with each other in casual conversation and in order to complete a short-term task (about 1/2-hour work period). Group members are expected to work together cooperatively; share space, materials, and tools; and be able to cope with limited competition. The occupational therapist is a leader who plans and presents the short-term task to the group and is available during the work period to support, assist, and guide individuals as needed. The goal of the group is to provide the participants with an opportunity for trial-and-error learning, for group interaction around a task, and for a balance of cooperative and competitive experiences. These experiences may be, for example, team sports and games, making holiday decorations, or planning and preparing a patient party.

EGOCENTRIC-COOPERATIVE GROUP

This is a group in which the participants come together to work on a task that is completed in one or two work sessions (1-hour per session). During the task, the group members learn to express their needs, acknowledge the needs of other members, ask for feedback, and give feedback to the others. The occupational therapist is a democratic leader that makes suggestions and allows the patients to choose and carry out the task and group plan. He or she is a resource for facilitating task completion and a support that promotes an atmosphere of acceptance and safety. The goal of the group is to have a task experience in which the members will learn to (1) identify group norms and goals, (2) use their own knowledge and skills to respond in the group, (3) experiment with different group roles, (4) identify themselves as a group member with rights, (5) respect the rights of other group members, (6) respond empathetically to group members' needs, and (7) gain satisfaction from participating in the group experience. Examples may include structured learning experiences such as assertiveness, communications skills, or stress management.

COOPERATIVE GROUP

This is a cohesive group in which individuals come together to express and share their needs, thoughts, and feelings, and in which they listen to each other. The task of this group is used to promote sharing and listening, and does not seek to produce an end product. The occupational therapist serves as an advisor rather than as a leader. He or she helps form the group and initiate the task experience, and then becomes a participant who freely shares his or her thoughts and feelings. The goal of the group is to provide an experience for the participants that helps them to share their thoughts, feelings, values, and common interests, and to gain pleasure and satisfaction from this shared experience.

Behavior change is not the focus of the group. Examples are art, music, poetry, or other creative experiences that facilitate the discussion of thoughts and feelings; another example is a values clarification group.

MATURE GROUP

This is a group experience in which participants independently select, plan, and complete a group task that is time limited and produces a specific end product. The occupational therapist is a group member and not the identified leader. During the task, the function of the group and group needs have priority over the needs of the individual. The task experience is processed in order to help the group members learn the social-emotional and task roles of the group. The goal of the group is to provide an activity that will allow the individual participant to put aside his or her needs for the betterment of the group, and to help the group accomplish its goal. During the task, from the group "process" discussion each participant will identify the social-emotional and task roles that he or she assumes. Examples of this are a community transition group or group in the community.

Note: Material used for these descriptions is adapted from Mosey A. (1970). *Three frames of reference for mental health* (pp. 201-206). Thorofare, NJ: SLACK Incorporated; and from Mosey A. (1973). *Activities therapy* (pp. 120-136). New York, NY: Raven Press.

Reprinted with permission from Bruce, M., & Borg, B. (1993). *Psychosocial occupational therapy: Frames of reference for intervention*. Thorofare, NJ: SLACK Incorporated.

Group Assessment Examples— Dynamic Interactional Model

Behavioral Rating Scale for Group Assessment: Completed Example

Patient _Mary Smith_   Week of ___June 10-14___

Activity	M	Tu	W	Th	F
	Orient at game I	Hockey ADL Quest	Role Play Level I	TENS	Muffin pizza
I. General Social Behavior					
1. Attendance	0	0	0	0	0
2. Level of Initiation	0	0	I	I	0
3. Affect	2	2	2	2	2
4. Social Interaction	2	I	2	2	I
5. Cooperative Team Behavior	3	2	2	3	2
6. Error Detection and Response to Feedback	2	I	2	2	2
7. Communication	I	I	2	I	I
II. Task Behaviors					
1. Keeps Track of Task Events	2	I	2	2	2
2. Goal Orientation	2	I	2	2	I
3. Modulates Speed of Response	3	2	3	3	I
4. Frustration Tolerance	2	I	2	3	I
5. Decision Making	I	I	2	2	I
6. Memory					
a. Names of Members	I	I	I	I	I
b. Previous Activity	I	2	I	I	I
c. Turn	I	I	I	2	I
d. Rules	I	I	2	2	I
7. Orientation					
a. Self _occupation/address_	X	0	0	X	X
b. Place _room #, floor_	I	X	X	X	I
c. Time _month_	I	X	I	I	X
d. Others _group member's names_	X	I	I	X	2

Comments: In this section please comment on behaviors which interfered with participation or performance in task (flexibility, rigidity, perseveration, confabulation, aggressiveness, etc.).

Mary continues to perform well in gross motor activities as their faster pace is not hindered by Mary's impulsivity. Activities which have more structure to them (Mon-Tues-Wed-Thurs activities) were more difficult.

I. General Social Behavior

1. Attendance
    0 = Attends willingly and on time.
    1 = Expresses interest in joining group but attends ____ minutes late.
    2 = Minimal encouragement required to join group.
    3 = Maximal encouragement required to join group.
    4 = Refuses to join group.

2. Level of Initiation
    0 = Participates freely and can work competitively.
    1 = Participates but needs persuasive cues 25% to 50% of time.
    2 = Participates but needs persuasive cues 50% to 75% of time.
    3 = Spectator. Works on fringe of group. Interaction is between patient and therapist.
    4 = Does not initiate. Isolates self from group.

3. Affect
    0 = Affect is appropriate to the situation or setting.
    1 = On occasion, demonstrates affect which is inappropriate to the situation or setting (such as laughing, crying); however, is able to independently gain control over emotions within a few minutes.
    2 = On occasion, demonstrates affect which is inappropriate to situation or setting; however, requires support and cues to control emotions.
    3 = Frequently demonstrates affect which is inappropriate to the situation or setting. Needs staff intervention and time-out from group to gain control over emotions.
    4 = Affect is inappropriate to the situation. Unable to gain control over emotions. Unable to continue participation in group.

4. Social Interaction
    0 = Interacts freely, consistently, and appropriately with both staff and patients.
    1 = Interacts appropriately with others 50% to 75% of group time.
    2 = Initiates appropriate interaction with others 25% to 50% of group time.
    3 = Appropriately interacts with others only when approached.
    4 = Unable to appropriately interact with others even when approached.

5. Cooperative Team Behavior
    0 = Able to offer assistance and encouragement to others.
    1 = Gives appropriate assistance 50% to 75% of group time or when cued.
    2 = Gives appropriate assistance 25% to 50% of group time.
    3 = Aware of others' needs but unable to offer appropriate assistance.
    4 = Self-centered. Concerned only with own needs. Does not attempt to offer assistance to others.

6. Error Detection and Response to Feedback
    0 = Able to recognize own errors and use constructive feedback without difficulty.
    1 = Able to recognize own errors the majority of the time (75%) and/or may occasionally require assistance to use feedback (25% or less of the time).
    2 = Inconsistently able to recognize own errors (50%) and/or may have difficulty using feedback (25% to 50%). Occasionally may respond with hostility or withdrawal.
    3 = Able to recognize own errors 25% of the time and/or may frequently (50% to 75%) have difficulty using feedback. May respond with hostility, withdrawal, or degrading of task value.
    4 = Unable to recognize errors or accept feedback. Consistently responds with hostility or withdrawal.

7. Communication
    0 = Expresses thoughts in a complete, well-organized manner and focuses on essential or appropriate factors.
    1 = Expresses thoughts in a complete, well-organized manner 75% of the time. Occasionally vague or tangential.
    2 = Expresses thoughts in a complete, well-organized manner 50% of the time. Frequently vague or tangential.
    3 = Expresses thoughts in a complete and well-organized manner only 25% of the time. Vague or tangential the majority of the time.
    4 = Thoughts are incomplete and tangential.

II. Task Behaviors

1. Keeps Tracks of Task Events
    0 = Consistently keeps track of all aspects of the task.
    1 = Able to keep track of 75% or more of relevant task details. Frequently omits important information or over-attends to non-essential details.
    2 = Able to keep track of 50% to 75% of relevant task details. Frequently omits important information or overattends to non-essential details.
    3 = Able to keep track of 25% to 50% of relevant task details. Omits important information or over-attends to non-essential details the majority of the time.
    4 = Over-attention to details and/or inability to keep track of ongoing essential information in group.

2. Goal Orientation

    0 = Able to stay focused and goal oriented without difficulty. Can work in an unstructured setting.

    1 = Occasional cues needed to focus on task (less than 25% of group time).

    2 = Requires cues to focus on task 25% to 50% of group time—does not lose track of goal of task.

    3 = Requires cues to focus and/or redirect attention to task 50% to 75% of group time. Needs a highly structured environment for task completion.

    4 = Needs consistent redirection to task (75% or more of group time). Displays a lack of goal-oriented behavior.

3. Modulates Speed of Response

    0 = Responds to information at appropriate speed (dependent upon task).

    1 = Responses are slow or impulsive less than 25% of group time; however, the patient can initiate self-monitoring of response speed.

    2 = Responses are slow or impulsive 25% to 50% of group time. The patient requires occasional structure to monitor own response speed.

    3 = Responses are slow or impulsive 50% to 75% of group time. The patient requires constant cuing to control speed of response.

    4 = Consistently demonstrates inability to monitor speed of response.

4. Frustration Tolerance

    0 = Handles all tasks without signs of frustration.

    1 = Demonstrates occasional signs of frustration by withdrawing from group, making faces, changing tone of voice, etc.; however, the patient is able to independently deal with frustration.

    2 = Demonstrates occasional frustration by withdrawing from group, raising voice, displaying anger, etc. Requires staff intervention to control this behavior.

    3 = Demonstrates frustration through verbal or physical outbursts. Requires staff intervention to control this behavior. With support is able to continue group participation.

    4 = Easily frustrated to the point of being unable to continue participation in the group despite support and staff intervention.

5. Decision Making

    0 = Makes all independent decisions with ease. On group decision, is able to listen and support other's viewpoints. Willing to compromise to reach a decision.

    1 = Makes independent decisions easily but tends to be passive or aggressive in group decision making.

    2 = Hesitant in making decisions. Needs to check with others. Participation in group decision making is limited.

    3 = Makes occasional independent decisions but is easily dissuaded by others. Looks to others for decisions the majority of the time.

    4 = Unable to make any independent decisions. Consistently looks to others for a decision or is led by other members.

6. Memory

    0 = Recalls information spontaneously.

    1 = Requires verbal cues less than 25% of group time.

    2 = Requires verbal cues 25% to 50% of group time.

    3 = Requires verbal cues 50% to 75% of group time.

    4 = Requires constant verbal cues.

7. Orientation

    0 = Intact.

    1 = Requires one cue.

    2 = Requires two cues.

    3 = Requires three cues.

    4 = Unable to answer.

All information in this appendix reproduced with permission from Toglia, J. P., & Golisz, K. M. (1990). *Cognitive rehabilitation—Group games and activities* (pp. 60-61). Tuscon, AZ: Therapy Skill Builders.

Monthly Goal Record Example

Patient *Mary Smith*   Month: *June*

Goal 1: *Responds to information at appropriate speed*

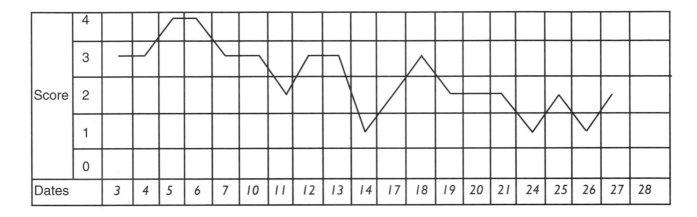

Goal 2: *Recognized errors—accepts feedback*

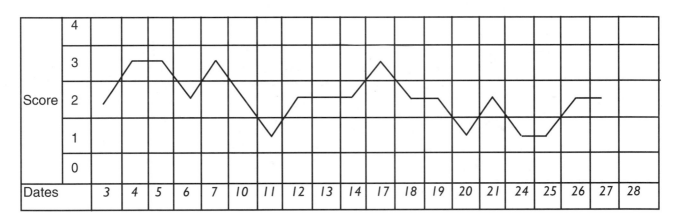

Goal 3: *Handles all tasks without signs of frustration*

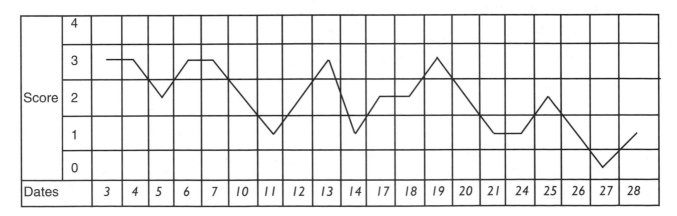

Index

BUILD *Your Library*

This book and many others on numerous different topics are available from SLACK Incorporated. For further information or a copy of our latest catalog, contact us at:

Professional Book Division
SLACK Incorporated
6900 Grove Road
Thorofare, NJ 08086 USA
Telephone: 1-856-848-1000
1-800-257-8290
Fax: 1-856-853-5991
E-mail: orders@slackinc.com
www.slackbooks.com

We accept most major credit cards and checks or money orders in US dollars drawn on a US bank. Most orders are shipped within 72 hours.

Contact us for information on recent releases, forthcoming titles, and bestsellers. If you have a comment about this title or see a need for a new book, direct your correspondence to the Editorial Director at the above address.

Thank you for your interest and we hope you found this work beneficial.